CLEFT PALATE SPEECH MANAGEMENT

A Multidisciplinary Approach

CLEFT PALATE
SPEECH MANAGEMENT
A Multidisciplinary Approach

ROBERT J. SHPRINTZEN, Ph.D.

Director
Center for Craniofacial Disorders, Montefiore Medical Center
Professor of Plastic Surgery and Otolaryngology
Albert Einstein College of Medicine, Bronx, New York

JANUSZ BARDACH, M.D.

Professor Emeritus of Plastic Surgery
Department of Otolaryngology-Head and Neck Surgery
Department of Surgery
The University of Iowa Hospitals and Clinics
The University of Iowa, Iowa City, Iowa

with 250 illustrations

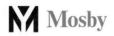 Mosby

St. Louis Baltimore Berlin Boston Carlsbad Chicago London Madrid
Naples New York Philadelphia Sydney Tokyo Toronto

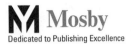

Dedicated to Publishing Excellence

Executive Editor: Martha Sasser
Associate Developmental Editor: Kellie F. White
Project Manager: Linda McKinley
Production Editor: Rich Barber
Cover Designer: Jeanne Wolfgeher
Manufacturing Supervisor: Linda Ierardi

Printed in the United States of America
Composition by Graphic World, Inc.
Printing/binding by Maple Vail Book Manufacturing Group

Mosby–Year Book, Inc.
11830 Westline Industrial Drive
St. Louis, Missouri 63146

Library of Congress Cataloging in Publication Data
International Standard Book Number 0-8016-6447-0

97 98 99 / 9 8 7 6 5 4 3

Contributor List

Janusz Bardach, M.D.
Professor Emeritus of Plastic Surgery
Department of Otolaryngology-Head and Neck
  Surgery
Department of Surgery
The University of Iowa Hospitals and Clinics
The University of Iowa, Iowa City, Iowa

Martin D. Cassell, Ph.D.
Department of Anatomy
University of Iowa
Iowa City, Iowa

George J. Cisneros, D.M.D., M.M.Sc.
Director, Postgraduate Program in Orthodontics
Montefiore Medical Center
Dental Director, Center for Craniofacial Disorders
Associate Professor, Pediatric Dentistry and
Orthodontics
Albert Einstein College of Medicine
Bronx, New York

Linda L. D'Antonio, Ph.D.
Loma Linda University School of Medicine
Surgery/Medical Group
Loma Linda, California

Hani Elkadi, M.D.
Department of Anatomy
University of Iowa
Iowa City, Iowa

Luigi Girolametto, Ph.D.
Assistant Professor, Graduate Department of
  Speech Pathology
Faculty of Medicine
Associate Member, School of Graduate Study
University of Toronto
Toronto, Ontario
Canada

Rosalie Goldberg, M.S.
Genetic Counselor
Center for Craniofacial Disorders and Human
  Genetics Center
Montefiore Medical Center
Associate, Plastic Surgery, Molecular Genetics,
  Pediatrics
Albert Einstein College of Medicine
Bronx, New York

Karen J. Golding-Kushner, Ph.D.
Clinical Director
Center for Craniofacial Disorders
Montefiore Medical Center
Assistant Professor of Plastic Surgery
Albert Einstein College of Medicine
Bronx, New York

Étoile M. LeBlanc, M.S.
Director of Communicative Disorders
Center for Craniofacial Disorders
Associate Plastic Surgery
Montefiore Medical Center
Albert Einstein College of Medicine
Bronx, New York

Kenneth E. Salyer, M.D., F.A.A.P., F.A.C.S.
Director, International Craniofacial Institute and
  Cleft Lip and Palate Treatment Center
Dallas, Texas

Nancy J. Scherer, Ph.D.
Associate Professor
Department of Communicative Disorders
East Tennessee State University
Johnson City, Tennessee

Robert J. Shprintzen, Ph.D.
Director
Center for Craniofacial Disorders, Montefiore
  Medical Center
Professor of Plastic Surgery and Otolaryngology
Albert Einstein College of Medicine, Bronx, NY

Eugene J. Sidoti, M.D.
Medical Director
Center for Craniofacial Disorders
Montefiore Medical Center
Associate Clinical Professor of Pediatrics
Albert Einstein College of Medicine
Bronx, New York

Karin Vargervik, DDS
Professor, Growth and Development
Director, Center for Craniofacial Anomalies
School of Dentistry
University of California
San Francisco, California

Mary Anne Witzel, Ph.D.
Associate Professor
Graduate Department of Speech Pathology
Faculty of Medicine
Member, Continuing, School of Graduate Study
University of Toronto
Toronto, Ontario
Canada

Speech distinguishes us from all other creatures. It not only allows us to communicate with each other, but it is integral to the development and expression of our distinctly human intellect and emotions. It is in recognition of the paramount importance of speech in the care of children with cleft palate that we offer this book.

ROBERT J. SHPRINTZEN, PH.D
JANUSZ BARDACH, M.D.

Preface

An enormous number of publications have been devoted to various aspects of the treatment of cleft lip and palate. However, very few texts have been designed to lead the reader into the practical intricacies of the field. The format of most of the books currently available is common to most academically oriented publications: the books are multi-authored, the subject matter is reviewed in detail, and long lists of references and summaries of what is known are supplied without necessarily providing strong opinion of the validity of treatment approaches by the authors.

Recently, a new surgical text has appeared on the market that is based entirely on the personal experiences of the authors and serves as an instructional guide for plastic surgeons. Nothing of the sort yet exists in the field of speech pathology in relation to cleft lip and palate. Realizing the need to guide speech pathologists into the "how to" aspects of diagnosing and treating disorders in patients with cleft lip and palate, we have designed a text book that will provide direct instruction and practical knowledge to speech pathologists for managing patients with clefts. Because speech is only one of many possible disorders in patients with clefts, we have also provided up-to-date information for other disciplines involved in the treatment of clefting.

Focusing on both academic presentation and practical guidance, the design of this text presents an alternative to existing books. Disorders of communication related to cleft lip and palate are emphasized in terms of the authors' clinical approach and the method of finding solutions to various problems faced in the treatment of children and adults with clefts. This book includes material not currently available in other publications, including exact descriptions of diagnostic and treatment protocols, the rationales for using them, the complications of various treatments, and the advantages of procedures applied to thousands of patients.

The interdisciplinary management of patients with cleft palate depends on the clinician's deep knowledge of both the field of speech pathology as well as other fields involved in the treatment of clefting. In other words, as is discussed in subsequent chapters, it is not only important for a team to be interdisciplinary in nature; the team members must all be transdisciplinary. Each team member should have a good foundation of knowledge of the other disciplines represented on the team. The speech pathologist should know as much as possible about surgery, orthodontics, genetics, otolaryngology, among other things. Similarly, the orthodontist and surgeon should be solidly versed in the problems faced by the speech pathologist and the language they use. This need for shared knowledge should apply to members of all disciplines.

A word about the authors. The contributors to this text are experts with many years of experience in the diagnosis and treatment of disorders associated with clefting. All of the authors have worked for many years in some of the largest cleft palate and craniofacial centers in the world. All have deep academic knowledge combined with valuable "hands on" experience. All of the authors have spent the majority of their careers in hospital-based programs, providing direct patient care on a daily basis while remaining academically active in their medical schools, dental schools, and hospital-based postgraduate programs. The authors of the text have published hundreds of articles and chapters, and several text books. They are all regarded as top specialists in their fields and are responsible for many innovations that have become accepted as the state-of-the-art. They represent internationally recognized clinicians and researchers, many of whom have exposed clinicians around the world to their expertise via hundreds, if not thousands of lectures in every inhabited continent. More than people who practice the state-of-the-art, this impressive group of authors have helped to establish the state-of-the-art. The reader will receive not only a presentation of the most current information, but also direct instruction guided by extensive clinical experience.

This text aims to describe what the clinician should do when treating a patient with a communicative impairment related to clefting. Several new concepts will be advanced and many tried and true procedures will be described. Along the way, several widely accepted procedures will be discredited. It is not the purpose of this text to give the reader a massive citation of literature, forcing the reader to go to other sources for information. Rather, the authors will suggest readings relative only to their own recommended procedures. We hope the material presented in this text will stand on its own so the reader can replicate the procedures described.

In summary, this text is meant to be a source readers will consult frequently throughout their working careers. While we would like this to be a tool of education, we would also like the book to be frequently used in the clinical setting. We hope the reader will approve of this novel approach. In our opinion, a proper education in the clinical sciences strongly relies on the expertise of practicing professionals.

ACKNOWLEDGMENTS

Very special words of gratitude and deep appreciation are directed to Kathleen Gleeson who helped immensely in the preparation of the surgical section of this book. Very special thanks also go to Hani Elkadi for the excellent illustrations, which have enhanced these chapters. Deep appreciation goes to the entire team at Montefiore Medical Center who have shared their knowledge, time, and kindness with their fellow colleagues who have written for this text. With over 60 team members at Montefiore, it is impossible to name them all, so a collective thank you is expressed to all of them. Special mention, however, must go to the Chairman of the Department of Plastic and Reconstructive Surgery, Dr. Berish Strauch, who provided his employees with the time, resources, and encouragement to pursue this project. Also critical to the successful completion of the text was the many hours of assistance from Lee Barker and Mary Cioffi, and the expert preparation and editorial assistance of Deborah Shprintzen. Appreciation is also given to the superb staff at Mosby, including Kellie White, Rich Barber, Amy Dubin, and Martha Sasser. Without them, this text would never have been completed.

Robert J. Shprintzen, Ph.D.
Janusz Bardach, M.D.

Contents

8   Communicative Impairment Associated with Clefting, 137

MARY ANNE WITZEL

9   The Evaluation and Remediation of Language Impairment, 167

LUIGI GIROLAMETTO

10 The Evaluation of Speech Disorders Associated with Clefting, 176

LINDA L. D'ANTONIO
NANCY J. SCHERER

11 Instrumental Assessment of Velopharyngeal Valving, 221

ROBERT J. SHPRINTZEN

12 The Use of Information Obtained from Speech and Instrumental Evaluations in Treatment Planning for Velopharyngeal Insufficiency, 257

ROBERT J. SHPRINTZEN

13 Secondary Surgery for Velopharyngeal Insufficiency, 277

JANUSZ BARDACH

17   Speech Bulbs, 352

KAREN J. GOLDING-KUSHNER
GEORGE J. CISNEROS
ÉTOILE M. LEBLANC

CLEFT PALATE SPEECH MANAGEMENT

A Multidisciplinary Approach

1 A New Perspective on Clefting

Robert J. Shprintzen

WHAT IS A CLEFT?

The simplest definition of a cleft is that it is an opening in an anatomical part that is normally not open. The lip is normally a solid structure spanning the entire distance from one corner of the mouth to the other corner. A cleft lip (which almost always refers to the upper lip; clefts of the lower lip are extremely rare) is an opening in the lip so that the lip is not contiguous. Similarly, a cleft of the palate, which is normally intact, is an opening in the palate such that there is a continuous passage between the mouth and the nose because the palate serves as both the roof of the mouth and the floor of the nose.

SHOW ME A CLEFT: WHAT DOES IT LOOK LIKE?

Clefts of the face may occur in many locations and for many reasons. Some are rare and occur in locations that do not correspond to embryonic fusion lines, such as near the eyes, the cheek, and even the corner of the mouth (the oral commissure). This book will not deal with these rare conditions, but rather will approach the management of the more typical clefts of the palate and lip. Though this text assumes a basic knowledge of anatomy and a knowledge of what a cleft is, it is possible that the reader has not yet had experience with newborns with clefts.

Cleft palate

Clefts of the palate occur in several variations and often occur in association with cleft lip. When cleft palate occurs without a cleft of the lip, the cleft always occurs posterior to the incisive foramen and is known as a cleft of the secondary palate. The secondary palate is formed from two embryonic halves, the maxillary processes (Fig. 1-1). These two halves grow towards the midline and fuse with the bony portion of the nasal septum (the vomer) at approximately the ninth to eleventh week of gestation. A cleft

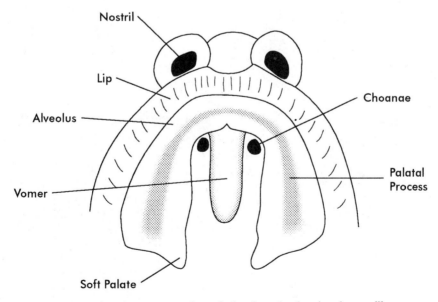

Fig. 1-1 The embryonic palate at approximately 7 to 9 weeks showing the maxillary processes, or palatal shelves, growing toward the midline.

occurs when these processes fail to fuse. Clefts of the hard palate may occur on one side (unilateral), or both (bilateral), of the nasal septum. Clefts of the soft palate (velum) are always in the midline because the vomer ends at the posterior border of the hard palate. Clefts may be of the soft palate only or of the soft and hard palate together (Fig. 1-2). The extent, width, and length of the cleft varies from case to case. In some cases, the clefts are very wide and U-shaped, a condition that accompanies a disorder known as the Robin sequence, which will be described in Chapter 2. Another variation of palatal clefting is the submucous cleft palate and occult submucous cleft palate (Fig. 1-3). In submucous cleft palate, there is a fusion of the skin (mucous membrane) of the palate, but the underlying muscle of the soft palate, and often the posterior portion of bone of the hard palate, are cleft (Fig. 1-3). The marker (i.e., clue) to the presence of a submucous cleft palate is a cleft of the uvula, or bifid uvula. A transparent area may be present in the midline of the palate in the most severe cases, known as a *zona pellucid*. A notch may also be felt with the finger in the posterior border of the hard palate. Almost all cases of bifid uvula are associated with a submucous cleft, but not all cases of submucous cleft palate are symptomatic for speech abnormalities (Shprintzen et al, 1985a). In fact, the majority of individuals with submucous cleft palate have normal speech (Shprintzen et al, 1985a). Occult submucous cleft palate is a term applied to submucous clefts that are not associated with bifid uvula or other abnormalities detectable on oral examination. Occult submucous cleft palate will be discussed in greater detail in Chapter 11.

Cleft lip

There are several types of clefts of the lip. Clefts occur along the lines of normal embryonic fusion (Fig. 1-4). It is generally accepted that the clefts occur because of a failure of the various embryonic elements to fuse. Cleft lip occurs infrequently as an isolated anomaly, occurring more frequently in association with cleft palate. Probably fewer than 5% of all cases of cleft lip occur without cleft palate (Shprintzen et al, 1985b).

The majority of clefts of the lip occur on only one side and thus are called unilateral clefts of the lip. Over three quarters of unilateral clefts of the lip occur on the left side; less than a quarter occur on the right. Bilateral clefts of the

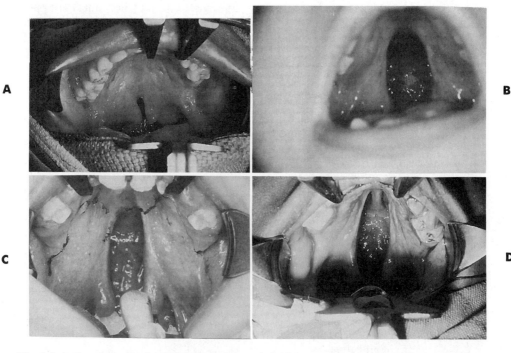

Fig. 1-2 A, A variety of palatal clefts including a cleft of the posterior border of the soft palate only. **B,** The entire soft palate. **C,** Soft palate and posterior border of the hard palate. **D,** Entire soft and hard palate to the incisive foramen

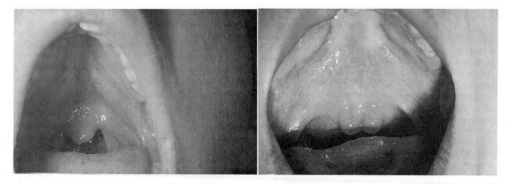

Fig. 1-3 Two examples of submucous cleft palate.

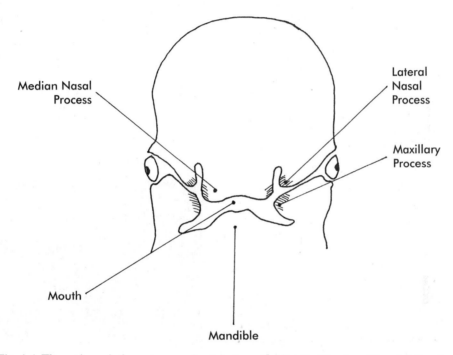

Fig. 1-4 The embryonic face at approximately 4 weeks after fertilization. The cross hatched lines mark where clefts occur in the lip.

lip are rare in the absence of accompanying cleft palate. Because isolated clefts of the lip are rare, and because they do not typically result in speech disorders, the following examples (and indeed the majority of the rest of the text) will address cleft lip within the context of the combined disorder of cleft lip and palate.

Unilateral cleft lip and palate. In unilateral clefts of the lip, the cleft extends from the base of the nostril (known as the alar base) through the lip at the point below the nostril (Fig. 1-5). Note that the vermillion of the lip extends into the floor of the nose (an issue to be addressed

in the subsequent chapter on lip repair) and that the nose is severely distorted, probably more than the lip (especially from the perspective of the surgeon). The underlying alveolar ridge is also cleft, which further distorts the floor of the nose because the maxillary alveolus comprises the anterior aspect of the nostril and nasal floor. Treatment outcomes for unilateral clefts, especially in males who may be able to mask lip scars with facial hair, are usually excellent.

Bilateral cleft lip and palate. While treatment outcomes in unilateral clefts are usually very good, the opposite is usually true for bilateral

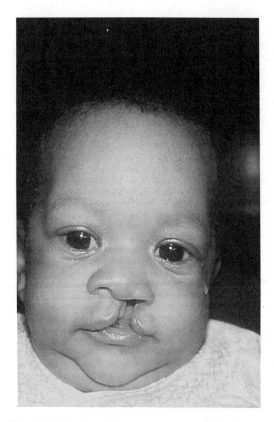

Fig. 1-5 An infant with a left sided unilateral cleft lip and palate.

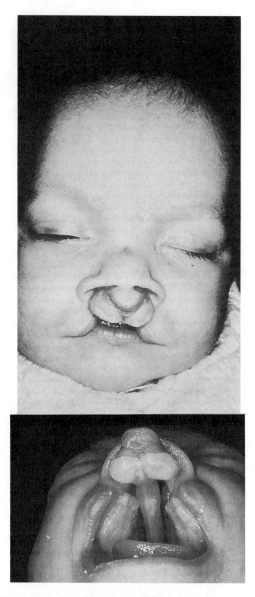

Fig. 1-6 An infant with a bilateral cleft lip and palate.

clefts. In bilateral cleft lip and palate (Fig. 1-6), there is a severe tissue deficiency in the middle of the face. Besides the fact that the lip and maxillary alveolus is cleft under both nostrils, the central portion of the lip and maxilla, referred to as the premaxilla, is positioned abnormally, at the tip of the nasal septum, often causing it to protrude at an abnormal angle (Fig. 1-6). The central cartilaginous structure of the nose, the columella, is almost always absent so that even after surgical repair, the nose is flattened with the tip essentially attached to the center of the lip. The alveolar clefts are almost always very large because of the severe anterior positioning of the premaxilla. As a result, there is a striking abnormality in the anterior oral cavity, which has a negative affect on speech production and both the appearance and function of the dental arches.

A NEW PERSPECTIVE

Though the reader is most likely a student or professional involved in the study and care of individuals born with clefts of the palate or lip and palate, I would ask for a brief change of roles. Imagine instead that you are a parent of a baby girl who has just been born with a cleft. For arguement's sake, let us imagine that the cleft is a bilateral cleft of the lip and palate (Fig. 1-6). The abnormality is frightening, and you have become overwhelmed with many concerns including how you are going to feed a baby with a huge opening in her face, impending surgery, what your daughter will look like after the surgery and even more importantly, what she will look like as an adult. What about her speech? Her teeth? Will this impair her ability to adjust in school? Is her intelligence going to be normal? You wonder if her life will be normal or perpetually haunted by the abnormality. You had wanted to have more children, so you are also concerned about the possibility that future progeny might also have clefts. And what about her children? The number of questions and doubts are enormous, and they are not necessarily abated by the early management of the baby in the hospital. There are problems in feeding. The nurses and resident doctors also seem overwhelmed. You are introduced to funny looking nipples and feeding contraptions. Someone suggests gavage feedings (passing a tube through the nose or mouth into the stomach), and you are immediately introduced to surgeons who give you more information than you can possibly absorb. You want the cleft repaired right away, but the surgeon says you must wait for a few months. Then you begin to wonder if this surgeon is "the best" or if there is someone elsewhere who has done more, done better, or has some magical technique not known in your community hospital. Who do you turn to for help? Confusion reigns and your anxiety heightens.

You might be introduced to a parent support group, or be contacted by a social worker. Someone mentions that clefts are typically managed by teams of professionals because babies with clefts may have speech problems, dental problems, and chronic middle ear infections with conductive hearing loss. A team sounds good to you because you will not be compelled to rely on a single doctor for advice. The representative from the parent group tells you comforting stories about their children, offers emotional support, and contradicts many of the things you were told by the nurses and doctors about feeding. If the doctors were so off base about the feeding, do they really know what they are talking about when it comes to treatment? Hope is restored, but confidence is still shaky.

In this scenario, the focus of attention has become the cleft. Professionals and other parents alike have given advice based on the "typical" child with a cleft. Teams have been structured to handle "the cleft palate child." Yes, there has been an enormous amount of research published on "the cleft palate child," including issues related to speech, facial growth psychology, and even learning problems. But is your daughter a "cleft palate child" or a child with a cleft? The difference is not merely semantic.

What is clefting and what causes it?

One of the first questions you may have as a parent of a child with a cleft is "Why me?" The real question the parent is asking, of course, is "What caused this? Did I do anything wrong? Is this my fault?" Very often, parents do not even know what a cleft is. They may have known of someone who had a "hare lip" when they were younger, but they do not understand clefting at all.

Stated simply, a cleft is a lack of union of embryonic oral and facial elements. There has been some argument as to whether this lack of fusion is caused by a failure of embryonic parts to grow toward each other (Fraser, 1961) or a rupture of already fused elements (Kitamura, 1991). However, the embryonic mechanism that made the cleft occur is not as important as understanding or identifying the etiology. In other words, the primary event or pathogen that caused the absence of union must be found. There are four different categories of etiologies representing hundreds of specific diseases that have cleft lip, cleft palate, or both as symptoms: chromosomal disorders, genetic disease, teratogenically induced disorders, and mechanically induced abnormalities. These different etiologies will be discussed in detail in Chapter 2. It is mentioned here, however, to point out that there is not a single cause for clefting. As such, clefting is not a single disease, but rather a clinical outcome of many possible diseases.

Readers familiar with the research on cleft palate understand that until recently the notion that clefting is not a specific disease, but rather a symptom of many possible disease processes has been lacking (Shprintzen, 1988). Regarding cleft palate as a specific disease has led many researchers and clinicians to speak about "the cleft palate child." By doing this, all children with clefting become equated in a sense. This has a serious effect on clinical research, especially with relation to outcome studies (studies assessing the outcomes of treatments). The results of clinical research and outcome studies are frequently applied to patient management.

There are several reasons why clefting has been regarded as a specific disease entity. The differentiation of etiologic factors is a relatively new consequence of the growth of the sciences of clinical and molecular genetics (discussed in Chapter 2) and has not yet become a routine component of evaluations among many teams that evaluate children with clefts (especially smaller teams not affiliated with major medical facilities).

Another reason is the obvious nature of clefting, which draws attention as the most significant abnormality in children with several other abnormalities, especially when those anomalies are minor. Another reason is the application of different models of thought prevalent in the health care professions. The biggest of these differences, the medical model versus the behavioral model, strikes to the heart of how the clinician defines exactly what a cleft lip and/or cleft palate is and how it should be managed. The use of one or the other of these models as a template for evaluation and treatment planning denotes a basic approach to problem solving, which will influence the entire process of patient management.

Medical versus behavioral model

In the management of children with cleft lip and cleft palate, a large number of specialties are usually required to fully assess the patient. In some more comprehensive centers, as many as 25 or more disciplines may be involved in the evaluation of patients with clefting and craniofacial anomalies. Among these many disciplines, there are basically two approaches to the management of human abnormality: the medical model versus the behavioral model. The majority of medical and dental disciplines utilize the medical model while speech pathology, audiology, psychology, social service, and other behavioral sciences follow the behavioral model. The difference between these two models is important.

In the medical model, the presenting problems are symptoms of a disease process. For example, a rash on the skin is not the disease, but rather an indication of an underlying problem that is causing the rash. Clinicians following the medical model will then determine if the rash is caused by allergy, viral infection, bacterial infection, or external mechanical irritation. The disease is often named by its cause. Therefore, a rash on the skin caused by the virus for "German measles" is called rubella, the name of the virus. A rash caused by an external mechanical or chemical irritant would be called a "contact dermatitis." The implication is that every symptom has an underlying cause and that physical manifestations that are considered to be abnormal are merely symptoms.

The behavioral model, on the other hand, equates the symptom with the disease. For example, in speech pathology, dysfluencies in speech called "stutters" are a sign of "stuttering." An inability to produce speech sounds correctly is known as an articulation disorder. In other words, the symptom is the disease. Causation, while it may be of interest to the clinician, is not necessarily important nor usually involved in the differential diagnosis of the disorder. It also follows that the cause may not be considered important to the treatment of the disorder.

Cleft lip and cleft palate have been studied largely by behavioral scientists who have had an enormous influence on how the problem is perceived. It is also true that some of the disciplines necessary to understanding clefting within the framework of a medical model did not exist at the time the first multidisciplinary teams were assembled to study the problem. For example, clinical genetics has become important only in the last decade, while the first cleft palate teams were assembled before World War II. As a result, a cleft lip and cleft palate have been regarded as specific disease entities rather than as a sign of an underlying disease process. Unfortunately, clefting is not a specific disease. As in the example just cited, stuttering becomes a disease entity named after and defined by its most noticeable symptom ("disease" is simply defined as an abnormality creating an aberrant state of structure or function). A similar circumstance occurred in children born with clefts in that their disease became named after the most obvious symptom (hence the "cleft palate child").

An illustration of how this appelation and adherence to the behavioral model can lead to erroneous decisions and treatment will help to clarify the difference in management. A child with a cleft palate is born at a hospital with a small cleft palate team. There are no other obvious abnormalities, and the child looks otherwise healthy. However, feeding is extremely difficult. Members of the team are called on to see the new "cleft palate baby" on the neonatal unit. It is immediately assumed that the feeding problem is related to the presence of the cleft. Feeding remains difficult, so gavage feedings (the use of an orogastric or nasogastric tube) are implemented for several weeks. With time, normal feedings are established. Two months later, it is noticed that the baby is small for its age and that the growth curve is consistently diminishing (i.e., not following a normal pattern of growth acceleration). It is again assumed that the problem was the difficulty with feeding, which is stunting the baby's growth. The pattern of growth deficiency continues, and it is finally noticed that the legs have an abnormal curvature and configuration. Radiographs (x-rays) of the legs are ordered and show a pattern of bone formation consistent with a genetic disease of short stature (previously called dwarfing) known as diastrophic dysplasia. Cleft palate is an occasional finding in this disorder. The feeding problem was related to the airway compromise often experienced in diastrophic dysplasia. Babies who have a marginal airway often have a difficult time exchanging air while feeding even though they may not have the problem at rest. The failure to follow the growth curve was the primary component of this genetic error (an autosomal recessive trait) and had nothing to do with lack of nutrition (feeding failure rarely results in decreased linear growth). Therefore, in this case, the failure to recognize clefting as a symptom of another primary disease (diastrophic dysplasia) led to errors in early management. By calling the child a "cleft palate baby," the natural conclusion is that all the problems seen are secondary to the assumed primary disease of clefting.

Differentiating cleft type

Even more fundamental than diagnosing syndromes, clinicians should be aware that clefts of the palate, unilateral clefts of the lip and palate, and bilateral clefts of the lip and palate are not equivalent. In reviewing the extensive literature on treatment outcomes in individuals with clefts, the reader will find that many investigations have included in their selection of subjects individuals who have only clefts of the palate together with individuals with clefts of the lip and palate, both unilateral and bilateral. Individuals with bilateral clefts of the lip and palate would be prone to speech problems not experienced by individuals with clefts of the palate only. While a cleft of the soft palate alone might predispose an individual to hypernasal speech and nasal air escape, individuals with bilateral clefts of the lip and palate will, in addition, encounter problems associated with abnormalities of the dental arch, missing teeth in the area of the cleft, and possible openings in the hard palate between the mouth and nose (fistulae). The abnormalities in the anterior portion of the oral cavity result in articulation disorders, which may be distinctly different from those found in individuals with clefts of the palate only. Therefore, treatments for these two conditions should not be the same even though both conditions may result in hypernasality. The various cleft types result in different aesthetic problems, lip mobility problems, and facial growth problems, all of which will affect the course of treatment, from speech therapy, to orthodontics, to surgery.

As previously discussed, one reason researchers have often lumped together the different cleft types in their studies is that they regard the cleft as the primary disease. Because the word *cleft* appears in both the bilateral lip and palate and palate only versions, these two distinctly different disorders have become in a semantic way homogenous. As a challenge to the reader, I would suggest going to the scientific literature on cleft palate, such as in *The Cleft Palate Craniofacial Journal* (known as the *Cleft Palate Journal* prior to 1990) and see how many articles published using a sample of individuals with clefts have mixed cleft types in the sample. However, as will also be discussed in Chapter 2, clefting of the lip and palate and clefting of the palate only are two completely different disorders with major differences in both etiology and embryonic timing. Cleft type also has major implications for syndromic diagnosis.

How etiology affects outcome

There are literally hundreds of conditions that can result in clefts in the newborn. In syndromes, the clefts are simply a manifestation of a more generalized pattern of malformation in the developing embryo. The mechanism that leads to the cleft is as specific as the gene, chromosome, teratogen, or mechanical factor, which was the primary etiology. These factors may have a more generalized effect on the growth of the embryo in general. Therefore, the cleft cannot be regarded as an isolated event, nor can the cleft be separated from the rest of the face, head, and craniofacial complex. This is not meant to be a trivial platitude, but rather a very important concept in understanding the future growth and development of the particular child who has a cleft of known causation.

If, for example, the cleft in a newborn is secondary to a genetic disorder in which the face is malformed as a result of a single gene, then both the cleft and the facial abnormality are a result of the gene. Many patients with clefts of the lip and palate are noted to have severe midfacial deficiency when they reach adulthood. Because nearly all patients with cleft lip and palate have early surgery to repair the clefts, the clinician may be tempted to correlate the early surgery with the subsequent failure in growth of the midface. This, again, is an example of using clinical observations to develop correlations, which then mislead clinical scientists into drawing cause and effect conclusions. One might be tempted to believe that the cause and effect relationship for midfacial growth deficiency and palate repair is a real one because there is a correlation coefficient of 1.0 between patients with clefts who have maxillary deficiency and palate repair early in life. This is a unidirectional relationship. Looking from the other direction, how many patients who have had palate repair end up with maxillary deficiency as adults? Certainly not all and possibly not the majority. Why is the observed correlation different when maxillary deficiency is the variable under initial observation rather than palate repair? Because of ascertainment bias.

Ascertainment bias

The manner in which clinical subjects enter studies as experimental observations can affect the outcome and conclusions. The observation of maxillary deficiency associated with cleft palate is a good case in point. The conclusion that patients who had early palate repair have growth impairment of the maxilla as a result of scarring was made after clinicians observed that many patients with clefts seen as adults had maxillary deficiency. All had had their palates repaired in infancy. The relationship between early repair and midface deficiency was nearly perfect (i.e., r = 1.0). However, the ascertainment of the patients almost predicts the resulting observations. For one thing, since the 1950s, the overwhelming majority of patients with clefts have had early palate repairs. It may also be presumed that the patients most likely to be seen as adults are the ones with the worst problems. It is also probable that throughout life, the patients with the best results are seen the least. Therefore, surgeons would be more likely to see a larger number of older patients with maxillary deficiency than those with normal maxillary growth. Furthermore, all or most of these patients will have had early palate repair.

The prevalence of hypernasal speech in individuals with submucous cleft palate is another good example. Clinicians who work at cleft palate centers have the impression that almost everyone with a submucous cleft of the palate is hypernasal. For example, an analysis of the clinical population at the Center for Craniofacial Disorders at Montefiore Medical Center with over 300 patients with submucous cleft shows that over 98% had hypernasal speech. The high prevalence of hypernasality in this type of clinical subpopulation should also be anticipated. Patients with submucous cleft referred to centers are referred specifically because of a problem. Stating this in another way, if someone with a submucous cleft palate had normal speech, what would be the reason for referral to

a center? Two studies have shown that the prevalence of submucous cleft in the general population is quite high and that a large majority of individuals with submucous clefts have normal speech, well over 90% (Stewart et al, 1972; Shprintzen et al, 1985a). In both these studies, subjects were ascertained from the general population with large samples being screened for bifid uvula and other signs of submucous cleft palate. In these studies, the ascertainment bias of specific referral was avoided. The reality is that many people with submucous clefts and normal speech never have them detected and the true prevalence of the disorder in the general population is not well understood.

What has the research shown us? What has it failed to show?

There is substantial literature in the area of clefting that examines many aspects of medical management, surgical outcomes, and human behavior. There have been literally many thousands of articles published in scores of journals covering essentially every topic germane to clinical and basic science (etiology, genetics, surgery, orthodontic treatment, speech and language development, facial growth, intellect, social factors, psychosocial adjustment, etc.). Because management of cleft disorders is undertaken by many disciplines, there is no shortage of clinical and basic scientists to study the phenomenon. For all of the study, where do we currently stand compared to 20, 30, 40 or even 50 years ago?

Without meaning to be excessively cynical, though there has been some progress in treating individuals with clefts, some of the same basic arguments vital to the very foundations of cleft care are, as yet, unresolved. Some of these issues seem so fundamental to the care of individuals with clefts that one must wonder why answers have not been forthcoming. Examining one such issue briefly may help to explain.

WHEN AND HOW TO REPAIR A CLEFT PALATE

This debate has raged on for as long as palates have been surgically repaired. Bardach will discuss the technical details and philosophy behind palate repair later in this text, and his view regarding timing is in concert with the goals of speech pathologists who are involved in the care of infants with clefts. However, many alternatives have been offered to Bardach's approach. In part, the problem is related to the interdisciplinary nature of care in individuals with clefts. The speech pathologists would obviously prefer to see the palate repaired as early as possible in order to intercept the normal development milestones of speech. Today, surgeons have relatively few constraints related to health and surgical morbidity constraints (early infant surgery is no longer considered to be terribly risky, nor are there many complications associated with palate repair), but in general, the procedure is technically easier when the child is larger. Orthodontists are concerned with normal occlusion and facial growth, and therefore prefer to see the hard palate untouched and unscarred so there will be no inhibitions on its growth nor changes in the position of the maxillary segments from scar contraction. Some of the options that have been implemented at various times and in various places are listed below with their rationales:

Delayed repair of the hard palate, but early repair of the soft palate

This approach was adopted because of the observation that people with complete clefts of the lip and palate who had palate repairs often had growth deficiencies in the midface. It was hypothesized that it was the surgery and scarring on the hard palate which caused maxillary deficiency by restricting the forward growth of the midfacial skeleton. Therefore, by not repairing the hard palate until late childhood or adolescence, the midface would be free to grow to "normal" dimensions. Some clinicians who advocated this approach suggested that the hard palate be obturated with a dental appliance; others suggested that it was not necessary and that the palate would actually close on its own by medial growth with increasing age.

In assessing this approach at face value alone, it makes little sense, both with regard to the purpose of palate repair and in relation to trying to make the quality of life as normal as possible for the patient. It is also true that within the framework of time (historical time), the concern regarding midfacial growth becomes less important.

Repairing the palate serves only one purpose; to try to provide normal speech production for the patient. It is essentially impossible to produce normal speech with a continuous opening between the mouth and nose. Besides excessive nasality in the individual's speech, normal articulation would be difficult to achieve because of the absence of normal oral landmarks and because the production of normal sounds would not occur even if the correct placement of the articulators was achieved (see the chapters by Witzel and Golding-Kushner for excellent descriptions of the problems associated with articulation). By leaving the hard palate unrepaired, normal speech would be very difficult to achieve, even if the cleft were obturated (i.e., covered). Obturators are rarely "air tight," the fit changes with growth, and an acrylic appliance is a poor substitute for normal oral tissues.

Because speech is likely to be impaired (usually severely), the patient will require long-term speech therapy. The patient's speech will be unintelligible to many of his or her peers, and social adjustment will be affected by the inability to communicate with proficiency. If an obturator is used, there will be frequent trips to the dentist to have the appliance adjusted or remade when it gets too small. Compared to one surgical intervention to repair the palate, the intensity and frequency of treatment with an unrepaired hard palate is far greater, causing increased financial and emotional cost.

The current availability of highly effective skeletal surgery to put deficient facial bones into normal position should negate the excessive worry over maxillary deficiency. Today, maxillary advancement and similar orthognathic surgical procedures are done with little risk or morbidity and excellent results. Normal facial profile and dental occlusion can be achieved with only a few days in the hospital, relatively short-term orthodontic therapy to "set up" the operation, and relatively little discomfort or pain. Prolonged efforts to avoid skeletal surgery while dooming the patient to long-term speech and dental therapies and unintelligible speech makes little sense.

Very early repair of the soft palate (2 to 6 months of age) with later repair of the hard palate (1 to 2 years of age) or two stage repair of the palate, soft palate first, hard palate second

There are clinicians and researchers who have advocated the early repair of the soft palate, deferring hard palate repair until 1 or 2 years. Often referred to as *two stage palate repair,* this approach has been more popular in European centers than in North America, but some centers in the United States have adopted this approach. The basic premise behind the very early repair of the soft palate followed some time later by hard palate repair is essentially to provide a working muscular palate while preventing the anterior scarring on the hard palate which some clinicians believe impairs midfacial growth. Reports of this two stage approach presume that the reconstruction of the soft palate allows normal palatal movement and stimulates the velum to move normally for speech (Randall et al, 1983). The presumption that simply repairing the velum will prompt it to move normally is clearly erroneous and has never been demonstrated clinically or experimentally. To the contrary, all logic relative to speech acquisition would contradict the ability of the soft palate to move normally if the hard palate remained unrepaired.

Speech is a learned activity that is dependent on the normal mechanisms of learning. During infancy, children begin to experiment with their speech mechanisms by making a variety of random sounds. Initially, they lack the coordination for sophisticated speech production, but more importantly, they lack the ability to understand and use language. The sounds they make are simply vocal play and initially consist mainly of vowels and prolonged nasal consonants (most frequently /m/). At the same time the infant is making the normal random movements of the lips, vocal cords, and tongue, eventually the velopharyngeal valve will close as well. This chance occurrence of both velopharyngeal closure and, for example, closure of the lips, will result in the production of a nonnasal consonant sound such as /p/ or /b/. This will create a whole new class of sounds for vocal play for the infant which, by itself, will be reinforcing. If this is done in the presence of the parents, additional reinforcement will be provided by the parents repeating the sounds (as they often do), or by their obvious signs of delight. The reinforcement of the /p/ or /b/ sound will teach the infant to continue to utilize velopharyngeal closure as a part of his or her vocal play. If there is an opening in the anterior palate, even if the velum were to successfully close the velopharyngeal port, air would still escape into the nose so that the sound could not be recognized as a nonnasal consonant. Consequently, velopharyngeal closure could not be reinforced. Therefore, two-stage palatoplasty at any age, cannot be expected to result in normal function of the velopharyngeal valve. In subsequent chapters, it will be shown how anterior openings in the palate also cause major problems with the normal development of articulation and velopharyngeal function. Therefore, repairing the soft palate prior to hard palate repair is not in the best interest of the child when one considers the development of speech. Furthermore, clinicians must be aware that there is only one reason to repair the palate; the development of normal speech. Feeding is not an issue (see Chapter 4), middle ear disease is not an issue, and general health is not an issue. Therefore, every effort must be made to assure that the initial surgical approach to palate repair is a successful one.

Repair of the hard palate at the time of lip repair with subsequent repair of the soft palate

Some centers have advocated repairing the hard palate at the time of lip repair (Semb, 1991; Trigos and Ysunza, 1988). The rationale for this approach is that the hard palate can be repaired in a relatively atraumatic manner by utilizing the skin of the nasal septum (the vomer) as a local flap for separating the nasal cavity from the oral cavity anteriorly (a procedure known as a vomer flap). The advantage of this approach, besides the early separation of the nasal cavity and oral cavity, is that the subsequent repair of the soft palate can be done without worrying about repair of the anterior defect. Fistulae caused by breakdowns of the repair are less likely to occur using this type of approach, which increases the likelihood of a positive speech outcome. Any procedure that will result in complete closure of the palate without leaving fistulae should produce normal speech in most cases.

Early complete repair, late complete repair, and all variations in between

A major debate has been joined by professionals around the world with regard to the proper timing of palate repair. It has already been stated that complete closure of the palate must be the goal and that no anterior defects should be left in the palate. Small defects in the maxillary alveolus are not problematic for speech, but defects posterior to the incisive foramen almost always result in compensatory changes in articulation, which can both cause velopharyngeal insufficiency and impair intelligibility (Isberg and Henningsson, 1987). The effect of age at repair on successful speech outcome would seem to be obvious. Logic would dictate that the earlier complete repair of the palate is affected, the more likely the child will be to learn normal patterns of velopharyngeal movement. Some data have supported this common logic (Dorf and Curtin, 1982). An analysis of the patient population at the Center for Craniofacial Disorders at Montefiore Medical Center reported at the International Congress on Cleft Palate and Related Craniofacial Disorders in Jerusalem in 1989 found that age was not a factor as long as repair was completed prior to 18 months of age (Hall et al, 1989). An analysis of 500 cases operated by a single surgeon using the same basic technique for all cases was accomplished using perceptual speech evaluation, nasopharyngeal, and multi-view videofluoroscopy. Because the timing of palate repair was often affected by scheduling difficulties with the surgeon, illness, frequency of middle ear disease (patients with frequent otitis were often scheduled for earlier surgery so myringotomy with tube placement could be accomplished), the 500 cases were distributed over a 1-year period for age at surgery. Some cases had surgery as early as 6 months of age, others not until 18 months. Surprisingly, no significant difference was found in the speech outcomes of the surgical results. Children completing repair at 18 months were as likely to have normal speech as those having repair complete at 6 months. However, a small sample of children having repair deferred until 2 years of age or later was also studied and found to have much worse speech outcomes than the group having surgery prior to 18 months. Therefore, there may be some type of threshold effect (perhaps 18 months of age), but there does not appear to be any significant advantage to very early surgery. The reasons for this result are not known, but suffice it to say that the process by which children learn to produce normal speech after palate repair is not as simple as it may seem and may be influenced by many factors. Some of these factors will be explored in subsequent chapters.

Repair without attempts to lengthen the soft palate, repairs with attempts to lengthen the soft palate, repairs to reconstruct the palatal muscles, repairs which do not reconstruct the muscles

Surgical technique has also been discussed as a contributor to successful outcome for palate repair. Some surgeons believe that lengthening the palate provides an advantage, others feel that careful repair of the muscles of the palate (intravelar veloplasty) is important. Results from numerous studies are contradictory. Is the type of operation of the palate very important? In the sense that complete closure must be attained and careful technique which avoids severe scarring is important, the answer is yes. However, to date, many centers have reported excellent results with a variety of primary repairs that meet these criteria. Centers using a variety of procedures have reported that 70 to 85% or more of their patients undergoing primary palate repair develop essentially normal speech without need for secondary surgery. It may be that technique, while somewhat important, is not as important as other factors that cannot be controlled by the surgeon, such as the child's learning ability, the size of the pharynx, the size of the adenoids, and the type of speech interaction the child has with his or her parents.

The example of the many approaches to palate repair is but one example of the many sources of disagreement among professionals who treat and research the problems associated with clefting. The volumes of literature on clefting are enormous with many thousands of articles having been published.

Should parents be encouraged that so much has been studied and written about children with clefts? Perhaps, but only if this large body of research had resulted in a consensus regarding treatment approaches to this large clinical population. Unfortunately, it has not. There is a profusion of possible approaches to treatment such as the timing of lip repair ranging from a few days of life to 6 months of age; early palate repair no later than 6 months of age to deferred repair of the hard palate until 12 years of age; speech therapy for resolving certain types of velopharyngeal insufficiency versus the philosophy that physical management (i.e., surgery or prosthetic treatment) must precede speech therapy; early orthodontics in the primary dentition versus waiting until the mixed dentition stage at approximately 8 years of age; and myringotomy and tube surgery for all children undergoing palate repair versus myringotomies only for children who have fluid at the time of surgery. From this author's perspective, it often seems as if the areas of disagreement outnumber those of agreement. However, it must also be said that as in many of life's endeavors, there is probably not a single treatment protocol that will achieve success. There may be several or many protocols that accomplish essentially the same final outcome. If this is the case, then what should the goals of a team be in managing the care of a child with a cleft? In my opinion, the goal should be the maximum result for the most minimal intervention. In other words, professionals should do as little as possible for the patient to achieve the best quality of life.

What is the best result?

Because each child with a cleft may be managed by many different professionals, each of whom have a different point of view that is influenced by their education and practice, it is likely that each of these professionals will define the outcome differently. For example, if a child has normal speech, but a malocclusion, the speech pathologist is likely to be more pleased than the orthodontist during the course of evaluation. Similarly, if the child has a normal occlusion but a heavily scarred lip, it is the plastic surgeon who is likely to be more upset. Is there a standard by which all children with clefts can be judged to have a good outcome of their treatment?

TEAM CONCEPT

As stated at the outset of this chapter, it is axiomatic that team management of clefting and craniofacial disorders is necessary. However, no one has ever defined just what a team is, or how comprehensive it should be. Does the composition and philosophy of a team make a difference in how patients are managed for diagnosis and treatment? Without a doubt.

The management of cleft lip and palate by many different professionals is tacitly assumed to be advantageous for both diagnosis and treatment. It is logical to assume that having many different professionals with a variety of areas of expertise examining a child with a cleft will yield more information than a single specialist from a single perspective. Though there has been no research done to confirm this conventional logic, the advantage of management by multiple professionals is so obvious as to be axiomatic. Of course, not all "team" management is equivalent. In addition, the management by multiple professionals could be "interdisciplinary" or "multidisciplinary"; these are not the same. This distinction will be discussed later in this chapter and is an important one to consider, as is the notion of "transdisciplinary" teams.

Obtaining a variety of opinions on cleft disorders can result in differences of opinion from different specialists. Some of the differences of opinion might be related to the disparate treatment approaches of each specialist. Surgeons are trained to operate, speech pathologists to do speech therapy, prosthodontists to make dental appliances. Each of these treatments certainly have a place in the management of clefts, but picking the right one for each patient becomes a challenge in the decision making process.

Why a team?

It is well recognized that individuals born with clefts of the lip and palate or palate only will face a number of interrelated problems. In the earliest days of team management of clefts, clinical observations led to the recognition that children with cleft lip and palate (including a cleft of the maxillary alveolar arch) required the services of a reconstructive surgeon to repair the clefts, a speech pathologist to address issues of velopharyngeal function and articulation, and a dental specialist to address problems associated with occlusion and congenitally missing teeth.

Centers were often built around these treatment specialists because of their long-term involvement with patients with clefts. Many teams did not have pediatricians (even though the majority of patients were children), or otolaryngologists (even though most patients had chronic middle ear disease). In its early advocacy of teams, the American Cleft Palate Association (ACPA) indicated that a proper team must have at a minimum a plastic surgeon, a speech pathologist, and an orthodontist. Would a team that had only these specialties be able to qualify as a comprehensive center? As the medical, dental, and behavioral sciences expanded, new subspecialties were born to address problems that could not even be detected four decades ago. Subspecialties such as human genetics and neuroradiology are recent additions to medicine, and specialty tests such as nasopharyngoscopy, multiview videofluoroscopy, and 3-D CT scans were not widely available before the 1980s. As a result, organizations such as ACPA have recognized that minimal standards may no longer be valid, and centers will need to be more comprehensive in order to meet a patient's needs. How comprehensive should a team be?

Table 1 lists the specialists who would have an interest in children with clefting or craniofacial anomalies along with the reason for that interest. Would patient care be compromised if any of these specialists were omitted? Correct diagnoses could go undetected. Proper treatments known only by certain specialists could go unadministered.

Interdisciplinary versus multidisciplinary

There has also been a tacit assumption that all groups of professionals who have banded together under the generic title "team" or "center" are somehow equivalent. Centers may utilize as few as three professional disciplines or may utilize as many as 30. In some centers, each discipline may be represented by only one professional, while at others there may be multiple members. The structure of the center is also extremely important. The majority of centers are directed by surgeons or other professionals who provide treatment for patients. Other centers may be directed by "generalists" who will actually never directly manage the surgical or dental care of the cleft. Do these issues make a difference in terms of the effectiveness of the team?

No one knows. No research has been done to explore the efficacy of how various models of centers function. Just as the term *cleft* has been shown to be nonspecific, the same is true of the concept of "team" or "center." There are two different models of teams, which will be described next.

Table 1 Specialists who should be included on a craniofacial team and the reason for their presence. When "pediatric" appears in parentheses, the implication is that the majority of patients are pediatric cases and should require pediatric subspecialization.

Specialty	Reason for inclusion
Medical specialists	
Plastic Surgery	Reconstruction of clefts and structural management of VPI
Pediatrics	"Medical manager" for the child
Neurology (Pediatric)	At least 10% of children with clefts have CNS anomalies
Endocrinology (Pediatric)	Approximately 20% of children with clefts are of short stature
Ophthalmology (Pediatric)	Frequent eye anomalies, especially in Stickler syndrome (5% of cleft palate)
Cardiology (Pediatric)	Frequent heart anomalies (at least 10% of children with clefts)
Otolaryngology (Pediatric)	Very frequent association of middle ear disease and airway disorders
Radiology/ Neuroradiology	Videofluoroscopy, CT, MR as frequent diagnostic modalities
Neurosurgery (Pediatric)	Frequency of craniosynostosis and need for intracranial surgery
Pulmonology (Pediatric)	Frequent association of airway related problems
Anesthesiology (Pediatric)	Difficult intubations common in children with craniofacial anomalies
Genetics/ Dysmorphology	Very high frequency of associated syndromes and genetic etiologies
Psychiatry	Need to assure psychological well being of children undergoing frequent surgery
Dental specialists	
Oral Surgery	Frequent facial skeletal surgery
Orthodontics	Universal need for orthodontic therapy in children with cleft lip/palate
Prosthetic Dentistry	Need for tooth replacement in many cases of complete clefts
Pediatric Dentistry	Need to maintain good dental health and prevent against tooth loss
Behavioral specialists	
Speech Pathology	Very frequent speech/language disorders in children with clefts
Social Service	Social adjustment problems, hospital related problems, funding problems
Psychology	Assessment and management of self-image and adjustment at home and in school
Neuropsychology	Psychometric assessment frequently required
Audiology	Very frequent hearing loss associated with clefting
Child Life Specialist	Frequent hospitalizations require attention
Other specialties	
Nursing	Frequent hospital services (in- and outpatient)
Nutritionist	Low weight a common associated anomaly
Computer Programmer	Data base management essential to learning about treatment outcome

"Carousel teams"

Many teams function by having all of the professionals involved in evaluation together in a room or clinic. The patients come to this clinic and are seen by each of the professionals during the course of a morning or an afternoon. The patients leave and their cases are then discussed by the professionals and decisions reached regarding their treatment. This is called a "carousel" approach because the patient rotates from professional to professional within a single day. Objections to this particular model of evaluation include the fact that comprehensive diagnostic tests cannot be administered within this atmosphere. Complete speech and language evaluations, thorough dentofacial evaluations, full audiometric assessments, and other diagnostic tests that require an hour or more of time individually would be impossible to apply in this type of setting. Therefore, decisions made under these circumstances are often based on incomplete information. It may also be true that the single day that the patient is seen is not necessarily representative of the patient at all times. Variation in speech quality, middle ear status, and general health may vary from day to day, and a single assessment at a finite period in time may mislead the professionals so that they conclude that this is the permanent or typical state of the patient.

"Triage" system

In the triage system, the patient first makes contact with a "gatekeeper," who makes an initial assessment of the patient's needs for evaluation. This method of triage allows the gate keeper to refer patients for extensive diagnostic batteries on an outpatient basis and allows the professionals involved to take as much time as required to reach diagnostic impressions. The group of professionals would then meet separately at a later time to discuss the case for treatment recommendations. Objections to this type of system might be that patients would need to make multiple visits to the center, which could be logistically difficult. This type of system can also incur enormous costs on the care providers, which cannot be recouped unless the patient is billed for potentially thousands of dollars.

Team director

Who should be the director? Does the person who directs the center have an impact on the outcome of both treatment recommendations and treatment results? Most certainly. Very often, the directors of teams are those individuals at a particular institution with the dominant personality. It may be that other team members find it difficult to challenge the authority of the dominant personality. It may also be true that the dominant personality can more easily sway the opinions of other team members. It is also certainly true that representatives of certain disciplines carry much more "weight" then those of other professions. For example, a plastic surgeon with an M.D. degree and extensive postgraduate training, often up to 10 years, has a greater perceived authority than a speech pathologist who has had one and a half or 2 years of postgraduate study to earn a masters degree. It is very often true that speech pathologists have difficulty in challenging the authority of someone with higher levels of training and seniority. Therefore, when discussions of case management are begun, the arguments of those with the more dominant attitude and greater longevity may have more power.

It is also true that the discipline of the dominant authority may affect the treatment protocols adopted by the center. For example, in institutions where dental practitioners are the

team directors, dental treatments may be given greater priority over surgical treatments. This may result in an approach to palate repair that includes deferred hard palate repair (in order to avoid scarring the dental-bearing tissue), neonatal or infant maxillary orthopedics, or early orthodontic intervention. In institutions where surgeons direct the team, it may be found that surgical recommendations are given precedence over other areas of management, including speech therapy or orthodontics.

Though it must be emphasized that no hard data exists to demonstrate the differences in the recommendations of various team models or team approaches, one cannot presume that different models will result in the same treatment outcomes. This particular area of patient management demands attention, but the research that would need to be done would be extremely difficult to implement.

Interdisciplinary versus multidisciplinary

The distinction between interdisciplinary and multidisciplinary may seem to be a semantic one, but it is not. Multidisciplinary teams would be those that have representatives from many disciplines, but they do not necessarily function in a cooperative or interactive manner. As mentioned previously, dominant personalities may dominate a team so much that the opinions of other specialists may not have as important an impact on patient management. In interdisciplinary teams (which are also, obviously, multidisciplinary), each specialist is given equivalent status in order to negotiate a treatment plan that is the best for the patient. The disciplines interact *with* each other rather than *at* each other. Rather than a competetive interaction, there is a cooperative interaction.

THE TRANSDISCIPLINARY APPROACH: BEYOND INTERDISCIPLINARY

This author was recently introduced to a new concept by LeBlanc (1994). The multidisciplinary approach, while better than individual management of a patient, is inferior to the interdisciplinary approach because the interaction between specialists may not necessarily be cooperative. Truly interdisciplinary teams function to the benefit of the patient by reaching treatment decisions based on a collaborative process where one professional becomes cognizant of another's treatment priorities. In the transdisciplinary approach, team members not only become aware of other discipline's priorities, they also learn about them. By being truly cooperative, transdisciplinary teams try to impart as much knowledge as possible about their disciplines to each other. It is desirable for the surgeon to understand as much as possible about speech and vice versa. If the speech pathologist understands what a surgeon can accomplish and exactly how specific operations can improve (or impair) speech, then the speech pathologist is in a better position to make treatment recommendations in a manner that is not completely independent of the surgeon's priorities.

TAKING THE CHALLENGE
Practical science and innovation

The purpose of this chapter has been to challenge some of the preconceptions regarding clefting and to introduce concepts that will ultimately help in delivering better patient care. In the chapters to follow, much of the information will do the same. The attempt is to expose the reader to practical aspects of care that are not typically presented in textbook form. The purpose of this text is not simply to provide the reader with interpretations of previous authors' works. The authors in this text represent true innovators and instruments of advancement of the state-of-the-art. They have been instructed by the editors to provide the reader with all of the practical knowledge they will require to assess and treat communicative problems associated with cleft lip and cleft palate. The techniques and treatment options described in the chapters to follow are based firmly in advanced scientific method and have been put to the test clinically in large centers across North America. For the experienced reader, some of the material presented in this text may seem contrary to other materials that have previously appeared in print.

REFERENCES

Dorf DS, Curtin JW: Early cleft palate repair and speech outcome. *Plast Reconstr Surg* 70:74-79, 1982.

Fraser FC: *The use of teratogens in the analysis of abnormal developmental mechanisms*. First international conference on congenital malformations, Philadelphia, 1961, Lippincott.

Hall CD, Golding-Kushner KJ: Long term follow-up of 500 patients after palate repair performed prior to 18 months of age. Paper presented at the 6th International Congress on Cleft Palate and Related Craniofacial Anomalies, Jerusalem, 1989.

Isberg A, Henningsson G. Influence of palatal fistulas on velopharyngeal movements: a cineradiographic study. *Plast Reconstr Surg* 79:525-530, 1987.

Kaplan EN: The occult submucous cleft palate, *Cleft Palate J* 12:356-368, 1975.

Kitamura H: Evidence for cleft palate as a postfusion phenomenon, *Cleft Palate J* 28:195-210, 1991.

Randall P, LaRossa DD, Fakhraee SM, Cohen MA: Cleft palate closure at 3 to 7 months of age: a preliminary report. *Plast Reconstr Surg* 70:624-629, 1983.

Semb G: A study of facial growth in patients with unilateral cleft lip and palate treated by the Oslo CLP team, *Cleft Palate-Craniofacial J* 28:1-21, 1991.

Shprintzen RJ: *A critic's look at the state-of-the-art in cleft palate and craniofacial disorders: where we have been, where we need to go*. In Gerber SE, Mencher GT, editors: International perspectives on communicative disorders. Washington, DC, 1988, Gallaudet University Press: 138-149.

Shprintzen RJ, Schwartz R, Daniller A, Hoch L. The morphologic significance of bifid uvula, *Pediatrics* 75:553-561, 1985a.

Shprintzen RJ, Siegel-Sadewitz VL, Amato J, Goldberg RB: Anomalies associated with cleft lip, cleft palate, or both, *Am J Med Genet* 20:585-595, 1985b.

Shprintzen RJ: *Hypernasal speech in the absence of overt or submucous cleft palate: the mystery solved*. Chapter in Diagnosis and Treatment of Palato Glossal Malfunction, Ellis R and Flack R, editors. College of Speech Therapists (London), 1979.

Stewart JM, Ott JE, Lagase R: Submucous cleft palate: prevalence in a school population, *Cleft Palate J* 9:246-250, 1972.

Trigos I, Ysunza A: A comparison of palatoplasty with and without primary pharyngoplasty, *Cleft Palate J* 25:163-166, 1988.

2 The Genetics of Clefting and Associated Syndromes

Robert J. Shprintzen and Rosalie Goldberg

Interdisciplinary teams caring for individuals with clefts have been accessible for over four decades. Without question, advances in the care of children with clefts have mirrored the rapid progress in technology and surgical technique, which have typically been rapidly absorbed by teams. Advances in instrumentation and technique are recognized as having a direct impact on patient care and treatment outcome and therefore must be utilized if teams are to remain current and competitive. This chapter will review what is currently known about the etiology of clefting, including the more common syndromes of cleft lip and/or cleft palate; theories of multifactorial causation; autosomal dominant, autosomal recessive, X-linked dominant, and X-linked recessive inheritance; contiguous gene deletion syndromes; mechanically induced anomalies; teratogens; and chromosomal aneuploidies. The concept of syndromic clefting will be discussed within the context of the etiologic heterogeneity of clefting. This information will be discussed in a framework that the nongeneticist will understand and find useful when working with families who have members with congenital anomalies of the face, lip, and palate.

Many teams, however, have been somewhat slow to respond to the area of science that is advancing at a more rapid pace than any other—human genetics. The breakthroughs in understanding the basic mechanisms of human malformation have been little less than amazing over the past several years, and the progress to come in years to follow should be even more astonishing. Worldwide, scientists are in the process of fully decoding the human genome. Genes resulting in human disease are being characterized, mapped to specific locations on chromosomes, and their mechanism of action and effect are being studied. The future will hold exciting discoveries regarding the action of genes, which scientists hope will result in the ability to cure disease and interrupt and correct abnormal developmental processes.

Though interdisciplinary teams are offering genetic services in growing numbers, the number of teams that have geneticists who see every patient are still very few in number. It may be that clinicians believe that most children with clefts have them as isolated anomalies. This belief was supported initially by the report of Fraser (1970), which cited that the overwhelming majority of clefts occurred as isolated anomalies and were not part of a syndrome with multiple anomalies. Fraser reported that 3% of clefts were features of multiple anomaly syndromes, a contention later refuted by reports from several centers where all patients were seen by clinical geneticists (Rollnick and Pruzansky, 1981; Shprintzen et al, 1985; Jones, 1989). However, many clinicians still postulate that most clefts are not syndromic. In a recent publication, Gorlin (1993) reported that only 5% of clefts were syndromic. Rollnick and Pruzansky (1981) reported that 44% of 2512 cases at the Center for Craniofacial Anomalies at the University of Illinois Medical Center in Chicago had multiple anomaly syndromes in association with their clefts. Shprintzen and colleagues reported on 1000 consecutive patients from The Center for Craniofacial Disorders of Montefiore Medical Center in New York and found 53% to have multiple anomaly syndromes. Jones (1988) reported that over 30% of 428 consecutive patients from the Cleft Palate Program at Children's Hospital in San Diego had multiple anomaly syndromes. The highest percentage of associated anomalies in all three studies occurred in individuals with cleft palate but no cleft lip. Though the percentages of associated syndromes in these three studies vary somewhat, the relatively high percentage in all three reports signifies that the notion that few children with clefts have associated anomalies or syndromes is mistaken.

16

THE ASSOCIATION OF CLEFTING WITH MULTIPLE ANOMALY SYNDROMES

One outcome of the report by Fraser (1970) that fewer than 3% of children with clefts had associated syndromes was the converse conclusion that 97% of children with clefts had the cleft as an isolated anomaly, or, in other words, as a specific disease. Furthermore, it was assumed that 97% of children with clefts were otherwise "normal." If the majority of children with clefts are otherwise normal, differences seen between children with clefts might be caused by the cleft itself or by the outcome of their treatments. For example, deficient growth of the midface would be blamed on the type of palate repair or language delay on the timing of palate repair. Because nearly all children with clefts born in the industrialized world are treated during infancy, it may be natural to assume that problems that show up in the child after treatment are caused by the therapeutic approach.

At the time of Fraser's early report, only a small handful of syndromes associated with clefting had been delineated, largely because genetics was a field in its infancy. Over the past 20 years, many new syndromes with clefting as a symptom have been described, thus resulting in an improved ability to differentiate the causation of clefts. As an example, in 1971, Gorlin and colleagues catalogued 72 syndromes in which clefting was found as a feature. In 1978, Cohen reported 154 syndromes associated with clefting. In a more recent report, Cohen and Bankier (1991) found 342 syndromes to be associated with clefting. In other words, as clinical genetics grew as a discipline and as advanced diagnostic tests became available, new syndromes became delineated that were found to have clefting as an associated finding. The frequency of clefting was not increasing, but within the population of children with clefts, many cases were found to be syndromic rather than isolated cases of clefting alone. In these cases, clefting was not a specific disease, but merely a symptom of some generalized pattern of malformation.

Is the frequent association of syndromes of any concern to clinicians who are treating patients with clefts? Yes, it is extremely important. The reality is that each syndrome that is treated represents a different disease. In the case of clefts associated with multiple anomaly syndromes, treatment outcomes may be affected by other symptoms of the syndrome, and problems that develop later in life may not be caused by management errors, but by problems intrinsic to the child. The dental, aesthetic, speech, and functional problems found in a particular pa-

tient may be related to syndromic features other than the cleft. Some examples are provided later in this chapter. Data are now showing that certain speech disorders in children with clefts may be syndrome specific (Golding-Kushner, 1991). For example, the pervasive use of glottal stop substitutions has been found to be a nearly universal finding in children with velo-cardio-facial syndrome (the most common syndrome of clefting), but less common in children with isolated clefts or other syndromes (Golding-Kushner, 1991).

To illustrate the issue, an example of a typical error in clinical judgment is appropriate here. A patient is born with a unilateral cleft of the lip and palate and a normal birth weight. Early attempts at feeding the baby boy prove unsuccessful. The baby chokes, cries, and becomes upset during the feedings. At the particular hospital where this baby is born, there is no clinical geneticist, nor does the "cleft palate team" have anyone experienced in dysmorphology. A general examination of the baby fails to reveal any obvious problems. This is simply a "cleft palate child," and the baby's failure to thrive is seen as a problem secondary to the cleft. In other words, the professionals involved in the baby's care have seen the correlation between clefting and poor feeding and have fallen into the trap of believing that a correlation represents a cause and effect relationship. This seemingly natural conclusion actually represents very bad science. Two things that occur together may or may not be causally related, and if they are, the direction of causation is not necessarily evident.

For example, Monday and Tuesday have a perfect correlation. Monday always precedes Tuesday, Tuesday always follows Monday. Does Monday make Tuesday happen? Or does Tuesday cause Monday to happen? In this case, neither. Though Monday and Tuesday have a 1.0 correlation, they are not causally related. Rather, they are both caused by a third event — the calendar.

Getting back to the baby in the previous paragraph, the professionals attack the problem by trying all types of "cleft palate nipples" and feeding devices. The problems persist, the baby loses weight, and it becomes necessary to gavage feed him. For the professionals involved, the episode has reinforced how difficult it is to feed babies with clefts. Continued efforts to feed the baby fail, and even with gavage feedings, the baby loses weight, does not show linear growth at the normal rate, and continues to be irritable. The clinicians relate the irritability to the baby's "frustration" at the failed feeding attempts.

Weeks go by and eventually, with difficulty, oral feedings are accomplished, but the baby remains irritable, gains weight poorly, and grows very little. The baby's developmental milestones are delayed. The clinicians conclude that this is from prolonged hospitalization and weakness from poor weight gain. However, the clinicians decide that the parents may be able to do better at home. The baby is discharged to two overwhelmed parents who spend the next month trying to make the baby grow, enjoy his feedings, and gain weight. None of these things happen. They finally seek another opinion from a more comprehensive center. The baby is examined by the dysmorphologist who notices that by measurement, the baby's eyes are too close together, even though facially he is not very unusual in appearance. However, the association of close set eyes and cleft palate makes the dysmorphologist suspicious. A battery of tests is performed, including blood work, a karyotype (chromosome analysis), and MRI (*M*agnetic *R*esonance *I*maging) of the brain. The MRI shows a lack of complete separation of the brain's hemispheres with communication between the lateral ventricles. The forebrain and cerebral cortex are small, and the olfactory bulbs are absent. The blood work reveals diabetes insipidus. The conclusion is obvious to the dysmorphologist. The baby has a condition known as holoprosencephaly, or DeMyer sequence. Cleft lip and palate is often associated with this disorder, as is irritability, failure to thrive, and even early death. All of these problems, including the diabetes insipidus and lack of growth, are caused by the brain malformation. The pituitary gland is absent, as are other midline brain structures, such as the corpus callosum. Finally, the karyotype comes back showing a small deletion from the short arm of chromosome 18. This chromosome abnormality is known to cause holoprosencephaly and all of the symptoms described in this baby, including the cleft lip and palate. Therefore, the feeding problems and failure to thrive were not secondary to the cleft. The cleft, the feeding problems, the short stature, and the developmental delay were all caused by a third event; the deletion of a portion of chromosome 18.

The clinicians who focused on the cleft in this case failed to recognize that clefting is not a specific disease. They made assumptions about the baby, which led to unsuccessful treatment, failed diagnosis, and parental anguish. Bad science was utilized in decision making. Unfortunately, the scenario described above is not fictitious, nor is it unique. The conclusion from it must be, however, that clefting is not a specific disease. It is merely the symptom of a disease process of which the primary disease must be identified.

WHY IS IT IMPORTANT TO DIAGNOSE ASSOCIATED SYNDROMES?

There is often a tendency for people to want to avoid labels because they may stigmatize a child with a "self-fulfilling prophecy." However, there are three important factors revealed by proper diagnosis, which will result in better patient care: the phenotypic spectrum, natural history, and prognosis of the disorder.

Phenotypic spectrum refers to the range of findings that are known to be associated with a particular syndrome. This includes not only obvious physical findings, such as cleft palate or microtia, but also behavioral abnormalities (such as mental retardation, language impairment, or learning disabilities). How does the phenotypic spectrum improve patient care? By providing the clinician with the full range of anomalies that are known to occur in association with a particular syndrome, but also by providing a list of all anomalies that *could* be associated with the syndrome. For example, Stickler syndrome is one of the most common syndromes associated with cleft palate and is also among the most common genetic syndromes involving connective tissue. Though there are relatively few anomalies associated with Stickler syndrome (Fig. 2-1), several of

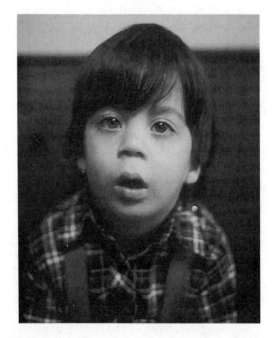

Fig. 2-1 Characteristic facial appearance in Stickler syndrome.

them require specific tests for identification. A particularly important anomaly often associated with Stickler syndrome is severe myopia, which is often a warning sign of vitreal degeneration and possible retinal detachment. Most children, and certainly nearly all infants, do not have full eye examinations with dilation and fundoscopic assessment. It would therefore be easy to miss congenital or progressive myopia in infancy and childhood until the problem were so severe as to be obvious.

Children with Stickler syndrome also may have minor anomalies of the growth centers of the long bones (the epiphyses) and minor spine anomalies. While these problems are not debilitating, they can result in arthritic type pains at an early age. If the source of these pains were not understood within the context of the phenotypic spectrum of Stickler syndrome, elaborate and even painful assessment procedures might be utilized in a search for a more common source of joint pains: juvenile rheumatoid arthritis. If the source of the pains is understood, or even anticipated, proper radiographic examinations can be employed (Fig. 2-2), the problem identified, and appropriate treatment recommended.

Children with Stickler syndrome also have a slightly increased risk for high frequency sensory hearing loss. The loss is usually mild and could potentially be masked by the chronic middle ear disease often found in children with clefts. Knowing that approximately 15% of children with Stickler syndrome and palatal clefts have a sensory hearing disorder, a more intensive search can be utilized for identifying the sensory hearing loss, if present.

Therefore, by understanding the phenotypic spectrum of a syndrome, clinicians can save time, expense, and trouble (for both the patient and the clinician) in the search for an accurate diagnosis and proper treatment. A precise definition of the mutant phenotype will help to elucidate the related genotype. Because the entire spectrum of disorders has been defined for other patients and the success of treatments confirmed, better patient care will be a direct outcome of knowing the phenotypic spectrum.

Natural history refers to the effect of the syndrome over time. For example, cleft lip and palate occur in approximately 10% of individuals with Robinow syndrome (Fig. 2-3), an autosomal dominant genetic disorder characterized by facial, limb, and genital anomalies

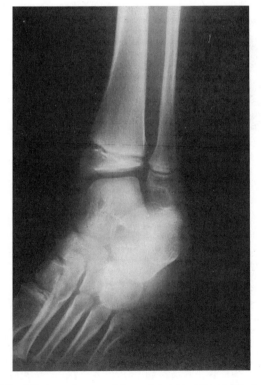

Fig. 2-2 Appearance of the epiphyses at the ankles in Stickler syndrome.

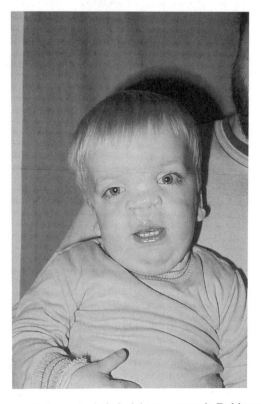

Fig. 2-3 Characteristic facial appearance in Robinow syndrome.

including hypertelorism, wide palpebral fissures, short arms and fingers, and micropenis in affected males. Though affected infants with clefts may not be very different from other newborns with cleft lip and palate, with time the facial appearance becomes more obvious and characteristic (Fig. 2-3). Head circumference often increases excessively with time, but not because of excessive brain growth or hydrocephalus. The bones of the skull may become sclerotic (excessively thick and calcified) with increasing age (Fig. 2-4). Also a part of the natural history is a failure for the micropenis to resolve, even after puberty. As a result of this knowledge base, testosterone treatments have been applied with positive results. Other examples of syndromic natural history would be the possible development of various neoplasias or tumors, such as nephroblastoma (in Beckwith-Wiedemann syndrome as well as the decreasing prominence of facial nevus flammeus in that same syndrome), late onset of psychiatric disorders in velo-cardio-facial syndrome, and late closure of the cranial sutures and fontanelles in cleidocranial dysplasia. One of the more interesting instances of how the natural history of a syndrome can lead to better patient care is illustrated by Prader-Willi syndrome. Speech in Prader-Willi syndrome, a

disorder associated with obesity, developmental delay, hypotonia, and cryptorchidism, is often hypernasal. However, with time, hypernasality often spontaneously resolves as hypotonia decreases. If the natural history of this disorder were not known, individuals with Prader-Willi syndrome might be referred for surgery to resolve the speech disorder. In fact, this surgery might prove to be life-threatening because another feature of the natural history of Prader-Willi syndrome is the development of obstructive sleep apnea (intermittent cessation of breathing during sleep), which can be exacerbated by pharyngeal surgery.

Each syndrome also has a well established prognosis. Unfortunately, in some syndromes, life span is decreased, and premature senility with mental deterioration may be a finding. Other factors may contribute to a bleak outlook. In such cases, professionals may be forced to make difficult decisions regarding the advisability of treatments, especially if no appreciable benefit is to be obtained by applying the treatment. What may appear to be humane and necessary treatment for most patients may prove to be wasted effort, time, and money in individuals with a poor prognosis. For example, patients with severe cases of holoprosencephaly (Fig. 2-5, *A*) have such abnormal brains that

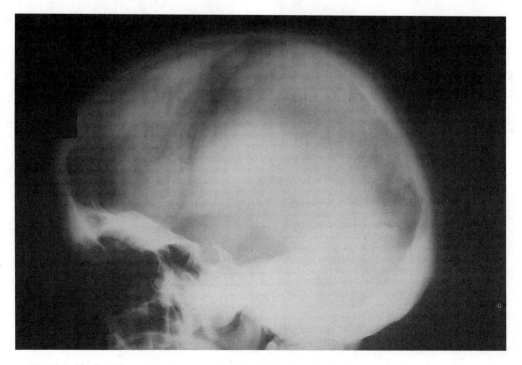

Fig. 2-4 Skull radiographs showing sclerosis of the bone in Robinow syndrome.

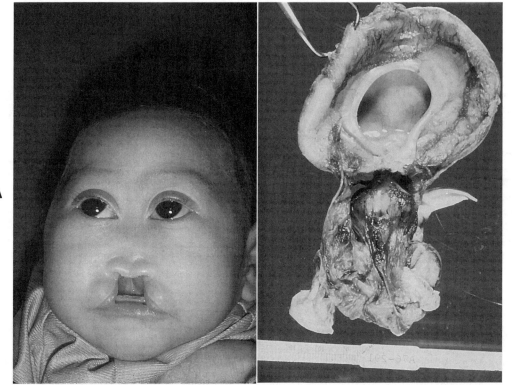

Fig. 2-5 Facial appearance of premaxillary agenesis type holoprosencephaly (**A**) and appearance of the brain (**B**) showing lack of differentiation of the hemispheres.

their central nervous systems are incompatible with life (Fig. 2-5, *B*). Though clefts of the lip are common (including true median cleft lip in premaxillary agenesis type holoprosencephaly as shown in Fig. 2-5, *A*), repair of the lip may be contraindicated if death is imminent. Many, if not most babies with this disorder, have central apnea, diabetes insipidus, poor temperature control, and seizures with essentially no intellectual development.

Conversely, some disorders may present with severe malformations but excellent prognoses if treatment is applied. For example, severe facial clefts and limb anomalies can be caused by early tears in the amnion (see discussion later in this chapter). Though severely disfigured, if the brain is unaffected, the prognosis for normal development is excellent.

Therefore, syndromic diagnosis can be a pivotal component in making appropriate treatment decisions regarding the patient. Diagnostic work-ups can be focused on the established phenotypic spectrum, the timing of needed treatments can be appropriately anticipated based on a defined natural history, and proper counseling for long-term outcome can be provided based on the prognosis. Treatments can be chosen on the basis of known outcomes in a particular syndrome as published by professionals who have had experience with the disorder. Finally, the parents of children whose problems might have seemed mysterious to them before diagnosis may take some comfort in the establishment of a name for the condition. It signals that the professionals are dealing with a known entity that they understand and can manage better.

SYNDROMES OF CLEFTING

Clefting is currently associated with over 400 multiple anomaly syndromes. This number of multiple anomaly conditions does not include children who have multiple anomalies not consistent with any known syndrome, but which apparently do represent a syndrome unique to that child. A simple definition of a syndrome is appropriate here. A syndrome may be defined as the presence of multiple anomalies in a single individual with all those anomalies having one primary cause. For an excellent text that details the principles of syndromology, the reader is referred to *The Child with Multiple Birth Defects* (Cohen, 1982). The following classification system was proposed by Cohen (1982) and represents an excellent method for the study and delineation of syndromes. There are two broad categories of syndromes that may, in turn, be further subdivided. The first category is *known genesis syndromes* (Cohen, 1982). Known genesis syndromes are those where the primary etiology can be identified. The second category is *unknown genesis syndromes* (Cohen, 1982). Unknown genesis syndromes are those that result in multiple anomalies, but the exact etiology cannot be identified. However, the multiple anomalies in the child did not occur by chance and do represent a syndrome. Known genesis syndromes may be caused by four basic groups of etiologies:

1. Chromosome abnormalities.
2. Genetic disorders.
3. Teratogenic influences.
4. Mechanical factors.

CHROMOSOME DISORDERS

The nucleus of most human cells has 46 chromosomes, which are arranged in sets. One set is given to the child by each parent. Each set has 23 single chromosomes—22 autosomes and an X or Y sex chromosome. The chromosomes contain roughly equal parts of DNA and protein and can be seen under a light microscope. When they are stained with certain dyes to enhance the analysis, alternating bands of light and dark regions become visible. The study of the size of these small regions of chromosome allows small segments of each chromosome to be well visualized (Fig. 2-6). The chromosomes carry the majority of human genetic information, including those genes that form the structure of the developing embryo. Abnormalities in the structure, number, and integrity of the chromosomes can be visualized during cell division. A karyotype, or gross chromosome analysis, is done by drawing blood, growing the cells in a culture medium, and looking at the white blood cells during cell division, photographing the chromosomes, and arranging these photographs so that the chromosomes can be paired and the structure assessed (Fig. 2-6). In most laboratories, karyotyping is aided by a computer. By applying various stains to the sample being analyzed, small pieces of chromosomes can be better visualized as bands of different shading, which correspond to known areas on the chromosome that regulate specific functions (Fig. 2-6). New techniques of chromosome analysis,

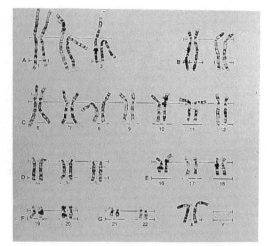

Fig. 2-6 High resolution female karyotype.

high resolution karyotyping and molecular cytogenetics, allow extremely small chromosome abnormalities to be detected. Sometimes very minute deletions can be classified as contiguous gene deletions. There are two classes of contiguous gene deletion syndromes; those with and those without visible chromosome defects. It is suspected that many genes can be deleted in a specific critical region and can be represented on a karyotype as a very small visible chromosome defect.

In the center of each chromosome is a circular structure known as a centromere. The shorter portion of the chromosome extending from the centromere is known as the short arm, or p arm of the chromosome, while the longer portion extending from the centromere is known as the long arm, or q arm of the chromosome (Fig. 2-6).

Most changes in DNA are too subtle to be detected by routine karyotyping, which shows rather large changes in chromosome structure. A newer technology that is becoming more commonplace in clinical assessment is molecular cytogenetic analysis. It will be discussed later in this chapter.

Abnormalities of the chromosomes are usually suspected in individuals with multiple malformations, especially when a newborn is very small, has severe malformations, has developmental delay or mental retardation, and severe heart or limb abnormalities. Abnormalities of the chromosomes may include the absence of an entire chromosome (monosomy), an extra chromosome (a trisomy), the absence of a piece of a chromosome (deletion), or the duplication of a piece of a chromosome (partial trisomy). Because many genes are usually located on a microscopic piece of chromosome material, individuals with chromosome abnormalities usually have severe problems, are often very small, and are usually mentally retarded. In many instances, conditions associated with chromosome abnormalities are incompatible with life. In fact, a high percentage (probably close to 60%) of miscarriages consist of fetuses with chromosome abnormalities. One of the birth defects common to individuals with chromosome disorders is cleft palate or cleft lip and palate.

GENETIC DISORDERS

Genes are submicroscopic and are strung along the chromosomes like beads on a necklace. Each molecule of DNA contains many genes. The chromosomes contain thousands of genes. A gene is a specific sequence of nucleotide bases whose order carry the information required for constructing proteins, which provide the scaffolding of cells, tissues, and enzymes. Human genes vary in length. Only about 10% of the human genome is known to include the protein coding sequences (exon) of genes. Interspersed within many genes are intron sequences, which have no coding function. Of primary importance, the genetic information contained in the genes determines the manner in which embryos develop. By the 1960s, the genetic code had been broken. Many scientists were involved in genetic experiments that were found to support the hypothesis that the genetic messages of DNA are conveyed by its sequenced order of base pairs, which comprise the genes. By 1966, the complete genetic code was established, and the building blocks of proteins, enzymes, and tissues were found to be dependent on the order of chemicals arranged by the code. A gene that is in some way abnormal (i.e., the action of the gene results in a developmental process different than the action of the normal gene) is said to be a mutant gene. Gene mutations occur frequently in human beings. Most mutations are extremely detrimental, and many result in nonviable individuals. Other mutations may result in congenital malformations that are not incompatible with life. Allelic mutations are different changes in the same gene. Allelic mutations can result in the same phenotype in two different individuals, or completely different phenotypes even though the same gene is mutated (though the change, or mutation, in the gene is different). Allelic heterogeneity can account for a range of different phenotypes even within the same monogenic condition. Sometimes intrafamilial phenotypic differences in the same syndrome are due to allelic mutations. Factors that may account for intrafamilial differences include modifying genes and environmental influences.

An individual's full complement of genes comes directly from the parents; half from the mother, half from the father. Genes may act in either a dominant or recessive manner, a concept that will be discussed in detail later in this chapter. Genes located on the X chromosome will result in traits known as X-linked traits. At present, the majority of syndromes associated with cleft lip and cleft palate are genetic in etiology. Of the 342 syndromes of clefting discussed by Cohen and Bankier (1991), nearly two thirds were of single gene causation. This represents an enormous number of conditions, which would result in a cleft in association with other congenital anomalies.

A comprehensive genetic evaluation should be provided for every patient born with a cleft lip, cleft palate, or both, preferably during the first visit to the center where treatment will be provided. The evaluation should begin with a detailed prenatal history, including any evidence of exposure to known or suspected teratogens, such as alcohol, cocaine, retinoids, phenytoins, or viruses (to be discussed in further detail). At the same time, a detailed family history will be taken and a pedigree constructed. A pedigree is a pictorial representation of family traits, including health information for parents, grandparents, aunts, uncles, and cousins (Fig. 2-7). Because children inherit 50% of their genes from each parent and clefting can be inherited genetically (but can skip one or more generations), it is essential to obtain as detailed a history as possible about as many family members as possible.

To understand how genes are inherited, models have been developed to fit observed patterns from pedigree information, which have been confirmed by what is known about the transmission of chromosomes and genes from parent to child. One form of inheritance is known as *autosomal dominant.* If one parent has a dominant gene for a particular disorder on one of the autosomes, each child has a 50% chance of inheriting this gene and developing the disorder (Fig. 2-8). There are many syndromes that have clefting as a feature and are inherited in an autosomal dominant manner, including van der Woude syndrome, Stickler syndrome, EEC syndrome, Treacher Collins syndrome, Apert syndrome, Rapp-Hodgkin ectodermal dysplasia syndrome, Robinow syndrome, and cleidocranial dysplasia syndrome, to name a few. According to Cohen and Bankier (1991),

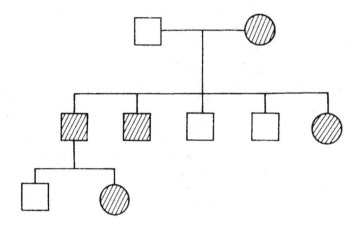

Pedigree of a family affected by Stickler Syndrome

◩ Affected male members
◪ Affected female members

Fig. 2-7 An example of pedigree.

over 20% of syndromes of clefting are inherited in an autosomal dominant manner.

Autosomal recessive inheritance requires the gene for the disorder to be inherited from both parents. If both parents carry a mutant recessive gene on one of the autosomes, each of their children has a 25% chance of inheriting both mutant genes and expressing the disorder (Fig. 2-9). Similarly, each child has a 25% chance of inheriting two normal genes and a 50% chance of inheriting one normal and one mutant gene (Fig. 2-9). Individuals who have only one mutant copy of the gene will not express the trait, but they are called carriers because they do have the possibility of passing on the trait to their children if their mate is also a carrier. According to Cohen and Bankier (1991), nearly one third of all syndromes of clefting are autosomal recessive.

Clefting can also be inherited in an *X-linked* or *sex linked* manner. Normal females have two X chromosomes, while normal males have one X and one Y chromosome. An apparently normal mother can carry a mutant gene on one of her X chromosomes, but because the mutant gene is recessive, the trait will not be expressed. Male children will have a 50% chance of inheriting the X chromosome with the abnormal gene (Fig. 2-10). Because the male child does not have a normal gene on a corresponding X chromosome (he will have a Y chromosome that

carries no corresponding gene at all) he will therefore express the trait. Female offspring of a carrier mother and unaffected father cannot express the trait because they will always have a normal X chromosome gene to cancel the effect of the mutant gene (recessive). A father, even if affected, cannot transmit the disease to his sons because his sons will never inherit his X chromosome; they will inherit his other sex chromosome (the Y). However, an affected father's daughters have a 50% likelihood of being carriers (Fig. 2-10). According to Cohen and Bankier (1991), there are a small number of X-linked syndromes of clefting comprising approximately 5% of all clefting syndromes. There are some traits that are *X-linked dominant* disorders. In the case of X-linked dominant traits, female children of affected fathers can express the disorder (Fig. 2-11), as can female children of affected females.

It is also possible for traits to be caused both by genetic and environmental factors. These are known as multifactorial effects, and in previous publications, the majority of clefts were thought to be caused by multifactorial effects (Fraser, 1970).

A final category of genetic disorders are newly recognized because of technology emanating from the study of molecular genetics. *Contiguous gene* syndromes, a term coined by Schmickel (1986) are caused by the deletion or duplication

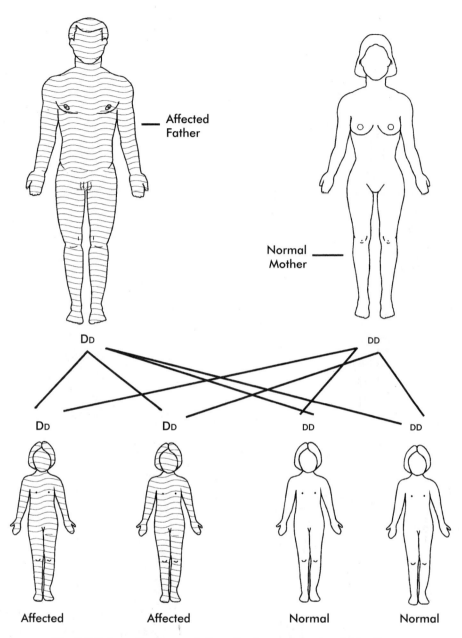

Fig. 2-8 Schematic representation of autosomal dominant inheritance.

of a string of genes located in a very small area on a single chromosome. Included among this type of syndromes are Prader-Willi syndrome, Beckwith-Wiedemann syndrome, and Rubin-stein-Taybi syndrome, which may have visible changes in the chromosomes, but which may also not be visible, observable only using molecular techniques. The most common syndrome of clefting, velo-cardio-facial syndrome,

may possibly be a contiguous gene syndrome involving a string of genes at the q11 region of chromosome 22. Contiguous gene syndromes most often involve deletions or duplications, which are too small to be seen under a microscope and can only be detected using molecular probes (to be discussed in more detail below).

An important concept to explain at this point

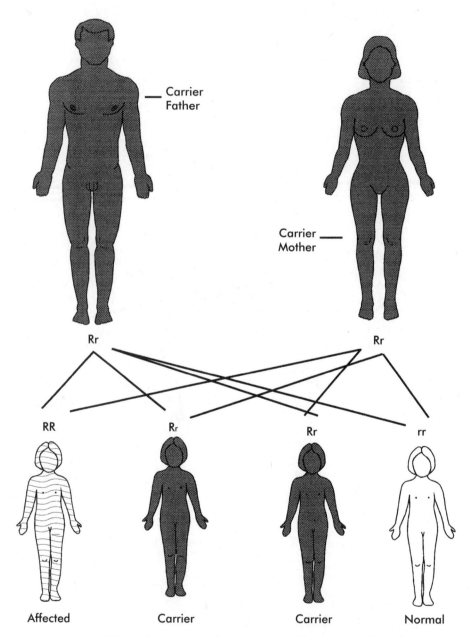

Fig. 2-9 Schematic representation of autosomal recessive inheritance.

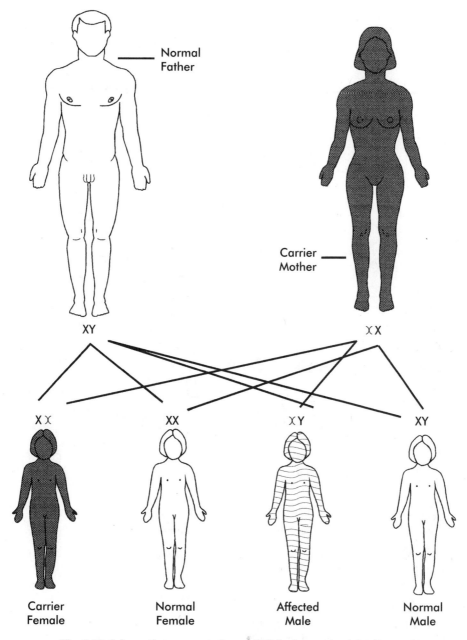

Fig. 2-10 Schematic representation of X-linked recessive inheritance.

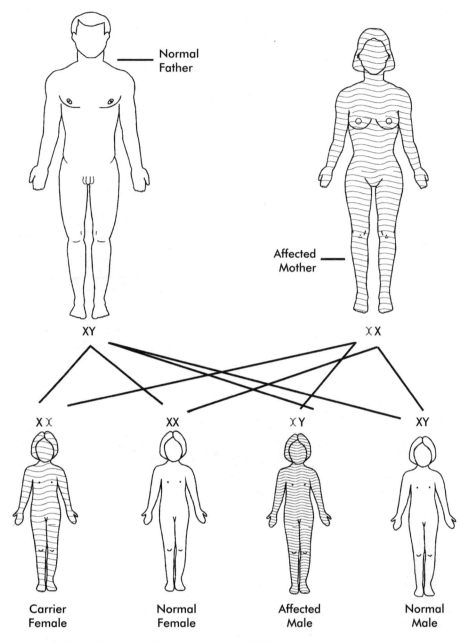

Fig. 2-11 Schematic representation of X-linked dominant inheritance.

is *variable expression.* Gene inheritance can be predicted, but gene effect cannot yet be predicted. Variable expression refers to the fact that two individuals who have inherited the same mutant gene may show varying degrees of severity of the disorder. However, more complex mutations may account for a wide variation in phenotype. Though there are basic similarities in all individuals who have the syndrome, not every individual with the syndrome may have

the same number or severity of anomalies, even within the same sibship.

For example, Treacher Collins syndrome is a very distinctive disorder with anomalies isolated to the craniofacial complex. Cleft palate is a frequent finding in Treacher Collins syndrome, and cleft lip can also occur as a syndromic feature, though less frequently than cleft palate. Some individuals with Treacher Collins syndrome have severe bilateral grade III microtia, while others have almost normal appearing ears with only a mild conductive hearing loss (Fig. 2-12). Some have cleft palate, others do not. Variable expression represents a diagnostic dilemma to even the most experienced clinicians.

TERATOGENIC DISORDERS

Teratogenic disorders, or environmentally induced conditions, are those congenital anomalies that are the result of the direct or indirect action of an agent external to the genetic material of the fetus. Teratogens may include medicinal drugs, nonmedicinal drugs and psychoactive substances (such as alcohol and cocaine), viruses, and some natural occurring substances in the environment. Relatively few teratogens result in cleft lip and/or cleft palate. According to Cohen and Bankier (1991), fewer than 3% of all clefts are caused by known environmental agents. However, one teratogen, alcohol, does result in many infants with clefts in addition to other anomalies (Shprintzen et al, 1985b). We have found alcohol to contribute both to clefting of the lip and clefting of the palate. As with most teratogens, which are substances taken by the mother, there are several factors that will influence the expression of the disorder: the timing of the delivery of the teratogen, the amount taken, and the mother's metabolism. Other potent teratogens include many of the anticonvulsant drugs (phenytoins), nontopical acne medications (retinoids), and most of the illegal psychoactive drugs, such as cocaine.

MECHANICALLY INDUCED CLEFTS

Mechanical factors that cause clefts are those that directly impinge on the developing embryo inside the uterus. Intrauterine crowding, tears in the amnion, the presence of a twin, the presence of a uterine tumor, or an abnormal uterus can all result in clefts. In many cases, especially when amniotic ruptures cause clefts, the malformation is in a sense accidental and sporadic with no pattern of inheritance. Though mechanical factors account for only a small percentage of all clefts, clefts caused by amniotic ruptures are relatively common (Fig. 2-13). In mechanically induced clefts, the presumption is that the developing fetus is otherwise normal (i.e., intrinsically normal) with the abnormality being induced by a factor extrinsic to the fetus.

UNKNOWN GENESIS SYNDROMES

In some cases, children have multiple anomaly disorders where the etiology is not known (hence, unknown genesis syndromes). There are two types of unknown genesis syndromes: recurrent pattern and provisionally unique (Cohen, 1982).

Recurrent pattern unknown genesis syndromes are those multiple anomaly disorders that have been seen, described, and reported previously, but they do not have an identifiable cause. No chromosome anomaly has been found, there is no history of teratogenesis, and no history of a similar occurrence in the family exists. It is possible that the disorder represents a spontaneous mutation of a dominant gene, or it could be a recessively inherited trait; however, without firm evidence of a mutant gene (by pedigree analysis or molecular analysis of DNA), it is impossible to know if there is a genetic cause. Because the disorder is one that has been seen and reported before, it has a recurrent pattern, and therefore it is possible to know something about the course of the disorder. It is often true that syndromes of this nature have many serious problems, such as mental retardation or major physical anomalies, so that reproduction by that individual is less likely, making confirmation of a genetic etiology difficult.

There are several well-recognized disorders that are unknown genesis recurrent pattern syndromes.

One syndrome that is quite common is often associated with cleft lip and/or cleft palate, yet still is of unknown genesis is oculo-auriculo-vertebral dysplasia, also known as hemifacial microsomia or Goldenhar syndrome. This disorder is associated with facial asymmetry, conductive hearing loss related to ossicular and middle ear anomalies, eye anomalies, and spine abnormalities. Though there have been some cases of apparent dominant inheritance, the overwhelming majority of cases are sporadic and etiology remains unknown. A familiar syndrome that was until recently of unknown genesis is Williams syndrome.

Until recently, there was no known cause of this distinctive disorder, but the rapid progress of molecular genetics has led to the discovery of a genetic deletion from the long arm of chromosome 7 at the 7q11.23 locus (Ewart et al., 1993). Perhaps one of the most familiar syndromes to speech-language pathologists is Williams syndrome, a disorder with a characteristic craniofacial pattern, but not cleft lip or palate. Individuals with Williams syndrome are cognitively impaired, yet have very sophisticated language usage. They are known to be very loquacious and gregarious. They also may have hypercalcemia and congenital heart disease. Their faces are characterized by thick lips, a

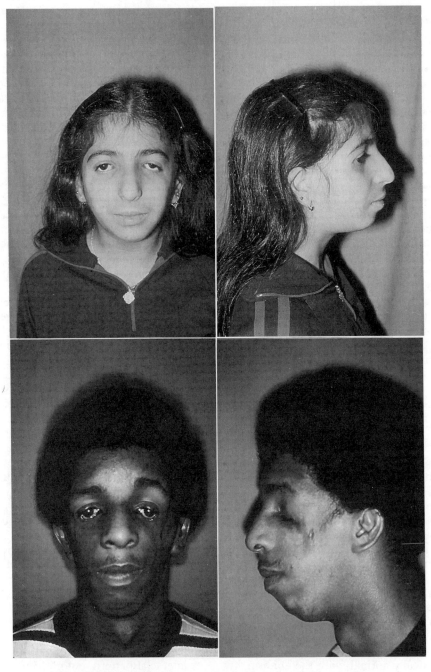

Fig. 2-12 Variable facial expression in Treacher Collins syndrome.

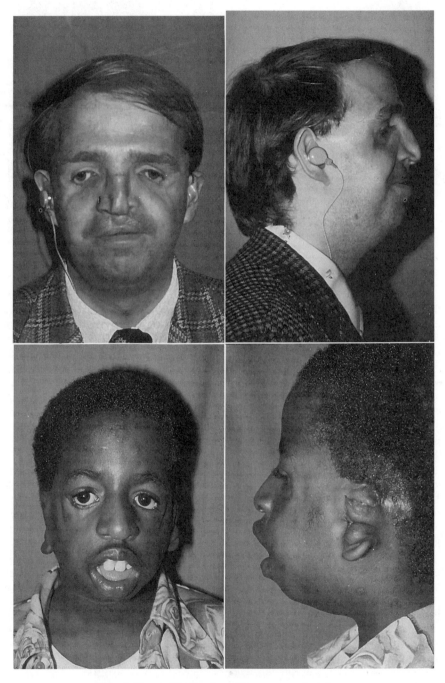

Fig. 2-12, cont'd. For legend, see opposite page.

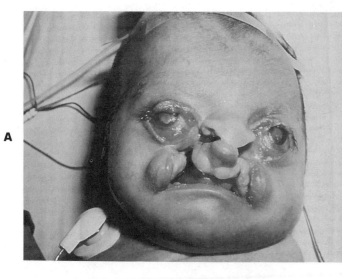

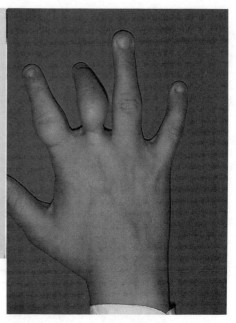

Fig. 2-13 Facial (**A**) and hand (**B**) anomalies in amnion rupture (ADAM) sequence.

large mouth, depressed nasal root, and puffiness around the eyes.

Many children with clefts have multiple anomalies that do not fit any pattern of syndromes that have been described, nor has the pattern been described before. Cohen (1982) describes such apparently unique disorders as "provisionally unique." Though the clinician may scour the literature, consult learned colleagues, and scan computer data bases, no similar patient is found (hence the "unique" nature of the syndrome). However, the condition is *provisionally* unique because the individual with the condition may reproduce and have a child with the same disorder (hence making it a recurrent pattern **known genesis** syndrome). In addition, someone may find an unrelated child with the same disorder (thus delineating a recurrent pattern **unknown genesis** syndrome).

SEQUENCE

Not all multiple anomaly disorders are syndromes. Some are called a *sequence*. A sequence is the occurrence of multiple anomalies in a single individual where one of the anomalies has led to the development of all the other anomalies. But the one primary anomaly may have multiple possible causes. The perfect model for the illustration of a sequence is the disorder that has incorrectly been named "Pierre Robin syndrome." This disorder is now correctly labeled *Robin sequence*. The disorder bearing the name of the early twentieth Century French stomatologist is typically regarded as the triad of findings of micrognathia, a wide U-shaped cleft palate, and upper airway obstruction. In Robin, both the cleft palate and upper airway obstruction occur secondary to the micrognathia. Embryologically, the palate begins forming at approximately 8 weeks postfertilization. At that time, the palatal shelves are vertical in orientation, and the embryonic tongue sits between these shelves flush against the base of the skull (Fig. 2-14). As the mandible grows, the oral cavity enlarges and the tongue is free to descend into the floor of the mouth, thus removing it from between the palatal shelves. The palatal shelves then flip into a horizontal orientation and begin growing toward the midline, where they ultimately fuse by 10 or 11 weeks postfertilization (Fig. 2-14). In infants born with Robin sequence, micrognathia prevents the mandible from enlarging sufficiently so that the tongue cannot descend in the oral cavity. The tongue stays between the palatal shelves as the skull continues to expand laterally, but the palatal shelves are prevented from growing by the physical obstruction. When the tongue finally does descend, the distance the palatal shelves would need to traverse to fuse is in excess of their growth potential, thus resulting in a U-shaped cleft palate, which has been molded by the tongue's presence. At birth, infants are

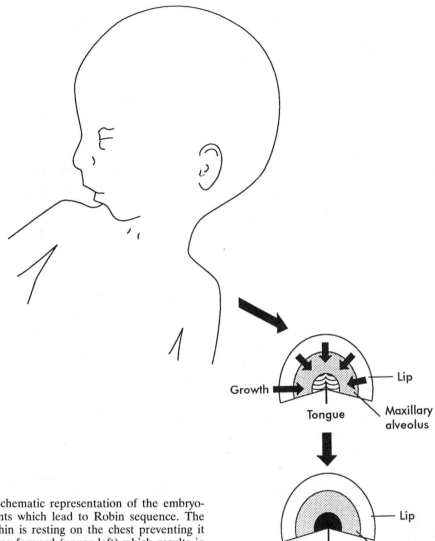

Fig. 2-14 Schematic representation of the embryological events which lead to Robin sequence. The embryo's chin is resting on the chest preventing it from growing forward (upper left) which results in the tongue being unable to descend from between the palatal shelves (center) resulting in a U-shaped palatal cleft (bottom).

obligate nose breathers (a reflexively determined respiratory pattern). With the mouth closed and the tongue sitting in the palatal cleft, the airway is obstructed by the tongue (known as glossoptosis). Therefore, the micrognathia is the primary anomaly, which is the direct cause of both the palatal cleft and airway obstruction; hence the term *sequence,* which accurately represents a sequence of events that would not have occurred without the micrognathia. However, micrognathia can have many possible causes. Micrognathia is a common occurrence in many chromosomal disorders, genetic disorders, teratogenic effects, and may even be secondary to mechanical factors. As an example, Robin

sequence can occur in the chromosomal deletion syndromes del(4q) and del(6q); the genetic disorders Stickler syndrome, velo-cardio-facial syndrome, and diastrophic dysplasia; and the teratogenic disorders fetal alcohol syndrome and fetal hydantoin syndrome. It should therefore be obvious that it is possible to have both a syndrome and a sequence in the same individual, because one of the anomalies caused by that syndrome may trigger a secondary chain reaction such as micrognathia in the Robin sequence. Mechanically induced Robin sequence is thought to be caused by physical compression of the chin by positional constriction of the mandible. This could be caused by the presence of a twin, or more commonly by a condition known as oligohydramnios where the mother has an abnormally small amount of amniotic fluid. The chin becomes wedged against the very prominent developing heart, thus physically deforming it and preventing it from growing forward. In this last case, the Robin sequence is most appropriately called the Robin deformation sequence because the mandible is deformed externally by mechanical forces, rather than malformed as it would be in the case of a malformation syndrome such as Stickler syndrome (which would result in the Robin malformation sequence). In the case of mechanically induced deformations, significant "catch-up" growth of the mandible might be expected after birth because the physical restraint is removed. In malformation syndromes, "catch-up" growth would not be anticipated because the mandible in intrinsically abnormal.

In a comprehensive study of 100 cases of Robin, Shprintzen (1992) reported that 83% of Robin cases represented malformation syndromes, the most common being Stickler syndrome (34% of all Robin cases) and velo-cardio-facial syndrome (11% of all Robin cases).

GENETIC COUNSELING

It should be obvious to the reader by now that there are many possible etiologies for clefting and that identifying the etiology (and hence the syndrome) leads to better patient care. A major component to that process is obtaining precise data regarding family history and possible roles of teratogens or mechanical factors. Once these factors, genetic or otherwise, have been identified, recurrence risk counseling (usually referred to as genetic counseling) can be given. Recurrence risk counseling allows people to make appropriate reproductive decisions and is an important component of care extending from the patient to the entire family.

DO NOT EQUATE CLEFT LIP AND CLEFT PALATE

As previously mentioned in Chapter 1, cleft lip and palate is a completely different disorder than cleft palate without cleft lip. Though cleft lip is almost always accompanied by cleft palate, cleft palate is often not accompanied by cleft lip. The lip is formed from different embryonic elements than the palate, but even more importantly, lip formation is temporally separated from palate formation by several weeks. In embryonic terms, this is a very long time and events that occur 2 weeks apart are unlikely to be affected by the same abnormal process. Gene effects tend to be of rather short duration, and

teratogens would affect both the lip and palate if they were in continuous use for an extended period of time.

Why is the differentiation of cleft lip and cleft palate so important? For two reasons. The first concerns diagnosis, and the second concerns research data collected in cleft palate centers.

In nonsyndromic cases of clefting, clefts of the lip and palate and clefts of the palate only do not occur together in the same family. In families with multiple affected individuals, there may be two or more members with cleft lip and palate, or several with cleft palate only, but there would not be one individual with a cleft lip and palate, and another with cleft palate only. However, in syndromic cases of clefting, this is not true. In several syndromes, cleft type can mix within a single pedigree. In cases of genetic syndromes, the variable expression of the gene may account for different cleft type, while in teratogenic syndromes, the timing, amount, and duration of the teratogen's presence can account for variability in severity. The most common genetic syndrome where this phenomenon occurs is van der Woude syndrome (cleft lip and/or cleft palate with mounds or pits of the lower lip) (Fig. 2-15). This actual pedigree of a large family with many affected members shows several sibships with mixing of cleft type (Fig. 2-16). Other syndromes where this might occur include Treacher Collins syndrome, Robinow syndrome, Rapp-Hodgkin syndrome, EEC syndrome, and fetal alcohol syndrome.

The issue of research problems caused by mixing of cleft type was addressed in more detail in Chapter 1. The effects of cleft lip and palate on facial growth, speech, appearance, and psychological status may be very different than the effects of cleft palate alone. These two conditions should not be equated simply because both disorders are "clefts" and both are treated in the same centers.

THE NEW BIOLOGY: MOLECULAR GENETICS

The state-of-the-art thinking on the genetics of clefting has changed dramatically over the past 20 years. Reading the current literature on the genetics of clefting requires the professional to be conversant with the terminology of the "New Biology," which barely resembles past concepts. The rapid advances in technology have opened entire new fields of investigation, the most promising of which is molecular genetics.

Geneticists have been speculating on the inheritance of clefting for over 50 years with modest consensus. In the past, observations of the clinical prevalence of clefting were matched to

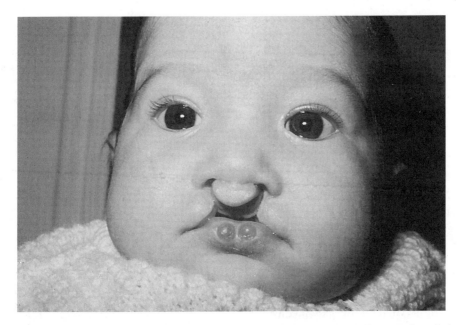

Fig. 2-15 Facial appearance of van der Woude syndrome with prominant lip mounds and pits.

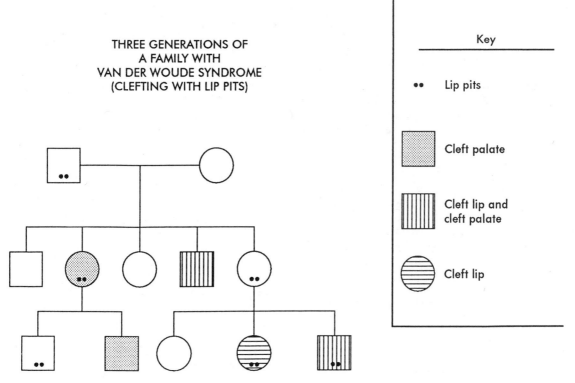

Fig. 2-16 Pedigree of a family with van der Woude syndrome showing the variable expression of the gene.

speculative models of inheritance. For example, in families with cleft lip and palate, all family members would be examined to see if minor expressions might be present, such as hypernasal speech, anomalous lateral incisors, or a characteristic face shape. If supposedly minor expressions were detected, they were considered to be expressions of a dominant gene, and a recurrence risk of 50% was given. Today, more sophisticated scientific assessments of gene expression are used. The rate at which disease-causing genes are being located and described is unprecedented in the history of medical science's efforts to unravel human illness.

In the past several years, it has been impossible to avoid articles in the science sections of newspapers describing the latest developments in DNA testing, *The Human Genome Project,* chromosome testing, candidate genes, genetic counseling, or the future promise of gene therapy. A professional not directly involved in genetics needs a primer in molecular biology to keep up with the progress that has occurred in genetics in the 1990s.

New theories of clefting have implicated genetically linked loci such as transforming growth-factor alpha (TGFA) and retinoic acid receptor loci (RARA). The TGFA association with clefting is particularly intriguing because TGFA is thought to be the embryonic form of epidermal growth factor. Epidermal growth factor is hypothesized to regulate the migration, proliferation, and differentiation of palatal epithelial cells. A gene that regulates the movements of embryonic tissues at a time in fetal development when the tissues of the lip (35 to 40 days postfertilization) or palate (8 to 10 weeks postfertilization) are fusing is a possible *candidate gene* for involvement in the process of clefting. The importance of candidate genes and single major loci is in understanding the cases of clefting that appear to be nonsyndromic. Until recently, it was universally accepted that nonsyndromic cleft lip and palate, which is responsible for clefts in 1 per 1000 live births, followed a multifactorial pattern of inheritance. However, study of the predicted frequencies of cleft lip and palate in nonsyndromic families was found to be incompatible with a multifactorial model. Single major gene loci became suspect as causative factors and subsequent studies of associated anomalies and linkage have begun to confirm these suspicions.

UNDERSTANDING DNA TESTING

New ways to test for certain inherited traits use a person's DNA. DNA is a structure found in the nucleus of almost every human cell. A DNA molecule consists of two strands that wrap around each other to resemble a twisted ladder; the sides are made of sugar and phosphate molecules, and the rungs of the ladder are made of *bases* (Fig. 2-17). Each DNA molecule

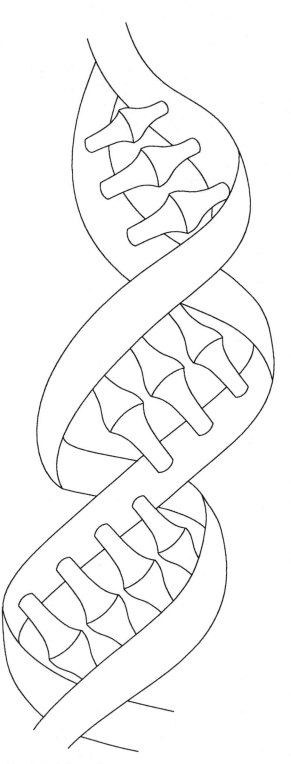

Fig. 2-17 Schematic representation of a DNA molecule.

contains many genes. A gene is a specific sequence of bases. The genes are the units of heredity and carry the message for constructing and running the organism. The complete set of instructions for making the organism is called its *genome,* which is coded by the DNA message found in the cell nucleus. This code is deciphered during the development of the fetus and is responsible for the normal structure and function of the organism.

There are two types of DNA analyses: direct and indirect. Direct analysis is the best method of DNA study, but it is available for only a few diseases; cleft lip and palate is not one of them. To use this type of study, it is necessary to know what type of change has occurred in the structure of the DNA and exactly where on the chromosome this change is located. An international initiative has been implemented known as *The Human Genome Project.* A large number of researchers have compiled the most comprehensive map of the human genome. This map, known as a genetic linkage map, contains specific molecular markers (over 1400) that cover over 90 percent of the genome. These maps are useful in the hunt for individual genes. The job is enormous because there are an estimated 100,000 genes comprised of 3 billion base pairs in the human genome.

In the search for genes that might cause clefting, indirect analysis has been used, because the exact location or the precise changes in the gene (or genes) that produces the developmental problem is not known. Genes are small pieces of information that are hooked together in a long chain of DNA on the chromosome. Genes or DNA regions that are close together are usually inherited together. In other words, they are *linked.* To use linkage analysis, it is necessary to study families that have normal variations in their DNA makeup. These variations are called *polymorphisms* or *markers.* The polymorphisms that are close to the suspected problem gene can be used as landmarks to study a family. The procedure is as follows:

1. Positional cloning. A family is identified in which a single mutant gene is sufficient to cause a particular disease, such as in families who show evidence of dominant inheritance of a particular trait or disease.
2. Identification of a DNA marker, or *probe* that is genetically linked to the disease phenotype. Polymorphisms are sought in family members who have the particular disease phenotype.

If the chromosomal location of the mutant gene is found, then the probes can be used as a test for biomolecular confirmation of the clinical diagnosis in new patients and provide an excellent test for the isolation of the gene causally related to the syndrome. Even more exciting, however, is the possibility of determining gene effect to understand the biological mechanism that causes the disease, thereby eventually resulting in a treatment specific to the gene effect.

Cleft lip and palate is a paradigm for the problems that prevent the application of direct gene analysis. Clefting is etiologically heterogenous, not all cases are genetically based (as in teratogenic or mechanically induced syndromes), and there may be many major gene loci involved in nonsyndromic clefting. Several gene loci have been suspected as candidate genes and have been studied in humans and in mouse models, including:

1. TGFA (transforming growth factor alpha). This gene has been mapped to the short arm of chromosome 2 in humans.
2. Adrb-2. This gene is located on chromosome 18 in the mouse and on the long arm of chromosome 5 (5q) in humans.
3. Pax 7. This gene is located on chromosome 4 in the mouse and the short arm of chromosome 1 in humans (1p).
4. Igf2 (insulin growth factor 2). This is located on mouse chromosome 4 and the short arm of chromosome (11p) in humans.
5. RARA (retinoic acid receptor). RARA is located on mouse chromosome 11 and the long arm of chromosome 17 (17q) in humans. It has long been known that intrauterine exposure to retinoic acid can result in cleft palate so that an abnormality in the retinoic acid receptor may be a candidate gene for clefting.

The advances in molecular biology hold great promise for the understanding of human disease. Animal models are used in laboratories allowing scientists to breed species with specific genes and then measure the outcome for the presence or absence of malformations. Sequences of genes are conserved throughout the animal kingdom. In other words, a gene that serves a particular purpose in a mouse will serve the same purpose in a human, but because humans and mice do not have the same number or form of chromosomes, a gene located on chromosome 1 in the mouse will probably not be on chromosome 1 in humans. Because breeding humans is not possible to determine gene effect, the inbreeding of mice and other animals is used as a successful substitute.

Molecular genetic analysis has provided a

powerful mechanism for defining the human genome. It is still necessary, however, to develop clinical suspicions of the presence of specific syndromes or genetic disorders in order to know which test to apply. The interaction between clinicians and basic scientists is becoming more and more frequent and increasingly fruitful in unraveling the mystery of what causes clefting to occur. Of critical importance for clinicians and clinical researchers is the realization that cleft lip and/or palate is not a single disease, but many diseases with many possible causes. Can the fact that clefting is etiologically heterogeneous have an effect on management?

THE INTERACTION OF ETIOLOGY AND ASCERTAINMENT

Patients are referred to "cleft palate children" specifically because of their clefts and not because they have a trisomy, fetal alcohol effects, or a genetic mutation. Once the label "cleft" has been attached to an affected child, a further diagnostic search may end. Therefore, the initial point of ascertainment may result in the diagnostic label, which will follow the child from that point forward. Without the recognition that the identification of a primary etiology is important, treatment decisions made for a "generic" child with a cleft may be wrong for a specific child. Because syndromes may comprise over half of children with clefts, the effects on treatment outcome are obviously significant.

A brief description of a single disorder, velo-cardio-facial syndrome, will illustrate the interaction of etiology and ascertainment and how this interaction affects treatment planning. Velo-cardio-facial syndrome has been described as the most common syndrome associated with cleft palate (Shprintzen et al, 1981; Shprintzen, 1990). The etiology of this disorder has been isolated to a microdeletion on chromosome 22 (Kelly et al, 1992). Over 30 clinical features caused by this microdeletion have been described. Included among the features in velo-cardio-facial syndrome are pharyngeal hypotonia, which results in severe hypernasality, language impairment, learning disabilities, personality disturbances, and relative small stature (Shprintzen et al, 1981; Golding-Kushner et al, 1985; Shprintzen et al, 1992; Goldberg et al, 1992). All of these findings have at one time or another been incorrectly linked to cleft palate in a cause and effect manner.

It has been reported that velo-cardio-facial syndrome comprises approximately 4.5% of all patients with clefts referred to cleft palate or craniofacial centers (Shprintzen et al, 1985).

Even more significantly, because cleft lip is not a clinical feature of velo-cardio-facial syndrome, but cleft palate is, approximately 8% of all children with cleft palate or submucous cleft palate (including occult submucous cleft) have been reported to have velo-cardio-facial syndrome (Shprintzen et al, 1985). Failure to detect this syndrome in a clinical population could significantly affect (in the statistical sense) the outcome of clinical research projects or even casual observations by clinicians, which result in determining treatment plans.

For example, a clinician wishes to determine the outcome of long-term treatment in patients with cleft palate only. The clinician finds that nearly 10% of patients treated from birth grow up with language impairment and short stature. A large number of them also have severely hypernasal speech and impaired articulation (Golding-Kushner, 1991). In applying statistical method to the data, the clinician sets a "significance level" at the arbitrary, but commonly accepted, 0.05. This level of significance, or level of confidence, actually represents a level of experimental error, which the researcher finds tolerable. In other words, it is understood by all researchers that no experiment is perfect. It is also understood that within an experiment, there are many possible sources of error. Measurement tools, the process of measurement itself, and sample selection are just a few of the possible sources of error in an experiment. By selecting 0.05 as a level of significance, the researcher is essentially indicating his or her acceptance that 5% of the data could be erroneous as a result of experimental or chance error and might affect the outcome of the experiment. But what if 8% of the sample population has velo-cardio-facial syndrome? For just this one syndrome, the researcher has encountered a source of error greater than 5%. There are several features of velo-cardio-facial syndrome that could affect the outcome of the experiment, but the researcher has failed to "weed out" subjects who have disorders associated with their clefts, which define them as something other than a child with just a cleft. Just as it is assumed there are multiple sources of error in an experiment, it is also assumed that the experimenter tries to control all sources of error. By not assuring as homogeneous a sample as possible, the experiment has been rendered invalid. However, because the researcher is not aware of the source of data contamination, he or she assumes that the results are valid. It is therefore conceivable that the experimenter could conclude that the treatment resulted in a high rate of speech abnormalities, that the feeding methods were not effective because so many of the patients were small, that the failure for the subjects to have normal velopharyngeal function resulted in language impairment and subsequent learning disabilities, and that as a result of being stigmatized by abnormal speech during their childhood, they developed a personality disorder including feelings of inferiority and persecution. Of course, all of these findings are actually the direct effect of the genetic error that causes velo-cardio-facial syndrome and are not causally related to cleft palate.

If this scenario seems too contrived, the reader must be assured that this is not the case. All one need do is to go to the literature and carefully read studies that have reported problems in children with cleft palate that are assumed to be caused by the cleft. A careful review of the Methods sections in these articles will reveal that the subjects were not examined by a dysmorphologist, geneticist, or syndromologist to rule out the possibility that the cleft was secondary to multiple anomaly disorder. There are many examples of articles that link cleft palate to small size or low weight, to developmental delay or intellectual impairment, to language impairment, and to personality disorders or maladjustment. In the majority of cases, authors have stated or implied that the cleft itself in some way contributed to these problems. In nearly all these publications, there was little or no attempt to maintain population homogeneity. Without prospective examination of all patients by an experienced clinical geneticist or dysmorphologist, the results of these studies cannot possibly be regarded as valid. Very few centers have geneticists who see all registered patients. Furthermore, very few geneticists are members of the American Cleft Palate-Craniofacial Association (less than 1% of the total membership of ACPA are geneticists). It is not the intent of this chapter to cite all these articles nor to criticize the authors for the research design. It is preferable that the reader recognizes the problem so that review of the literature can be made within an appropriately critical framework. An understanding that the so-called "cleft palate child" is a nonentity is essential to gaining the new perspective on the problem advocated by this chapter.

Several anecdotal cases are described next, which point out the necessity of having genetics as a principal component of a team, as well as having as comprehensive a team as possible.

Case 1

Jenny was referred to a "cleft palate clinic" at the age of 6 years with hypernasal speech, which has been present since the onset of verbal language. As an infant, she gained weight poorly and was slightly "floppy," but developmental milestones were grossly within normal limits. Her first word, "ma-ma" was noted at 12 months of age, but few recognizable words followed. Some words were evident at 3 years of age, but they were largely unintelligible. Jenny had frequent ear infections, several episodes of bronchitis, and two bouts of pneumonia. Her pediatrician had noted a heart murmur in infancy, which eventually disappeared. Jenny's speech and language evaluation showed severely disordered articulation, a high pitched voice, and a mild language impairment. Her palate was normal in appearance on peroral examination. Her face was long and had been described as "adenoid facies." During Jenny's preschool years, her mother would question her pediatrician frequently about Jenny's lack of intelligible speech development. The pediatrician would always say, "Don't worry. She'll outgrow it. Some kids don't talk at all until they're 3 years old!" However, the constant middle ear disease prompted referral to a local otolaryngologist. She was also noted to have "allergic shiners" (suborbital congestion of the tiny blood vessels under the eye giving the skin a deep reddish-purple appearance). This made both the pediatrician and otolaryngologist think that Jenny had chronic nasal obstruction, as do many children with chronic allergies. In fact, the combination of her long face, open mouth posture, allergic shiners, and chronic middle ear disease led the otolaryngologist and pediatrician to conclude that an adenoidectomy was necessary at the age of four. An adenoidectomy was performed, and Jenny's speech, though hypernasal before the operation, worsened afterward.

After her adenoidectomy, Jenny began kindergarten. At school, she underwent nearly 2 years worth of speech therapy without benefit. Therapy was provided twice a week in a group where traditional articulation procedures were applied. Her hypernasality did not diminish, and her speech remained nearly completely unintelligible. Glottal stops were substituted for essentially every consonant, but in the reports from the public school speech pathologist, these substitutions were described as "omissions." Though the adenoidectomy had been done to relieve her upper respiratory and otologic illnesses, Jenny continued to have recurrent otitis media, bronchitis, frequent colds and another episode of pneumonia. She was noticeably shorter than her classmates, and her teacher noted that her fine motor coordination was poor. She also was immature compared to her peers and tended to keep to herself, rarely playing with classmates. Her teacher attributed this to her speech problem and her inability to communicate with other children effectively.

The otolaryngologist continued to follow Jenny for her middle ear disease and was concerned that her speech had worsened and was showing no signs of improvement. The otolaryngologist had heard of the work with nasopharyngoscopy at the large academic medical center in a nearby city and referred Jenny for evaluation to see if there were any structural problems he had not detected. At age 6, with Jenny in first grade, her parents brought her to the Craniofacial Center.

Jenny's first contact at the Craniofacial Center was with the geneticist. Even at first glance, Jenny's appearance registered with the geneticist, who had seen many children like this before. The "gestalt" of Jenny's facial appearance, her allergic shiners, her developmental history, her medical history, her immaturity and personality pattern, and her distinctive speech pattern were all consistent with the diagnosis of velo-cardio-facial syndrome, a genetic syndrome of clefting related to a microdeletion of chromosome 22 (Scambler et al, 1992). The source of all Jenny's problems, the cause of which had previously been a mystery to both her parents and her doctors, was now perfectly clear.

A cardiac evaluation showed that Jenny had had a small ventriculoseptal defect of her heart, which spontaneously closed shortly after birth. However, a chest x-ray, echocardiogram, and ECG showed that Jenny also had a right-sided aortic arch. This was asymptomatic, but an unusual heart anomaly. There were also some other anomalies of the cardiovascular system, which were asymptomatic. A metabolic evaluation showed that Jenny had transient hypocalcemia. An eye examination showed tortuous retinal blood vessels. Her frequent pneumonias led to an immunologic assessment, which showed diminished thymic hormone and decreased populations of T lymphocytes. All of these findings are consistent with the diagnosis of velo-cardio-facial syndrome.

Jenny's hypernasality was a frequent feature of velo-cardio-facial syndrome contributed to by more than one component. Nearly all individuals with velo-cardio-facial syndrome have clefts of the palate (the lip is not involved), but in many cases, the clefts are not overt. Submucous cleft palate or occult submucous cleft palate have been reported to occur more frequently in this syndrome than over cleft palate. Occult submucous cleft palate cannot be detected by oral examination (Kaplan, 1975; Croft et al, 1978; Shprintzen, 1979). The diagnosis is dependent on endoscopic observation of the nasal surface of the soft palate (Croft et al, 1978; Shprintzen, 1979) which reveals absence of the musculus uvulae (Fig. 2-18), an important muscle to normal velopharyngeal closure (Lewin et al, 1980).

Pharyngeal hypotonia is also a common finding in velo-cardio-facial syndrome. As a result, absence of movement of the pharyngeal and palatal muscles necessary for velopharyngeal closure has been reported in the majority of cases. Another contributor to velopharyngeal insufficiency in velo-cardio-facial syndrome is an abnormally voluminous pharynx. The pharynx is suspended from the cranial base, and in velo-cardio-facial syndrome, the cranial base is flatter than normal (Arvystas and Shprintzen, 1984). Because the placement of the posterior pharyngeal wall in relation to the palate is in part determined by the position of the posterior cranial base, a flat cranial base (known as platybasia) draws the posterior pharyngeal wall further away from the velum (Fig. 2-19). An increase in pharyngeal volume makes it more difficult for the palate and pharyngeal walls to traverse the space necessary to close the velopharyngeal orifice.

All of these factors could have been contributing to Jenny's hypernasality, so it became critical to determine exactly which of them was actually in effect. Furthermore, it has been found that individuals with velo-cardio-facial syndrome have abnormalities of the internal carotid arteries, which can be detected on nasopharyngoscopic examination (MacKenzie-Stepner et al, 1987). This finding may be a contraindication to certain types of pharyngeal surgery, such as pharyngeal flap, in cases where the internal carotid is in the surgical field (Fig. 2-20).

Even the characteristic articulation disorders in velo-cardio-facial syndrome are a consistent finding (Golding-Kushner, 1991). Not all individuals with palatal clefts develop glottal stop articulation patterns, but nearly all children with velo-cardio-facial syndrome with clefts do. When combined with the language impairment that has been reported in velo-cardio-facial syndrome (Golding-Kushner et al, 1985), the prognosis for children with velo-cardio-facial syndrome is very different than that for other individuals with clefts. While

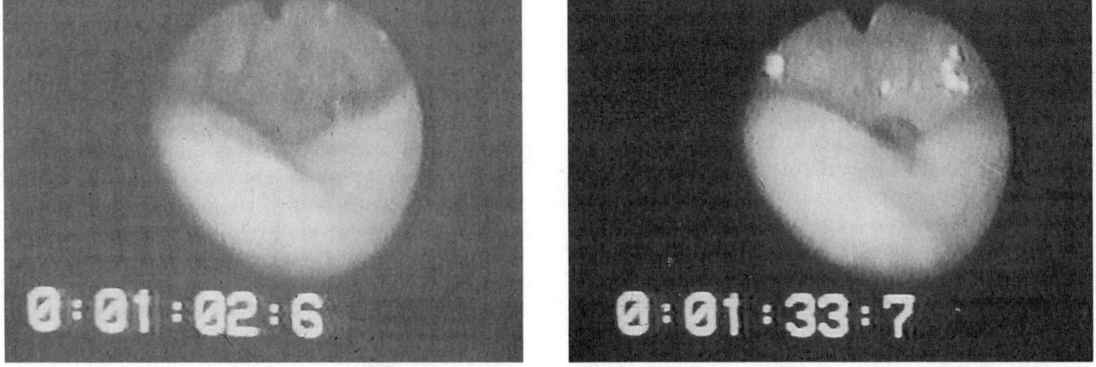

Fig. 2-18 Nasopharyngoscopic appearance of an occult submucous cleft palate with a midline concavity in the nasal surface of the velum at rest (**A**) and during speech (**B**) showing a central gap in velopharyngeal valve.

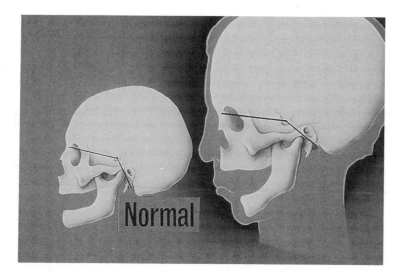

Fig. 2-19 Artistic representation of platybasia (flattening of the skull base) in VCF in relation to a normal skull.

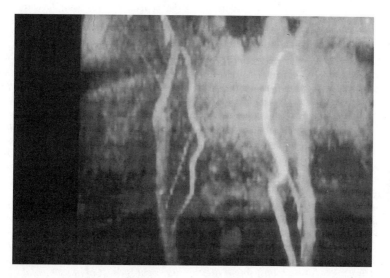

Fig. 2-20 Magnetic resonance angiography of abnormal internal carotids in velo-cardio-facial syndrome showing a medial displacement of the vessels.

the majority of children with nonsyndromic cleft palate develop normal speech after palate repair, this is true of few if any children with velo-cardio-facial syndrome. Follow-up and intervention for speech disorders needs to be more aggressive and frequent. Counseling of parents needs to be suited specifically to the types of disorders children with velo-cardio-facial will almost certainly develop.

Perhaps the most significant aspect of the natural history of velo-cardio-facial syndrome is the possible development of severe personality disturbance in ado-

lescence and adulthood. A percentage of individuals with velo-cardio-facial syndrome develop psychosis (Shprintzen et al, 1992; Goldberg et al, 1993), including schizophrenia, paranoid delusions, and other dysfunctional behavior patterns. Thus, it can be seen that in a syndrome caused by a single genetic defect, multiple areas of anatomy and physiology can be affected, ranging from cleft palate to heart anomalies to cognitive deficiencies to personality disturbance. The growth, performance, and treatment outcome are largely predicted by the diagnosis. The multiple disorders displayed *in these cases are not caused by the cleft but are simply part of a symptom complex that includes the cleft.*

The number and types of specialists required to assess the problems associated with velo-cardio-facial syndrome extend far beyond those typically associated with cleft palate or craniofacial teams. It becomes essential in velo-cardio-facial syndrome to have the services of a pediatric cardiologist, pediatric endocrinologist, psychiatrist, neuropsychologist, pediatric ophthalmologist, molecular geneticist, clinical geneticist, and neuroradiologist (for MR angiography detection of the internal carotid anomaly). Furthermore, it is essential that the other specialists have specific knowledge of the syndrome in order to find some of the more obscure features and provide proper treatment. It might be reasonable to ask why an entire team should be restructured and expanded just to accommodate one syndrome. For one thing, this single syndrome probably comprises a large percentage of the patients in most centers. Secondly, this is only one syndrome of hundreds. Each syndrome has its own phenotypic spectrum, natural history, and prognosis. It is therefore unlikely that teams that are not comprehensive will be able to adequately meet the needs of their patients.

Case 2

Joe was an 8-year-old boy with a left-sided unilateral cleft lip and palate who had had his lip repaired at 3 months of age and his palate at about 18 months of age. His developmental milestones were all within normal limits, including the onset of speech and language. His aesthetic result from the early repairs was poor. The lip was short and tight and the nose severely collapsed. His eyes looked as if they were very close together. He was a good student in school but was having trouble making friends because he was so much smaller than his peers. His parents had been told that his small size was probably the result of early feeding difficulties because of his cleft. His speech was hypernasal and his dental occlusion was abnormal with severe collapse of the maxilla with a class III malocclusion (where the lower jaw protrudes beyond the upper jaw). Joe's parents were dissatisfied with his appearance and speech, so they sought the opinion of a more comprehensive center.

One of the things that struck the clinical geneticist and orthodontist was the congenital absence of one of Joe's maxillary central incisors. The orthodontist found that the absence of the central incisor was accompanied by a smaller than normal maxilla. The geneticist found that the distance between the eyes was much smaller than normal, and examination of the genitals showed that Joe had a micropenis. A growth hormone study was done and it was found that Joe was not producing sufficient growth hormone. A CT scan was done to see if the pituitary gland was normal, and it was found that the pituitary was very small and nearly absent, which also explained the lack of normal growth and genital development. In addition, some of the normal communicating tracts between the cerebral hemispheres were absent. The olfactory bulbs were also smaller than normal leading to a test of olfaction. It was found that Joe had a reduced sense of smell.

The small pituitary, small stature, single central incisor, reduced olfaction, and maxillary deficiency led to a diagnosis of DeMyer sequence (also known as holoprosencephaly sequence). This disorder is related to a lack of complete differentiation between the cerebral hemispheres and deficiency in the embryonic median nasal process so that midline structures of the head and face may be absent or smaller than normal. In its most severe form, these midline deficiencies can result in cyclopia, true median cleft lip (premaxillary agenesis), and complete absence of the normal ventricular system in the brain with only a large single central ventricle and no hemispheric differentiation (Fig. 2-5, B).

Without knowing where to look for the possible anomalies associated with this disorder (the phenotypic spectrum), the natural history of the problem would not have been understood. The administration of growth hormone and testosterone helped Joe grow and develop normal sexual characteristics. Had the window of opportunity been lost to apply these needed treatments, the outcome would have been less satisfactory.

Case 3

Peter was born at a community hospital with a complete right sided unilateral cleft lip and palate. He was noted to have a small ear tag near his right ear, which was removed in the delivery room. When seen by the local cleft palate team, he was considered to have an isolated cleft lip and palate and treated in the routine manner for this disorder. His lip and palate were repaired without problem, but his speech developed with significant hypernasality. He had chronic otitis media with a persistent conductive hearing loss in his right ear. He seemed to have a constant infection in the right ear and eventually developed a perforation in the right tympanic membrane. He was given a hearing aid to manage the chronic moderate conductive hearing loss.

As a result of his hypernasality, the local team, which did not have access to nasopharyngoscopy or videofluoroscopy, recommended a standard, centrally placed pharyngeal flap. The operation failed with no improvement in Peter's hypernasality.

Because of the failure to resolve Peter's speech problem, the local team referred him to a center where nasopharyngoscopy and videofluoroscopy were available. It was found that Peter had an asymmetric pharynx and that the air was leaking through the nasopharynx on the right side (Shprintzen et al, 1980). The chronic hearing loss in the right ear was also explored and it was found that even though Peter did have a perforation and chronic infections, the degree of the loss was related to an ossicular anomaly, fixation of the footplate of the stapes. The pharyngeal asymmetry, stapes fixation, and the previously removed ear tag confirmed the diagnosis of oculo-auriculo-vertebral spectrum, or hemifacial microsomia. In hemifacial microsomia, one side of the face is smaller than the other, but it has also been found that there are internal asymmetries. The palate and pharynx are anatomically and physiologically asymmetric (Shprintzen et al, 1980). Hemifacial microsomia is frequently associated with cleft lip and palate, or cleft palate only. Approximately 15% of patients with hemifacial microsomia have clefts (Gorlin et al, 1990). Had the appropriate diagnosis been established prior to applying treatments, failures could have been avoided.

These anecdotes represent three genuine cases from a single center. Rather than these cases being exceptions, they are actually the rule. This same center reported that over 50% of all of its cleft cases had multiple anomaly syndromes (Shprintzen et al, 1985). In all three cases, the identification of the syndromes that caused their clefts was essential to proper management of their cases. Correct diagnosis would not be possible unless the proper personnel examine every patient. But because many interdisciplinary teams still do not have geneticists examine every patient, all clinicians should be aware of the importance and possibility of multiple anomaly syndromes among patients at cleft palate centers.

REFERENCES

Arvystas M, Shprintzen RJ: Craniofacial morphology in the velo-cardio-facial syndrome, *J Craniofac Genet Devel Biol* 4:39-45, 1984.

Cohen MM Jr. *The child with multiple birth defects,* New York, 1982: Raven Press.

Cohen MM Jr, Bankier A: Syndrome delineation involving orofacial clefting, *Cleft Palate J* 28:119-120, 1991.

Croft CB, Shprintzen RJ, Daniller AI, Lewin MI: The occult submucous cleft palate and the musculus uvuli, *Cleft Palate J* 15:150-154, 1978.

Ewart AK, Morris CA, Atkinson D, Jin W, Sternes K, Spallone P, Stock AD, Leppert M, Keating MT: Hemizygosity at the elastin locus in a developmental disorder, Williams syndrome, *Nature Genetics* 5:11-16, 1993.

Fraser FC: *The use of teratogens in the analysis of abnormal developmental mechanisms.* First international conference on congenital malformations, Philadelphia, 1961, Lippincott.

Fraser FC: The genetics of cleft lip and cleft palate, *Am J Hum Genet* 22:336-352, 1970.

Goldberg R, Motzkin B, Marion R, Scambler PJ, Shprintzen RJ: Velo-cardio-facial syndrome: a review of 120 cases, *Am J Med Genet,* 45:313-319, 1992.

Golding-Kushner KJ, Weller G, Shprintzen RJ: Velo-cardio-facial syndrome: language and psychological profiles, *J Craniofac Genet* 5:259-266, 1985.

Golding-Kushner KJ: Craniofacial morphology and velopharyngeal physiology in four syndromes of clefting. Unpublished doctoral dissertation. The Graduate School and University Center, City University of New York, 1991.

Gorlin RJ: *Development and genetic aspects of cleft lip and palate.* Chapter in Moller KT, Starr CD, editors: Cleft Palate: Interdisciplinary Issues and Treatment. Austin, TX: Pro-Ed, pp. 25-48, 1993.

Gorlin RJ, Cohen MM Jr, Levin LS: *Syndromes of the head and neck,* New York, 1990, Oxford University Press.

Kelley D, Goldberg R, Wilson D, Lindsay E, Carey A, Goodship J, Burn J, Cross I, Shprintzen RJ, Scambler PJ: Velo-cardio-facial syndrome associated with haploinsufficiency of genes at chromosome 22q11, *Am J Med Genet* (in press), 1992.

Jones MC: Etiology of facial clefts: prospective evaluation of 428 patients, *Cleft Palate J* 25:16-20, 1988.

Kaplan EN: The occult submucous cleft palate, *Cleft Palate J* 12:356-368, 1975.

Lewin ML, Croft CB, Shprintzen RJ: Velopharyngeal insufficiency due to hypoplasia of the musculus uvulae and occult submucous cleft palate, *Plast Reconstr Surg* 65:585-591, 1980.

MacKenzie-Stepner K, Witzel MA, Stringer DA, Lindsay WK, Munro IR, Hughes H: Abnormal carotid arteries in the velocardiofacial syndrome: a report of three cases, *Plast Reconstr Surg* 80:347-351, 1987.

Rollnick BR, Pruzansky S: Genetic services at a center for craniofacial anomalies, *Cleft Palate J* 18:304-313, 1981.

Scambler PJ, Kelly D, Lindsay E, Williamson R, Goldberg R, Shprintzen RJ, Wilson DI, Goodship JA, Cross IE, Burn J: Velo-cardio-facial syndrome associated with chromosome 22 deletions encompassing the DiGeorge locus, *Lancet* 339:1138-1139, 1992.

Schmickel RD: Contiguous gene syndromes: a component of recognizeable syndromes, *J Pediatr* 109:231-240, 1986.

Shprintzen RJ: *Hypernasal speech in the absence of overt or submucous cleft palate: the mystery solved.* Chapter in Diagnosis and Treatment of Palato Glossal Malfunction, Ellis R and Flack R, editors. College of Speech Therapists (London), 1979.

Shprintzen RJ: *A critic's look at the state-of-the-art in cleft palate and craniofacial disorders: where we have been, where we need to go.* In Gerber SE, Mencher GT, editors: *International perspectives on communicative disorders.* Washington, DC, 1988, Gallaudet University Press: 138-149.

Shprintzen RJ: *Velo-cardio-facial syndrome.* In "Birth Defects Encyclopedia." Dover, MA, 1990, Center for Birth Defects Information Services, pp. 1744-1745.

Shprintzen RJ: The implications of the diagnosis of Robin sequence, *Cleft Palate J* 29:205-209, 1992.

Shprintzen RJ, Croft CB, Berkman MD, Rakoff SJ: Velopharyngeal insufficiency in the facio-auriculo-vertebral malformation complex, *Cleft Palate J* 17:132-137, 1980.

Shprintzen RJ, Goldberg R, Golding-Kushner KJ, Marion R: Late-onset psychosis in the velo-cardio-facial syndrome, *Am J Med Genet* 42:141-142, 1992.

Shprintzen RJ, Goldberg RB, Young D, Wolford L: The velo-cardio-facial syndrome: a clinical and genetic analysis, *Pediatrics* 67:167-172, 1981.

Shprintzen RJ, Siegel-Sadewitz VL, Amato J, Goldberg RB: Anomalies associated with cleft lip, cleft palate, or both, *Am J Med Genet* 20:585-595, 1985.

3 Anatomy and Physiology of the Palate and Velopharyngeal Structures

Martin D. Cassell and *Hani Elkadi*

The notion that the human soft palate and pharynx are parts of the same structure has found little recognition in modern anatomical texts. The pharynx is usually depicted as a relatively vertical muscular tube into which the oral and nasal cavities open anteriorly. The upper part of the pharynx is divided into a region lying behind the nasal cavity, the *nasopharynx,* and a part lying behind the oral cavity, the *oropharynx.* In the context of this description, the soft palate is usually represented as a musculomembranous flap that contributes to the closure of the area between the nasopharynx and the oropharynx. Though this type of description illustrates, to some extent, the intimate relationship between the soft palate and pharynx, it ignores several factors that are important to understanding the concept of the velopharyngeal mechanism. The oral cavity in humans is a direct continuation of the pharynx, a fact that has been obscured by the forward displacement of the head to accommodate the upright posture. This continuity can be better appreciated in most other mammals since the long axis of the oral cavity is usually in line with the axis of the pharynx (Fig. 3-1). The passage connecting the oral cavity and the pharynx, the *oropharyngeal isthmus,* is surrounded by a continuous ring of tissue that consists of the dorsal surface of the tongue inferiorly, the anterior and posterior pillars of the fauces (or palatoglossal and palatopharyngeal arches) laterally, and the soft palate superiorly. Behind this ring of tissue is the upper attachment of the pharynx. The uppermost circular muscle of the pharynx, the superior constrictor, is attached to the buccinator muscle that forms the lateral wall of the oral cavity. Below, the superior constrictor is attached to the mandible and tongue. Above, the attachment of the pharynx to the oral cavity is represented by the attachment of the soft palate to the hard palate. The soft palate thus represents the superior wall, or roof, of the pharynx, and its posterior free border, including the uvula, forms the anterior boundary of an aperture in the roof of the pharynx, the *nasopharyngeal hiatus.* The continuity of palate and pharynx is clearly evident when the soft palate is in its elevated position. In this position, the oral surface of the soft palate is continuous with the posterior and lateral walls of the pharynx. Conceptually then, the soft palate is involved in closing an aperture (the nasopharyngeal hiatus) in the superior wall of the oropharynx. The region above the soft palate, conventionally but erroneously termed the *nasopharynx,* is the posterior limit of the nasal cavities, and the term *posterior nasal cavity* will be used here to describe it.

The continuity between palate and pharynx is embodied in our use of the term *velopharynx.* As defined here, the velopharynx is a complex, musculomembranous valve that surrounds both the oropharyngeal isthmus and nasopharyngeal hiatus. The velopharynx, as defined here, includes the structures associated with the anterior and posterior pillars of the fauces, as well as the soft palate and the lateral and posterior walls of the oropharynx.

At the simplest level, the velopharynx acts as a valve closing off the nasal part of the upper respiratory tract, a function that it performs during both deglutition and respiration. However, the ability of the velopharynx to regulate the movement of air through and between the oral and nasal cavities gives it a prominent role in the production of oral and nasal speech sounds. From a mechanistic perspective, the action of the velopharynx in deglutition, respiration, and phonation resembles a sphincter. This sphincteric action can be reduced to two basic sets of movements: elevation and depression of the soft palate and movements of the lateral and posterior pharyngeal walls.

45

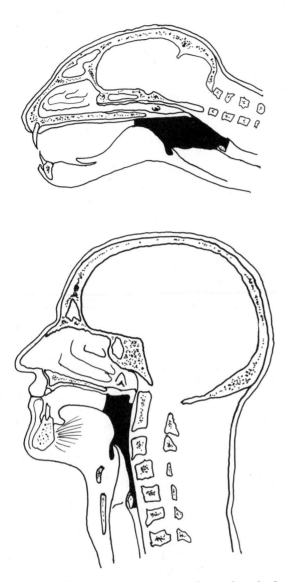

Fig. 3-1 Diagrammatic representations of sagittal sections through the head of a cat *(top)* and human showing the extent of the true pharynx *(black area)* with the soft palate elevated. Note that in the cat the long axis of the oral cavity is normally in line with the long axis of the pharynx. In humans, this continuity is clearly apparent when the soft palate is elevated. In both species, elevation of the soft palate closes the pharynx off from the posterior nasal cavity ("nasopharynx").

BONY COMPONENTS OF THE PALATE AND VELOPHARYNX

Though solely composed of soft tissues, the velopharynx is anchored to the surrounding regions of the skull, specifically the hard palate and inferior parts of the sphenoid and temporal bones. The shape of the hard palate is a determining factor in the resonance character-istics of the oral cavity and consequently the tonal properties of the voice.

Hard palate

The hard palate is a plate of bone that forms the roof of the oral cavity and the floor of the nasal cavity. It is curved in both its longitudinal and transverse axes and thus defines a dome-shaped space in the upper part of the oral cavity, termed the *palatal vault.* Because of the great individual variability in the curvatures of the hard palate, particularly in the transverse axis, the contribution of the palatal vault to the resonance of the oral cavity varies widely. The anterior three fourths of the hard palate is formed by the *palatine processes of the maxillae,* the posterior one-fourth by the *horizontal plates of the palatine bones* (Fig. 3-2). The palatine processes arise laterally from the alveolar processes of the maxillae. In front of the second molar, they pass horizontally to meet at the median *intermaxillary palatine suture.* In Northern Europeans, a prominent longitudinal ridge, the *palatine torus,* is commonly found on the oral surface along the margins of the suture. The nasal aspect of the intermaxillary palatine suture is marked by the two *nasal crests,* which form a groove for approximation with the *vomer,* which forms the lower portion of the bony nasal septum. Anteriorly, the nasal crests are prolonged to form the *anterior nasal spines,* which can be felt at the junction between the upper lip and the nasal septum. Behind the incisor teeth, the palatine suture is depressed to form a prominent hollow, the *incisive fossa.* In the lateral walls of the incisive fossa are the openings of the *incisive canals* and in the median aspects of its floor are occasionally found the *anterior* and *posterior incisive foramina.* These openings transmit branches of the greater palatine artery and the nasopalatine nerves supplying the palatine mucous membrane.

The posterior border of the maxillary contribution to the hard palate forms a U-shaped notch into which the *horizontal plates of the palatine bones* almost completely insert (Fig. 3-2), forming the *palatomaxillary suture* and completing the hard palate. Anteriorly and medially, the junction between the palatine and maxillary bones is demarcated by the palatomaxillary suture, but this suture is generally obliterated laterally.

The medial borders of the horizontal plates meet at the median *interpalatine suture,* whereas the anterior and lateral borders articulate with the palatine processes of the maxilla. The posterior borders of the horizontal plates form the posterior edge of the hard palate and at the

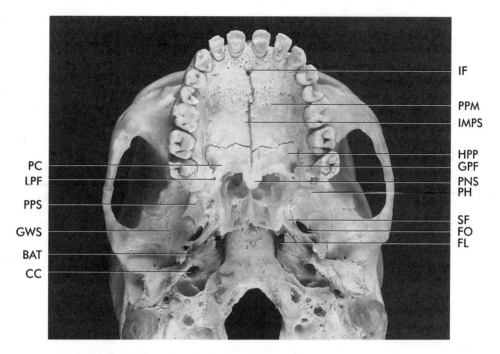

Fig. 3-2 Photograph of the base of an adult male skull showing the bony structures associated with the velopharynx. Abbreviations: *BAT:* - bony part of auditory tube; *CC:* - carotid canal; *FL:* - foramen lacerum; *FO:* - foramen ovale; *GPF:* - greater palatine foramen; *GWS:* - greater wing of sphenoid; *HPP:* - horizontal process of palatine bone; *IF:* - incisive fossa; *IMPS:* - intermaxillary palatine suture; *LPF:* - lesser palatine foramen; *PC:* - palatine crest; *PH:* - pterygoid hamulus; *PNS:* - posterior nasal spine; *PPM:* - palatine process of maxilla; *PPS:* - pterygoid process of sphenoid; *SF:* - scaphoid fossa.

midline project back as the *posterior nasal spine* (Fig. 3-2). At the junction between the horizontal plate and the pyramidal process, a smooth ridge of bone, the *palatine crest,* passes anteromedially. The lateral aspect of the palatine crest forms the medial edge of the *greater palatine foramen* (which transmits the greater palatine vessels and nerves) while medially the crest is continuous with the raised lip of the posterior border of the horizontal plate. The *lesser palatine foramina,* when present, are generally openings in the pyramidal process of the palatine bones (Fig. 3-2). The lesser palatine foramina transmit the lesser palatine vessels and nerves supplying the soft palate and uvula.

Sphenoid and temporal bones

Though they do not contribute directly to the composition of the hard palate, the inferior aspects of the sphenoid and temporal bones provide attachments for the levator and tensor veli palatini muscles. The projection of the inferior surface of the petrous part of the temporal bone that forms the floor of the carotid canal lies between the greater wing of the sphenoid bone and the occipital bone (Fig. 3-2). Anteromedially, this plate of bone forms the posterior aspect

of the foramen lacerum and posterolaterally forms the anterior lip of the opening of the carotid canal. Between these two boundaries, the bone is roughened and provides the bony attachment for the levator veli palatini (Figs. 3-2 and 3-3). The lateral edge of the inferior surface of the petrous temporal bone forms the posteromedial wall of the distal part of the canal containing the auditory tube. The attachment of the levator veli palatini continues across this edge to the auditory tube. Posterolaterally, the attachment of the levator is also continuous with the fascia of the carotid sheath that is attached to the margins of the aditus of the carotid canal (Fig. 3-3)

The *medial pterygoid plate* of the pterygoid process of the sphenoid bone forms an important bony attachment for velopharyngeal musculature. The medial pterygoid plate is a vertical plate of bone. At its inferior end is the knob-like *pterygoid hamulus* that provides a partial attachment for the superior constrictor and the tensor veli palatini (Fig. 3-2). A centimeter or so above this is the *processus tubarius* that supports the auditory tube. Where the posterior edge of the medial pterygoid plate merges with the body of the sphenoid, it splits into two ridges that bound

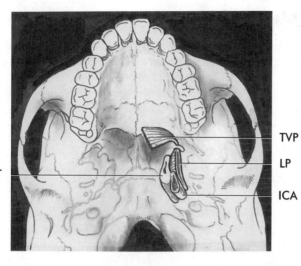

Fig. 3-3 Line drawing of the base of the skull showing the relationships between the attachment of the levator veli palatini *(LP)*, the tensor veli palatini *(TVP)*, the auditory tube *(AT)*, and the internal carotid artery *(ICA)*.

a rhomboid depression, the *scaphoid fossa,* that lies anteromedially to the foramen ovale. Part of the tensor veli palatini arises from the scaphoid fossa. The belly of the tensor lies in the wide *pterygoid fissure* located between the medial and lateral pterygoid plates.

The palatine aponeurosis

The palatine aponeurosis is the principal structural element within the velopharynx, providing flexibility and a degree of stiffness to the soft palate as well as an anchoring point for a number of velopharyngeal muscles (Fig. 3-4). The palatine aponeurosis is a diamond-shaped sheet of fibrous tissue extending backwards about 1 cm from the posterior edge of the hard palate. Along its attachment to the hard palate, the palatine aponeurosis is continuous with the periosteum and submucosal connective tissue covering both the oral and nasal surfaces of the hard palate. On either side, it is continuous around the pterygoid hamulus with the tendon

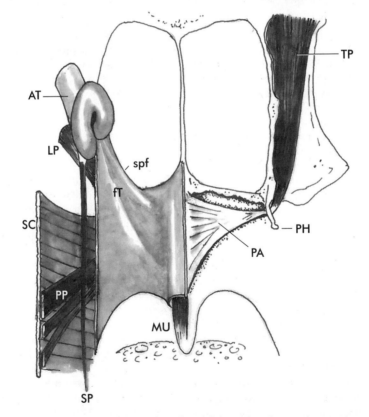

Fig. 3-4 Diagrammatic view of the nasal surface of the soft palate and posterior nasal cavity after removal of the posterior pharyngeal wall and the velopharyngeal mucosa. On the left, the velopharyngeal fascia *(grey area)* is shown passing from the pharynx and auditory tube *(AT)* onto the soft palate. Note the two thickened areas, the fascia of Troltsch *(fT)* and the salpingopalatine fascia *(SPF)*, and the splitting of the fascia to surround the musculi uvulae *(MU)*. On the right, the palatine aponeurosis *(PA)* and its continuity with the tensor veli palatini *(TP)* tendon is shown after removal of the levator palati, palatopharyngeus, and palatoglossus muscles. Abbreviations: *LP* - levator palati; *PH* - pterygoid hamulus; *PP* - palatopharyngeus; *SC:* - superior constrictor; *SP:* - salpingopharyngeus.

and fibrous sheath of the tensor veli palatini. More posteriorly, the palatine aponeurosis receives contributions from the *internal fascia* of the pharynx, the *salpingopalatine fascia* (ligament), and the *fascia of Troltsch* forming the membranous portion of the auditory tube. Along the midline, the palatine aponeurosis is at its broadest and receives contributions from the fibrous sheaths of the levatores veli palatini, the palatoglossi, and palatopharyngei muscles.

Velopharyngeal musculature

The essential function of the velopharyngeal musculature is closure of the nasopharyngeal isthmus through apposition of the velopharyngeal mucosa by elevation of the soft palate and movements of the pharyngeal walls. Extensive studies on the nature of this closure in normal individuals and individuals with clefts have revealed four basic patterns of apposition of velar and pharyngeal mucosa (Skolnick et al, 1973) (Fig. 3-5): a coronal type with a linear, coronally oriented line of apposition between the soft palate and posterior pharynx; a sagittal type where greater movements of the lateral pharyngeal walls results in a sagitally-oriented line of apposition; a circular type produced by equal movements of the velum and lateral pharyngeal walls; and a sphincteric type involving the presence of the so-called Passavant's ridge in the posterior pharyngeal wall. All of these patterns utilize two basic sets of movements: elevation of the soft palate, and inward movements of the pharynx. Consequently, the following description will classify the velopharyngeal muscles into those that affect velar movement and those that affect pharyngeal wall movement.

The musculature of the velopharynx can be viewed as consisting of several muscular slings formed by the paired *palatopharyngeus, palatoglossus, levator veli palatini* and *superior constrictor* muscles, and the paired *musculi uvulae.* The palatoglossal "sling" surrounds most of the oropharyngeal isthmus: the palatopharyngeal and superior constrictor "slings" form a complete ring around the nasopharyngeal hiatus. Associated with these primary velopharyngeal muscles are the *salpingopharyngeus* and *palatothyroideus* muscles (Fig. 3-6). Functionally, these muscles can be divided into those that move or alter the shape of the soft palate (levator veli palatini, palatoglossus, palatothyroideus, and musculi uvulae) and those involved in movements of the lateral and posterior pharyngeal walls (superior constrictor, palatopharyngeus, and salpingopharyngeus). The *tensor veli palatini* has been mistakenly associated

with movements of the soft palate but appears to be primarily involved in middle ear aeration and will not be considered here. The palatothyroideus muscle as described here represents the vertically oriented fibers running from the palate to the thyroid cartilage and classically described as being a component of the palatopharyngeus. We have reserved the latter term, however, for the more horizontally aligned fibers running from the palate into the pharynx that are often referred to as the "palatopharyngeal sphincter." Note that the nomenclature of velopharyngeal muscles used here generally follows that suggested by the 1983 Nomina Anatomica, as indicated by the suffix *N.A.*

Muscles involved in velar movements.

Levator veli palatini (N.A.). The levatores veli palatini (Figs. 3-7 to 3-9) arise from the base of the skull and pass onto the upper or nasal surface of the soft palate, forming a sling beneath the musculi uvulae. The origin of the levatores, which is remarkably constant even in clefting of the palate (Fig. 3-8), is by a tendon attached to the inferior surface of the petrous temporal bone, with a few fascicles arising from the adjacent carotid sheath and cartilage of the auditory (Eustachian) tube (Fig. 3-3). The fibers of the levatores pass downwards and medially parallel with the auditory tube, which lies superior to the muscle. Some of the anterior fibers of the levatores pass into the lower or oral surface of the palatine aponeurosis, while the bulk of the muscles pass beneath the musculi uvulae forming a sling that occupies the intermediate 40% of the soft palate. Here, muscle fibers from both levatores, and the palatoglossus and palatopharyngeus muscles intermingle (Figs. 3-9 and 3-10). Fibers from the levatores do not, however, pass into the uvula.

The levatores appear to be primarily involved in elevation and possibly posterior displacement of the soft palate. A close relationship between movements of the levatores and the production of oral sounds has been confirmed visually as well as electromyographically. Short bursts of electrical activity have been recorded from the levatores at the onset of swallowing. Though activity in the levatores is minimal at rest, detailed studies utilizing electromyographic recording and radiography indicate that the degree of velar elevation (and hence velar position) is a function not only of activity in the levatores but also in largely antagonistic muscles such as the palatoglossus.

Palatoglossus (N.A.). The palatoglossi are two thin fasciculi of muscle fibers passing from the soft palate to the sides and dorsal surface of the

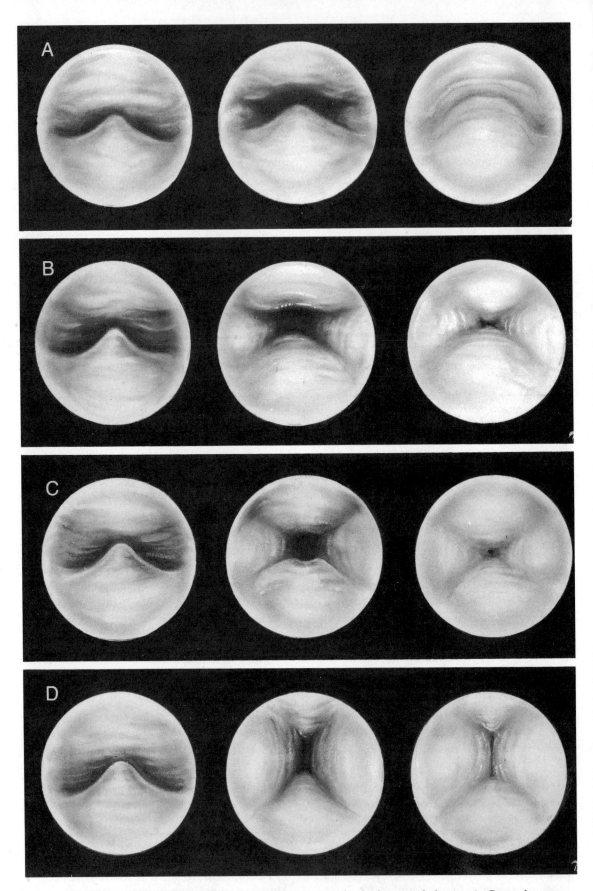

Fig. 3-5 Artist's rendering of the four basic patterns of velopharyngeal closure. **A,** Coronal pattern. **B,** Circular pattern. **C,** Circular pattern with Passavant's ridge. **D,** Sagittal pattern. (Reproduced with permission from *Pharyngoplasty.* J. Bardach, K.E. Salyer and I.T. Jackson. In *Surgical Techniques in Cleft Lip and Palate,* ed 2. by J. Bardach and K.E. Salyer, New York, 1991, Mosby.

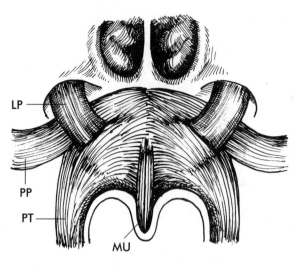

Fig. 3-6 Diagrammatic representation of the "muscular sling" arrangements of the velopharyngeal musculature as viewed from behind. *LP:* - levator veli palatini; *MU:*- musculi uvulae; *PP:* - palatopharyngeus; *PT:* - palatothyroideus.

tongue (Fig. 3-7). The fibers of the palatoglossi follow a curved course, the general direction of which is in an oblique plane that runs parallel to the orientation of the fibers of the levatores palati (Fig. 3-7). Hence, when considered as paired muscles, the levatores and palatoglossi are antagonistic. Because the fibers of both pairs of muscles converge on the middle of the soft palate, each palatoglossus is antagonistic to the contralateral levator (Fig. 3-10). The attachments of the palatoglossi along the sides of the tongue appear to be by the continuation of their fibrous sheaths into the lingual muscles. The palatal attachment of the palatoglossi is generally considered to be by two bundles: an inferior bundle that passes into the mucosa on the oral surface of the soft palate; and a superior bundle that pierces the palatal mass of the levator sling to end in connective tissue lateral to the musculi uvulae (Fig. 3-10). Neither bundle apparently reaches the midline nor do their fibers interdigitate with fibers from the contralateral muscle. In individuals with cleft palate, the

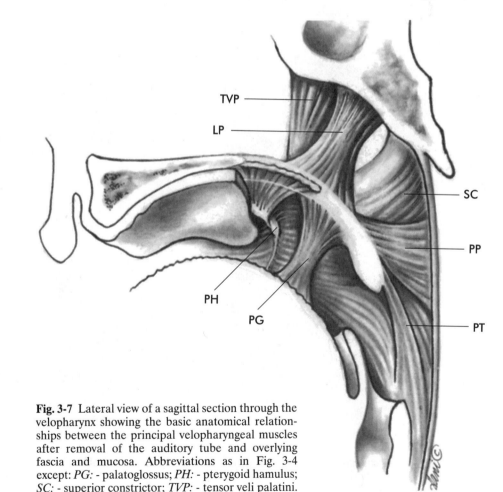

Fig. 3-7 Lateral view of a sagittal section through the velopharynx showing the basic anatomical relationships between the principal velopharyngeal muscles after removal of the auditory tube and overlying fascia and mucosa. Abbreviations as in Fig. 3-4 except: *PG:* - palatoglossus; *PH:* - pterygoid hamulus; *SC:* - superior constrictor; *TVP:* - tensor veli palatini.

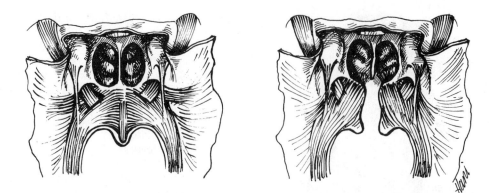

Fig. 3-8 Semi-diagrammatic representation of the velopharyngeal musculature viewed from behind in normal *(left)* and cleft palate *(right)* individuals.

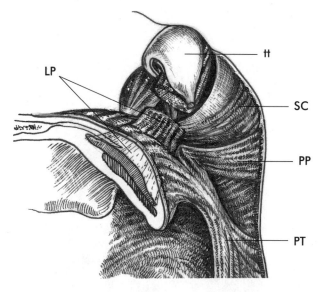

Fig. 3-9 Lateral view of the velopharyngeal musculature in the vicinity of the auditory tube showing the relationship between the levator and palatothyroideus muscles within the soft palate. Abbreviations as in Figs 3-4 and 3-5, except: *tt:* - torus tubarius.

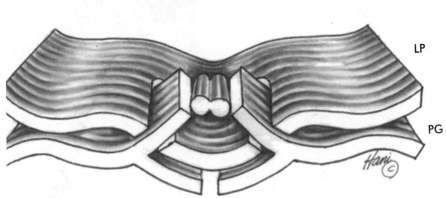

Fig. 3-10 Schematic representation of the arrangement of muscle fibers derived from the levator veli palatini *(LP)* and palatoglossus *(PG)* in the soft palate. Note that the fibers of the palatoglossus do not reach the mid-line.

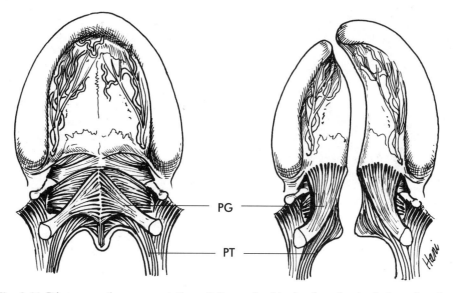

Fig. 3-11 Diagrammatic representation of the underside (oral surface) of the soft palate showing the attachment of the palatoglossus *(PG)* and palatothyroideus *(PT)* muscles in normal *(left)* and clefted *(right)* individuals.

palatoglossi generally insert into the posterior edge of the hard palate (Fig. 3-11).

The palatoglossal arches (anterior pillars of the fauces) are formed by the oral mucosa passing over the palatoglossi. The palatoglossal arches contain a prominent sheet of elastic fibers. These fibers, into which some fibers of the palatoglossi insert, extend from the soft palate to the tongue.

Consistent with their anatomical position as antagonists of the levatores, the palatoglossi appear to be active in velar lowering, particularly in relation to the production of nasal sounds and at the end of speech. However, it should be noted that velar position, whether produced by velar elevation or depression, is likely to be determined by the degree of activity in *both* the palatoglossi and levatores. The role played by the elastic fibers present in the palatoglossal arches in velar lowering remains uncertain, though they may assist in restoring the palate to its rest position. With the soft palate held fixed by contraction of the levatores, the palatoglossi can elevate the posterior part of the tongue. In addition, contraction of the palatoglossi straightens the curvature of the palatoglossal arches, bringing them toward the midline and reducing the oropharyngeal isthmus.

Palatothyroideus (M. palatopharyngeus, N.A.).
The palatothyroidei muscles (Fig. 3-7) each arise from the soft palate by two flat fasciculi that pass either side of the levator veli palatini. The smaller, anterolateral fasciculus arises from

the posterior border of the hard palate and the palatine aponeurosis immediately behind the posterior nasal spine. The posteromedial fasciculus is attached to the palatine aponeurosis and the palatine raphe (a somewhat vaguely defined midline band of connective tissue), though some fibers pass over the musculi uvulae. The two fasciculi merge at the posterolateral border of the soft palate and the resultant fasciculus descends in the posterior faucies, or palatopharyngeal arch, behind the tonsil. The most anterior fibers of the palatothyroidei insert into the superior cornu and posterior border of the lamina of the thyroid cartilage. Some fibers reportedly insert into the capsule of the tonsil and purportedly assist in raising the tonsil in deglutition. More lateral fibers merge with the internal pharyngeal fascia while the most posterior fibers reportedly insert into the midline pharyngeal raphe, though some cross over the raphe to merge with fibers from the opposite muscle.

Functionally, the palatothyroidei are involved in velar lowering in much the same way that the palatoglossi act. Electromyographic studies have recorded electrical activity in the palatothyroidei during both velar elevation and depression suggesting that, as in the case of the palatoglossi, the palatothyroidei act antagonistically with the levatores in determining velar position. Through their attachments to the larynx and lower pharynx, the palatothyroidei can assist in elevating the larynx and pharynx when the

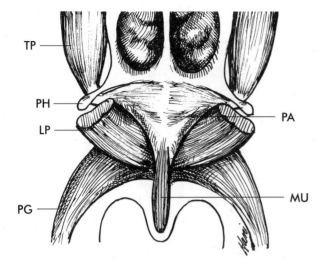

Fig. 3-12 Diagrammatic representation of the nasal surface of the soft palate with the mucosa and fascia removed revealing the attachments and relationships of the musculi uvulae. *MU:* Musculi uvulae; *TP:* Tensor palati m.; *PH:* Pterygoid hamulus; *LP:* Levator palati m.; *PG:* Palato glossus; *PA:* Palatine aponeurosis.

soft palate is fixed. The resultant changes in pharyngeal height may influence the resonant properties of the upper respiratory tract.

Musculi uvulae (N.A.). The musculi uvulae are two short muscles lying in an anteroposterior orientation along the midline of the soft palate (Figs. 3-12 and 3-13). Since little nonmuscular tissue is present between the two muscles, they have often been described (incorrectly) as a single muscle, the azygos musculus uvulae. The musculi uvulae arise largely from the nasal surface of the palatine aponeurosis close to its attachment to the posterior border of the hard palate (Figs. 3-12 and 3-13). Contrary to statements in many texts, the musculi uvulae do not arise from the hard palate nor from the posterior nasal spine. A distinct bundle of muscle fibers reportedly arises from the oral surface of the palatine aponeurosis (Fig. 3-14) and passes inferiorly to enter the oral or ventral surface of the musculi uvulae. The fleshy bellies of the musculi uvulae pass over the "levator sling" to enter the uvula where the muscles terminate among glandular and connective tissue. The posterior parts of the musculi uvulae

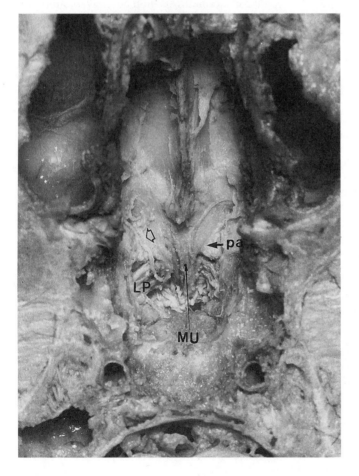

Fig. 3-13 Dissection of the musculi uvulae in a 49-year-old male cadaver. The view is identical to that shown in Fig. 3-10. Arrow indicates branches of the lesser palatine nerves running beneath the mucosa on the nasal surface of the soft palate.

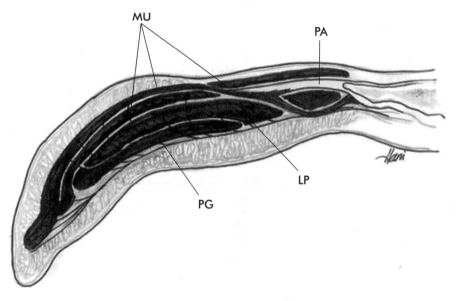

Fig. 3-14 Schematic representation of a mid-sagittal section through the soft palate showing the relationships between the muscle fibers of the musculi uvulae *(MU)* and other velopharyngeal muscles.

appear to be anchored to the soft palate by tendinous fibers of palatoglossus and palatothyroideus that pass over and into the muscles (Fig. 3-14). Furthermore, a connective tissue sheath completely surrounds the musculi uvulae. This sheath appears to be formed by the splitting of a sheet of fascia that descends from the upper surface of the levatores onto the soft palate.

The functional role played by the musculi uvulae in velar movement and phonation remains controversial. The most recent anatomical and physiological studies have proposed that the musculi uvulae act as a "flexible beam" that resists the distorting action of the levatores on the curvature of the soft palate in the coronal plane and straightens the sagittal curvature of the soft palate during velar elevation. It has been suggested that the musculus uvulae assists velopharyngeal closure by thickening during phonation, a result of its contraction, which shortens the muscle, adding bulk to the point at which it overlies the levatores. The actual contribution of the musculi uvulae to speech remains uncertain, however.

Muscles involved in movements of the pharyngeal walls

Though the pharynx is an integral part of the gastrointestinal tract, the arrangement of its muscular coats is the reverse of that found along the remainder of the digestive tube. The circular muscular layer, composed of the three (superior, middle, and inferior) pharyngeal constrictors and the palatopharyngeus, lies exterior to the longitudinal muscular layer, which is composed of the fibers of the stylopharyngeus, palatothyroideus, and salpingopharyngeus muscles. The present description will confine itself to those muscles primarily associated with the velopharynx (the superior constrictor, palatopharyngeus, and salpingopharyngeus).

Superior constrictor (M. constrictor pharyngis superioris, N.A.): The superior constrictors arise from a series of bony and fibrous attachments extending from the pterygoid hamulus superiorly to the posterior border of the tongue (Fig. 3-15). Because of this extensive origin, the superior constrictor is commonly divided into four parts named according to the specific origin of fibers. Other than this, there is no good reason for so dividing the superior constrictor. The most superior fibers of the superior constrictors (musculus pterygopharyngeus) arise from the pterygoid hamuli and very occasionally the adjacent part of the medial pterygoid plates. Below this attachment, the major part of the superior constrictors (musculus buccopharyngeus) is continuous with the whole posterior border of the buccinator muscles (Fig. 3-16) though the existence of a tendinous band at this continuation, the so-called pterygomandibular raphe (Fig. 3-16) is unlikely. The most inferior fibers of the superior constrictors arise from the posterior edge of the mylohyoid line of the mandible (musculus mylopharyngeus) and the posterolateral aspect of the tongue (musculus glossopha-

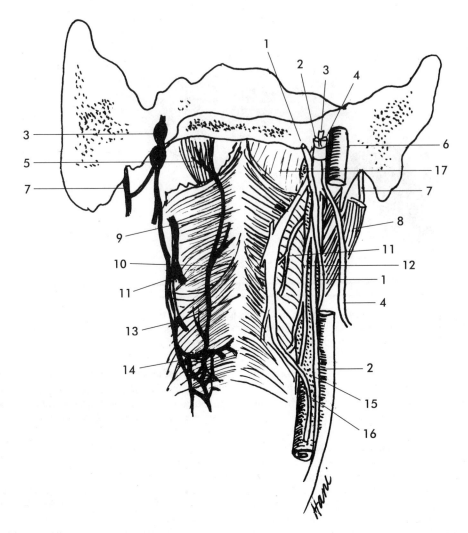

Fig. 3-15 Schematic representation of posterior pharynx showing the interrelationships between the cranial nerves associated with motor innervation of the velopharynx. On the left side *(drawn in black)* are the branches of the vagus and glossopharyngeal nerves providing the bulk of the motor innervation to velopharyngeal muscles. Key.: *1* Hypoglossal nerve; *2* vagus nerve; *3* glossopharyngeal nerve; *4* Spinal accessory nerve; *5* Levator veli palatini; *6* Jugular bulb; *7* Facial nerve; *8* Digastric muscle; *9* Superior constrictor; *10* Nerve to the levator; *11* Pharyngeal branches; *12* Superior laryngeal nerve; *13* Middle constrictor; *14* Pharyngeal plexus; *15* Common carotid artery; *16* Sympathetic trunk; *17* Pharyngobasilar fascia.

ryngeus) where they interlace with fibers from styloglossus and hyoglossus.

The muscle fibers of the superior constrictors curve posteriorly and laterally in an upward direction (Figs. 3-16 and 3-17), inserting into a tendinous, midline raphe formed by a thickening of the internal fascia of the pharynx. The most superior fibers may insert into the pharyngeal tubercle on the underside of the basilar part of the occipital bone.

Palatopharyngeus (M. palatopharyngeus, N.A.). The existence of well-defined bands of muscle

fibers running almost horizontally from the posterolateral border of the soft palate into the superior pharynx has been well documented (Fig. 3-9). Unfortunately, these fibers have been grouped either with the vertically oriented fibers of palatothyroidei running from the palate to the pharynx or with the superior constrictors. These fibers are functionally distinct from the palatothyroidei since they are poorly arranged to participate in velar lowering and are anatomically distinct from the superior constrictors, being separated by the internal pharyngeal

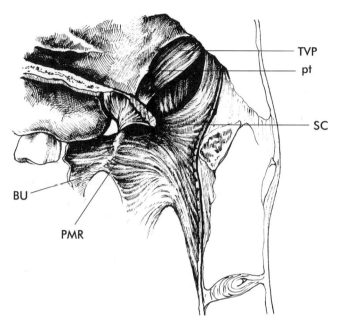

Fig. 3-16 Lateral view of the velopharynx after removal of the levator, palatoglossus, and palatothyroideus muscles showing the attachments of the superior constrictor. *BU:* - buccinator; *PMR:* - pterygomandibular raphe; *pt:* - processus tubarius.

fascia and a branch of the ascending palatine artery. These horizontal fibers will be referred to here as the palatopharyngei muscles.

The palatopharyngei are two thin, triangular laminae of muscle fibers that pass in a vertical plane from the lateral surface of the soft palate to insert into the pharyngeal raphe (Figs. 3-9 and 3-17). The general orientation of the muscle fibers of the palatopharyngei is downward and lateral, that is, at almost right angles to the fibers of superior constrictor, which pass upward and medial (Fig. 3-17). In the anatomical position, most fibers of the palatopharyngei pass down at roughly 30° to the horizontal plane, though their uppermost fibers are almost horizontally aligned (Fig. 3-17). The palatopharyngei arise from the superior surface of the palatine aponeurosis either in front of, behind, or on either side of the levatores. The fibers appear to insert into the pharyngeal raphe.

Salpingopharyngeus (M. salpingopharyngeus, N.A.). The salpingopharyngei are two vertically oriented fascicles of muscle fibers running from the auditory tube to the laryngopharynx and larynx (Fig. 3-17). Inferiorly, the fibers of the salpingopharyngei blend with fibers of the palatothyroideus and stylopharyngeus muscles. The superior attachment of the salpingopharyngei is along the whole length of the posterior lamina of the tubal cartilage. The muscles, each consisting of between one and five distinct fascicles, run downward beneath the salpingopharyngeal fold that is largely produced by underlying connective and glandular tissue.

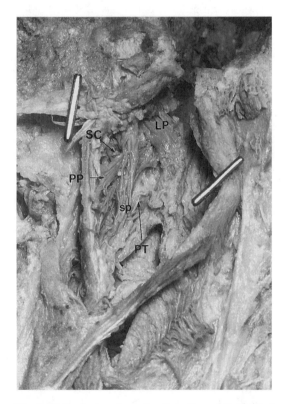

Fig. 3-17 Posterior view of a dissection of the lateral pharyngeal wall in a 49-year-old male cadaver showing the relationship between the palatopharyngeus *(PP)*, salpingopharyngeus *(SP)*, and superior constrictor *(SC)* muscles. Note that the fibers of the palatopharyngeus muscle are oriented at right angles to the fibers of superior constrictor.

It has been well established that movements of the lateral and posterior pharyngeal walls contribute to closure of the velopharynx, but the exact mechanisms by which such movements are achieved are still uncertain. As mentioned at the beginning of this chapter, the soft palate and the lateral and posterior pharyngeal walls form a complete ring of tissue around the nasopharyngeal hiatus. Closure of the hiatus involves essentially simultaneous movements of these structures to the extent that velopharyngeal closure can be described as a "sphincteric" mechanism. According to most researchers, maximal lateral pharyngeal wall movements occur at or below the level of the hard palate, and the superior constrictor is the primary muscle involved in these movements. Contraction and shortening of the fibers of the superior constrictors moves the lateral, and posterior, walls of the pharynx inward, reducing the size of the nasopharyngeal isthmus. However, the uppermost fibers of the superior constrictors are attached to the pterygoid hamulus and the pterygomandibular raphe (Figs. 3-7 and 3-16) and do not continue onto the soft palate. The superior constrictors do not therefore provide the complete ring of muscular tissue characteristic of a sphincter. However, the horizontally aligned fibers of palatopharyngeus (Fig. 3-17) do pass from the nasal surface of the soft palate onto the lateral pharyngeal walls and, with the superior constrictors, complete the sphincter. Contraction of this ring of muscle fibers results in a reduction in the size of the whole extent of the nasopharyngeal hiatus.

Historically, there has been considerable disagreement about movements of the posterior pharyngeal wall in velopharyngeal function. These disagreements revolve largely around whether the so-called ridge of Passavant is present in normal speakers. Passavant's original description of a prominent ridge appearing during speech was made in a patient with a cleft palate. Though the ridge is present in cleft and repaired-cleft speakers as often as it is in normal subjects, there is still disagreement as to whether the ridge of Passavant contributes to closure of the velopharynx. What muscle is responsible for its production remains more uncertain. Some authors have suggested that it is produced by contraction of all or part of the superior constrictor while others have specifically implicated the palatopharyngeus.

A clear functional role for the salpingopharyngei muscles has yet to be defined. Involvement of the salpingopharyngei in lateral pharyngeal wall movement has been denied, although nasoendoscopic examination of velopharyngeal closure in normal subjects has suggested that in many cases the salpingopharyngeal folds fill a potential defect in the lateral limit of soft palate apposition with the lateral pharyngeal walls. What role activity in the salpingopharyngei muscles plays in this phenomenon remains uncertain, particularly since it has been suggested that the salpingopharyngeal folds are in fact pulled into position by contraction of the palatopharyngeus. The underlying superior constrictor may also cause a passive medial motion of the folds. The anatomical relationship of the palatopharyngeus and salpingopharyngeus muscles clearly supports this suggestion (see Fig. 3-17).

Neuroanatomy of the velopharynx

Motor supply: Like all muscular systems, the motor innervation of the velopharynx is derived from motorneurons located within the central nervous system — in this case the medulla — which are influenced by muscle afferents and sensory fibers, as well as descending systems originating at higher levels of the brain. This innervation provides for a range of operation for the velopharynx extending from the subtle movements required for effective speech production to the gross "valvelike" movements associated with deglutition and respiration. The present review will make no attempt to describe the central nervous system structures involved in control of velopharyngeal movements and will focus solely on the anatomy of the peripheral components of the nerve supply of the velopharynx. However, in view of the controversy over exactly which cranial nerves provide motor innervation to the velopharynx, a brief description of the central location of motor neurons innervating this structure is warranted.

Studies in several species of experimental animals using the retrograde neuronal tracer horseradish peroxidase (HRP) report a consistent organization of velopharyngeal motor neurons in the medulla. Following injections of HRP into velopharyngeal muscles, including the palatopharyngeus and levator veli palatini, labeled neurons are found mostly in the nucleus ambiguus and nucleus retrofacialis. Neurons in these medullary nuclei project peripherally through the glossopharyngeal (IX) and vagus (X) nerves. Injections into the tensor veli palatini muscle produce labeled neurons in the motor nucleus of the trigeminal (V) nerve. Injections of HRP into the palatoglossus muscle label neurons in the nucleus ambiguus and hypoglossal (XII) nucleus.

Taken together, these findings clearly associate the motor innervation of the velopharynx with the motor neurons of the glossopharyngeal, vagus, and hypoglossal nerves. The controversy arises, however, when considering the peripheral courses of the fibers arising from these neurons. For example, the levator veli palatini has consistently been reported to receive innervation from the facial nerve, and complex routes have been devised to explain the course of motor fibers running from the facial nerve to the levator. Yet experimental studies have consistently failed to identify neurons in the facial nerve nucleus that innervate the palate. The problem is compounded in humans by the close relationship between palatine sensory fibers and the greater petrosal branch of the facial nerve in the pterygopalatine ganglion, and the presence of rami interconnecting the facial, glossopharyngeal, and vagus nerves both within the temporal bone and as they (as well as the hypoglossal nerve) emerge from the skull (Fig. 3-15). Thus, the following description, which is based on reports in the literature and the authors' gross dissections of cadaver specimens, refers only to the peripheral courses of motor nerve fibers innervating the velopharynx. It should not be regarded as definitive concerning the specific cranial nerve of origin of these fibers.

Classically, the motor supply of the velopharynx has been described as arising from the so-called pharyngeal plexus. This plexus, which is particularly well developed in humans, largely overlies the posterior and lateral surfaces of the middle pharyngeal constrictors and is derived from the pharyngeal branches of the glossopharyngeal and vagus nerves as well as the cervical sympathetic chain (Fig. 3-15). However, nerve fibers entering the levator veli palatini, superior constrictor, and palatothyroideus muscles generally can be followed grossly back to the pharyngeal branch of the vagus nerve. In six cadaver specimens examined by one of this chapter's authors (M.D. Cassell), the nerve to the levator (Fig. 3-18) was clearly visible as a single, slender trunk arising from the pharyngeal branch of X as it crossed the border between the superior and middle constrictors. The nerve to the levator passed obliquely upward across the exterior surface of the superior constrictor to pierce the pharyngobasilar fascia before entering the posterior surface of the levator (Fig. 3-18). In each of these specimens, between three and six slender filaments arose from the pharyngeal branch of X after the origin of the nerve to the levator and

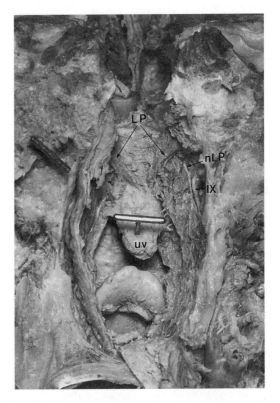

Fig. 3-18 Posterior view of a dissection of the exterior pharynx in a 49-year-old male cadaver, showing the nerve to levator veli palatini *(nLP)* and the glossopharyngeal nerve *(IX)*. The sling formed by the levatores *(LP)* in the soft palate can be clearly seen following removal of the musculi uvulae.

entered the superior constrictor, presumably supplying that muscle. In three specimens, it was possible to follow at least one of these filaments through the superior constrictor into the vertically running fibers of palatothyroideus. No filaments running into the palatopharyngeus or salpingopharyngeus could be seen. The presence of a ramus of the pharyngeal branch of X entering the palatothyroideus by passing between the middle and superior constrictors, as has been reported, could not be confirmed. At this level, the pharyngeal branch of X had dispersed into a number of filaments that merged with the pharyngeal plexus on the posterior surface of the middle constrictors.

The glossopharyngeal nerve reportedly sends filaments into the palatothyroideus. In the material examined, a pharyngeal branch arising from the glossopharyngeal nerve as it passed across the lateral border of stylopharyngeus was consistently observed, but its fibers appeared to disperse across the posterior surface of the middle constrictor, and no fibers could be followed into any velopharyngeal muscles. In the tonsillar bed, however, two slender filaments were seen consistently entering the fascicles of the palatoglossus. It should be noted, however, that clinical studies of patients with intracranial lesions of the glossopharyngeal nerve generally report no *motor* disturbances of velopharyngeal function.

In view of the reported tracing of fibers from the hypoglossal nucleus to the palatoglossus, the hypoglossal nerve was dissected in the floor of the mouth in two specimens. No direct branches were observed entering the palatoglossus from the hypoglossal nerve as it travelled across the hyoglossus muscle, but the possibility that filaments entered the tongue before passing to the palatoglossus could not be ruled out.

It is generally reported that the musculi uvulae receive their motor supply from the lesser palatine nerves. Such fibers were observed in the material dissected here (Fig. 3-13), but whether they were motor fibers or merely sensory fibers innervating the velar mucosa remains unknown. Interestingly, earlier studies have reported that fibers from the nerve to levator palati can be followed into the soft palate.

In summary, the motor supply to the velopharyngeal musculature appears to be derived from brain stem nuclei associated with the vagus and glossopharyngeal nerves, and their peripheral fibers appear to run largely in the pharyngeal branches of these nerves. In view of the interconnecting rami present between the facial, glossopharyngeal, vagus, and hypoglossal nerves, notably in the vicinity of their exit foramina from the skull, the possibility that a portion of the peripheral fibers of brain stem neurons innervating the velopharynx pass through other cranial nerves remains viable.

Sensory supply. The sensory nerves innervating the velopharynx are primarily concerned with mediating pain, temperature, touch, and vibration from the overlying mucosa and the periosteum of the hard palate. Unlike the remainder of the respiratory and digestive systems, these sensory modalities are consciously perceived. Since taste buds appear to be absent from the soft and hard palates in adult humans, the question of gustatory afferents arising from the velopharynx will not be addressed. The existence of proprioceptive afferents conveying information concerning such things as muscle tension and velar position has been poorly addressed. Muscle spindles have been identified in the levator and palatoglossus muscles, but their presence in the remaining

velopharyngeal musculature is still unclear. Before describing the gross anatomy of the sensory innervation of the velopharynx, two issues need to be addressed. First, it is very difficult to describe specific regional sensory innervation patterns in the velopharynx as both anatomical and clinical data indicate considerable overlap in the regions supplied by different branches of a particular nerve and even different cranial nerves. Second, the central fibers of primary sensory neurons innervating the human velopharynx all appear to terminate in the spinal nucleus of the trigeminal nerve even though their peripheral fibers may run in the facial, glossopharyngeal, and vagus nerves.

The palatine nerves. The bulk of the sensory supply of the hard and soft palates appears, at least grossly, to be provided by the greater (anterior) and lesser (middle and posterior) palatine nerves with a small contribution in the region of the incisive fossa from the nasopalatine nerves (Fig. 3-19). The greater and lesser palatine nerves arise from the maxillary division of the trigeminal nerve in the pterygopalatine fossa and descend in the palatine canal to emerge by the greater palatine and lesser palatine foramina, respectively. The greater palatine nerves run along the lateral border of the hard palate almost to the incisors, supplying palatine and gingival mucosa (Fig. 3-19). While still in the palatine canals, the greater nerves give off several small filaments that pierce the walls of the canals to supply the nasal surface of the hard palate and the lower part of the lateral walls of the nasal cavity. The lesser palatine nerves primarily supply the oral and nasal surfaces of the soft palate and uvula. Filaments supplying the nasal surfaces generally pierce the palatine aponeurosis and palatine musculature to reach the mucosa (Fig. 3-13).

The sensory innervation of the faucial and pharyngeal mucosa is generally described as being provided by the glossopharyngeal nerve either through direct branches arising in the tonsillar bed or through the pharyngeal plexus (Fig. 3-19). However, one characteristic finding in patients with the intracranial section of the glossopharyngeal nerve is analgesia not only over the lateral and posterior pharynx but also the soft palate as well. Anatomical studies in humans and non-primates have described fibers from the glossopharyngeal nerve ascending in the fauces from the tonsillar bed to the soft palate. Clearly, some revision of the usual description of the sensory innervation of the soft palate as being solely by the lesser palatine nerves may be in order.

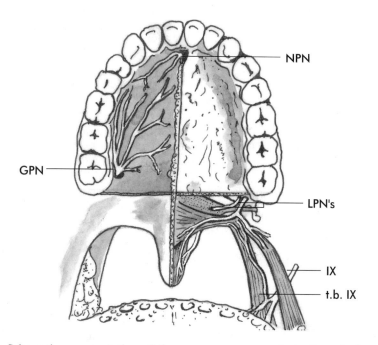

Fig. 3-19 Schematic representation of the sensory nerve supply to the velopharynx. The innervation of the hard palate by the nasopalatine *(NPN)* and greater palatine *(GPN)*) nerves is shown top left; the innervation of the soft palate and fauces by the lesser palatine *(LPN)* and tonsillar branches *(tbIX)* of the glossopharyngeal nerve *(IX)* is shown at bottom right.

In addition to its motor and sensory supply, the velopharynx receives a rich autonomic innervation. Sympathetic efferents arise from the superior cervical ganglion and enter the velopharynx via the pharyngeal plexus or via the interconnecting rami (e.g. the jugular nerve) passing from the superior cervical ganglion to the glossopharyngeal and vagus nerves. Sympathetic efferents appear to be largely vasomotor. Parasympathetic efferents, which are largely secretomotor to palatine and pharyngeal mucous glands, run in the palatine nerves and the glossopharyngeal nerve. The cells of origin of these efferents are located in the pterygopalatine and otic ganglia.

In summary, the motor supply of the velopharynx appears to be primarily derived from brain stem nuclei that are associated with the glossopharyngeal and vagus nerves (i.e., the nucleus ambiguus and nucleus retrofacialis). The first order sensory neurons innervating the velopharynx are associated with brain stem components of the trigeminal system. However, the extracranial course of motor and sensory fibers is complicated by the presence of extensive interconnections between the trigeminal, facial, glossopharyngeal, vagus, and hypoglossal nerves to the extent that even tracing distinct branches into velopharyngeal muscles or mucosa is at best only suggestive.

Velopharyngeal mucosa. The velopharyngeal musculature is sealed off from the upper airway by a covering of mucosa of varying thickness. The mucosa covering the soft palate and adjacent parts of the pharynx is typical nonkeratinizing, stratified squamous epithelium that is continuous anteriorly with the similar oral mucosa. The mucosa over the oral surface of the soft palate is bordered by the keratinized epithelium of the hard palate. A similar abrupt transition occurs on the nasal surface of the soft palate with the ciliated, columnar epithelium lining the nasal cavity. This type of epithelium also lines most of the posterior nasal cavity (nasopharynx). Laterally and posteriorly, a band of transitional epithelium covers the levatores and the auditory tube, covers the lower part of the posterior nasal cavity, and demarcates the upper limit of the pharynx.

In the living subject, the velopharyngeal mucosa appears smooth and continuous except where it is thrown into folds by the underlying structures. Below the soft palate, the anterior and posterior pillars of the fauces are formed by the underlying palatoglossus and palatothyroideus muscles, respectively. Under nasoendoscopic examination, the folds produced by the mucosa passing over the cartilage of the auditory tube *(torus tubarius),* the levator veli palatini *(torus levatorius),* the salpingopalatine ligaments *(salpingopalatal fold)* and the salpingopharyngeus *(salpingopharyngeal fold)* can be clearly seen. The salpingopharyngeal fold appears to be produced by an accumulation of mucous glands and not the salpingopharyngeus muscle.

SUMMARY

This chapter has attempted to give a comprehensive overview of the normal functional anatomy of the velopharynx as it relates to speech production. While a considerable amount of detailed information is available in the literature, a vast amount of work remains to be done, particularly in regard to biomechanical modeling of the velopharyngeal valve, correlation of velopharyngeal movements with the underlying anatomy, and the neurobiology of velopharyngeal control.

SUGGESTED READING

Bell-Berti F: An electromyographic study of velopharyngeal function in speech, *J Speech Hear Res* 19:225, 1976.

Broomhead IW: The nerve supply of the muscles of the soft palate, *Br J Plast Surg* 4:1, 1951.

Calnan J: Movements of the soft palate, *Br J Plast Surg* 5:286, 1955.

Croft CB, Shprintzen RJ, Rakoff S: Patterns of velopharyngeal valving in normals and cleft palate subjects: a multi-view videofluoroscopic and nasoendoscopic study, *Laryngoscope* 91:265, 1981.

Fritzell B: The velopharyngeal muscles in speech, *Acta Otolaryngol* Supp 250, 1969.

Gairns FW: The sensory nerve endings of the human palate, *Q J Exp Physiol* 40:40, 1955.

Harrington R: A study of the mechanism of velopharyngeal closure, *J Speech Hear Disord* 9:325, 1944.

Isberg AM, Henningsson GE: Intraindividual change in the occurrence of Passavant's ridge due to change in velopharyngeal sphincter function: a videofluoroscopic study, *Cleft Palate J* 27:253, 1990.

Keller JT, Saunders MC, van Loveren H, Shipley M: Neuroanatomical considerations of palatal muscles: tensor and levator veli palatini, *Cleft Palate J* 21:70, 1984.

Kriens O: Anatomy of the velopharyngeal area in cleft palate, *Clin Plast Surg* 2:261, 1975.

Kuehn D: Velopharyngeal anatomy and physiology, *Ear Nose Throat J* 58:316, 1979.

Kuehn D, Folkins J, Cutting C: Relationships between muscle activity and velar position, *Cleft Palate J* 19:25, 1982.

Shprintzen RJ, McCall G, Skolnick L: Selective movement of the lateral aspects of the pharyngeal walls during velopharyngeal closure for speech, whistling and blowing, *Cleft Palate J* 12:51, 1975.

Skolnick ML, McCall GN, Barnes M: The sphincteric mechanism of velopharyngeal closure, *Cleft Palate J* 10:286, 1973.

Wood Jones F: The nature of the soft palate, *J Anat* 74:147, 1940.

4 Pediatric Care and Feeding of the Newborn with a Cleft

Eugene J. Sidoti and Robert J. Shprintzen

The birth of a child with a cleft lip and cleft palate, or with just a cleft palate, whether associated with a multiple anomaly syndrome or not, is quite a shock to parents who are expecting the delivery of a "bundle of joy." Besides the disappointment that might attend the birth of a child with a congenital anomaly, there is the fear accompanying the unknown and the concern for the baby regarding surgery. All future considerations, however, soon take a back seat to the need to feed the baby.

There may be no more compelling need for both baby and parent than the feeding process. Today, many mothers look forward to nursing their babies. Unfortunately, babies born with clefts seem to present insurmountable problems for normal feeding, especially nursing. If the oral cavity cannot be separated from the nasal cavity, how can the baby suck (i.e., create suction)? Is it necessary to modify feeding procedures in babies with clefts? Do special bottles, nipples, or devices need to be used? At a time when emotions are running high for the parents of infants with clefts, information should be readily available to make life as normal as possible. The purpose of this chapter is to describe feeding procedures that have been utilized for over 30 years in over 3000 infants with clefts and to discuss the role of the pediatrician in the management of patients with clefts.

FEEDING IN NORMAL INFANTS

The feeding process in newborns and infants is a fascinating physiological event, which is disrupted by the presence of a cleft palate. Cleft lip alone has little or no effect on the feeding process. If the palate is intact, it is not essential for there to be a lip seal around the nipple in order to suckle. This is because the "suction" occurs behind the tongue, not anteriorly. Therefore, it is the palate that is the more important anatomical structure for sucking. In order to create a seal posterior to the tongue, the palate must be intact.

It is also important for the infant to be able to maintain normal respiration during feeding. It is the norm for infants to breathe through the nose while feeding orally. This is done by an anatomical and physiological process unique to infants, which is subsequently lost to older children and adults. In infants, the pharynx is short in its vertical dimension and is angled more horizontally than in adults (Fig. 4-1). As a result of the short vertical airway dimensions, the top of the epiglottis sits in close proximity to the base of the soft palate (velum) even at rest. During the feeding process, the epiglottis elevates slightly and hooks around the back of the velum, thus allowing the nasal airway to be in direct contact with the glottis, thus providing a continuous airway from the nose to the lungs (Fig. 4-1). During feeding, the oral contents are deflected laterally around the epiglottis into the esophagus, while the infant is able to maintain a normal nasal respiratory process.

The mechanism of normal feeding involves expressing a bolus of milk from a nipple (bottle or breast) and conveying that bolus from the anterior portion of the mouth to the oropharynx where it can then be transported to the esophagus and stomach (Fig. 4-2). After the nipple is taken into the front of the infant's mouth, the tongue elevates to squeeze the nipple against the hard palate as the lips create a seal around the nipple. The tongue then sweeps backward, thus enlarging the volume between the lips and the tongue-palate contact (Fig. 4-2). By enlarging the space in the anterior oral cavity without allowing air into it (because it is sealed anteriorly at the lips and posteriorly at the tongue-palate contact), a small negative pressure, or suction, is created. The milk is expressed from the nipple by a combination of the tongue squeezing out the contents of the breast and the negative pressure created in the oral cavity by sucking the milk into the mouth.

After the oral cavity fills (which may take several sucks), the tongue sweeps the bolus of milk posteriorly into the oropharynx and around

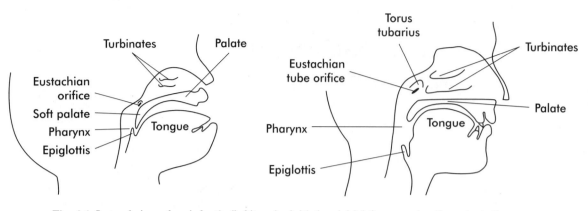

Fig. 4-1 Lateral view of an infant's (left) and adult's head (right) comparing the orientation and anatomy of the airway and the ability for the infant epiglottis to hook around the velum.

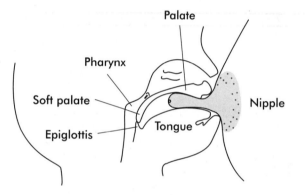

Fig. 4-2 Lateral view of an infant's head to show the mechanism of feeding.

the connection between the epiglottis and velum. The milk is prevented from escaping through the nose by the velum. After the milk enters the pharynx, it is swallowed and the tongue is returned anteriorly to repeat the process. The relatively airtight seal allows the baby to nurse without swallowing much air, but some will be swallowed during the feeding procedure, which may precipitate either some burping, or, if the amount of air is relatively large, some regurgitation of some formula with a large release of air.

The process continues until the baby is satiated (usually when the stomach is full and can no longer accept additional fluid). The process of feeding is the same regardless of the food source (breast or bottle). The difference between breast and bottle relates largely to the rate of flow, in addition to the psychological and physiological parameters that jointly affect mother and baby. In general, the flow from a

bottle is faster, though this is affected by the type of bottle, the type of nipple, the size of the hole in the nipple, and the technique used by the mother. The flow of milk from a mother's breast is also affected by a number of factors, but the most important is the mother's ability to lactate, which is not uniform among all women. Though the selection of the feeding source may appear on the surface to be one of personal preference, in the case of babies with clefts, both parents and clinicians must be continuously cognizant of the need to provide the infant with adequate nutrition.

FEEDING IN INFANTS WITH CLEFTS

Though the cleft lip is the far more visible defect, it is the palatal cleft that is more troublesome relative to feeding in babies with clefts. Though a cleft lip may be problematic for creating an anterior seal around the nipple, an anterior closure can still be obtained with the tongue tip and alveolar ridges. A cleft of the palate, however, completely prevents a seal posteriorly. The oral cavity becomes continuous with the nasal cavity, preventing the ability to create a negative pressure, thus eliminating one of the mechanisms the infant has for extracting milk from the breast or bottle. Even more problematic is the absence of the connection between the epiglottis and velum. If the velum is cleft at its posterior end, the epiglottis cannot hook around its back and create a separation between the nasal respiratory route and the oral feeding route. Therefore, the infant's ability to coordinate breathing and eating is impaired and milk may escape through the nose. This factor alone will significantly lengthen the feeding period and nasal regurgitation may reduce intake. It is typical in babies with clefts of the palate to suck at the nipple until a bolus has been extracted, swallow, and then stop feeding to take several breaths. Therefore, rather than respiration and nursing occurring together, they occur consecutively, which will cause the feeding period to be at least twice as long as in a noncleft infant.

Clefts of the hard palate (but not clefts of the soft palate) also present an obstacle to the normal tongue-pressing component of the phase of feeding where milk is extracted from the nipple. If the hard palate is cleft and the nipple is held straight into the infant's mouth, then as the tongue elevates to press the nipple to the hard palate for the purpose of squeezing milk out of it, the nipple may be pushed into the cleft (Fig. 4-3). This causes two problems. First, the nipple cannot be pressed flat against the palate so that little or no milk may be extracted as a result of the tongue activity. Second, whatever milk is extracted may be directed into the nasal cavity rather than the oral cavity. If the milk enters the nose, the tongue will not be able to sweep it posteriorly into the esophagus. Instead, it may come out of the front of the nose, where there is no obstacle to its escape. Because less milk will be extracted with each suck, the feeding process is once again lengthened.

Therefore, the structural anomaly of the palatal cleft can present major problems to the normal feeding process. However, it should be pointed out that infants with clefts who are otherwise normal (especially with regard to neurological integrity) have the same reflexive drive to suck and feed as noncleft infants. It is typical, therefore, to see babies with clefts vigorously sucking at a nipple without having much success at actually feeding. The less success encountered by the baby, the higher the anxiety of the adults who are care providers, including parents, grandparents, and even pediatricians and nurses. Weight will start to decline, or weight may be maintained without significant gain. The lack of success with feeding in infants with clefts has led to the development of a number of irrational approaches to the problem, including the use of various devices, special nipples and bottles, and even the use of alternative feeding methods, such as gavage feeding or gastrostomy. These methods should be reserved only for the most severely neurologically impaired babies. As will be discussed later in this chapter, very minor modifications in the feeding process can easily resolve feeding problems in babies with clefts.

LENGTH OF THE FEEDING PERIOD

The increased length of time in the feeding process in babies with clefts can cause a number of problems. They include weight loss or inadequate weight gain, disruption of feeding schedules affecting hunger, and parental frustration caused by lack of success and being tied down to the baby for inordinate lengths of time. Perhaps the major goal of the clinician in instructing the parents in proper feeding technique is to reduce the amount of time it takes to get adequate nutrition for the baby.

When a baby takes too long to feed, he or she expends many more calories in the feeding process than he or she should. The muscle activity involved in sucking, especially if the sucking is unsuccessful and not met with a flow of caloric intake, will result in the baby burning off more calories than he or she is consuming. It is typical for young babies to fall asleep after a feeding. It is during this sleep period that the baby's metabolism slows down, which allows weight gain. In addition, a proportionately larger amount of pituitary growth hormone is secreted during sleep than during wakefulness. It is therefore likely that staying awake longer (hence, sleeping less) will reduce the baby's opportunity to grow and gain weight normally. Staying awake longer also means that the baby will burn more calories than he or she would if asleep, which will also limit weight gain. Therefore, the feeding period should not be extended beyond a reasonable time period.

A newborn should not take more than 20 to 30 minutes to finish a bottle or nursing session, regardless of the amount consumed. For example, newborns may only require 1.5 to 2 ounces of formula to support a weight of 7 pounds, while a larger baby might require 6 or 7 ounces of formula per feeding. A larger baby is capable of taking larger amounts of milk in a

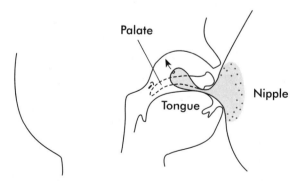

Fig. 4-3 Lateral view of a cleft infant's head showing the tongue pushing the nipple into the cleft.

shorter time period (the baby is stronger and the mouth larger) so that consuming larger amounts of formula should not lengthen the feeding.

Another negative aspect of extending the feeding period beyond 20 to 30 minutes is that the time period between feedings is shortened. It is preferable to keep newborns with clefts on a 3 hour feeding schedule. It is suggested that babies be given feedings at 6 AM 9 AM, 12 noon, 3 PM, 6 PM, 9 PM, and midnight. If the baby sleeps through the night, missing the 3 AM feeding would be permitted. When the feeding period is extended to nearly an hour, it means that the time period until the next feeding is reduced to only 2 hours, which may not be sufficient time for the baby to get hungry. Reduced hunger would mean a subsequent unsuccessful feeding and reduced caloric intake. By keeping the feeding period to 30 minutes or less, the time period between feedings is closer to 3 hours, which allows time for hunger, sleep, and things other than eating. By keeping the feeding periods short, parental bonding to the baby is a pleasant one, without the frustration involved in a protracted and difficult feeding session. Parents are able to sleep while the baby sleeps, and there is time for play, which further strengthens parent-child bonding.

Is it necessary to make major modifications in the feeding process in order to reduce feeding time to the recommended 20 to 30 minutes? Stated simply, not at all.

RECOMMENDED FEEDING PROCEDURE

The procedure we are about to describe is not unique. There are probably many other centers that employ the same type of technique with perhaps minor variations. We have successfully applied this procedure to literally thousands of babies with clefts of the palate or lip and palate. Based on this experience, it can be stated unequivocally that unless there is a complicating factor, any baby with a cleft can be successfully bottle fed with only minor modifications.

Complicating factors

As discussed in Chapter 2 of this text, clefting is often one of several clinical findings in children with multiple anomaly syndromes. Many multiple anomaly syndromes have airway compromise and/or neurological complications. In cases where feeding is extremely problematic, airway and neurological problems should be ruled out as contributing factors.

Airway disorders. In order to feed, newborns must be able to exchange air simultaneously to avoid asphyxiation. Airway protection is given primary importance in the infant's physiological functioning. If the airway is too small or anomalous to support both respiration and feeding simultaneously (as is the normal situation as previously discussed), infants will do everything they must do to assure adequate ventilation. This is often at the expense of feeding. Babies with marginal airways will often cough, cry, seem irritable, or start to suck but then will stop in order to maintain respiration. Therefore, feedings become long, almost agonizing procedures because the baby seems fussy and unwilling to eat. Weight decreases or the infant does not gain ample weight in relation to linear growth. This is often referred to as "failure to thrive." In our experience, the majority of babies with failure to thrive have airway problems. Resolution of the airway problems will alleviate the feeding problem.

At particular risk for airway related feeding problems are babies with Robin sequence and its associated syndromes. As described in Chapter 2, Robin is an etiologically nonspecific grouping of clinical features including micrognathia, cleft palate (many clinicians specify that the cleft must be wide and U-shaped), and airway obstruction, usually thought to be caused by glossoptosis (the tongue falling back into the airway). Many cases of Robin sequence require surgical management of their airway problems, such as glossopexy (Argamaso, 1992) or tracheotomy. Other babies with Robin have initial difficulties with respiration that are managed nonsurgically for a brief period of time. Positioning and nasopharyngeal tubes have been used for several days or weeks to temporize respiration so that with growth and increased neurologic integrity, normal respiration can be maintained (Sadewitz, 1992; Singer and Sidoti, 1992). In such cases, the airway is often barely adequate to maintain normal respiration. During quiet breathing, the airway is easily maintained, and the baby appears well. However, when the respiratory mechanism is stressed, obstruction or partial obstruction of breathing becomes evident. Feeding can stress the airway because food occupies the same pharyngeal space as air in the baby with a cleft. If the airway is structurally small or compromised by a small jaw or glossoptosis, then it becomes impossible for the infant to coordinate breathing and eating. Other sources of airway stress would include an upper respiratory infection and vigorous crying where deep inspirations can cause negative pressure within a small airway. There are certain clues to the presence of airway compromise under these circumstances. One is a pectus excavatum (Fig. 4-4). A pectus excavatum (often referred to simply as a pectus) is a

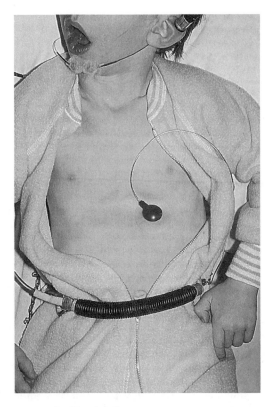

Fig. 4-4 Pectus excavatum.

deep indentation at the base of the sternum, which becomes even deeper on inspiration. In babies with constant airway obstruction, the pectus will be prominent even during quiet respiration. In babies with marginal airways, the pectus may not be present during normal respiratory effort. However, during periods of airway stress, such as when feeding, during an upper respiratory infection, or on deep inspirations when crying or screaming, the pectus will become very pronounced. The appearance of a pectus in association with failure to thrive is a certain sign of airway compromise leading to feeding difficulties. Babies with Robin sequence frequently have failure to thrive and show poor weight gain or even marked weight loss. Of the syndromes associated with Robin sequence, many have structurally small airways, such as Stickler syndrome, spondiloepiphyseal dysplasia syndrome, and Larsen syndrome.

A major airway concern is the possibility of aspiration; that milk will be inappropriately diverted into the lower airway (i.e., trachea, bronchi, or lungs) because of an inability to direct the flow properly. Aspiration occurs very infrequently in babies with clefts. When it does occur, it should not be assumed that aspiration is the result of the cleft malformation. In fact, the presence of aspiration almost always signals the presence of a more serious anomaly, such as a tracheo-esophageal fistula (T-E fistula), malformation of the larynx (such as a cleft larynx), or severe anomalies of the central nervous system leading to impaired coordination of even the autonomic process of reflexive swallowing. In our experience, babies who are neurologically intact and who have no other structural anomalies of the upper or lower airway do not aspirate, and the process of feeding should not be modified to avoid aspiration.

Neurological anomalies. Neurological disorders are also often associated with syndromes of clefting. One of the major sequelae of neurological anomalies is hypotonia. Hypotonia will cause laxity of the muscles involved in feeding, resulting in a weak suck or weak tongue press of the nipple, which will slow the rate of flow and lengthen feeding time. Hypotonia may also weaken the muscles of the airway, predisposing the baby to airway collapse and obstruction. One example of a syndrome with hypotonia associated with cleft palate is velo-cardio-facial syndrome (see Chapter 2). Velo-cardio-facial syndrome is the most common syndrome of clefting and makes up approximately 5% of the population of all children seen at cleft palate centers and 8% of all babies with cleft palate without cleft lip (Lipson et al, 1989; Shprintzen et al, 1985). Early failure to thrive is common in velo-cardio-facial syndrome, with several components contributing to the feeding problem. Feeding may be compromised by pharyngeal hypotonia, by a weak suck, by the palatal cleft, by the association of Robin sequence in approximately 17% of velo-cardio-facial syndrome cases, and by congenital heart anomalies, which can cause overall weakness and decreased vigor.

A number of clefting syndromes have such severe brain malformations that many physiological functions, feeding included, are impaired. In newborns with severe brain malformations, the feeding problems have nothing to do with the cleft. Even if the cleft were not present, infants with severe brain anomalies would have problems feeding and would be categorized as failure to thrive. In such cases, alternatives to normal feeding procedures, such as gastrostomy or nasogastric feedings, must be employed.

Unfortunately, gastrostomy is frequently performed on children with failure to thrive in association with airway problems. A cycle of failure is established in many infants, especially those with airway related disorders and mild neurological impairment. Infants who initially demonstrate poor feeding are often managed temporarily with gavage feedings by nasogastric or orogastric tube. Initiation of alternative feeding methods may be commenced very shortly after birth in order to prevent dehydration in babies who fail oral feeding. Therefore, this type of infant may have little or no opportunity to establish normal oral feeding patterns. If gavage feeding persists for a week or more, it becomes difficult to establish oral feeding because the infant has adapted to the alternative feeding procedure. While not initially pleasant, gavage feedings are quick and efficient. The passage of a tube, or leaving a tube in place for a period of time does not significantly distress most babies. They learn that feeding can be rapid, and the comfort of a full stomach is reached with essentially no effort on the baby's part. Even after the airway obstruction is resolved or neurologic maturity allows better muscle tone, it becomes difficult to make the baby work for its food. It takes perseverance and major effort on the part of the caregiver to get babies to feed by mouth because the baby has never established the entire process of feeding, including the physical contact with the parent, sucking, swallowing coordination, and the pleasure of simultaneous oral stimulation and parental affection. Initial attempts to establish oral feedings are almost always met with resistance, screaming, crying, and obvious expressions of displeasure and annoyance. Caregivers must learn to tolerate these behaviors and persist until oral feeding can be established. Unfortunately, after several of these unhappy feeding episodes, many clinicians feel that oral feeding is an impossibility, and a permanent surgical solution is sought, such as gastrostomy. A gastrostomy is a surgical entry into the stomach through an opening in the abdominal wall, which is maintained by a tube with a removable lid. This allows caregivers to pour milk or liquified food directly into the stomach. This, too, is a quick and efficient technique for feeding, but regrettably, one which is utilized inappropriately in far too many cases. Among the thousands of babies managed at our center, only one has required gastrostomy because of a severe brain malformation and subsequent institutionalization. Gastrostomy should be utilized only in cases where the neurological abnormalities are so severe that the baby cannot even reflexively respond to the oral stimulation of food. Gastrostomy should not be utilized in infants with airway obstruction. In cases of obstructive respiratory disorder, resolution of the breathing problem will lead to the ability to learn oral feeding (though not without effort).

Therefore, when feeding difficulties are encountered in babies with clefts, the cleft itself may simply be a "red herring." In other words, the cleft is often part of a symptom complex that presents other problems to the feeding process that are far more difficult to overcome than the cleft. Essentially all babies with clefts who do not have severe neurologic or airway problems can be fed orally with little difficulty and without unusual feeding implements.

FEEDING TECHNIQUE

There are several basic principles important to successfully feeding babies with clefts, which are applicable in essentially all cases. First, the baby should be kept in a relatively upright position. This is actually a good suggestion for all babies. In an upright position, gravity will assist the proper flow of milk. In babies with clefts, it is also thought that horizontal feeding will contribute to flooding of the Eustachian tube orifices with milk, leading to retrograde reflux into the middle ear and contamination of the middle ear space with milk and bacteria. This notion has never been convincingly demonstrated in scientific literature. The rationale for feeding upright is simply that this is a much more natural position for babies (and adults).

A second principle, as detailed previously, is to confine the feeding period to 20 minutes, certainly no more than 30 minutes. Minor modifications in technique and feeding implements will be helpful to prevent a prolonged feeding period.

Feeding devices

A large number of implements designed for feeding infants with clefts have been devised, but none have been universally accepted. All these devices have been designed in some way to accommodate for the cleft based on the same working hypothesis; that infants with clefts have

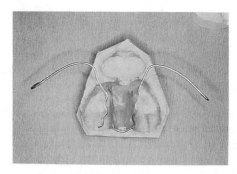

Fig. 4-5 Feeding plate.

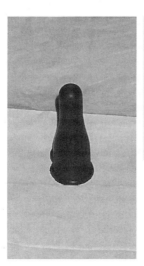

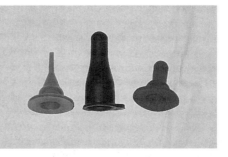

Fig. 4-6 Lamb's nipple (left) and the comparison of all three types of nipples (above).

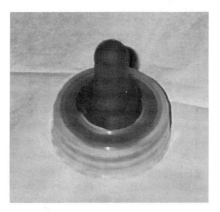

Fig. 4-8 Red premie nipple.

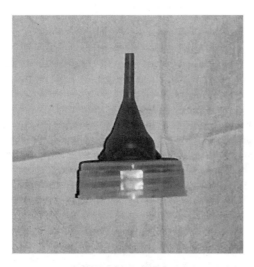

Fig. 4-7 Ross cleft palate nipple.

difficulty feeding. We will show that this underlying hypothesis is simply not true and that special devices are not necessary in most babies with clefts. To reiterate a point elaborated before, it is only babies with multiple anomaly syndromes with structural anomalies of the airway or severe brain abnormalities who require special devices or techniques.

The use of feeding plates has been advocated by some clinicians. There are a number of types of feeding plates, all with a common purpose; to obturate the cleft (Fig. 4-5). Again, the assumption is that babies with clefts cannot successfully prevent food from coming out of the nose unless an artificial palate is placed. The assumption is erroneous, and feeding plates are not at all necessary. Feeding plates usually consist of an acrylic plate molded to the infant's maxilla.

They must be remolded with growth. Keeping them in place may be troublesome, and they must be periodically cleaned. Furthermore, they send a clear message to parents that the cleft anomaly is a serious problem that cannot be easily overcome by more conservative means. This is a disconcerting message to parents who are already upset at the birth of a less than "perfect" baby. Our approach has been to keep things as simple and "normal" as possible.

Bottle and nipple. Many different types of nipples have been devised and recommended for use by babies with clefts, ranging from lamb's nipples (Fig. 4-6) to specially shaped nipples (Fig. 4-7). All of them achieve some degree of success for one primary reason; they all have large holes. Some of these nipples are very long, the intent being to deliver the formula into the back of the throat and bypass the cleft in the anterior portion of the mouth. In our opinion, this makes little sense and would only tend to cause the baby to gag and have an uncomfortable feeding. A simple modification to a normal shaped nipple is all that is required. Our preference is to use a "red premie" nipple (Fig. 4-8). These nipples, designed for premature babies, are readily available in most hospitals, pharmacies, or surgical supply stores. Fig. 4-5 shows the nipple made by Ross Laboratories, though other brands, such as Enfamil, make similar nipples that are also readily available. We suggest making a large cross-cut in these nipples with a scissor, razor blade, or scalpel (Fig. 4-9). The cuts, crossed like an X, should each be approximately 5 mm long. When the bottle is held upside down, drops of milk should dribble out slowly. The advantage of the premie nipple is that it is thinner and softer than standard nipples so that tongue pressing action is more likely to express milk. Standard nipples can also be used with large cross-cuts; boiling standard nipples several times will soften them. Another advantage of using the premie nipples is that their shape is much more natural and fits the baby's mouth well. The nipple will also appear like a normal nipple and therefore not stigmatize the mother or baby by having an unusual device evident to even casual observers.

The position in which the nipple is held in the mouth is important. Because babies with clefts feed by tongue press, as the tongue elevates, the nipple must be squeezed on a shelf of something rigid in order to express the milk. In babies with complete clefts of the palate or lip and palate where the cleft extends anteriorly, the midline of the palate is open. If the nipple is held straight into the mouth, when the tongue elevates, the nipple will be pushed into the cleft, and the nipple will not be flattened completely so that the contents cannot be fully extracted. Furthermore, if the nipple is in the cleft, the contents of the nipple will be injected into the nasal cavity rather than the oral cavity. This will increase the likelihood that milk will be extruded through the nose rather than swallowed. Therefore, the nipple should be held in the mouth so that it is underneath a shelf of bone. In babies with unilateral complete clefts, the nipple should be held underneath the noncleft side of the palate either by introducing the bottle in the noncleft side of the mouth, or by introducing it into the cleft side, but angling the tip of the nipple across the mouth towards the noncleft side of the hard palate. Therefore, the elevated tongue will always press the milk-bearing portion of the nipple against an intact portion of the hard palate, squeezing out the full contents and keeping the milk in the mouth. In complete bilateral clefts, the infant's mouth should be examined to see which palatal shelf is more substantial; that side should be chosen for the placement of the nipple (Fig. 4-10). The same would be true for complete clefts of the secondary palate. In incomplete clefts of the secondary palate or clefts of the soft palate only, the nipple can be positioned in the center of the mouth as in any other baby. Positioning the nipple laterally in the mouth of a baby with a cleft will have no adverse consequences. There is certainly no rule regarding where a nipple should be placed,

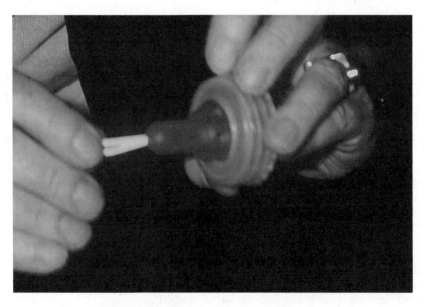

Fig. 4-9 Making a cross-cut in the nipple.

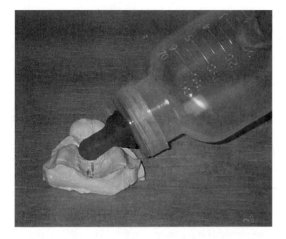

Fig. 4-10 Method of positioning the nipple in babies with clefts. The tip of the nipple is shown against a portion of the bony palate using a dental impression of an infant with a bilateral cleft lip and palate.

and the infant simply does not care. The success of this procedure belies the logic of using very long nipples, such as lamb's nipples, or other unusual feeding devices.

We prefer to use plastic bottles rather than glass. Another way the feeding can be held to within 20 to 30 minutes is to keep the flow of milk continuing even if the baby has stopped during the feeding session without finishing the formula. This can be accomplished by gently squeezing a pliable plastic bottle to inject some milk into the baby's mouth. Obviously, large amounts of formula should not be introduced during crying when a baby might aspirate on a deep inspiration. In combination with the cross-cut nipple, a soft squeeze on a plastic bottle will inject sufficient formula into the baby's mouth to require swallowing without running the risk of aspiration. Special bottles have been devised specifically for this purpose, such as the Mead Johnson nurser (Fig. 4-11), but these are not essential. Any plastic bottle that can be squeezed and has even a small amount of yield to the sides will assist in the process. We recommend the Evenflow frosted plastic bottles as having adequate pliability.

The third principle is to keep air out of the stomach. If the stomach fills with too much air, there are three problems that compromise the feeding session. One is early satiation caused by air occupying space that would better be filled with milk. If the infant feels full, then additional formula will be refused or vomiting will occur if more is forced. The second problem will be discomfort and cramping (perhaps mistakenly diagnosed as colic) caused by the gas bubbles. If

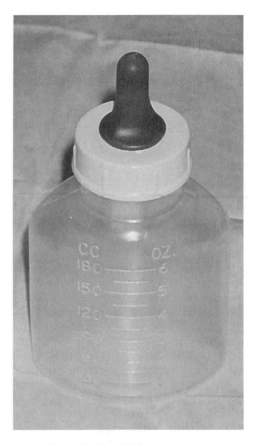

Fig. 4-11 Mead Johnson nurser.

the baby is irritable from pain caused by entrapped gas, the feeding will be terminated with unpleasant crying and a frustrated and irritated caregiver. The third potential problem is vomiting caused by a sudden release of entrapped gas at the end of the feeding. If too much gas is released all at once, then some proportion of the milk will be expelled with the air, resulting in the possibility of the loss of a portion of the nutritional value of the feeding.

In order to avoid the problems associated with excess air in the stomach, babies with clefts should be burped more frequently than noncleft babies. In noncleft babies, it is typical to burp them several times during the feeding and once at the end. Babies with clefts should be burped more frequently, at least every 5 minutes.

Is it possible to nurse?

Many mothers would prefer to nurse their babies, and there are sound reasons for wanting to do so. For one thing, the bonding between mother and infant is often regarded as a major advantage of breastfeeding. The close physical contact required during nursing is a powerful reinforcement of the normal maternal feelings a mother has toward her infant. It is also believed that there are many health advantages to nursing, though much of the data are far from conclusive. However, if the mother wishes to nurse her baby, it is of paramount importance that every attempt be made to comply with that desire. Unfortunately, it is not always possible for mothers to nurse babies with clefts. One of the biggest problems is the rate of milk flow. Some mothers have a much more vigorous flow of milk and with minor modifications in the feeding process can manage to feed their babies within the prescribed time period. However, many mothers cannot provide a strong enough flow of milk to feed the baby within 20 or 30 minutes, so the feeding period may be long and frustrating. Emotional stress created by the birth of an infant with a visible defect can seriously interfere with a mother's attempts to initiate breastfeeding. Furthermore, mother's milk tends to satiate babies more rapidly than cow's milk formula. As a result, infants who are nursed may not react to hunger after a feeding where insufficient formula was taken to gain weight. They will satiate and not become fussy and irritable even if their stomachs are less than full. An additional major drawback of nursing is that there is no way to monitor the amount of milk the baby has consumed. If a baby's weight is not monitored very closely, it would become possible for the baby to dehydrate within a day or two (depending on its size and a number of other factors, such as the ambient temperature). Without careful observation of the amount of milk consumed, it is nearly impossible to tell if an infant is at risk for the potentially life-threatening consequences of dehydration. It is virtually impossible to determine how much milk has been consumed during nursing. If a prime concern is for the baby to have mother's milk, one alternative to nursing is for the mother to express her milk using a breast pump and to store it for bottle feeding (the milk can be refrigerated or frozen and stored, if necessary). This way, consumption can be observed carefully, and the baby can have the full benefit of mother's milk. Of course, the physical component of nursing is missing, which may be a major detraction for many mothers. However, the baby's health and well being must be of primary importance. Some proponents of nursing insist that any mother can successfully nurse any baby. This is simply not true. A cleft represents an extraordinary circumstance that calls for dili-

gence and common sense in maintaining the baby's welfare. It is obvious that the process of nursing should not be considered more important than the goal of providing a baby adequate nutrition for health and growth.

Other concerns about feeding

Before the time clinicians understood about the etiologic heterogeneity of clefting, problems encountered in the feeding process were mistakenly attributed to the cleft. Because other structural anomalies might go undetected at birth, whereas the cleft is an obvious anomaly that is difficult to overlook, it became convenient to blame difficulties on the cleft. Besides the immediate concern of "thriving," pediatricians and parents are both concerned about overall growth and development.

Weight gain versus linear growth

Clinicians often confuse two issues that relate to a baby's size; weight gain and linear growth. In reality, the only issue relevant to feeding is weight gain. Linear growth is rarely ever effected by malnutrition, especially in the modern industrial world where routine medical care can be supplied to babies who are not thriving. If a baby's "size" is adversely affected by poor feeding, it will become immediately obvious in a disproportion between body weight and linear growth. There are tables that are available to every pediatrician that plot weight versus height (i.e., linear growth). These tables should be checked routinely, especially in babies with clefts, to assure that sufficient nutrition is being delivered.

Deficiencies in linear growth (height) are almost always related to problems that are not the result of feeding difficulties. The most important factor tends to be the association of multiple anomaly syndromes, which have short stature as a clinical symptom. Shprintzen et al (1985) reported that over 20% of individuals with clefts have short stature as a part of a multiple anomaly syndrome. Many of the most common syndromes of clefting have short stature as a common clinical finding, including velo-cardio-facial syndrome, Stickler syndrome, and fetal alcohol syndrome which, when combined, comprise at least 10% of all babies with clefts. Many other syndromes also have the association of short stature and clefting, including spondyloepiphyseal dysplasia syndrome, Larsen syndrome, diastrophic dysplasia syndrome, DeMyer sequence, and fetal hydantoin syndrome. Any syndrome that might have a hypoplastic or absent pituitary gland would almost certainly result in short stature and reduced linear growth. Syndromes with pituitary abnormalities also usually involve anomalies of the brain and other midline abnormalities, including midline clefts. Linear growth is also often affected by metabolic abnormalities, which may be associated with a number of syndromes of clefting as well.

Linear growth may also be disturbed by severe obstructive sleep apnea. Apnea is defined as a temporary cessation of breathing. Apnea will be discussed in greater detail in Chapter 5. Briefly, there are three basic types of apnea: obstructive, central, and mixed (a combination of obstructive and mixed apnea). In obstructive apnea, the effort to breathe is continuous, but air is not exchanged in and out of the lungs because of an obstruction at some point in the airway. Therefore, the baby looks as if it is breathing (the chest and abdomen move as if air is being exchanged), but air does not pass in or out of the mouth and/or nose. In central apnea, all efforts to breathe cease for brief periods of time. Not only is air not passing into the lungs, but there are no chest or abdominal movements. In mixed apnea, both central and obstructive elements are present. The episodes of breathing stoppages may begin as obstructive and end as central or vice versa. The reader is urged to see Chapter 5 for a detailed description of a common problem in babies with clefts and craniofacial anomalies that could have potentially dangerous consequences.

Apnea leads to a reduction of linear growth because of a disturbance of the normal distribution of sleep. A major percentage of growth hormone is secreted by the pituitary gland during deep sleep. Infants with obstructive sleep apnea are almost always on the verge of wakefulness and spend little or no time in deep sleep. As a result, there is a marked reduction in growth hormone secretion and decreased linear growth (Goldstein et al, 1985).

Reduced linear growth should be a source of concern to clinicians following babies with clefts. Rather than immediately turning attention to feeding difficulties as the source of the growth reduction, clinicians should instead turn their attention to more serious medical problems as a source of the deficiency. Today, feeding problems are often managed by nonmedical personnel, such as speech pathologists or occupational therapists. There may be a tendency among clinicians inexperienced with the medical complications giving rise to linear growth reduction to believe that any problem with a baby's "size" is the result of a feeding problem. If the problem is not detected and

managed properly, the consequences could be serious or even life-threatening.

THE ROLE OF THE PEDIATRICIAN

A review of the membership of the American Cleft Palate-Craniofacial Association shows that relatively few pediatricians are members of the organization. This may reflect the early emphasis on surgical, dental, and speech needs for patients with clefts, while more general concerns such as growth and development were secondary to the more immediate needs of repair of the lip and/or palate. In our opinion, the pediatrician should play an integral role in the management of patients with clefts and craniofacial malformations.

As mentioned in Chapter 1, the direction of overall patient care may depend, in large part, on the influence of the director of the team managing the patient. If the director and dominant personality on a team is someone who treats the cleft and related anomalies, the direction of patient management may be dictated based upon a disciplinary bias (surgeons are more likely to recommend surgery, dentists are more likely to be concerned about occlusion, speech pathologists about speech, etc.). In our opinion, the pediatrician has a different "bias" than treaters. Pediatricians are trained to be "generalists." Their approach is one of overall development of the child and, as such, treatment recommendations must fit a cohesive plan for management, which will show both short- and long-term benefits to the child. Though few pediatricians belong to the American Cleft Palate-Craniofacial Association, in our opinion, they should play pivotal roles as team directors or "mediators" for teams. It would seem advantageous to have the pediatrician serve as an impartial patient ombudsman; to act as a liaison between the highly specialized concerns of the team professionals who provide treatment and the broader concerns of the parents. In other words, there may be an advantage to the patient having someone medically "neutral" in helping to negotiate an overall treatment plan.

Children with clefts require overall medical management in combination with treatment of their malformations. Team members who specialize in treating specific problems may be unaware of more basic medical needs for their patients. Concerns about growth, development, immunizations, feeding, and general health maintenance should not be left to specialists focusing on the cleft. These are issues that must be placed in a much broader context in overall patient care. Without the involvement of a pediatrician, it is possible to make decisions about surgery that may make sense to the surgeon, but could be detrimental to the overall health and welfare of the child.

It is also important to have a pediatrician involved in the care of the patient during the many hospital stays required for reconstructive procedures. Patients with clefts require specific types of postoperative care, and the potential complications must be anticipated by a general medical specialist experienced in pediatric medicine. We have found it advantageous to have specified pediatric specialists managing our patients in the hospital, which has certainly reduced the number of serious complications.

In summary, the focus of treatment and management of children with clefts is on their many special needs. We must not, however, lose sight of the fact that these patients are first and foremost children. Besides their special needs, they also have all of the routine needs of any other child. Therefore, the presence of a pediatrician on any team becomes imperative.

REFERENCES

Argamaso RV: Glossopexy for upper airway obstruction in Robin sequence, *Cleft Palate-Craniofacial J* 29:232-238, 1992.

Goldstein S, Shprintzen RJ, Wu RHK, Thorpy MJ, Hahm SY, Marion R, Sher AE, Saenger P: Correction of deficient sleep entrained growth hormone release and obstructive sleep apnea by tracheostomy in achondroplasia, *Birth Defects* 21(2):93-101, 1985.

Lipson AH, Yuille D, Angel M, Thompson PG, Vanderwood JG, Beckenham EJ: Velo-cardio-facial syndrome: An important syndrome for the dysmorphologist to recognize, *J Med Genet* 28:596-604, 1991.

Sadewitz VL: Robin sequence: changes in thinking leading to changes in patient care, *Cleft Palate-Craniofacial J* 29:246-253,

Shprintzen RJ, Siegel-Sadewitz VL, Amato J, Goldberg R: Anomalies associated with cleft lip, cleft palate, or both, *Am J Med Genet* 20:585-596, 1985.

Singer L, Sidoti EJ: Pediatric management of Robin sequence, *Cleft Palate-Craniofacial J* 29:220-223, 1992.

5 Complications Associated with Clefting and Craniofacial Disorders

Robert J. Shprintzen and Eugene J. Sidoti

Clinicians tend to be tightly focused on the outcomes of their treatments in children with craniofacial anomalies. Success may be easily defined based on the expected results of, for example, the elimination of hypernasality by pharyngeal flap, correction of misarticulations by speech therapy, or eradication of a cross-bite by maxillary expansion. All treatments have a certain risk associated with them. Clearly, surgical risks represent the more serious complications associated with treatment, though not the only ones. Many of the risks associated with surgery are those that would be common to any surgical procedure where general anesthesia is used, or where blood loss becomes a factor. However, there are a set of surgical complications that are especially characteristic of surgery in individuals with clefts, and while not necessarily unique, they do represent causes for concern, because most surgery in children with clefts is elective (i.e., not essential for the prolongation of life). The purpose of this chapter is to describe the complications of special concern in individuals with clefts and certain common clefting syndromes. The possibility of these complications makes careful evaluation using state-of-the-art diagnostics essential in the preoperative assessment of all patients with clefts.

TYPES OF COMPLICATIONS

It is easy to think of complications only in terms of surgically based problems. The problems commonly anticipated by the lay public, and of concern to surgeons, include anesthesia risks, bleeding, and infection. Though each of these complications is quite rare in the majority of surgical procedures associated with clefting, they are nonetheless the ones that probably cause the most concern among the majority of patients and their families. These problems will be discussed within the context of specific operations later in this chapter, but clinicians should be aware that other surgical complica-

tions are much more common and potentially more dangerous than these. Airway related problems are, in particular, the most worrisome complications in patients with congenital malformations of the head and neck.

However, not all complications are related to surgery. We will also discuss complications that may arise from inappropriate dental and speech treatments and complications that may arise from poorly timed treatments in all areas of management. In other words, one of the biggest challenges in team management of children with clefts is the coordination of needed treatments to avoid two potential problems: "bridge burning" and missed opportunities.

"Bridge burning"

Clinicians do not want to burn any bridges behind them. This colloquialism refers to avoiding the application of treatments, which may then present problems for subsequent essential treatments. As an example, surgeons would like to avoid introducing a scar in an area where they subsequently need to perform additional surgery because healing may be compromised. This issue will be discussed in relation to the issue of maxillary bone grafting and pharyngoplasty.

Missed opportunities

Conversely, there are critical time windows for the application of some treatments that will help to avoid subsequent problems. Because many patients with clefts require the staged management of their structural anomalies, it may be true that failure to provide adequate correction at one stage will present major problems for the successful completion of the next stage. The occurrence and repair of fistulae will illustrate this type of problem later in this chapter.

SURGICAL COMPLICATIONS

Though major life-threatening complications related to surgery in individuals with cleft lip and/or palate are unusual, there are certain "red flags" that must be heeded in order to avoid problems. Surgical risks increase dramatically when patients have conditions in association with the cleft that might contribute to potential complications. Blood disorders that might lead to increased risk of hemorrhage or bleeding are infrequent syndromic findings associated with clefting, but it is always possible that they may be inherited separately. Obviously, the routine blood analyses required by hospitals before admission for surgery would likely detect any of these disorders. More problematic would be other structural or metabolic anomalies, which could precipitate unanticipated surgical crises. Examples of these types of problems will be presented next in the context of particular procedures.

Essentially all patients with cleft lip and palate will require lip repair, palate repair, nasal surgery, myringotomy and tube surgery, and probable lip and nose revisions. In addition, maxillary bone grafting and pharyngoplasty are done in a high percentage of cases, depending on the philosophy of treatment at the particular center. All patients with isolated cleft palate require palate repair, most require myringotomy and tube surgery, and many will require pharyngoplasty. Complications for most of these procedures are unusual.

The following section will discuss specific complications within the context of individual operations. Not all operations are discussed because the number of possible procedures that can be applied to individuals with clefts are numerous and diverse in the method of application. Lip and palate repair are discussed even though complications are rare, especially in light of the frequency of each of these operations. The other operations discussed are the ones with the higher complication rates (specifically pharyngoplasty and maxillary bone graft).

Lip repair

Complications during lip repair are very unusual for the experienced surgeon. There is little blood loss, and infection is unusual. The major concerns the surgeon has after lip repair relate to scar formation and contraction around the scar line. Total dehiscence (pulling apart) of the repair is also very unusual, though partial dehiscence may occur in a small percentage of cases, especially in the hands of inexperienced surgeons. Partial dehiscence may result in a lack of union of the lip muscles causing a visible depression underneath the skin (Fig. 5-1), which will require another repair at a later date.

The most common complication of lip repair is abnormality in the appearance of the lip

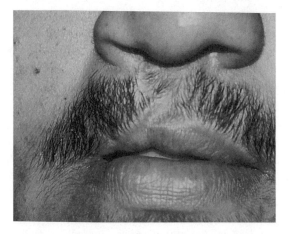

Fig. 5-1 Lack of muscle union under skin.

vermillion, such as the so-called whistle tip deformity or redundancy of the vermillion (Fig. 5-2). These problems point out, in part, that healing is always an unknown factor that is difficult, if not impossible, to anticipate from person to person. Other complications associated with lip repair are rare.

Palate repair

As in lip repair, major life-threatening complications in palate repair are rare. Bleeding problems are slightly more frequent in palate repairs because there are more major vessels located in tissue that is somewhat more difficult to handle. Though palate surgery is done inside the mouth, there is usually very little swelling, which could contribute to airway obstruction.

One potential problem in palate surgery, which is also true in pharyngoplasty and several other operations, is related to the need for hyperextending the patient's neck. There are several syndromes that have spinal anomalies that would make hyperextension a problem and could result in damage to the spinal cord. The most common syndrome associated with clefting that would have a risk of spinal cord injury is oculo-auriculo-vertebral dysplasia, or OAV (also known as hemifacial microsomia, Goldenhar syndrome, lateral facial dysplasia, and first and second branchial arch syndrome). This etiologically nonspecific disorder has many clinical features, but the distinguishing characteristics include facial asymmetry related to varying degrees of mandibular and soft tissue deficiency, ear tags or pits, conductive hearing loss related to middle ear anomalies, and dermoid cysts of the eye (called choristomas) including epibulbar dermoids. Cervical spine anomalies are common in OAV and may

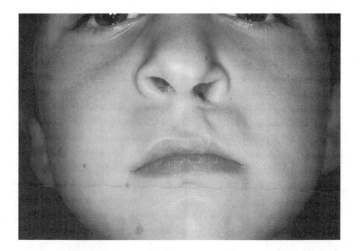

Fig. 5-2 Whistle tip deformity and vermillion redundancy.

include vertebral fusions, hemivertebrae, and spina bifida occulta. Cleft palate is common in OAV. Cleft lip, though less common than cleft palate, is underdetected in OAV. Many cases of unilateral cleft lip and palate, especially those with ear tags or marked facial asymmetry, may represent OAV. In patients with ear tags, ear pits, dermoid cysts in the eye, limitation of head rotation, or marked facial asymmetry, spine radiographs are indicated to rule out anomalies of the spine, which could modify positioning on the operating room table.

Down syndrome has a prevalence of cleft lip and/or cleft palate greater than that of the general population, but there is a relatively low frequency anomaly in the syndrome. Approximately 20% of individuals with Down syndrome have atlantoaxial and/or occipitoatlantal instability, which may lead to subluxation of the craniocervical joint during hyperextension and could cause spinal cord injury.

By far, the most common surgical complication of palate repair actually occurs in the postoperative period: oronasal fistulae. Fistulae are small openings in the repair line and may occur because of poor healing, excessive tension on the repair, or poor surgical technique. Though fistulae may be very small, no bigger than a pencil point, they are extremely troublesome in relation to speech development. It has been reported that fistulae are causally related to both velopharyngeal insufficiency (VPI) and compensatory articulation errors as described in Chapters 8, 10, 12, and 16 in this text and elsewhere (Hoch et al, 1987; Isberg and Henningsson, 1987). Therefore, though a small fistula may seem a minor complication of palate

repair, they are actually a major source of concern because they will lead to an additional operation in order to resolve the speech problems they cause. Because patients with fistulae also have cleft palate and almost always have some degree of VPI, it is impossible to know if the VPI is related only to the fistula, or if it is also related to the anatomical abnormality of the palate. The problem is exacerbated by the fact that fistulae also cause articulatory compensations, which are also related to VPI in a causal manner. This presents a treatment dilemma to the team and the surgeon who must decide if the VPI should be treated simply by fistula repair, or by fistula repair combined with pharyngoplasty. Obturating the fistula with chewing gum or dental wax may not completely answer the question, because the compensatory articulation errors will still be present and may contribute to the presence of the VPI. Therefore, in our opinion, when fistulae are detected, they should be repaired at the earliest possible opportunity, even before the time pharyngoplasty might be recommended (see Chapter 12). For example, if it is evident that a fistula is present within months after the palate repair, the fistula should be closed as soon as possible to prevent the infant from developing abnormal articulation patterns and to minimize the possibility of VPI. In some cases, fistulae are not obvious. They may look like small slits with the margins of the palatal halves seemingly in approximation. In such cases, the collapse of the palatal shelves that occurs in many patients with clefts prevents easy detection of the fistulae but they are present nonetheless. However, the patient's articulation patterns will probably indicate the presence of a fistula. The presence of mid-dorsal lingual contacts for normally lingua-alveolar sounds would be clear evidence for the presence of a fistula. Even if the fistula is detected in this manner at age 2 or 3 years, they should be surgically closed and speech therapy initiated immediately after surgery. Therefore, it can be seen that the complication of an oronasal fistula is actually quite serious, because it inevitably leads to additional operations.

It should be mentioned that fistulae detected immediately after palate repair can be closed nonsurgically (Berkman, 1978). We have found that by covering newly formed fistulae with a dental appliance, the relatively fresh opening will often close by spontaneous formation of fibrous scar tissue. It is therefore critical to carefully examine patients with frequency after palate repair. The first time a fistula is detected, it should immediately be covered with an appliance in order to keep the opening free of fluid, food, and air, which will tend to keep it open.

Pharyngoplasty

The procedure with the highest rate of complications is pharyngoplasty. The term *pharyngoplasty* here is utilized to indicate any operation involving the pharynx done to eliminate hypernasality in patients with hypernasal speech. The generic term *pharyngoplasty* encompasses many types of procedures, including pharyngeal flaps, sphincter pharyngoplasty (Orticochea or modified Orticochea), Hynes pharyngoplasty, and implants (either homologous tissues, alloplastic substances, or injectable substances). Actually, each of these separate categories of pharyngoplasties are generic in that there are many different types of pharyngeal flaps and implants. There is also probably enough variation in how individual surgeons do each operation that no two pharyngoplasties are exactly alike. As a result, it is likely that some surgeons experience more complications than others, even with the same generic technique. However, even in the best of hands, airway and bleeding complications are far more common in pharyngoplasty than in other operations for patients with clefts.

Types of airway complications

Airway complications following pharyngoplasty may be either temporary (limited to the immediate postoperative period), short-term or long-term. In general, the airway complications caused by surgery in the pharynx are related to some type of obstruction. Obstructions may be partial or complete. Partial obstructions would be predictable in an operation where swelling in the upper airway is likely to occur, or when swelling in the lower airway may result from endotracheal intubation for anesthesia during surgery. Partial obstructions that resolve within several days or a week of surgery are of no major significance or risk. One sign of a long-term partial obstruction is postoperative snoring. Snoring is a common complication of some types of pharyngeal flap surgery and should not be dismissed as insignificant. It is not normal for children to snore unless they have a cold, tonsillitis, or some other contributory acute illness. Snoring is indicative that inspirations are passing through a constricted opening during sleep when the muscles of the pharynx usually relax. If air is to be collected into the lungs through a more constricted opening, there may need to be greater respiratory effort (often noted as a struggle to breathe or as restless sleep). Another possibility is that insufficient air will enter the lungs, causing the blood to store excess amounts of carbon dioxide. These partial obstructions are called hypopneas, and their presence may indicate a possibility that more severe obstructions (apneas) may occur subsequently. It is also possible that with age the partial obstructions will resolve. It is therefore important to monitor postoperative respiratory and sleep behaviors very carefully.

The most severe complication of pharyngoplasty is postoperative sleep apnea. Apnea is simply defined as a temporary cessation of respiration. Apnea may occur during wakefulness, in which case it is quite severe and requires immediate attention. More common is the occurrence of apnea during sleep, hence the appellation *sleep apnea.*

There are three basic types of sleep apnea: obstructive apnea, central apnea, and mixed apnea. Obstructive sleep apnea (OSA) implies that the effort to breathe continues, but there is an obstruction of airflow in the upper airway, lower airway, or both. The obstruction could be a physical one or a functional one. Physical obstructions could be caused by foreign bodies or by anatomical structural anomalies. Examples of physical obstructions not specifically related to pharyngoplasty include blockage of the nasal passage by choanal atresia or stenosis, enlarged tonsils or adenoids, enlarged tongue, small lower jaw, hypertrophic palate, swollen epiglottis, laryngeal web, collapsing larynx or trachea (laryngomalacia or tracheomalacia), compressed trachea or bronchus from an abnormal major blood vessel, or abnormal cartilaginous support of the trachea or bronchi. Even chronic mucus secretion can cause an obstruction of the airway, as is often the case in syndromes where there is constant hypersecretion, such as the lysosomal storage diseases (Hurler syndrome, Hunter syndrome, Morquio syndrome, etc.). These problems are not mutually exclusive and may occur in patients being considered for pharyngoplasty. Any contributors to obstructive apnea should be considered carefully before recommending surgery because the additional airway obstruction caused by the pharyngoplasty may add the additional risk necessary to cause significant obstructive apnea.

In obstructive apnea, casual clinical observation of the patient might indicate to the examiner that the patient is breathing. The chest moves up and down, the mouth may be open, and there is usually silence, especially in young children and infants. Snoring may occur during sleep in some cases, but snoring is usually more indicative of a milder degree of obstruction (or more appropriately, chronic constriction). Careful observation of patients with obstructive apnea who appear to be breathing can include placing a stethoscope at the patient's nose and mouth, which would fail to show evidence of air flow. In other words, the drive to breathe is present, but some type of blockage obstructs the airway. Some signs of a struggle to breathe may be evident. Struggle is not as common in infants who are typically very weak from prolonged oxygen deprivation and failure to thrive, but in children, some type of movement or struggle (including vigorous tossing and turning) is quite common. Biochemically, the patient will start to store excessive carbon dioxide in the blood, and oxygen levels will drop. The heart will have to work harder during the struggle to breathe so that initially, heart rate speeds up (tachycardia). As more carbon dioxide builds up in the blood and oxygen saturation decreases, the heart slows down (bradycardia). If this pattern continues for a long time, the right ventricle of the heart will become enlarged as the lungs fail to oxygenate the blood and the flow backs up into the heart from the pulmonary artery. In the most severe cases, prolonged and excessive right ventricular hypertrophy can eventually lead to cor pulmonale and congestive heart failure.

Functional obstruction of the airway occurs most frequently in syndromes with hypotonia where the inherent muscular strength of the pharyngeal muscles is weak. Syndromes such as velo-cardio-facial syndrome, Down syndrome, and others with some form of central nervous system impairment are often characterized by hypotonic upper airways so that the induction of

any negative pressure in the upper airway will cause it to collapse. Central apnea is the cessation of breathing accompanied by the absence of effort to breathe. In other words, there is no chest or abdominal movement, no struggle, and no exchange of air. This type of apnea is called *central* because in almost all cases, it is caused by some type of abnormality in the central nervous system. In infants, central apnea is common in disorders that have brain malformations, or in very premature neonates who have less mature central nervous systems. In older children, central apnea is almost always associated with some type of brain malformation. Because of the severe brain malformations that cause central apnea (and the intellectual impairment that usually accompanies such brain anomalies), it is unlikely that patients with central apnea would be recommended for pharyngoplasty. Conversely, pharyngoplasty would not be likely to cause central apnea because of the lack of effect on the brain.

Mixed apnea is the co-occurrence of components of both central and obstructive apnea. This is actually quite common in infants and young children, in part because many children with abnormalities of the central nervous system also have anomalies of structure or function of the upper airway. For example, in velo-cardio-facial syndrome, there are brain anomalies (Mitnick et al, 1994) in association with hypotonia of the pharynx (Shprintzen et al, 1981). The DeMyer sequence (also known as holoprosencephaly) has major brain malformations in association with absent or severely constricted nasal passages.

In mixed apnea, there are two possible scenarios. The apneic episode may begin with a central event. As the central apnea becomes more prolonged, more carbon dioxide builds up in the blood causing the baby to become more hypotonic from lack of adequate oxygen to the brain. With increasing hypotonia, the muscles of the pharynx become more likely to collapse when the central component ceases and active breathing is restarted. The hypotonia of the pharyngeal muscles causes a functional collapse of the airway during respiration, resulting in an obstructive event. The other scenario for mixed apnea begins with an obstructive component. As the obstructive apnea progresses, the blood builds up larger amounts of carbon dioxide, which eventually reaches the brain and triggers central apneas.

Apneas associated with pharyngoplasty are typically obstructive, though they may be mixed. Central apnea is much less common in patients undergoing pharyngeal flap, though central apnea is not uncommon among infants with craniofacial anomalies, especially those associated with concomitant central nervous system anomalies.

Why are airway complications so common in pharyngoplasty? Collapse of the upper airway resulting in obstructive apnea is often induced by the introduction of a negative pressure in the pharynx. For example, it is well known that the presence of hypertrophic tonsils and adenoids can induce obstructive apnea because the blockage of the upper portion of the pharynx causes a negative pressure to be induced beneath the point of maximum constriction (the Bernoulli effect). Pharyngoplasty reduces the overall size of the upper portion of the pharyngeal airway and can induce the same type of negative pressure as hypertrophic tonsils and/or adenoids. However, there are multiple factors that cause reduction in size of the airway with essentially all types of pharyngoplasties.

Pharyngeal flap, in particular, has attracted the majority of attention in relation to sleep apnea. In large part, pharyngeal flap has drawn the majority of attention because far more pharyngeal flap operations have been done than any other type of pharyngoplasty. In fact, it is probable that many more pharyngeal flaps have been done than all other types of pharyngoplasties combined. Because of this, complications have been observed more frequently and studied in more detail. The literature has hundreds of papers published on the outcome of pharyngeal flap surgery, but only a small number are devoted to other types of pharyngoplasties. To date, though it is tacitly assumed that pharyngeal flap is the riskiest of pharyngoplasties, there is no data whatsoever to validate this assumption.

The contribution of pharyngeal flap to obstructive apnea has been studied in detail (Shprintzen, 1988; Shprintzen et al, 1992). It has been found that the factors leading to OSA can be avoided and that pharyngeal flap, in particular, can be made relatively risk-free (Shprintzen, 1988; Shprintzen et al, 1992). This notion is very important because many clinicians have abandoned the pharyngeal flap operation because of fears of obstructive apnea (OSA in particular). The concerns regarding pharyngeal flap are well founded in that the potential dangers of complications have been reported to result in occasional mortality (Kravath et al, 1980). However, rather than abandon an operation that has proven useful in the treatment of hypernasality, it should be determined how the operation can be made safe without sacrificing effectiveness. Furthermore, there is no evidence that other operations for the treatment of

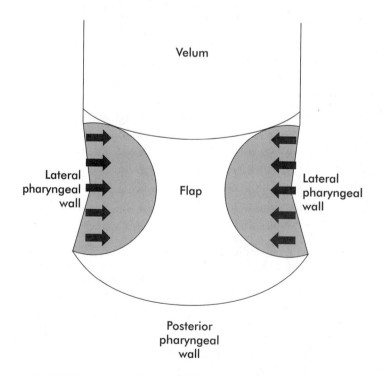

Fig. 5-3 Diagram of pharyngeal flap function as seen from above.

hypernasality have a lower rate of complications, airway or otherwise.

As will be discussed in subsequent chapters, pharyngeal flap surgery is an operation designed to obturate the nasopharynx in order to prevent nasal escape and hypernasal resonance during speech. The design of the operation is to raise a flap of mucous membrane and muscle from the posterior pharyngeal wall and insert it into the palate to create a tissue bridge between the palate and pharynx (Fig. 5-3). Following surgery, the movements of the lateral pharyngeal walls close the openings on either side of the flap, thus eliminating nasal escape during speech (Fig. 5-3).

Pharyngeal flap surgery can prompt the development of OSA because three of the direct effects of the operation will act to decrease total airway size and therefore increase negative pressure:

1. Obstruction of nasal respiration.
2. Decrease in the oropharyngeal and nasopharyngeal respiratory space.
3. Permanent alteration of the habitual respiratory pattern.

Obstruction of the nasal airway. It has been assumed by many clinicians that obstruction of the nasal airway is the primary problem created by pharyngeal flaps, which causes OSA. In part, this assumption is based on the observation that newborns with nasal obstruction from choanal atresia or stenosis develop severe obstructive apnea. However, this phenomenon is isolated to newborns who are obligate nose breathers. With increasing age, children are able to shift successfully to oral respiration without developing significant apnea. However, because pharyngeal flaps do obstruct the nose, the correlation has led investigators to assume a cause and effect relationship between nasal obstruction and OSA. In reality, nasal obstruction alone is rarely sufficient to precipitate obstructive apnea even in young children. In an investigation of the prevalence of OSA following pharyngeal flap surgery, Shprintzen (1988) found that there was no relationship between the postoperative width of a pharyngeal flap and the presence of OSA. In other words, patients with very narrow pharyngeal flaps that caused essentially no nasal obstruction were as likely to have postoperative OSA as patients with pharyngeal flaps that obstructed the entire nasopharynx.

Nasal obstruction can, however, be a contributing factor to the development of OSA by increasing negative pressure in the pharyngeal airway, particularly in children who have been exclusively nose breathers until the time of the flap. This is a more significant complication in the immediate postoperative period. When recovering from the procedure, the patient may still be groggy from the anesthesia and may be attempting to maintain the habitual nasal respiration pattern. They will therefore take breaths through the nose, which is now blocked at least partially by the pharyngeal flap. In the immediate postoperative period, the blockage is more severe because of swelling (edema) related to the operation. Therefore, as the patient tries to breathe in through a largely or completely obstructed nose, the resistance caused by the flap and edema results in a negative pressure being built up below the flap in the oropharynx and hypopharynx. In addition, the twilight state induced by the recovery from anesthesia results in laxity of the pharyngeal muscles, which could prompt some degree of airway collapse. As edema recedes and the effects of anesthesia are no longer present, the contribution of nasal obstruction to OSA becomes minimal. It is therefore advisable to carefully monitor respiration in the immediate postoperative period and, if possible, to keep the nasal airway patent to permit nasal respirations.

Decrease in the oropharyngeal and hypopharyngeal respiratory space. There are multiple sources contributing to a decrease in the total volume of the respiratory space in the oropharyngeal and hypopharyngeal airway below the pharyngeal flap. With the nose partially or fully obstructed by the flap itself, reduction in size of the airway below the flap only further exacerbates the development of significant negative pressure in the pharynx resulting in collapse and OSA.

The first source of narrowing of the pharynx is the flap itself. In pharyngeal flap surgery (see Chapter 13), a rectangular flap is raised from a donor site on the posterior pharyngeal wall (Fig. 5-4). The donor site is then either closed with a few sutures, or left raw (Argamaso, 1990). Some clinicians believe that closing the donor site with suturing reduces discomfort after surgery, but this has never been demonstrated in the literature or research. Whether sutured or left raw, the donor site heals by circumferential narrowing (Shprintzen, 1988; Shprintzen et al, 1992) (Fig. 5-5). Thus, the diameter of the pharynx is narrowed by the width of the flap for the entire vertical height of the donor site. Many surgeons (perhaps the majority) harvest the flap from the full width and height of the posterior pharyngeal wall. In other words, the flap consists of a muco-muscular rectangle of tissue incorporating the entire posterior pharyngeal wall from the nasopharynx to the vallecula. As a result, assuming that the pull of air from the lungs

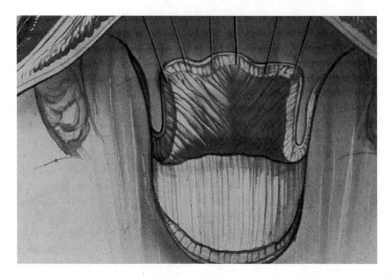

Fig. 5-4 Pharyngeal flap donor site.

remains constant (which it must because the lungs have not become smaller or decreased their capacity), the same amount of air must pass through a smaller pharyngeal opening. This increases the speed with which the air must pass through the pharynx. When air passes through a smaller opening, a phenomenon known as the Bernoulli effect occurs. Bernoulli's Law states that when air passes through a constricted opening (resulting in an increase in speed), it leaves a vacuum (negative pressure) in its wake. Therefore, circumferential narrowing of the pharyngeal airway causes an induction of negative pressure in the oropharynx and hypopharynx resulting in possible collapse and OSA.

The second cause of narrowing of the airway beneath the flap is the presence of tonsils. Tonsils normally sit between the faucial pillars in the oral cavity, not the pharynx (Fig. 5-6). As a result, with nasopharyngoscopy in an individual with normally placed tonsils, the tonsils are not visible as the endoscope is passed into the oropharynx and hypopharynx (Fig. 5-7). When tonsils are in this normal position in someone requiring pharyngeal flap surgery, the tonsils do not interfere with respiration and will not contribute to OSA unless they are extremely large (3+ or 4+ on the standard 4 point scale used by otolaryngologists to rate tonsil size). However, it has been our observation that many individuals with clefts have abnormal positioning of the tonsils. It has been observed that the tonsils often intrude behind the posterior tonsillar pillars into the oropharyngeal airway. If the tonsils are hypertrophic, they may even be seen extending upward into the nasopharynx or downward into the hypopharynx (Fig. 5-8). When the tonsils extend into the pharynx, their position places them into or just below the lateral ports or openings on either side of a pharyngeal flap. Therefore, not only does their presence decrease the volume of the oropharyngeal or hypopharyngeal airway, they also obstruct whatever nasal airway is left in the nasopharynx.

Tonsils also contribute to increased negative pressure in the airway by adding a curved surface in the respiratory space. In addition to the Bernoulli effect just described, there is another phenomenon known as the Coanda effect. The Coanda effect describes the consequence of placing a curved surface beneath a constricted opening. When air passes over a curved surface, the negative pressure is greater than if the surface were straight. Therefore, the presence of tonsils beneath the constricted opening under a pharyngeal flap will cause a larger vacuum to occur in the pharynx on inspiration.

How to avoid complications following pharyngeal flap

In a questionnaire and clinical study of 200 patients who had pharyngeal flap surgery with careful attention paid to the development of OSA, the postoperative prevalence of sleep apnea was 10% with all but two cases resolving within a week (Shprintzen, 1988). As part of that same study, a smaller group of 50 patients were studied with preoperative and postoperative

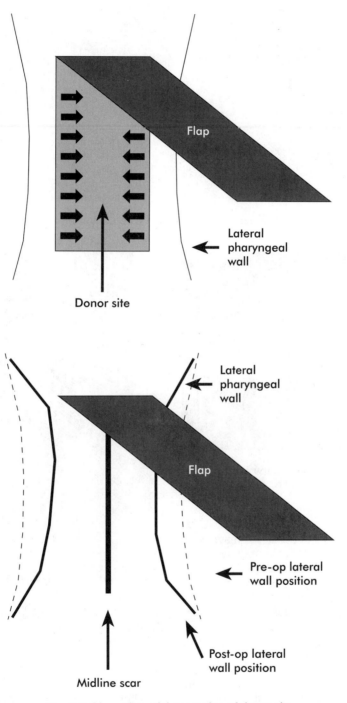

Fig. 5-5 Circumferential narrowing of donor site.

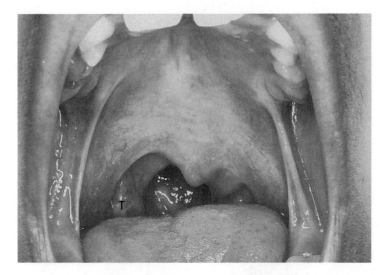

Fig. 5-6 Normal tonsil position between the tonsillar pillars.

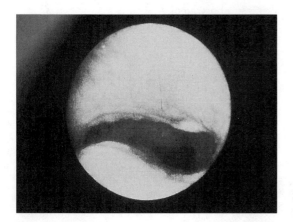

Fig. 5-7 Endoscopy of a normal airway showing no evidence of tonsils in the pharynx.

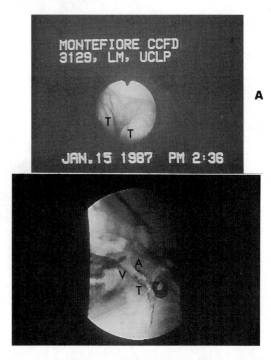

Fig. 5-8 Nasopharyngoscopic (**A**) and videofluoroscopic (**B**) view of tonsils posteriorly positioned in the pharynx. The tonsils are labelled T, the adenoids A, and the velum V in (B).

all-night polysomnograms (PSG). A PSG is regarded as the "gold standard" for diagnosing OSA. Briefly, a PSG is a multichannel recording of parameters that measure sleep stage, heart rate, arterial oxygen saturation, movement, and air flow. The preoperative studies did not predict the development of postoperative OSA. Some patients with completely benign PSGs preoperatively were found to develop OSA postoperatively, while several others with occasional apneas preoperatively had completely benign postoperative studies. It was found that the best predictor of the development of OSA was the association of syndromic patterns or specific anomalies, such as velo-cardio-facial syndrome (because of pharyngeal hypotonia), micrognathia, and congenitally small pharynx (as might be found in Treacher Collins syndrome).

There are "red flags" that should preclude pharyngeal flap. These would include a history of obstructive apnea, severe micrognathia, significant neurologic impairment, which might result either in pharyngeal hypotonia or abnormal respiratory patterns, and other structural anomalies that cause airway constriction, such as lower airway anomalies (tracheal constriction, laryngeal web, etc.) or skull base anomalies that cause pharyngeal constriction (Shprintzen, 1982). For example, babies with a history of Robin sequence with severe obstructive apnea should be carefully assessed to see if pharyngeal flap or other pharyngoplasty is absolutely necessary, and if so, the airway and sleep patterns should be assessed as thoroughly as possible.

Tonsils and tonsillectomy

The importance of the use of nasopharyngoscopy as a diagnostic tool is emphasized frequently elsewhere in this book, including chapters 11, 12, and 16. Not only is this diagnostic technique useful for obtaining information that can ensure a successful speech outcome, but it may even be important for ensuring the health and well-being of the patient postoperatively. As discussed above, tonsils can be positioned posteriorly in the pharynx. When positioned in this manner, they may fill the lateral ports of the flap, resulting in total obstruction of the nasal airway (Fig. 5-9) while also constricting the oropharynx medially. Therefore, it is recommended that in cases where the tonsils are seen endoscopically within the pharyngeal airway, they should be removed at least 6 weeks before pharyngeal flap surgery. There is another advantage of preceding pharyngeal flap with tonsillectomy. It has been noted in several investigations that tonsils may actually cause velopharyngeal insufficiency when positioned posteriorly in the pharynx (Shprintzen et al, 1987; MacKenzie-Stepner et al, 1987a) by inhibiting movement of the palate and/or lateral pharyngeal walls. In cases where the tonsils obstruct the movement of the velopharyngeal structure, tonsillectomy alone has been noted to resolve the problem (Shprintzen et al, 1987;

MacKenzie-Stepner et al, 1987a). Therefore, it is possible, if not likely, that tonsillectomy done before pharyngeal flap may eliminate the need for pharyngeal flap in at least some cases.

The tonsils should not be removed at the same time as pharyngeal flap surgery. Though simultaneous tonsillectomy and pharyngeal flap was recommended in a single publication (Reath et al, 1987), this approach was strongly opposed by a large number of experts (Argamaso et al, 1988) on airway complications because:

1. One of the most common complications of both tonsillectomy and pharyngeal flap is bleeding. If postoperative bleeding occurred, because of the proximity of the surgical fields, the surgeon would have a difficult time in knowing the source of the problem, thus making resolution that much more difficult.
2. Tonsillectomy alone may resolve the hypernasality and velopharyngeal insufficiency.
3. The reported complication rate from the combined procedure far exceeded the complication rate from either tonsillectomy alone or pharyngeal flap alone.

Protocol for avoiding postoperative complications

Based on observations of the contributing factors to OSA following pharyngeal flap, a protocol covering the preoperative, intraoperative, and postoperative period was described, which has essentially eliminated the complication (as well as reducing bleeding, discomfort, and hydrating problems) (Shprintzen, 1988; Shprintzen et al, 1992). The protocol is as follows:

Preoperative assessment of tonsils and tonsillectomy. If the tonsils are large or occupying any

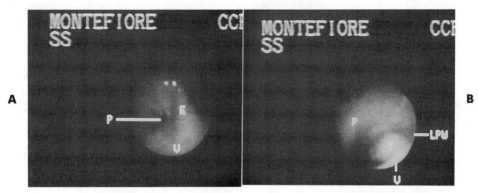

Fig. 5-9 Tonsils intruding into the lateral port of a pharyngeal flap.

portion of the oropharynx, they should be removed at least 6 weeks before pharyngeal flap. Therefore, it is essential to evaluate all cases with nasopharyngoscopy and multi-view video-fluoroscopy before pharyngeal flap.

Shorter pharyngeal flaps. As described by Argamaso (1990) and Shprintzen et al (1992), reducing the length of the donor site for the pharyngeal flap reduces both respiratory and bleeding complications. Argamaso (1990) described raising a short flap so that only a small portion of the posterior pharyngeal wall is left raw. The majority of the oropharynx and the entire hypopharynx is left untouched. This eliminates a major bleeding site, and prevents the circumferential healing, which could prompt airway obstruction and OSA (Shprintzen et al, 1992). In addition, there is much less postoperative discomfort (such as neck stiffness or pain), hospital stays are shortened, and drinking becomes much less of a problem because there is relatively little postoperative pain.

Placing a nasopharyngeal tube. Shprintzen (1988) found that the large majority of respiratory complications following pharyngeal flap occurred in the immediate postoperative period. It was found that apnea often occurred in the first postoperative day when children had localized edema from the flap, which blocked the nose. If they were habitual nose breathers before surgery, they would be attempting to breathe through the nose against a closed system after surgery. This would induce a negative pressure in the airway which, in combination with muscle hypotonia induced from the twilight state following anesthesia, could prompt collapse of the airway and obstructive apnea. Therefore, Shprintzen (1988) and Argamaso (1990) have suggested placing a 3.5 mm nasopharyngeal tube through one nostril to maintain a patent nasal airway in the immediate postoperative period (24 to 48 hours). A standard endotracheal tube is used as the nasopharyngeal tube and is cut short so that it just bypasses the flap but does not reach the glottis. The tube also provides access to the pharynx for suctioning. It has been recommended that the patient be kept in an intensive care unit while the tube is in place so that he or she can be carefully monitored for apnea.

It was found that using this protocol completely eliminated postoperative apnea in a large series of prospectively studied cases (Shprintzen, 1988; Shprintzen et al, 1992). If complications from pharyngeal flap surgery can be so dramatically reduced and the operation proves effective when properly executed, then objections to the use of pharyngeal flap surgery should be eliminated.

Other possible pharyngeal flap complications

Three other possible complications that are common in certain multiple anomaly syndromes may present significant risk. They are abnormal pharyngeal vasculature, cervical spine malformations, and malignant hyperpyrexia (malignant hyperthermia).

Pharyngeal vascular anomalies. Normally, the major vessels that travel from the heart to the brain go through the neck in the most lateral area of the pharynx, quite deep and away from the donor area for the flap. However, an abnormal course and position of the pharyngeal vessels has been noted in velo-cardio-facial syndrome (VCF), the most common syndrome of clefting. Because hypernasal speech is so common in this syndrome, it is likely that patients with abnormal neck vessels will be having pharyngeal flap surgery with high frequency. An abnormal position of the internal carotid arteries in VCF was reported by MacKenzie-Stepner et al (1987b) based on CT scans using contrast, prompting them to recommend that pharyngeal flap might be contraindicated in select cases. Using magnetic resonance angiography, Mitnick et al (1994) found a wider range of anomalies in VCF, which included abnormal course of the vertebral arteries, tortuosity of the vertebrals and internal carotids, and low bifurcations of the carotid arteries from the common carotid. Though medial displacement of the internal carotids was found in several patients, none of the cases studied had arteries that would have been risks for the type of surgery utilizing short superiorly based pharyngeal flaps (Argamaso, 1990). However, because anomalies of the pharyngeal vessels are clearly common in at least 8% of cases of cleft palate (Shprintzen et al, 1985), preoperative assessment of the pharyngeal vasculature is recommended in cases of VCF (Mitnick et al, 1994).

Cervical Spine Anomalies. Another common multiple anomaly disorder that has cleft palate or cleft lip and palate as a common finding is oculo-auriculo-vertebral dysplasia, or OAV (also known as hemifacial microsomia, Goldenhar syndrome, lateral facial dysplasia, and a number of other appellations). As mentioned above, cervical spine fusions, hemivertebrae, and other spine anomalies are common in OAV. As mentioned in the section on palate repair, hyperextension of the patient on the operating room table could cause permanent spinal cord injury. Other syndromes, such as Down syndrome and syndromes with Klippel-Feil anomaly, would also present as a risk for hyperextension. Therefore, in patients where spine anomalies may occur, neck radiographs should be obtained to rule them out because they may present a risk for paralysis secondary to spinal cord injury.

Malignant hyperpyrexia. Some neuromuscular diseases present as special risks for any type of pharyngoplasty because of an unusual response to general anesthesia. Patients with many of the muscular dystrophies, such as Steinert syndrome (myotonic dystrophy), develop severe and rapid elevations of body temperature known as malignant hyperpyrexia or malignant hyperthermia. This intraoperative complication can prove fatal if not detected and treated immediately. However, it is possible to avoid the problem if knowledge of the condition and diagnosis exists before the administration of anesthetic gases. Specific anesthetic agents and techniques can avoid the complication completely. This is an important complication to acknowledge because many of the muscular dystrophies have hypernasality as a possible clinical finding, and surgery has been recommended in many cases. It is also possible that clefting can accompany neuromuscular disease, especially as a secondary consequence of Robin sequence, which has been reported to occur in association with myotonic dystrophy (Cohen, 1978). Clinicians, especially those affiliated with cleft palate or craniofacial centers, who do not typically see patients with neuromuscular disease, should be aware that the frequent occurrence of hypernasality in the muscular dystrophies may bring such patients to their facilities for treatment.

Other pharyngoplasties

Data are not available for complications from other forms of pharyngoplasty. This is, in part, because other operations have been done far less frequently than pharyngeal flap. However, several complications are known to occur with other types of pharyngoplasty, including sphincter pharyngoplasty and implant procedures (posterior wall augmentations).

Sphincter pharyngoplasty. In sphincter pharyngoplasty procedures, the risks are essentially the same as in pharyngeal flap, but the frequency of bleeding and airway problems is as yet unknown. In sphincter pharyngoplasty, a short pharyngeal flap is raised and the posterior tonsillar pillars are dissected away from their original locations. Instead of a midline flap of tissue with bilateral openings between the nasopharynx and oropharynx, there is a single small central opening with a circumferential ridge of tissue around the entire pharynx. There has, as yet, been no investigation of the frequency of postoperative OSA with sphincter pharyngoplasty, nor has there been a study of

short-term complications. However, because the circumference of the airway is reduced in sphincter pharyngoplasty, there is no reason to presume that patients having this operation will be immune to OSA.

One potential objection to sphincter pharyngoplasty is that it may prove to be a "bridge burner." Success rates for the operation have not yet been computed for a large number of cases, as has been done for pharyngeal flap. It can be said, however, that no operation is successful in all cases. Therefore, an "escape route" must be available for salvaging an unsuccessful result. In pharyngeal flap surgery, revisions have proven to be fairly easy and effective (Barone et al, 1994). Because there is a permanent ridge of tissue along the posterior pharyngeal wall, revision of a sphincter pharyngoplasty may be more problematic. No data currently exist to demonstrate a large experience with sphincter pharyngoplasty revisions.

Implants. Posterior wall implants have always had appeal as a way of treating small midline gaps in the velopharyngeal valve. Unfortunately, substances used to date have all had complications, which render them unacceptable for routine use. Teflon paste, cartilage, Proplast, and silicone have all been suggested as implants, but wide acceptance has been hampered by complications and/or lack of approval by the FDA. Injectable Teflon, though approved for use in the vocal cords, is not approved by the FDA for pharyngeal injection. Pharyngeal implant of Teflon runs the risk of inadvertent injection into one of the major pharyngeal vessels, such as the internal carotid or vertebral arteries.

Proplast is a porous carbon filament that has been advocated for pharyngeal implant (Wolford et al, 1989). The procedure is not widely applied because of rejection or fracture of Proplast implants, complications that would both compromise the speech result and require some secondary care of the surgical site. Complications from the use of silicone have received a significant amount of attention in relation to breast prostheses and are therefore unlikely to gain wide acceptance for use in the pharynx.

Cartilage implants have also not gained wide acceptance because of rejection, infection, and, if homologous (i.e., taken from the rib), the need to find and operate on a donor site elsewhere in the body.

Posterior wall augmentation has also been accomplished by rearranging local tissues, as in the Hynes pharyngoplasty. As with other infrequently used procedures, the frequency of complications is unknown, as is the effectiveness of the operation.

Maxillary bone graft

Maxillary bone grafting has become a commonly accepted method for creating a contiguous maxillary arch and allowing a bony matrix for the canine teeth to erupt into the dental arch (Bergland et al, 1986). There has been some debate over the source of bone (Sadove et al, 1990), but in general, the majority of maxillary bone grafts have come from the iliac crest. The complications of maxillary bone grafting include loss of the graft, bleeding, infection, and discomfort. These complications are essentially the expected problems that might occur in association with an operation of this type. More important is the timing factor in maxillary bone grafting with respect to missed opportunities. The majority of centers today believe that the ideal time for bone grafting is just before eruption of the maxillary canine tooth, which would normally erupt into the cleft site. The bone graft is necessary to maintain that tooth so that the root does not become exposed and the tooth lost. When radiographic evidence shows that the root of the canine is approximately 50% formed, this is considered to be the ideal time for maxillary alveolar grafting. If the graft is placed too late, then there is a better chance that the tooth will be lost or not maintained within the arch. If the graft is placed too early, there is no tooth to erupt into the graft. As a result, the bone may not be maintained and the graft will reabsorb, which may require subsequent regrafting. Even when the procedure is done properly, the timing of the procedure becomes critical, and complications can be avoided by not missing the opportune time for the operation.

DENTAL COMPLICATIONS

If treatment is to be truly interdisciplinary, all therapy applied must have a common goal. This means that all dental treatments (pediatric, orthodontic, prosthetic, and surgical) must be in concert with overall management goals: normal speech, aesthetically pleasing appearance, and normal function and occlusion of the jaws, among other things. For example, surgeons would like the patient to have a normal profile. Good projection of the midface is dependent in part on full dentition in the maxillary arch to maintain as much alveolar bone as possible. Some orthodontists might, however, be tempted to extract teeth in a crowded maxillary arch in order to get the teeth aligned edge-to-edge.

While the extractions might achieve a short-term goal of normal occlusion and dental alignment, in the long term, it may be a real "bridge burner" by preventing normal maxillary growth and constricting a dental arch by reducing the total number of teeth contained within it.

Similarly, if maxillary bone grafting is not utilized at a particular center, then the patient must have prosthetic tooth replacement. Successful maxillary bone grafting usually eliminates the need for tooth replacement by allowing the normal canine to erupt through the graft, orthodontically moving it into the region of the congenitaly missing lateral incisor, and filing it to make it look like an incisor. The rest of the teeth are aligned orthodontically and the maxillary arch can be completed without a prosthesis of any type (Bergland et al, 1986). Therefore, the concepts of "burned bridges" and missed opportunities as outlined above should play a major role in the planning of dental treatment, especially in relation to long-term surgical management.

SPEECH COMPLICATIONS

The same concepts of "burned bridges" and missed opportunities is applicable to speech pathology services. We have found that it is not difficult to recognize when an infant is beginning to develop "compensatory" articulation patterns, such as glottal stops and pharyngeal fricatives. As stated later in this text (Chapter 16), it becomes important to intercept these patterns at the first possible opportunity to make sure that they do not become pervasive and result in inactivity in the velopharyngeal valve. Therefore, delaying speech evaluation and treatment beyond infancy and early childhood could be a major missed opportunity that could result in extended treatment at a later date, the need for secondary pharyngoplasty, and years of unintelligible speech.

It is also possible to burn a bridge or two by applying therapeutic services that are contrary to the development of speech and language acquisition. There is a common, but highly regrettable philosophy among some speech pathologists that children who have unintelligible speech be provided with an alternative communication system, such as sign language. Because many children with clefts develop pervasive glottal stop articulation patterns (see Chapters 8, 10, and 16), which are largely unintelligible to most listeners, we have encountered many instances where these children have been taught to sign. Our experience has shown the following drawbacks to this approach:

1. The reliance on an alternative language system retards the development of normal expressive language. Children with gross articulatory errors who rely on spoken language do not experience the same extent of expressive language problems.
2. Since a very limited number of people are conversant in sign language, there are very few opportunities for the child to communicate.
3. Family members must also learn to sign, thus causing disruption of the lives of many people in order to introduce a language system that serves a very limited purpose.

The delays caused by this approach may set the patient back by years in overall management toward a normal life.

SUMMARY

Though many complications are regarded as unexpected events during the course of surgical management, every treatment applied (or withheld) should be reviewed carefully to make sure that the consequence of that action do not harm the patient. True interdisciplinary treatment is highly dependent on not missing opportunities and not taking actions that will cause irreversible damage. When such caution is taken, complications can be limited to unexpected surprises, which in the great majority of cases represent only a temporary setback.

REFERENCES

Argamaso RV: The pharyngeal flap in cleft lip and palate. In Kernahan DA, Rosenstein SW, editors: *Cleft lip and palate: a system of management,* Baltimore, 1990, Williams & Wilkins.

Argamaso RV, Bassila M, Bratcher GO, Brodsky L, Cotton RT, Croft CB, Greenberg LM, Laskin R, MacKenzie-Stepner K, Meyer CM III, Rakoff SJ, Ruben RJ, Sher AE, Shprintzen RJ, Sidoti EJ, Singer L, Strauch B, Stringer D, Witzel MA: Tonsillectomy and pharyngeal flap should not be performed simultaneously, *Cleft Palate J* 25:176-177, 1988.

Barone CM, Shprintzen RJ, Strauch B, Sablay LB, Argamaso RV: Pharyngeal flap revisions: flap elevation from a scarred posterior pharynx. Plast Reconstr Surg 93:279-284, 1994.

Berkman MD: Early non-surgical closure of postoperative palatal fistula, *Plast Reconstr Surg* 62:537-541, 1978.

Bergland O, Semb G, Åbyholm FE: Elimination of residual alveolar cleft by secondary bone grafting and subsequent orthodontic treatment, *Cleft Palate J* 23:175-205, 1986.

Cohen MM Jr: Syndromes with cleft lip and cleft palate, *Cleft Palate J* 15:306-328, 1978.

Hoch L, Golding-Kushner KJ, Sadewitz V, and Shprintzen RJ: Speech Therapy. In BJ McWilliams, editor: *Seminars in speech and language: current methods of assessing and treating children with cleft palates,* New York, 1986, Thieme Inc.

Kravath RE, Pollak C, Borowiecki B, Weitzman ED: Obstructive sleep apnea and death associated with surgical correction of velopharyngeal incompetence, *J Pediatr* 96:645-648, 1980.

Isberg A, Henningsson G: Influence of palatal fistulas on velopharyngeal movements: a cineradiographic study, *Plast Reconstr Surg* 79:525-530, 1987.

MacKenzie-Stepner K, Witzel MA, Stringer DA, Laskin RI: Velopharyngeal insufficiency due to hypertrophic tonsils. A report of two cases, *Int J Pediatr Otorhinolaryngol* 14:57-63, 1987a.

MacKenzie-Stepner K, Witzel MA, Stringer DA, Lindsay WK, Munro IR, Hughes H: Abnormal carotid arteries in the velocardiofacial syndrome: a report of three cases, *Plast Reconstr Surg* 80:347-351, 1987b.

Mitnick RJ, Bello JA, Shprintzen RJ: Brain anomalies in velo-cardio-facial syndrome, *Neuropsych Genet* (in press) 1994.

Mitnick RJ, Bello JA, Shprintzen RJ: Pharyngeal vascular anomalies in velo-cardio-facial syndrome detected by MR angiography, *Plast Reconstr Surg* (in press) 1995.

Reath DB, LaRossa D, Randall P: Simultaneous posterior pharyngeal flap and tonsillectomy, *Cleft Palate J* 24:250-253, 1987.

Sadove AM, Nelson CL, Eppley BL, Nguyen B: An evaluation of calvarial and iliac donor sites in alveolar cleft grafting, *Cleft Palate J* 27:225-228, 1990.

Shprintzen RJ: Palatal and pharyngeal anomalies in craniofacial syndromes, *Birth Defects* 18(1), 53-78, 1982.

Shprintzen RJ: Pharyngeal flap surgery and the pediatric upper airway, *Int Anesthesiol Clin* 26:74-83, 1988.

Shprintzen RJ, Goldberg RB, Young D, Wolford L: The velo-cardio-facial syndrome: a clinical and genetic analysis, *Pediatrics* 67:167-172.

Shprintzen RJ, Sher AE, Croft CB: Hypernasal speech caused by tonsillar hypertrophy, *Int J Pediatr Otorhinolaryngol* 14:45-56, 1987.

Shprintzen RJ, Siegel-Sadewitz VL, Amato J, Goldberg RB: Anomalies associated with cleft lip, cleft palate, or both, *Am J Med Genet* 20:585-595, 1985.

Shprintzen RJ, Singer L, Sidoti EJ, Argamaso RV: Pharyngeal flap surgery: postoperative complications, *Int Anesthesiol Clin* 30:115-124, 1992.

Wolford LM, Oelschlaeger M, Deal R: Proplast as a pharyngeal wall implant to correct velopharyngeal insufficiency. Cleft Palate J 26:119-126, 1989.

6 Cleft Classification and Cleft Lip Repair

Janusz Bardach and Kenneth E. Salyer

The wide variety of cleft forms presents a serious diagnostic and treatment problem. Because clefts differ in so many parameters, precise diagnoses must be established so that proper treatment procedures may be selected. Many classification systems are used to describe and define cleft deformities. Among these systems, perhaps the most appropriate one was described by Otto Kriens in 1990 and presents a documentation system for all forms of clefting including complete unilateral and bilateral clefts, partial clefts, minor lip anomalies, combined complete clefts, and combinations of complete and partial clefts. Kriens' system is expressed by the symbols *LAHSHAL*, which represent the anatomic areas affected by cleft lip (L), alveolus (A), and the hard (H) and soft (S) palate. The paramedian cleft regions (LAH) are projected on a line with the median S, resulting in the LAHSHAL formula (Fig. 6-1).

Another classification system used at the Iowa Cleft Palate Center includes five groups of clefts:

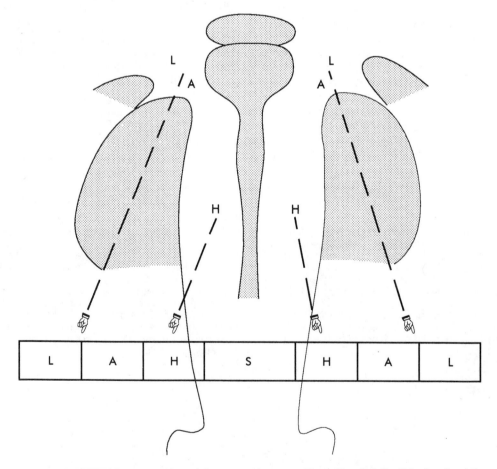

Fig. 6-1 LAHSHAL, an acronym of the anatomic areas affected by cleft lip *(L)*, alveolus *(A)*, and hard *(H)* and soft palate *(S)*. The paramedian cleft regions LAH are projected on a line with the median *S*, resulting in the LAHSHAL formula, designed by Kriens.

Group 1: Cleft lip only, unilateral and bilateral, partial and complete

Group 2: Cleft lip and alveolus, unilateral and bilateral, partial and complete

Group 3: Cleft palate only, submucous, partial, and complete

Group 4: Complete cleft of the lip, alveolus, and palate, unilateral and bilateral

Group 5: Combined cleft forms, which may represent various combinations of complete and partial clefts (for example, partial cleft of the right lip and alveolus, and complete left unilateral cleft of the lip, alveolus, and palate).

No single, widely accepted classification system serves as a basis for obtaining uniform information in all cleft centers. It may be that each center should adopt a system most appropriate to its needs, and consistently use it to facilitate the data gathering and retrieval needed to assess the validity of different treatment modalities. The classification of clefts is only one segment of the coding form that must be introduced in each cleft palate center to document diagnosis, multidisciplinary treatment procedures, and the outcome following completion of treatment. This information is valid for all specialists within the same institution, especially when transferring patients to another institution; it can be efficiently used for analysis and research purposes.

Clefts of the lip without clefting of the alveolus and palate require an entirely different approach to management than cleft lip associated with cleft of the alveolus and palate. In the treatment of an isolated cleft lip, surgical procedures suffice. The treatment of cleft lip, alveolus, and palate requires a multidisciplinary approach with active involvement of multiple members of the cleft palate team, such as the surgeon, speech pathologist, various dental specialists, otolaryngologist, psychologist, and others.

Cleft lip is usually associated with nasal deformity so that most cases of surgical treatment involve primary lip repair and correction of the nasal deformity. In the large majority of cases, cleft lip is associated not only with nasal deformity but also with cleft of the alveolus and palate. In unilateral complete cleft of the lip, alveolus, and palate, the maxilla is divided into two unequal segments: the larger and the smaller maxillary segments. In bilateral complete clefts of the lip, alveolus, and palate, the maxilla is divided into three segments: two lateral maxillary segments and the medial segment including the premaxilla attached to the

vomer. In unilateral cleft lip, the lip itself is divided into two uneven segments: the larger segment, which includes the philtrum and one philtral column; and the smaller lip segment. In bilateral clefts, the lip is divided into three portions: two lateral lip segments and a medial segment called the prolabium.

The severity of the cleft lip depends on:
1. Cleft type
2. Width of the cleft
3. Position of the maxillary segments
4. Congenital dysmorphogenesis

CLEFT TYPE

In the mildest form, cleft lip may be expressed as subcutaneous cleft or partial cleft involving only the vermilion. Subcutaneous cleft usually appears as a vertical groove indicating partial or total clefting of the orbicularis oris muscle, while the skin and mucosa remain intact (Fig. 6-2). Though there is no disruption of lip continuity with regard to skin and mucosa, the divided muscle creates aesthetic and functional problems. During lip function, the divided lip segments bulge at the margins of the cleft. Separation of the muscle also leads to nasal distortion, which is expressed by malpositioning of the alar base on the cleft side and deformity of the nasal ala and nasal tip on the same side. This nasal asymmetry is typical for unilateral cleft lip, and its severity depends on the extent of the cleft. Subcutaneous unilateral cleft lip requires surgical correction, which must include exposure of the separated muscle and joining both segments to assure proper appearance and functioning of the reconstructed lip.

Partial cleft lip is more common than subcutaneous cleft lip. Partial cleft lip may be unilateral or bilateral. The cleft may extend into the vermilion only or into one third or two thirds of the lip height. In some cases of partial cleft lip, the orbicularis oris muscle may remain intact in the upper portion of the lip where there is no clefting. Partial cleft may also be combined with a subcutaneous cleft that extends into the nasal sill. This type of cleft lip leads to the same nasal deformity as previously described. In partial clefts, it is not uncommon to find a bony deficiency in the maxilla in the cleft area, which indicates the presence of maxillary hypoplasia. When the divided orbicularis oris muscle extends into the entire height of the lip, it contributes to nasal deformity by distorting the base of the ala that is displaced laterally (Fig. 6-3). This displacement results in distortion of the ala, which becomes elongated and changes the orientation of the nostril from oblique to

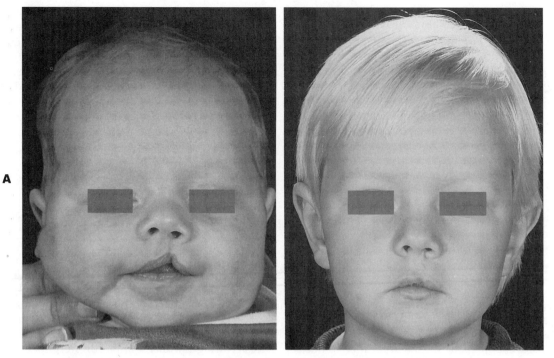

Fig. 6-2 A, Partial cleft of the lip involving the lower third of the lip. A submucous cleft extends into the upper two-thirds of the lip. Minimal nasal deformity. **B,** After lip-nose repair using rotation-advancement technique (Salyer's modification).

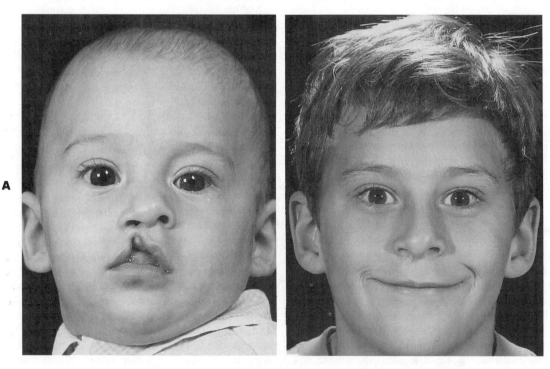

Fig. 6-3 A, Partial cleft of the lip and complete cleft of the alveolus and palate. Marked nasal deformity. **B,** Following lip-nose repair using rotation-advancement technique (Salyer's modification).

horizontal. It is also associated with nasal tip asymmetry and displacement of the lower lateral cartilage on the cleft side. The muscle imbalance following division of the orbicularis oris muscle may lead to growth disturbances even in partial cleft lip.

Complete cleft of the lip may be unilateral or bilateral. In the large majority of cases, unilateral complete cleft of the lip is associated with unilateral cleft of the alveolus and palate. Bilateral complete cleft is also usually associated with cleft of the alveolus and palate. In unilateral cleft, the asymmetric division of the orbicularis oris muscle leads to functional imbalance that influences the position of the maxillary segments. The larger maxillary segment, including the premaxilla, is influenced by the larger portion of the facial muscles and thus may be rotated outward and upward. The smaller segment, affected by the less functional facial muscles, tends to rotate inward and medially. On some occasions, the lesser segment may appear severely collapsed. The sooner muscle equilibrium is established, the better the chance to improve the alignment of the maxillary segments and thus create conditions for normal facial growth and development. In unilateral cleft of the lip, alveolus, and palate, nasal distortion is always present, but its degree of severity varies depending on cleft width and position of the maxillary segments. The wider the cleft, the more distorted the nasal features will be. With increased displacement of the lesser maxillary segment, more severe nasal deformity will occur (Fig. 6-4).

In unilateral complete cleft lip, the nasal deformity has characteristic features but varies in degree of severity. The columella is usually shorter on the cleft side and is positioned obliquely with its base deviated toward the noncleft side. The ala is S-shaped because of the deformity of the lateral crus of the lower lateral cartilage; the lateral crus is longer on the cleft side than on the noncleft side. The lower lateral cartilage on the cleft side is displaced in frontal and horizontal planes, causing distortion of the nasal tip and ala. Flattening of the nasal ala creates a horizontal orientation of the nostril. The base of the nostril may be displaced in three dimensions, laterally, posteriorly, and inferiorly. The nasal floor is absent. During primary lip repair, some correction of the nasal deformity is highly beneficial because it decreases the severity of the nasal deformity, and may result in final correction (Fig. 6-5).

In unilateral complete cleft of the lip, it is important to realize that the muscles are not only divided but are also malaligned curving upward along the edges of the vermilion. Because this malalignment must be corrected to achieve normal lip function, during lip repair the muscles are realigned into a normal horizontal position and sutured so that normal anatomy and function are reestablished. The vermilion curves upward, becoming thinner as it extends further toward the floor of the nose. On the noncleft side of the lip, the highest point of the Cupid's Bow is easily detectable, while on the cleft side, this point has to be established through measurement. The philtral column and the dimple of the philtrum are defined only on the noncleft side.

Complete bilateral cleft lip is commonly associated with cleft of the alveolus and palate

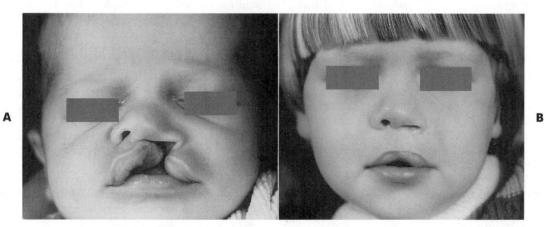

Fig. 6-4 A, Complete unilateral cleft lip, alveolus, and palate with severe nasal deformity. **B,** Following triangular flap repair (Bardach's modification). Note that there is still marked nasal deformity.

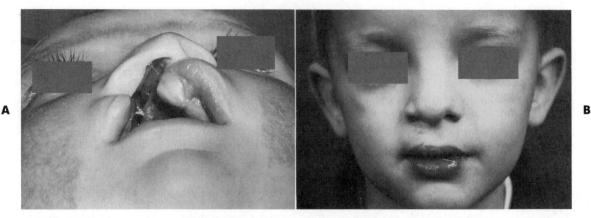

Fig. 6-5 A, Complete unilateral cleft of the lip, alveolus, and palate. **B,** Following triangular flap repair (Bardach modification). Note symmetry of the lip and nose.

and may be symmetric or asymmetric. Because the lip and maxilla are divided in three segments, two lateral and one medial, the relationship between segments varies. When the cleft is symmetrical, the two lateral segments of the lip and maxilla are similar, while the medial segment that includes the premaxilla and prolabium may be positioned within the maxillary segments or displaced. Displacement of the premaxilla also varies in severity and position. It can be displaced anteriorly, inferiorly, or laterally, or in all of these dimensions simultaneously. The size of the premaxilla and prolabium is also variable. The premaxilla may be larger than the space between the maxillary segments; in this case, it cannot be inserted into the alveolar arch. When the premaxilla is smaller than the distance between the maxillary segments, it can be moved within the alveolar arch by using presurgical orthopedics if this is considered to be beneficial. No matter how small the prolabium is, it must be utilized for construction of the midportion of the lip. It is a mistake to use the prolabium for lengthening of the columella or for reconstruction of only the upper or middle portion of the lip while using the lateral lip segments for reconstruction of the lower portion of the lip because the prolabium has little or no muscle, while the lip segments do contain muscle. Inclusion of the prolabium into the reconstructed lip leads to asymmetric lip growth. This condition definitely requires corrective surgery.

Nasal deformity is probably the most serious problem in bilateral complete clefts of the lip, alveolus, and palate. The columella is short, the nasal tip flattened, and alar bases are laterally displaced creating a horizontal orientation of the nostrils. In this type of deformity, the lower lateral cartilage has a very short medial crus, while the lateral crus is largely elongated. At the time of primary lip repair, an attempt can be made to correct this deformity. In the majority of cases, a secondary operation is necessary to achieve an adequate appearance of the nose.

CLEFT WIDTH

The width of the cleft lip is an important factor in assessing and treating unilateral and bilateral clefts. Cleft width contributes to the severity of this congenital anomaly with increased displacement of the lip, maxilla, and nose. The wider the cleft, the more severe are the problems encountered in planning and multidisciplinary treatment. Surgical treatment is more difficult with wide clefts because there is increased tension when suturing the lip segments together. This increased tissue tension is transferred as pressure to the maxillary complex and may inhibit anteroposterior maxillary growth. Partial clefts of the lip are usually accompanied by nasal deformity and, in some cases, hypoplasia of the underlying bony skeleton in the cleft. In the majority of cases, the lip and nasal deformity can be successfully treated with surgical procedures designed to establish simultaneous lip and nose repair, or by repairing the lip and improving the nasal deformity in the same operation, while delaying final correction of the nasal deformity to a later age.

A wide cleft is defined as one in which the distance between the edges of the maxillary segments is more than 1 centimeter. The distance between the edges of the lip segments is usually greater because of muscle contracture on each side. In severe cases, the distance between the maxillary segments may exceed 2 centimeters. This condition creates lateral displacement of the base of the ala causing severe nasal deformity with flattening of the ala and severe deformity of the nasal tip. Absence of the nasal floor in wide clefts is a serious problem, because reconstruction of the nasal floor is an integral part of treatment of complete clefts. Wide palatal clefts may be considered inoperable by less experienced specialists. However, when preoperatively assessing the morphology of a wide cleft, it is necessary to realize that these conditions will change dramatically following primary cleft lip repair. After cleft lip repair, the tension of the repaired lip will bring together the maxillary segments and in a very short period of time, the segments will be so close together that closure of the alveolar defect can be performed with no difficulties. Approximation of the maxillary segments also results in dramatic narrowing of the palatal cleft, which facilitates palate repair. It is also important to realize that following lip repair, there may not only be a change in the approximation of the maxillary segments, but the position of the lesser maxillary segment may improve, creating a more equal skeletal platform for the base of the ala leading to improvement of nasal appearance.

It is understandable that closure of narrow and medium-size clefts results in less tension in the reconstructed lip, while closure of a wide cleft produces increased tension. Many surgeons and orthodontists are of the opinion that using presurgical orthopedic treatment reduces cleft width and improves the conditions for lip repair with less tension. The width of the cleft may be a factor in the selection of the technique for lip repair. In narrow and medium-size clefts, rotation-advancement technique may be successfully used as well as triangular flap technique. In wide clefts, rotation-advancement technique produces too much tension, which may lead to an undesirable result in the form of small nostril. For this reason, it is preferable to use triangular flap repair in all wide clefts since this technique allows for equal distribution of tension throughout the entire height of the lip, while the rotation-advancement flap creates the area of maximal tension at the upper portion of the lip.

POSITION OF THE MAXILLARY SEGMENTS

The position of the maxillary segments plays an important role in designing and executing primary cleft lip repair. In partial cleft of the lip, unilateral and bilateral, the maxilla is not affected, while in complete unilateral and bilateral cleft, the maxilla is divided into two or three segments, respectively. In unilateral complete

cleft of the lip, alveolus and palate, the position of the maxillary segments may vary because the division is asymmetrical, leading to the creation of one larger and one smaller segment. The larger segment, which includes the premaxilla and the lip on the noncleft side, is influenced by more muscle forces than the lesser segment. The pull of muscle forces on the larger maxillary segment may be rotated upward and outward.

The smaller maxillary segment is less influenced by muscle forces, and therefore, more often it may be displaced downward and medially. Displacement of the lesser maxillary segment may be so severe that it is positioned behind the larger segment. This condition is described as collapse of the lesser maxillary segment. Asymmetry and displacement of the skeletal platform results in asymmetry of the nasal structures and especially the base of the ala, which is displaced laterally, backward, and downward, causing severe distortion of the nasal ala and nasal tip.

Malposition of the maxillary segments may lead to malocclusion, which could necessitate long-term orthodontic treatment. To improve the position of the maxillary segments before cleft lip repair, some surgeons and orthodontists suggest presurgical orthopedic treatment, active or passive, which corrects the position of the segments, brings them into better alignment, and thus creates better conditions for primary cleft lip repair and correction of the nasal deformity.

The primary goal of presurgical orthopedic treatment is to realign the maxillary segments to achieve a more normal position of the alveolar arch as well as a more symmetric skeletal base before primary lip repair. Presurgical orthopedic treatment improves proper positioning of the maxillary segments before lip repair, which contributes to greater facial symmetry. It also improves the balance of the skeletal base and creates a better condition for growth and development. Correction of the nasal deformity is easier when the skeletal base is symmetrical. Despite these advantages of presurgical orthopedic treatment, not all surgeons and orthodontists view this treatment as necessary. Many studies performed by highly experienced specialists indicate that proper surgical management with careful orthodontic treatment during the stage of mixed dentition leads to similar results in terms of facial growth and occlusion as compared to cases in which presurgical orthopedic treatment is applied.

Presurgical orthopedic treatment in bilateral clefts of the lip, alveolus, and palate deals primarily with the maxillary segments and the premaxilla. In the case of a protruding premaxilla, the maxillary segments may be collapsed medially, thus preventing retropositioning of the premaxilla within the alveolar arch. In such situations, the goal of presurgical orthopedics is to expand the maxillary segments and simultaneously reposition the premaxilla. Because the premaxilla may be displaced anteriorly, inferiorly, laterally, and sometimes simultaneously in all three dimensions, positioning of the premaxilla within the alveolar arch or close to it may present serious difficulties. When the premaxilla is displaced only anteriorly, it has been assumed that by applying pressure it can be moved backward within the maxillary segments to achieve proper positioning and to assure proper occlusion; however, only on rare occasions can this be easily and successfully achieved. Because the premaxilla is attached to the tip of the nose, it is not really possible to "move" it. Rather, orthopedic forces tend to torque the bottom portion of the premaxilla backward, thus bending it at an angle.

Some surgeons and orthodontists apply presurgical orthodontic treatment in the form of a special device that expands the lateral maxillary segments, creating space for the premaxilla, which is forcefully moved within the space between the lateral segments. This technique seems more successful than external pressure applied by various bands. External pressure usually bends the premaxilla not only backward but forces it downward, which complicates an already difficult situation. There are plastic surgeons and orthodontists who prefer to allow unrestricted midfacial growth when there is a protruding premaxilla, delaying surgical intervention until 6 years of age. At about 6 years of age, the premaxilla is surgically retropositioned and stabilized within the alveolar arch with bilateral bone grafting and a dental plate wired for 3 months to immobilize the premaxilla.

Currently, the issues of presurgical orthopedic treatment in unilateral and bilateral clefts as well as the problem of surgical repositioning of the premaxilla remain open to interpretation. For this reason, the choices made in particular cleft centers are based on the specialists' experience according to their own treatment protocol.

CONGENITAL DYSMORPHOGENESIS

Congenital dysmorphogenesis is a factor that must be considered in every case of unilateral and bilateral cleft. However, its expression may vary from minimal to very substantial. Dysmorphogenesis expressed as hypoplasia of the soft and hard tissues may affect the lip and the maxillary complex. More often, hypoplasia is expressed within the skeletal base, although at the edges of the cleft it is also evident in the soft tissue. The degree of hypoplasia can be described but cannot be measured. Therefore, when hypoplasia is evident, we may assume that maxillofacial growth may be affected not only because of the failures in surgical treatment, but also because of intrinsic factors related to dysmorphogenesis.

GOALS OF PRIMARY CLEFT LIP/NOSE REPAIR IN UNILATERAL AND BILATERAL CLEFTS

The general goals of lip/nose repair in unilateral and bilateral clefts are basically the same: to reconstruct the lip as close to its normal anatomical and functional features as possible and to correct the nasal deformity to minimize the severity of secondary deformities. Because there is a large difference between unilateral and bilateral cleft lip, alveolus, and palate, and different approaches and surgical procedures may be applied, we will discuss each deformity separately.

Reconstruction of the unilateral cleft lip/nose includes positioning both sides of the lip at equal height to obtain balance and symmetry. The Cupid's Bow must be reconstructed because its presence is essential to enhancing an optimal aesthetic result. On both sides of the cleft edges, the orbicularis oris muscles are maldirected and malpositioned, with abnormal attachments. These muscles must be released on both sides, redirected, and sutured in a normal horizontal position to assure normal lip function. One of the most difficult problems in primary lip repair is construction of a symmetrical vermilion without notching and without discrepancies in volume and thickness. It is also important to reconstruct a deep buccal sulcus to assure proper mobility of the lip and facilitate future orthodontic treatment.

Closure of the nasolabial fistula constitutes an important part of the primary cleft lip repair and can be successfully completed in the majority of the patients, excluding very wide clefts. Fistulae may occur after surgery, but may be masked by collapse of the maxillary segments so that an opening is not apparent. Unfortunately, during orthodontic treatment and maxillary expansion, these hidden fistulae become evident due to the forces applied to achieve adequate expansion and proper occlusion. The presence of a nasolabial fistula is an indication for surgical closure because its presence leads to both speech disorders and leakage of fluids and air, creating a place for retention of food particles.

During primary repair, correction of the nasal deformity can be conservative or radical. Bardach prefers a conservative approach, limited to medial approximation of the alar base in a position symmetrical to the opposite side, strengthening of the columella, and most importantly, creating a symmetrical skeletal base to support the nasal framework. As mentioned, this can be obtained through presurgical orthopedic treatment by repositioning the maxillary segments as well as an appropriate surgical procedure in which repositioning of the maxillary segments is directed by the muscle pull. Other surgeons prefer a more radical approach to the correction of nasal deformity at the time of primary lip repair. This approach includes repositioning of the lower lateral cartilages and especially the lateral crura into a more symmetrical position, as well as the use of stent sutures to ascertain the position of the cartilages and the newly molded shape of the nostrils and nasal tip. Some Japanese surgeons very effectively use a molding intranasal stent that is inserted in both nostrils after surgery, allowing the healing process to create symmetrical shapes of the nostrils.

Correction of the secondary cleft lip deformity will be discussed separately from secondary cleft nasal deformity, because each of these operations is usually performed independently. In the majority of cases, primary cleft lip/nose repair does not lead to the optimal aesthetic and functional result; also, various lip and/or nose distortions or deformities may remain and require further correction. However, in some patients, primary lip repair is also the final repair because the aesthetic and functional results are excellent and no secondary correction is required. Following primary lip repair, the appearance and function of the lip will improve with time, while the existing nasal distortions will remain the same or worsen. For this reason, it is prudent to not hurry with correction of the secondary lip deformity because its appearance and function may improve to the degree that no surgery is needed. This improvement is always related to constant function of the lip and molding pressure from the lower lip. The secondary nasal deformity requires correction, and the timing of the correction is crucial since it is more advantageous to correct the deformity before the time when children attend school rather than waiting until they are adolescents. If indicated, we intend to correct the secondary lip deformity before school age, and in cases of severe nasal deformity, we also operate at 5 to 6 years of age. The decisive factor in establishing the timing for

nasal correction is the growth and development of the lower lateral cartilages. When the cartilages are firm enough and may produce the necessary support for the reconstructed nose, the surgery is performed at approximately 6 years of age. If the cartilages remain thin and weak, we do not recommend performing nasal reconstruction, since adequate support cannot be created using these cartilages. There are many more varieties related to the bilateral cleft lip, alveolus, and palate, and each one requires very careful preoperative analysis to establish the sequence of surgical and orthodontic treatments as well as the involvement of other specialists.

The goals of primary cleft lip/nose repair in bilateral clefts are more complex and definitely more difficult than in unilateral clefts because the majority of cases have some degree of asymmetry. This asymmetry, combined with a cleft that divides the lip into three segments, requires a different approach than those used for unilateral clefts. The main problem lies with the prolabium and the premaxilla. The prolabium may not only vary in size, but it also represents a portion of the lip that has little or no vermilion or muscle. Even with these differences between the anatomical structure of the prolabium and the lateral lip segments, the prolabium must be used for reconstruction of the entire midportion of the lip, except the vermilion, which is brought to this area from the lateral lip segments. The premaxilla complicates reconstruction of the lip in bilateral clefts, especially in cases when it protrudes in front of collapsed maxillary segments. The size and the position of the premaxilla may vary to a great degree. The premaxilla may be malpositioned in three dimensions, forward, downward, and laterally. The premaxilla may be larger than the distance between the maxillary segments, which means that even by pushing the premaxilla backward, it cannot be inserted within the alveolar arch where it belongs. For these reasons, some surgeons and orthodontists expand the maxillary arches in infancy, attempting to place the protruding premaxilla within the alveolar arch before cleft lip repair. This practice must be critically analyzed because maxillary expansion at this age is done without any guidance for the occlusal relationship and may lead to an exceedingly wide maxilla compared to the normally developed mandible. Some surgeons and orthodontists hold the opinion that allowing for undisturbed maxillary growth, even with a severely protruding premaxilla, may establish a normal growth pattern in the first 5 to 7 years of age and that surgical retropositioning of the premaxilla at this age may be beneficial if performed simultaneously with bilateral bone grafting to stabilize the premaxilla and close oronasal and nasolabial fistulas.

Another problem that distinguishes bilateral cleft lip repair from unilateral repair relates to the staging of lip repair. In cases when the bilateral cleft is symmetrical, which occurs most often in incomplete clefts of the lip, simultaneous lip repair seems perfectly justified and successful.

Asymmetrical bilateral clefts of the lip, alveolus, and palate are more common than symmetrical cases. The asymmetry is related to the size and position of the premaxilla and nasal septum and the position of the maxillary segments. The nasal septum and the premaxilla may be deviated to one side, thus creating a very wide cleft on one side and a narrow cleft on the other side. The nasal deformity in this case is also asymmetrical and more severe on the side of the wide cleft. Asymmetry of bilateral clefts may also result from a difference in cleft form on each side. For example, on one side there may be a complete cleft lip and alveolus, while on the other side there may only be partial cleft of the lip without an alveolar cleft, although the palatal cleft may be bilateral (Fig. 6-6).

Asymmetrical bilateral clefts present much more difficult treatment problems than symmetrical bilateral clefts so that the expectations for a successful outcome must be regarded with caution. Additional surgical procedures are usually required to obtain a successful result and more involvement of other specialists may be necessary in the course of treatment. Asymmetry associated with bilateral clefting stimulates many surgeons to use two-stage cleft lip-nose repair instead of simultaneous bilateral cleft lip repair. The first operation repairs the more severely affected side with the wider cleft. This selection to close the wider side first will transform the bilateral asymmetrical cleft into a unilateral one that will be subsequently closed 6 to 8 weeks later. It is usually assumed that closure of the second side using the same surgical technique will result in better symmetry of the reconstructed lip and nose. These expectations are not always fruitful. In the majority of cases, secondary correction of the lip and nose is needed and on many occasions, more than one corrective procedure is performed on the lip, and at least one more corrective procedure is performed on the nose.

When performing primary and secondary surgery in cases of bilateral cleft lip, alveolus,

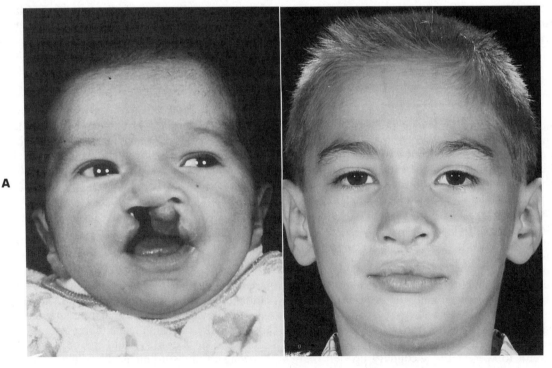

Fig. 6-6 A, Asymmetrical bilateral cleft of the lip. Unilateral cleft of the alveolus and palate. **B,** Following lip-nose repair using rotation-advancement technique (Salyer modification). Both sides are closed simultaneously.

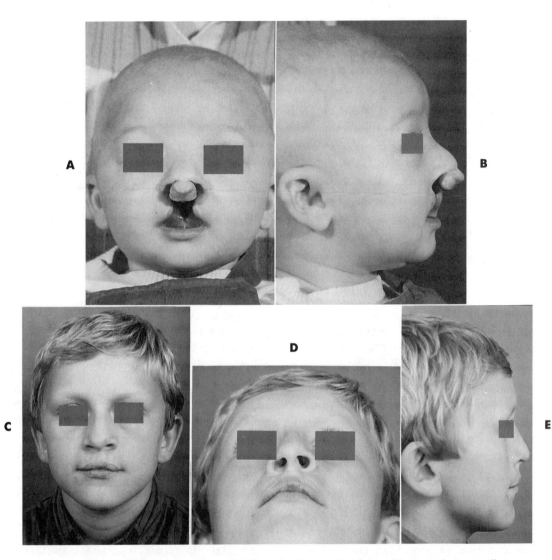

Fig. 6-7 A-E, Bilateral complete cleft lip, alveolus, and palate with severely protruding premaxilla. Note the position of the premaxilla and prolabium attached to the nasal tip. Since the cleft was perfectly symmetrical, cleft lip repair was performed in one stage using straight-line closure technique. Corrective lip surgery was performed at 3 years of age. Correction of the nasal deformity was performed at 7 years of age (Bardach's technique).

and palate, there are several special points that require a careful and attentive approach. One involves deciding how to deal with the protruding premaxilla, which may not only protrude forward, but also may be displaced downward and laterally. Presurgical orthopedic treatment aimed to reposition the misplaced premaxilla into the alveolar arch is considered the treatment of choice by some surgeons and orthodontists. Pressure devices are also considered for replacement of the premaxilla. However, the results are not always successful. Bardach and Olin consider surgical repositioning of the premaxilla at 6 to 7 years of age as the most

appropriate treatment of choice because it allows the establishment of a pattern of normal facial growth and repositioning of the premaxilla within the alveolar arch with stabilization by bilateral bone grafting (Fig. 6-7).

In bilateral clefts, correction of the nasal deformity during primary lip repair is more difficult than in unilateral clefts because in many cases, the size and the position of the prolabium and the premaxilla severely interferes with nasal reconstruction. In bilateral clefts, the columella may be very short and almost nonexistent with the prolabium pulled almost to the level of the nasal tip. In these cases, it is impossible to lengthen the columella during primary cleft lip repair, and this procedure must be performed at a later age. Without lengthening the columella, reconstruction that includes changing the shape of the nostrils from horizontal to oblique cannot be performed because the nasal tip is pulled downward and the nose is very wide in this area. Repositioning the alar bases is helpful, but does not constitute a decisive change in the appearance of the nose. In cases when the columella has adequate length, correction of the nasal deformity can be successfully performed during primary lip repair by repositioning the lower lateral cartilages as is done with unilateral clefts and securing the cartilages in a new position with stent sutures.

The secondary lip and nasal deformities in bilateral clefts require correction in the great majority of cases. It is desirable to have all surgical treatment of the lip and nose completed before the child enters school; however, it is very difficult to achieve a final successful result at this age, especially with respect to the nose. In most cases, correction of the lip deformity is related to the prolabium and to asymmetry of the vermilion in the midportion of the lip. Most secondary lip deformities occur in the form of short prolabium, whistle deformity, and notch in the vermilion; these can be successfully corrected before 5 to 6 years of age. The existing nasal deformity cannot be easily corrected at that early age since weak lower lateral cartilages cannot be properly rearranged to support the new shape of the reconstructed nose. For this reason, it is often necessary to wait until 8 to 12 years of age to perform the final correction and create an appealing nose. Most corrections of the nasal deformities are performed using open tip rhinoplasty, which allows for a direct approach to the lower lateral cartilages.

Advances in reconstructive surgery have permitted successful correction of primary and secondary bilateral lip and nose deformities. However, several surgical procedures are usually necessary to achieve a final successful result that pleases the patient and the surgeon. It is also necessary to remember that surgical treatment is performed in close cooperation with orthodontists, whose interventions are extremely important in establishing proper occlusion and monitoring facial growth.

SURGICAL TECHNIQUE

The surgical technique for primary unilateral cleft lip/nose repair accepted by many surgeons is based on the rotation-advancement method described by Millard. Another very popular technique is based on the concept initiated by Tennison, which includes the use of triangular flaps for lip reconstruction. Both techniques can be successfully used; however, selection must be made according to cleft type and severity. It is the author's personal preference to use rotation-advancement technique in partial cleft lip and triangular flap technique in cases of complete cleft lip. No matter which technique is used for primary cleft lip repair, it is important to follow basic principles. One principle is to try to save all of the lip tissue without discarding any of it, because there is a deficit of tissue in the area of the cleft and rearrangement of the lip segments to reconstruct a normal looking and functioning lip requires all available tissue. Another principle related to lip repair deals with obtaining the proper lip length on both sides, which results in a symmetrical and well-balanced lip. In the area of the cleft, the lip height is impaired; therefore, the use of the rotation-advancement technique or triangular flap technique is helpful in achieving proper height on both sides. It may be unfortunate to create a short lip, but it is worse when the lip is longer than normal, since correction of a longer lip is more difficult than correction of a short lip deformity. One more basic principle of lip reconstruction is creation of a normal Cupid's Bow and a symmetrical vermilion.

During primary lip repair, it is always important to ensure that no incisions in the buccal sulcus are performed on either side. According to our experience and experimental work, incisions in the sulcus and undermining of the soft tissue from the face of the maxilla may impair the growth and development of the midface. In every cleft lip repair, it is also important to attempt to create a deep normal sulcus which is important when orthodontic treatment is indicated. The presence of a deep sulcus enhances normal mobility of the upper lip.

As was discussed previously, primary cleft lip repair aims not only to create a normal-looking and functioning lip, but also to correct the existing nasal deformity as much as possible. To achieve this goal, it is necessary to use a surgical technique that corrects both the lip and nose simultaneously and aims to achieve an optimal result in the primary surgery. When using rotation-advancement or triangular flap lip repair, correction of the nasal deformity is incorporated in this procedure and can be performed in a conservative or more radical fashion. No matter which approach is used, reconstruction of the nasal floor is imperative and must be performed in a way that also closes the nasolabial fistula. The major goal is to minimize the existing deformity, thus creating better conditions for final correction. Final correction can be performed when the cartilages become firm enough to create a support for reconstructed nasal structures.

In bilateral clefts, the problem of lip and nose repair is more complex since in many cases of complete cleft, the nasal deformity becomes more severe after surgery due to shortage of tissue that prevents simultaneous successful reconstruction of the columella and philtrum. In bilateral clefts, it is much more difficult to achieve a well-balanced and symmetrical lip because most of the bilateral clefts are asymmetrical and there is always a tissue deficiency in the midportion of the vermilion that must be overcome by skillful approximation of vermilion flaps from both lip segments.

Advances in surgery for cleft lip and palate as well as multidisciplinary management of clefts by a team of specialists has significantly improved the outcome of treatment. Not all primary lip-nose repairs result in an optimal outcome necessitating corrective procedures for both the lip and nose in the large majority of cases. In our experience, one additional corrective surgery is usually needed to achieve an optimal aesthetic and functional result with the lip, and at least one more surgery is required for correction of the nasal deformity.

SUGGESTED READINGS

Bardach J, Salyer K: *Surgical techniques in cleft lip and palate,* St. Louis, 1991, Mosby.

Kriens O: *Documentation of cleft lip, alveolus, and palate.* In Bardach J, Morris H, editors: *Multidisciplinary management of cleft lip and palate,* Philadelphia, 1990, W B Saunders.

Millard DR Jr: *Cleft craft: the evolution of its surgery,* Boston, 1977, Little, Brown & Co.

Noordhoff MS: Bilateral cleft lip repair. In Bardach J, Morris H, editors: *Multidisciplinary management of cleft lip and palate,* Philadelphia, 1990, W B Saunders.

Randall P: Long-term results with the triangular flap technique for unilateral cleft lip repair. In Bardach J, Morris H, editors: *Multidisciplinary management of cleft lip and palate,* Philadelphia, 1990, W B Saunders.

Salyer KE: Unilateral cleft lip and cleft lip nasal reconstruction. In Bardach J, Morris H, editors: *Multidisciplinary management of cleft lip and palate,* Philadelphia, 1990, W B Saunders.

7 Cleft Palate Repair: Anatomy, Timing, Goals, Principles, and Techniques

Janusz Bardach and *Kenneth E. Salyer*

Cleft palate is a condition in which excessive communication between the oral and nasal cavities causes distorted speech production. The cleft may be isolated to the palate only, or it may be associated with unilateral or bilateral clefts of the lip and alveolus. Cleft palate is present in over 90% of the population affected with clefts; unilateral cleft lip, alveolus and palate comprises up to 50% of all clefts; bilateral complete cleft of the lip, alveolus, and palate comprises 15%; and cleft palate only comprises 25%. The remaining 10% includes cleft lip only and cleft lip and alveolus (the rarest form of clefting). This last category requires additional explanation since it may include, for example, both bilateral partial cleft of the lip and cleft of the soft palate. In this case, the patient qualifies to be listed in two groups: cleft lip only and cleft palate only. Another example of a cleft that qualifies for the mixed group is partial cleft of the lip on one side, and complete unilateral cleft of the lip and palate on the other. This cleft cannot be listed as unilateral complete cleft or as bilateral cleft.

Cleft palate, which may appear in a variety of forms, is often associated with other congenital conditions defined as syndromes. The treatment of cleft palate in patients with syndromes is presented extensively in Chapter 2. A great majority of palatal clefts result in speech distortions due to excessive communication between the oral and nasal cavities, impaired function of the muscles of the soft palate, and increased space between the posterior edge of the soft palate and the posterior pharyngeal wall.

Cleft palate may vary in terms of size, shape, and location. The mildest form of cleft involves cleft of the uvula only, which may have no effect on speech production. Submucous clefts, in which the muscles of the soft palate are split but the mucosa remains intact, are also considered a mild form of palatal cleft; however, as will be discussed later, submucous cleft may cause speech problems. Cleft of the soft palate only

may extend partially or completely, reaching the posterior edge of the hard palate. The most severe form of cleft palate only is complete cleft of the soft and hard palate, extending to the incisive foramen, with some shaped in a "horseshoe" form. Clefts of the hard and soft palate, without involvement of the alveolus, are quite common. Cleft palate, when associated with unilateral or bilateral cleft of the lip and alveolus, presents the most difficult problem in terms of multidisciplinary treatment. All of the forms of palatal clefts just mentioned will be described in more detail later in the chapter, with an indication and description of the appropriate surgical treatment.

A variety of factors must be considered when evaluating the patient with cleft palate. Cleft type is only one factor. Other factors to be considered include the severity of the cleft, the width of palatal cleft, the position of the maxillary segments, the inclination of the palatal shelves, the mobility of the soft palate, the length of the soft palate, the lateral pharyngeal wall movements, and the prominence of Passavant's ridge, when present.

Each cleft patient with speech impairment requires surgical treatment. The majority of these patients also require speech therapy. On some occasions, cleft palate surgery combined with speech therapy may prove to be inadequate for full speech rehabilitation. In these instances, further surgical treatment as well as further speech therapy is indicated. During the entire course of treatment, the involvement of both surgeon and speech pathologist is necessary for optimal speech rehabilitation.

A multidisciplinary approach is imperative in the management of patients with clefts. Close cooperation between surgeon and speech pathologist is essential to patient evaluation, diagnosis, treatment planning, and therapy. Postoperative care and long-term observations must be performed simultaneously by both specialists, with exchange of information and mutual agreement on further decisions regarding management when indicated. For this reason, speech pathologists participating in comprehensive treatment need to understand the surgeon's approach to clinical evaluation and the decision-making process that leads to surgical treatment. To help speech pathologists understand the anatomical and functional problems related to the cleft palate, the particular forms of palatal clefts will be described.

SURGICAL ANATOMY OF THE CLEFT PALATE
Submucous cleft of the palate

Submucous cleft, which may not be evident at birth, is the most inconspicuous cleft. It may involve only the posterior portion of the soft palate, one half of the soft palate, or the entire soft palate, including the posterior portion of the hard palate. In this form of cleft, the muscles of the soft palate are divided to some degree at the midline. The division of the muscles of the soft palate does not involve the mucous membrane on the oral and nasal sides; therefore, the muscles are separated but clefting does not actually occur, although the function of the soft palate may be impaired and speech production may be distorted to various degrees. Since the muscles of the soft palate are divided in the midline, the orientation is changed as well as the attachment to the posterior edge of the hard palate. Reorientation of the muscles of the soft palate along the edges of the cleft (from horizontal to oblique or even vertical) affects the function of the soft palate. It is interesting to note, however, that submucous cleft of the soft palate does not always result in impaired speech production. Impairment depends on the degree of the separation of the muscles, and the length and mobility of the soft palate. Some people with submucous cleft may live their entire lives unaware of the defect. Since it may be difficult to understand the variable effect or lack of effect of submucous cleft on speech production, in specific cases other factors may explain this relation. For example, in cases of submucous cleft with good mobility of the soft palate and the lateral pharyngeal walls, as well as a short distance between the posterior edge of the soft palate and the posterior pharyngeal wall, there may be no indication of distorted speech production. On the other hand, a submucous cleft of the same severity may cause serious speech problems when, in addition to the existing cleft, the soft palate is short and has poor mobility. These examples underscore the

importance of evaluating an entire set of factors in addition to the submucous cleft when determining its effect on speech production. There have been several reports that indicate that the majority of people with submucous clefts have normal speech.

Another form of submucous cleft palate is the occult submucous cleft palate. In occult clefts, the oral aspect of the palate appears normal with no evidence of bifid uvula, notched hard palate, or muscle separation. However, endoscopic examination of the palate shows muscle separation on the nasal surface of the palate, as well as absence of the musculus uvulae (Croft et al., 1979; Lewin et al, 1980).

It is very important to understand that, in contrast to all other forms of clefting, the diagnosis of submucous cleft does not always indicate surgery. However, in cases when submucous cleft results in speech distortions, no matter how small the cleft, surgery is necessary to improve the conditions for speech production. It may be summarized that the extent of the submucous cleft, the function of the soft palate, as well as other components must be assessed in the decision-making process for surgical intervention.

It is unfortunate that some surgeons as well as some speech pathologists consider the presence of submucous cleft an indication for surgery, insisting that surgical repair of submucous cleft be performed at the same time as cleft palate repair at 6 to 12 months of age. These specialists falsely assume that submucous cleft will cause speech impairment in every individual, but realistically, speech impairment at this age cannot be detected. Less experienced surgeons and speech pathologists may have difficulty establishing a proper diagnosis of submucous cleft in the infant as well as in the older child because clefting of the soft palate may not be evident, and submucous separation of the muscles may be hardly detectable. To properly diagnose submucous cleft when speech impairment is not evident, it is necessary to observe the action of the soft palate so that division of the muscles and their bulging at the cleft edges becomes more pronounced.

When submucous cleft extends the entire length of the soft palate, it is also important to palpate the soft palate and the posterior margin of the hard palate. In these cases, the posterior nasal spine in the hard palate usually cannot be detected, although the small indentation at the midline of the hard palate may be detectable. With appropriate lighting, some cases of submucous cleft can be diagnosed by observing the transparency of the mucous membrane between lateral segments of the soft palate. Again, it must be emphasized that the mere diagnosis of submucous cleft without evidence of an existing speech impediment is not indication for surgical repair. Surgical intervention and the choice of surgical procedure depends on the severity of speech impairment, the length and functioning of the soft palate, the lateral pharyngeal wall movements, the distance between the posterior edge of the soft palate and the posterior pharyngeal wall, and the age of the patient.

Two surgical approaches are usually considered when treatment of submucous cleft is indicated. Many surgeons advocate approaching the surgical treatment of submucous cleft in the same manner in which other forms of palatal clefts are treated. The techniques applied resemble those used for any other type of cleft palate only, and include raising mucoperiosteal flaps on the hard palate, detachment of the muscles of the soft palate from the posterior edge of the hard palate, reorientation of the muscles and suturing them together to restore their continuity and to ensure proper function.

Another group of surgeons advocates primary pharyngoplasty, which in the majority of cases, involves superiorly based pharyngeal flap technique. This concept is based on the belief that in many cases of submucous cleft, the primary cleft palate repair does not produce successful results in terms of speech production so that secondary pharyngoplasty is indicated. The fallacy of this approach is evident when one realizes that pharyngeal flap is indicated in only 20 to 30% of patients following primary palatoplasty. Applying pharyngoplasty in the remaining 70% of patients is not necessary because their speech will improve following palatoplasty only. Since palatoplasty creates definitely less secondary problems and complications than pharyngoplasty, it may make sense to initiate treatment of patients with submucous clefts by performing palatoplasty first; pharyngoplasty is performed only if palatoplasty proves to be unsuccessful and if the speech pathologist indicates a need for this procedure.

Cleft of the soft and hard palate

The mildest form of clefting of the soft palate affects only the uvula, may not be detected, and may not affect speech production. When evaluating the size of the cleft in the soft palate, it is usually acceptable to express it as a partial cleft of the soft palate (which may involve the posterior ⅓, ½, or ⅔ of the soft palate), or as a complete cleft of the soft palate (which involves the entire soft palate and may extend as a partial cleft of the hard palate). If the cleft further extends into the hard palate, reaching the incisive foramen, it is then considered a complete cleft of the soft and hard palate (the secondary palate). From this description it is evident that minimal clefts appear at the posterior edge of the soft palate and progress in size anteriorly, while more severe clefts extend across the entire palate.

In the large majority of cases of cleft palate only, the cleft is oblong in shape, with the tip directed toward the alveolar arch. Three dimensions must be considered when evaluating cleft shape and size: the anterior extension of the palatal cleft, its width, and the length of the soft palate. The extension of the palatal cleft is measured from the uvula to the alveolar arch. Depending on the extension of the cleft, the cleft is described as: partial cleft of the soft palate; complete cleft of the soft palate; complete cleft of the soft palate and partial cleft of the hard palate; and finally, as complete cleft of the soft and hard palate, which extends from the tip of the uvula toward the incisive foramen.

The muscles of the soft palate are divided in the midline so that their orientation is changed from horizontal to oblique and even vertical along the medial margin of the palatal cleft. Because attachment of the muscles to the posterior edge of the hard palate is also abnormal, it must be completely released during the operation to allow for reorientation of the entire muscular complex of the soft palate into a normal horizontal position to create the palatal sling. The width of the cleft in the palate varies in different areas and depends to a great extent on the length of the cleft. In cases where the cleft is limited to the soft palate only, the width may vary between 2 and 10 mm, with the narrower part at the anterior tip of the cleft and the widest part on the level of the uvula. In some cases, the cleft may be narrow enough so that both sides can be sutured together without tension. The separation of the segments of the soft tissue results from the contraction of the muscles of the soft palate. When the cleft enters the hard palate, it narrows toward the tip and becomes wider toward the posterior edge of the soft palate. Division of the musculature of the soft palate causes it to contract, which results in the shortening of both segments of the soft palate.

The length of the soft palate is measured in terms of the distance between its posterior edge and the posterior pharyngeal wall. This dimension is crucial in terms of normal speech production. The length of the palatal cleft, its width, and the length of the soft palate are important factors to consider when planning surgical repair.

The nasal septum is another feature that must be considered when analyzing the anatomy of the cleft palate and planning surgical repair. In complete clefts, the septum is projected at the midline, varying in length and in prominence in relation to the cleft. When the nasal septum is on the same level or very close to the level of the palatal shelves, the mucoperiosteal flaps from the septum may be used to create the nasal layer for closure of the palatal defect. When the lower edge of the nasal septum is higher than the level of the palatal shelves, it may be difficult to incorporate the mucoperiosteal flaps from the septum into the nasal layer of the reconstructed palate.

On extremely rare occasions, the shape of the palatal cleft is somewhat different than usual. With the so-called "horseshoe" shape, the cleft is widest in the area of the hard palate, and narrowest in the portion toward the uvula. This shape, which fortunately is so rare that some surgeons may never observe one in their lifetime, presents an extremely difficult problem for surgical repair due to the paucity of mucoperiosteal flap tissue for closure of the defect. Neither speech pathologists nor surgeons should exaggerate the importance of the "horseshoe" shape of palatal cleft, because it figures so minimally in the overall problem of cleft palate repair. Even more rare than the "horseshoe" shape of palatal cleft is clefting of the hard palate without clefting of the soft palate.

The anatomy of the palatal cleft is relevant when planning and performing surgical procedures. In clefts of the soft palate only, surgeons often falsely assume that this seemingly mild condition of palatal clefting can be easily repaired, with a high expectation of success. This approach is typical for less-experienced clinicians who do not realize that this form of palatal cleft requires serious attention and highly developed surgical skills to obtain a positive result.

Because clefts of the soft palate only may be very narrow and on many occasions may be repaired without raising the mucoperiosteal flaps or releasing the attachment of the muscles of the soft palate from the posterior edge of the hard palate, the repair results in a short and poorly mobile palate with poor speech production. The simplicity of this cleft form may therefore be deceptive.

The problem of the surgical treatment of cleft of the hard and soft palate may present serious difficulties depending on the cleft width and the position of the palatal shelves, which often have a sharp inclination. Also, the position of the lower edge of the vomer may be important in performing surgical repair. It is important to realize that each form of cleft palate only must be evaluated individually to assess all factors that may contribute to successful management in terms of closing the existing palatal cleft and creating adequate conditions for normal speech production.

Unilateral cleft of the palate associated with cleft of the lip and alveolus

The palatal cleft associated with a complete unilateral cleft of the lip and alveolus extends through the entire palate and joins the alveolar cleft. This type of cleft divides the maxillary complex into two uneven segments: the larger maxillary segment, which includes the premaxilla and the larger portion of the lip and palate; and the smaller maxillary segment. The larger maxillary segment, including the premaxilla, may be rotated upward and outward, while the smaller segment may be collapsed both medially and caudally (Fig. 7-1, A-C).

In the majority of cases of unilateral cleft lip, alveolus, and palate, the lower edge of the nasal septum is attached to the margin of the hard palate of the larger maxillary segment. This variation, in contrast to complete cleft of the palate only in which the lower edge of the septum is projected at the midline of the cleft, makes a great difference in planning surgical repair of the palatal cleft. In some cases the attachment of the lower edge of the nasal septum to the palatal edge in the area of the hard palate may be minimal or nonexistent. In these cases, mucoperiosteal flaps from the nasal septum cannot be used to create the nasal layer for closure of the palatal cleft, and a different surgical approach must be considered.

In unilateral palatal cleft, the following factors must be considered when planning surgical repair: extension of the palatal cleft into the alveolar cleft, the width of the palatal cleft, the width and angle of the palatal shelves, and the length of the soft palate. Since the palatal cleft extends into the alveolar cleft, closure of both clefts must be carefully planned.

Some surgeons and orthodontists believe that the alveolar cleft must be left intact to allow for repositioning of the maxillary segments into proper alignment. Only after achieving proper position of the maxillary segments and proper occlusal relationships is closure of the alveolar cleft performed with or without simultaneous bone grafting. On the other hand, some sur-

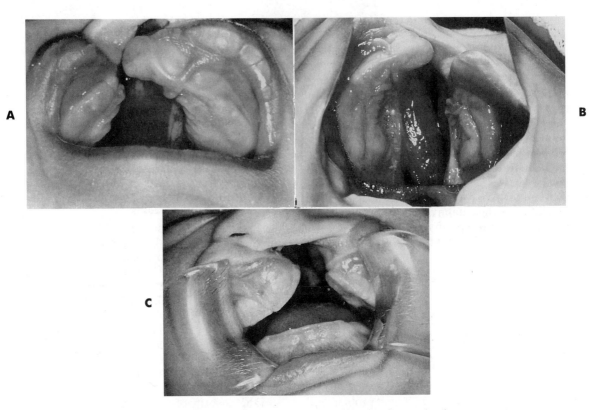

Fig. 7-1 Various forms of unilateral cleft lip, alveolus, and palate.

geons and orthodontists are of the opinion that the alveolar cleft must be closed from the labial side at the time of cleft lip repair, and from the lingual side at the time of cleft palate repair.

A small number of surgeons advocate primary bone grafting of the alveolar cleft at the time of lip repair. In some surgical techniques, closure of the alveolar cleft is performed in two stages. In the first stage, when the cleft lip is repaired, the alveolar cleft is closed in two layers on the vestibular side. In the second stage, when the cleft palate is repaired, the palatal portion of the alveolar cleft is completed. In this way the entire alveolar cleft is closed with mucoperiosteal flaps. Some surgeons advocate repairing the alveolar cleft with simultaneous bone grafting at this early stage. The majority of experienced cleft surgeons, however, strongly oppose this approach since it locks the maxillary segment in a position that may affect the normal maxillary-mandibular relationship and normal occlusion. It is more beneficial to close the alveolar cleft at the time of lip and palate repair while delaying alveolar bone grafting until 7 to 9 years of age.

The width of the palatal cleft is an extremely important factor in planning surgical repair, since very wide clefts are extremely difficult to close. It is important to note, however, that even the widest cleft can almost always be successfully closed with tissue from the palatal shelves and soft palate.

Preoperative evaluation of a patient with wide unilateral or bilateral cleft of the lip, alveolus, and palate serves only to assist in precise planning of the primary cleft lip or cleft lip-nose repair. At the time of this evaluation, no decisions must be made about management of the palatal cleft because of rapid and dramatic changes that occur following primary lip repair. Each specialist involved in the treatment of cleft patients must realize and remember that the conditions change dramatically following primary lip repair. The presence of a wide cleft in an infant often influences less experienced surgeons and orthodontists to believe that surgical repair of the wide palatal cleft is practically impossible and that the use of an obturator is required. This conclusion is based on the erroneous assumption that cleft width remains the same following cleft lip repair. In reality, one has to realize that after primary lip repair, approximation of the maxillary segments occurs as a result of lip tension which leads, in the vast majority of cases, to contact between the edges of the alveolar arches and to marked narrowing of the palatal cleft. For this reason, it is definitely premature to make any decisions about using an obturator in infants with wide clefts instead of proceeding with the accepted approach. The most widely accepted approach includes primary lip repair and creation of the nasal floor at approximately 3 months of age. In follow-up observation, changes are monitored in the positioning and approximation of the maxillary segments. After 3 to 6 months, even in cases of very wide clefts, contact occurs between the edges of the alveolar ridges, and marked reduction is seen in the cleft palate.

The inclination of the palatal shelves is an important factor that must be considered when assessing the width of the palatal cleft. The more vertical the position of the palatal shelves, the wider the palatal cleft will be. When assessing the inclination and width of the palatal cleft, consideration must also be given to the width of the palatal shelves since the mucoperiosteal flaps from the palatal shelves will be used to close the palatal cleft.

The use of an obturator in infants is thought by some to facilitate feeding and the development of speech habits (though this is unproven). However, there is one serious negative aspect: an obturator prevents approximation of the maxillary segments and palatal shelves following cleft lip repair, thus retaining the initial width of the palatal cleft, making palatoplasty extremely difficult at a later age. When choosing between

an obturator and surgical closure of the palatal cleft, the latter decision is always preferable and more beneficial for the patient.

Bilateral cleft of the palate associated with bilateral cleft lip and alveolus

Bilateral cleft of the palate is considered to be the most severe form of palatal cleft. The cleft extends through the entire palate. Anteriorly, there are two clefts from the lip through the posterior edge of the premaxilla, separating the premaxilla from the anterior part of the palate and from the lateral segments of the alveolar arches.

In bilateral clefts, the position of the premaxilla determines the relative ease of treatment. When the premaxilla is positioned within the alveolar arch, closure of the palatal and alveolar clefts can be achieved without presurgical orthodontic treatment and without additional surgery to move the premaxilla into the proper position. When the premaxilla is positioned anteriorly to the lateral segments of the alveolar arch, closure of the palatal cleft as well as closure of the alveolar cleft may be difficult. In this situation, additional surgical intervention may be necessary to reposition the protruding premaxilla, placing it within the alveolar arch to achieve normal occlusion (Fig. 7-2, A-B).

Managing the protruding premaxilla requires a complex surgical-orthodontic approach that must be properly planned, timed, and executed. At the Cleft Palate Center at the University of Iowa, surgical-orthodontic treatment was estab-

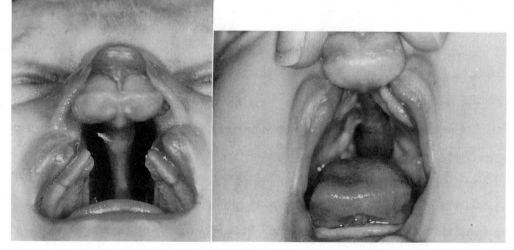

Fig. 7-2 Various forms of bilateral cleft of the lip, alveolus, and palate with severely protruding premaxilla. **A,** Note nasal septum in the midline and a wide distance between the maxillary segments and nasal septum. **B,** Premaxilla protrudes in front of the collapsed maxillary segments, which approximate the nasal septum behind the premaxilla.

lished and carried out by Bardach and Olin. The basic philosophy for the established protocol was to avoid interference with facial and maxillary growth until 6 years of age. The protruding premaxilla as well as the entire facial skeleton were allowed unrestricted growth, which often resulted in an unappealing appearance in children affected by severely protruding premaxillas. The authors believed that allowing unrestricted growth until the age of 6 created a normal growth pattern that would continue even with surgical intervention aimed at repositioning the premaxilla at a later age.

The arbitrarily established timing for surgical repositioning of the premaxilla is based on the desire to change a child's appearance before entering school. The surgical procedure that places and secures the protruding premaxilla in the optimal position within the aveolar arch is performed simultaneously with closure of oronasal and nasolabial fistulas, as well as with cancellous bone grafting. Long-term observations of patients treated at the Iowa Cleft Palate Center demonstrate that this approach does not interfere with normal maxillofacial growth, and in most cases allows for the achievement of proper occlusion.

In bilateral clefts, the lower edge of the nasal septum is usually positioned at the midline. The palatal defect may then be closed using the mucoperiosteal flaps from the septum, a technique that will be described in detail later in this chapter. In this type of cleft, the soft palate is usually short. Because the width of bilateral clefts vary, the position of the lower edge of the nasal septum greatly influences palatal closure. When the lower edge of the septum is on the same level as the palatal shelves, closure can be easily achieved because the mucoperiosteal flaps from the nasal septum can be used to construct the nasal layer and the mucoperiosteal flaps from the palatal shelves can be approximated medially to close the cleft.

The situation is different when the lower edge of the nasal septum is positioned above the level of the palatal shelves. Then the mucoperiosteal flaps from the septum cannot be incorporated into the construction of the nasal layer. In this case, it is necessary to create a nasal layer from the mucoperiosteal flaps of both palatal shelves. In some instances of extremely wide bilateral clefts, additional maneuvers may be required to achieve closure without tension.

TIMING OF CLEFT PALATE REPAIR

Cleft palate requires multidisciplinary treatment in which both surgeons and speech pathologists are primarily involved. The surgeon evaluates the patient and plans surgical treatment in all cases of cleft palate. The speech pathologist diagnoses speech disorders and when necessary, conducts preoperative and/or postoperative speech evaluation. In cases of unilateral and bilateral cleft lip, alveolus, and palate, the treatment team may also include orthodontists, otolaryngologists, audiologists, and psychologists, among others.

A variety of opinions are held regarding the timing of cleft palate repair. Controversies among surgeons, orthodontists, and speech pathologists are related to the timing of palatoplasty and the influence of this procedure on speech and maxillofacial growth. To understand these controversies, it is helpful to discuss the reasoning behind them. The different clinical objectives of the specialists involved in cleft palate treatment dictate different timing of palatoplasty for optimal results, and this is the source of conflict involved in the timing of surgical repair.

The goal of speech pathologists is to obtain normal speech production following cleft palate repair. On the other hand, plastic surgeons, although concerned with speech, are primarily concerned with complete closure of the palatal cleft, the creation of an adequately functioning soft palate, and the influence of their surgical technique on the growth of the maxillary complex (Fig. 7-3 A&B). Orthodontists are interested in securing undisturbed maxillofacial growth and normal occlusion. At the present time, there is no established protocol for the timing of palate repair that is universally and unconditionally accepted by all three specialties.

Even within each specialty, opinions vary regarding the timing of palate repair. Some speech pathologists believe that the earlier the palate repair is performed, the better speech production will be. Dorf and Curtin studied the speech results following cleft palate repair at approximately 6 months of age, and concluded that speech development in these children progresses better than in those in whom cleft palate repair was performed at a later age. Morris also has found that early palate repair is more beneficial for speech development than repair at a later age. At the same time, a large number of speech pathologists question the validity of early surgical repair of the palatal cleft, and suggest that cleft repair performed at 12 to 24 months of age also creates optimal conditions for normal speech production in the vast majority of cases.

Speech pathologists who express dismay about early cleft palate repair are influenced by

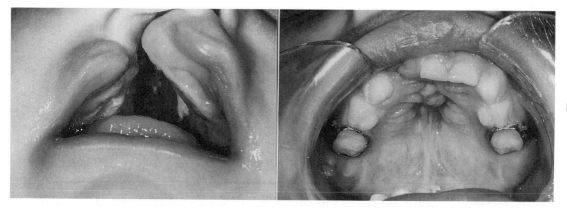

Fig. 7-3 A, Unilateral complete cleft of the lip, alveolus, and palate. **B,** following cleft lip repair and one-stage two-flap palatoplasty. Note complete closure of the palatal cleft and normal configuration of the palate and alveolar arch.

the widespread belief that early palate repair inevitably results in maxillary growth aberrations with subsequent secondary maxillofacial deformities. Since there are many controversies and misconceptions related to the influence of cleft palate repair on maxillofacial growth, this subject will be discussed in detail later in the chapter. Here is it sufficient to mention that the widespread opinion that cleft palate repair is the primary cause of maxillofacial growth aberrations has no solid scientific, experimental, or clinical basis.

Appropriately selected surgical procedures for cleft palate repair as well as properly and delicately executed techniques will assure complete closure of the palatal defect and the creation of an adequately functioning soft palate, without detrimental effects on maxillofacial growth. It is important to realize that opinions accepted in the past concerning the detrimental influence of cleft palate repair on maxillofacial growth may no longer be valid.

In addition to close cooperation between plastic surgeons and orthodontists, active participation of orthodontists in the multidisciplinary treatment of cleft lip and palate significantly decreases the possibility of severe secondary maxillofacial deformity and malocclusion. Constant monitoring of facial growth and occlusion by orthodontists allows for intervention at any stage of treatment and rehabilitation if there is any sign of growth disturbance or malocclusion.

It is reasonable to assume that the earlier the cleft palate is repaired and the muscles of the soft palate are joined and begin to function appropriately, the better the condition for the development of normal speech. Reconstructive surgery that eliminates the palatal cleft estab-

lishes more normal anatomical conditions, restores the functioning of the soft palate, and enhances development of normal speech at an early age.

Early surgery must be differentiated depending on the type and severity of the palatal cleft. When we discuss early surgery, it must be emphasized that we do not consider it necessary to perform palatoplasty earlier than 6 to 9 months of age. According to our investigations, in cases of unilateral and bilateral cleft lip and palate, cleft palate repair is more successful when performed after cleft lip repair. Clefts of the soft palate only can be successfully closed at 6 to 9 months of age without worrying about facial growth aberrations as a result of the surgical procedure. In the case of complete palatal cleft only, that is, cleft of the soft and hard palate reaching the incisive foramen with the alveolar arch and lip intact, we usually close the cleft at 9 to 12 months of age. We often repair palatal clefts associated with unilateral or bilateral clefts of the lip and alveolus at 12 to 18 months of age, with unique cases repaired at a later age.

This differentiation in timing has evolved from our clinical observations and from the results of our clinical studies that evaluate the efficiency of surgical treatment in relation to speech production. According to our studies, following this timing schedule for surgical repair of all types of palatal cleft allowed us to obtain 75 to 80% of normal speech production. These results were obtained at the Cleft Palate Center at the University of Iowa following the two-flap palatoplasty technique, which will be described later in this chapter. Our data indicates that 75 to 80% of cleft palate patients in our institution do not require secondary surgical intervention in the form of pharyngoplasty or pharyngeal flap. It also indicates that the timing of cleft palate repair followed in our institution results in highly satisfactory speech production. However, it should be added that the timing of surgery must be evaluated along with two other important factors that influence the result of surgical repair: surgical technique and the proficiency of the surgeon. These factors will be discussed later in the chapter.

SURGICAL EVALUATION OF PATIENTS WITH CLEFT PALATE

All patients with cleft palate must have surgical treatment; however, not all require speech rehabilitation. Treatment is applied only to patients demonstrating postsurgical speech problems. Cooperation between the surgeon and speech pathologist is crucial to achieving the primary goal of cleft palate repair, i.e., normal speech development. Evaluation of patients by both specialists and discussion of the findings is helpful in planning the timing of the cleft palate repair, the timing of speech therapy, and the technical aspects of cleft palate repair or pharyngoplasty.

The cooperation of an orthodontist is required when occlusal malformations or missing teeth may affect speech production. Children with cleft palate also require careful evaluation by otolaryngologists and audiologists, since many problems of middle ear effusion are related to the presence of cleft palate. Each specialist evaluates the patient to assess the conditions that are important within his or her specialty, while keeping in mind specific treatment techniques.

In surgical evaluation, various factors must be considered in designing a comprehensive treatment plan appropriate to the type and severity of the cleft. Among the factors that must be considered by surgeons, the following seem to be most important:

1. Type of cleft palate
2. Severity of cleft palate
3. Position of the maxillary segments
4. Position of the premaxilla and nasal septum
5. Width of cleft
6. Width of the palatal shelves
7. Inclination of the palatal shelves
8. Length of the soft palate
9. Symmetry of the soft palate
10. Mobility of the soft palate
11. Mobility of the posterior and lateral pharyngeal walls

Although these factors are of primary importance to surgeons, speech pathologists should also be familiar with them since the surgical techniques chosen for the specific palatal cleft will determine the outcome in terms of speech.

Type of cleft palate

Ranking cleft palates from the mildest to the most severe, submucous cleft of the soft palate is the least complicated form. This cleft presents a condition in which the muscles of the soft palate are partially or completely divided at the midline while the oral and nasal mucosa remain intact. Submucous cleft may not be clinically evident, depending on the extent of the cleft as well as other factors such as mobility of the soft palate, mobility of the lateral pharyngeal walls, and the presence of a Passavant's ridge. A more detailed description of the submucous cleft was presented earlier in this chapter.

Another mild expression of palatal cleft is cleft of the uvula only, which may or may not affect speech production. Further extension of the cleft into the soft palate almost always occurs at the midline and may involve part of or the entire length of the soft palate. Commonly, a complete cleft of the soft palate extends partially into the posterior edge of the hard palate; in these cases the posterior nasal spine is absent. Further extension of the cleft into the hard palate may involve part or all of the hard palate up to the incisive foramen. It is important to remember that embryologically, cleft palate originates separately from the cleft lip and alveolus and that the dividing point runs across the incisive foramen.

The most severe forms of cleft palate are associated with unilateral and bilateral cleft of the lip and alveolus. Unilateral cleft palate associated with cleft lip and alveolus may present a multitude of forms due to these factors: various positions of the maxillary segments; cleft width, length, and symmetry; mobility of the soft palate; inclination of the palatal shelves; and the position of the nasal septum and its relationship to the palatal shelf. Combined with other anatomical and functional conditions related to the lateral and posterior pharyngeal walls, these factors are essential to planning surgical repair to close the palatal cleft. In bilateral palatal clefts associated with cleft lip and alveolus, the position of the premaxilla and nasal septum may determine the surgical approach. There is no question that the type of cleft plays an important role in planning surgical treatment.

Severity of the cleft palate

The severity of the cleft palate must be evaluated from two standpoints: the surgeon must examine the palatal cleft to determine the extent of the morphological and functional changes and note any technical problems that may be encountered at the time of cleft palate repair.

Morphological changes depend on cleft form, which can be described as mild, moderate, and severe. Severity depends on several factors; most importantly, the extent and shape of the cleft. Mild forms of cleft palate include cleft of the uvula, submucous cleft, and partial cleft of the soft palate. Moderate palatal clefts involve complete cleft of the soft palate with partial cleft of the hard palate, and some forms of complete cleft of the soft and hard palate.

Additional factors that must also be considered when evaluating the severity of the cleft palate only include cleft width, inclination of the palatal shelves, the position of the vomer, and the mobility and length of the segments of the soft palate. In unilateral and bilateral complete clefts of the lip, alveolus, and palate, several other factors must be evaluated when planning surgical repair. The position of the maxillary segments plays an important role in determining the asymmetry of the maxillary segments, the inclination of the palatal shelves, the position of the vomer, and asymmetry of the segments of the soft palate. An asymmetrical palate presents a more difficult problem for repair than a symmetrical one. However, symmetry usually occurs in all forms of cleft palate only, and in some cases of bilateral cleft.

Determining the severity of the cleft is most important when choosing the surgical procedure as well as when deciding whether the surgeon who intends to perform the cleft palate repair is competent enough to achieve a successful outcome. When surgeons with limited experience are faced with a severe palatal cleft, they must be prudent when deciding whether to undertake surgical repair. It is more ethical to refer the patient to a more experienced surgeon than to jeopardize successful rehabilitation. It must be emphasized that primary palate repair provides unique and optimal conditions for a successful outcome, while every secondary operation on the palate is more and more difficult to perform, and the potential for success is less and less probable (Fig. 7-4, A-B).

Position of the maxillary segments

In unilateral clefts, the maxillary complex is divided into two uneven and asymmetrical segments. The larger segment includes the premaxilla, a major portion of the lip and alveolus, and the larger palatal shelf, which may be joined with the lower edge of the vomer. This segment may be rotated outward and upward due to large muscle forces influencing the segment. The smaller segment includes the narrower portion of the palatal shelf, a shorter alveolar arch, and a shorter portion of the lip. This segment may be rotated medially and backward. Collapse of this segment may occur

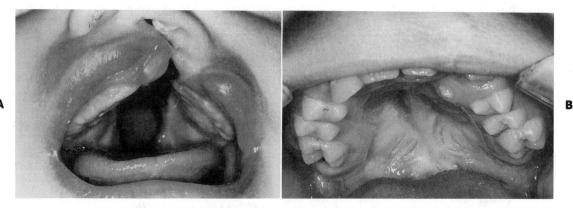

A   **B**

Fig. 7-4 A, Unilateral complete cleft of the lip, alveolus, and palate. Note that the palatal cleft is very wide, primarily due to the vertical position of the palatal shelf on the noncleft side. The large maxillary segment is rotated upward and outward. The lesser maxillary segment is collapsed, which determines the position of the alar base on a different level than on the opposite side. **B,** After one-stage two-flap palatoplasty, complete closure of the palatal and alveolar cleft. The cleft lip was previously repaired. Note normal configuration of the palate and alveolar arch.

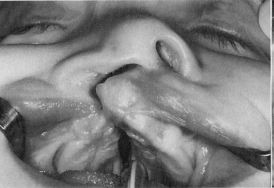

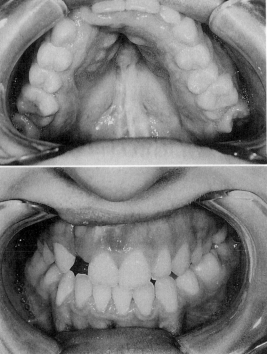

Fig. 7-5 A, Unilateral complete cleft of the lip, alveolus, and palate with severe collapse of the lesser maxillary segment and the premaxilla rotated upward and outward. **B,** After closure of the lip at 3 months of age and two-flap palatoplasty at 12 months of age. Note complete closure of the palatal cleft with normal configuration of the palate and alveolar arch. **C,** Occlusion before orthodontic treatment. Note repair of the alveolar cleft. There is a distortion in the midline position of the central incisors.

spontaneously or as the result of tight lip repair. The position of the maxillary segments in unilateral complete cleft is an important factor in planning closure of the maxillary and alveolar clefts, especially in cases where the segments of the soft palate are asymmetrical and the smaller segment is collapsed (Fig. 7-5, A-C).

In bilateral complete cleft of the lip, alveolus, and palate, the positions of the premaxilla and the vomer between the maxillary segments are important factors that must be taken into account in surgical evaluation. A detailed description of this problem is presented later in this chapter.

Position of the premaxilla and nasal septum

In bilateral complete cleft of the lip, alveolus, and palate, the premaxilla is isolated from both maxillary segments and remains attached only to the vomer. The position of the premaxilla varies: it may protrude in front of both maxillary segments; it may be positioned within the maxillary segments; or it may be positioned behind the alveolar arches. When the premaxilla protrudes in front of the maxillary segments, closure of the anterior portion of the palatal cleft may present serious difficulty, and in the vast majority of cases, the alveolar clefts and the

anterior position of the palatal cleft will remain open until the premaxilla is placed within the alveolar arch.

Some surgeons and orthodontists give preference to presurgical orthopedic treatment, which allows for the repositioning of the premaxilla within the alveolar arch or just in front of it. This treatment is usually performed before lip repair, and definitely before cleft palate repair. However, many surgeons and orthodontists object to presurgical orthopedic treatment because of uncertainty about the degree to which the maxillary segment may expand before causing serious disturbances in the occlusal relationship. This group of specialists advocates unrestricted growth of the premaxilla and the entire maxillofacial skeleton until 6 or 7 years of age when surgical retropositioning of the premaxilla is performed.

Width of the palatal cleft

When planning surgical repair, assessment of the palatal cleft width must be considered as one of the most important factors in choosing the appropriate management technique. This is especially true in complete unilateral and bilateral cleft of the lip, alveolus, and palate. The width of the palatal cleft is in direct relationship to the inclination of the palatal shelves. The more vertical the inclination, the wider the palatal cleft.

It is important to realize that the examination and assessment of the palatal cleft before lip repair cannot serve as the basis for planning surgical management of the cleft palate, or for prediction of speech problems. As was mentioned previously, each specialist participating in the treatment of children with clefts and especially the surgeons, speech pathologists, and orthodontists, must realize that the width of the cleft palate and the positioning of the maxillary segments will change following cleft lip repair. This change can be observed within 3 to 6 months after cleft lip repair as close approximation of the maxillary segments, particularly in the area of the alveolar processes, and in narrowing of the palatal cleft.

In cases of initial asymmetry of the palatal cleft, more symmetrical conditions of the palatal structures may become evident. To less experienced surgeons, a wide palatal cleft may seem to be the main obstacle preventing the successful outcome of surgery. Although surgical difficulty increases with wider clefts, an experienced surgeon should be able to completely close the existing cleft.

The major problem faced by surgeons when attempting repair of wide palatal clefts is excessive tension that occurs when closing the nasal or oral layer or both. This excessive tension results from incorrect design of the mucoperiosteal flaps for the nasal and oral layers, inadequate release and mobilization of the mucoperiosteal flaps, or inadequate approximation and stabilization of the oral and nasal layers.

All of this amounts to flaws in surgical technique, which may lead to impairment of the healing process, usually resulting in partial dehiscence and oronasal fistulae. Skillful and careful surgical techniques applied by an experienced surgeon allow for tension-free closure of the entire cleft with special attention paid to closure of the anterior portion of the hard palate and to close approximation of the oral and nasal layers. A wide palatal cleft can be closed using appropriate surgical techniques supplemented by experience.

Closure of moderate and narrow palatal clefts presents fewer difficulties than closure of wide clefts since ample tissue is available to close the gap. The most common complication in repairing palatal clefts lies in the development of oronasal fistulae. To prevent the development of fistulae, the undermining and transposition of

mucoperiosteal flaps must be carefully performed so that tension-free closure can be easily achieved.

Secondary surgery of the palate to close the fistula is always more difficult and causes more bleeding due to scar tissue between the mucoperiosteal flaps and underlying bone.

Width of the palatal shelves

The width of the palatal cleft is directly related to the width of the mucoperiosteal flaps needed for closure. Because mucoperiosteal flaps are raised from the palatal shelves, it is important to assess palatal shelf width before surgery and the possibility of using them to create mucoperiosteal flaps of adequate width. This problem is especially relevant in cases of complete unilateral and bilateral clefts of the lip, alveolus, and palate. In unilateral complete clefts, the width of the palatal shelves is uneven; the larger maxillary segment has a wide palatal shelf while that of the smaller maxillary segment is narrow. For this reason, in unilateral complete clefts, the width of the raised mucoperiosteal flaps is uneven, a fact that must be taken into consideration when planning and performing closure of the palatal cleft.

Inclination of the palatal shelves

Although the inclination of the palatal shelves plays a major role in many cleft forms, this factor is especially important in complete cleft of the palate only and in complete unilateral and bilateral clefts of the lip, alveolus, and palate. The position of the palatal shelves is seldom flat, occuring only in cases of cleft of the soft palate only. In all other cases of cleft palate, the palatal shelves are somewhat angular; the more vertical the inclination of the palatal shelves, the wider the cleft palate.

It is quite common, especially in unilateral complete clefts, for the angle of inclination to be different on each side. Usually, the palatal shelf on the smaller maxillary segment is more vertically positioned than its counterpart. Following surgical repair of the cleft, the inclination of the palatal shelves changes, becoming more horizontal. In contrast, when an obturator is even temporarily used to close a cleft, the inclination of the palatal shelves remains in the same position, and the width of the palatal cleft does not decrease.

Length of the soft palate

The length of the soft palate is an important feature related to speech production. Several surgical procedures aim at lengthening the soft palate in order to obtain velopharyngeal closure, resulting in improved speech. Since Dorrance's push-back palatoplasty, many surgeons have attempted to approximate the soft palate to the posterior pharyngeal wall. The Wardill-Kilner three-and four-flap palatoplasty is based on the concept of the push-back technique. Furlow double-reversing Z-plasty aims to lengthen the soft palate. Some surgical techniques, however, make no attempt to lengthen or approximate the soft palate to the posterior pharyngeal wall. For example, the von Langenbeck palatoplasty technique does not include lengthening of the soft palate, nor does our two-flap palatoplasty technique. Both of these surgical procedures are considered to be as effective as those in which the soft palate is lengthened.

Symmetry of the soft palate

In all forms of cleft palate only, both segments of the soft palate are symmetrical. Asymmetry of the soft palate usually occurs in cases of unilateral complete cleft of the lip, alveolus, and palate, with malpositioning of the maxillary segments. When one segment of the soft palate is longer than the other, it may be difficult to adjust both sides to equal lengths. On some occasions, the shorter segment of the soft palate can be lengthened by using an angular incision, which opens a gap and lengthens the side of the soft palate. Asymmetry of the soft palate must be assessed before surgery to plan for proper adjustment of the soft palate as well as undermining of the mucoperiosteal flaps from the hard palate.

Mobility of the soft palate

The mobility of the soft palate plays an important role in speech production. A long, immobile soft palate may not be adequate to secure velopharyngeal competence. The development of the muscles of the soft palate may be impaired, especially in cases of complete unilateral and bilateral clefts. It is also true that the longer the cleft palate remains unrepaired, the more impaired muscle function of the soft palate will be. Early closure of the soft palate stimulates better and more coordinated function, and in all probability contributes more to normal speech production than when the palate is closed at a later age. My concept of the functioning of the soft palate is related primarily to its mobility rather than its length.

Posterior and lateral pharyngeal walls

The posterior pharyngeal wall must be evaluated in terms of its relationship to the posterior edge of the soft palate and in terms of its ability to create a Passavant's ridge. Both aspects are important when considering velopharyngeal closure. They are also important when considering pharyngoplasty after palatoplasty has failed to produce the conditions for normal speech.

Good lateral pharyngeal wall movement may compensate for other impairments such as a short palate or the absence of the Passavant's ridge, and may contribute greatly to normal speech production. For this reason, careful evaluation of the posterior and lateral pharyngeal walls, especially in action, is very important when planning and performing cleft palate surgery.

PRESURGICAL ORTHOPEDIC TREATMENT

Many surgeons and orthodontists advocate presurgical orthopedic treatment as preparation for cleft lip and palate repair. In unilateral complete clefts, the larger, malpositioned maxillary segment is usually rotated outward and laterally, while the smaller malpositioned maxillary segment is rotated downward and medially. Malpositioning of the maxillary segments results in deformity of the alveolar arches and asymmetry of the hard and soft palates. In addition, collapse of the smaller maxillary segment contributes to severe nasal distortion due to displacement of the base of the ala on the cleft side.

Displacement of the base of the ala, which is usually directed backward, downward, and laterally, presents a difficult problem for surgical correction if the skeletal base remains asymmetrical and uneven as compared to the opposite side. Presurgical orthopedic treatment is designed to alleviate these problems by repositioning the maxillary segments in a more normal position and by approximating them, thereby narrowing the cleft and creating a better skeletal base for nasal reconstruction. Narrowing the cleft and improving the position of the maxillary segments can contribute to a more successful cleft lip repair.

There are two approaches that must be distinguished when applying presurgical orthopedic treatment: passive and active. According to Salyer, in passive treatment, the appliance consists of a plate that covers the palatal cleft and alters the position of the maxillary segments. This plate also protects the nasal septum during feeding. In active treatment, the appliance is designed to expand or retract the palate, depending on the position of the maxillary segments and the shape of the alveolar arch. Direct force is exerted, using pins or screws to secure the appliance in the hard palate, which move the segments into the desired positions. Some cleft palate centers use presurgical orthopedic treatment as an integral part of the multidisciplinary management of clefts. Surgeons and orthodontists in Zurich (Hotz, Gnoinski, Perko) and Dallas (Salyer, Genecov) as well as others advocate presurgical orthopedic treatment for the following reasons:

1. Proper alignment of the maxillary segments facilitates primary lip-nose repair
2. An improved position and symmetry of the skeletal base facilitates correction of primary and secondary nasal deformities associated with unilateral and bilateral clefts
3. An improved position of the skeletal base creates a more symmetrical and balanced condition for growth and development of the midfacial skeleton.

Although many surgeons and orthodontists use presurgical orthopedic treatment in cases of unilateral complete cleft of the lip, alveolus, and palate, there is evidence that similar results can be achieved without this type of management. The final results related to lip repair, palate repair, and growth of the midfacial complex achieved with presurgical orthopedic treatment are very similar to the results achieved without it.

The use of presurgical orthopedic treatment in bilateral clefts is more complex than in unilateral clefts because of the protruding premaxilla. Although advocates claim that a variety of appliances improve the position of a protruding premaxilla by pushing it back into place within the alveolar arches, these appliances have drawbacks. Devices that exert pressure on the premaxilla bend the premaxilla back and also move it downward, which creates additional problems for proper repositioning and distorts the shape of the premaxilla.

Appliances that are pinned into the palate effectively reposition the protruding premaxilla as well as expand the maxillary segments, but they do not always maintain a proper relationship between the shape of the alveolar arch of the maxilla and the mandible, which may later result in poor occlusion. There is little agreement among specialists as to which appliance is the most appropriate for presurgical orthopedic treatment in bilateral clefts with a protruding premaxilla.

In addition, a large group of surgeons and orthodontists deny the need for presurgical orthopedic treatment. These specialists permit unrestrained growth and the development of the maxillary segments and protruding premaxilla until the age of 6 or 7 years when surgical repositioning of the premaxilla is performed, along with closure of oronasal and nasolabial fistulas and bilateral bone grafting. In some centers, this approach has proved to be successful, as indicated in studies by Bardach and Olin at the Iowa Cleft Palate Center.

In very wide horseshoe-shaped palatal clefts, repair is more difficult because of a paucity of mucoperiosteal flap tissue. In these cases obturators may be applied. Unfortunately, obturators used over a long period of time retain the initial size of the cleft and the position of the palatal shelves, thus creating great difficulty in closing this cleft at a later age. Closure of a wide horseshoe-shaped palatal cleft may require a combination of mucoperiosteal flaps and a primary pharyngeal flap.

PRINCIPLES OF CLEFT PALATE REPAIR

At the present time, there are probably as many surgeons, speech pathologists, and orthodontists who advocate one-stage cleft palate repair as there are who advocate two-stage palatoplasty. Two stage palatoplasty here refers to repairing the velum first, leaving the hard palate unrepaired until a later date, ranging from several months to several years. The aim of one-stage palatoplasty is simple and straightforward: complete closure of the palatal cleft to create adequate conditions for normal speech. In the multidisciplinary treatment, advocates of one-stage palatoplasty are not concerned with the malpositioning of the maxillary segments nor with malocclusion since these problems can be corrected with proper postsurgical orthodontic treatment. Many speech pathologists (Morris, Shprintzen, Witzel, and others.) report more favorable speech results following one-stage palatoplasty than following the two-stage approach.

Advocates of two-stage palatoplasty, a concept presented by Schweckendiek in the late 1930s and early 1940s, prefer this approach because it was designed to achieve two goals simultaneously: the creation of a functional soft palate and unrestricted maxillary growth. According to this concept, which will be described in detail later in this chapter, primary soft palate repair is performed along with cleft lip repair at 6 months of age. The hard palate is not repaired until later so that its growth is unrestricted, which allows for proper positioning of the maxillary segments and the development of normal occlusion, thus preventing severe secondary maxillofacial deformities. Closure of the hard palate is performed at various ages, although according to Schweckendiek, the most appropriate timing is between 12 and 16 years of age. This technique is applied in complete clefts of the lip, alveolus, and palate, as well as in cleft palate only when it involves the hard and soft palate. I prefer one-stage palatoplasty since it closes the hard palate during primary repair, bypassing the need for secondary surgery, and achieves successful results. Other negative aspects of two-stage palatoplasty will be presented later in the chapter.

Goals of two-flap palatoplasty

Surgeons choose their techniques for cleft palate repair according to principles they have established based on experience. The diverse principles held by surgeons result in many different surgical techniques used for closure of the palatal cleft. Since there are few comparative studies and little information on the validity of particular surgical techniques, it seems practical to present the principles and surgical technique which, in my experience, results in complete closure of the palatal cleft and successful speech production. Through years of experience in the multidisciplinary management of cleft patients, and especially in the surgical treatment of clefts, I have established a set of principles as guidelines for the surgical treatment of cleft palate. Two-flap palatoplasty is the technique I developed based on these principles.

In two-flap palatoplasty, cleft palate repair is performed for two primary reasons:

1. To completely close the existing palatal cleft
2. To construct an adequately functioning soft palate

These two goals prevail during the entire program of surgical cleft palate treatment. Primary surgery offers the best conditions for successfully closing the cleft palate because the mucoperiosteal flaps can easily be undermined from the oral and nasal sides of the hard palate, and the soft palate can be dissected to allow for intravelar veloplasty. This procedure is important because by performing intravelar veloplasty, the muscles of the soft palate are redirected from the abnormal oblique and vertical position into a horizontal position that allows for normal functioning of the soft palate. Also, creation of the muscle sling by changing the position of the muscles results in lengthening of the soft palate, which may enhance velopharyngeal closure.

When planning surgical repair of the palatal cleft it is important to employ a surgical technique that will allow for complete two-layer closure of the hard palate and proper recon-struction of the soft palate. One cannot expect successful speech results when complete closure of the cleft is not achieved. The two-layer technique ensures complete and secure closure of the hard palate. The soft palate is closed in three layers: nasal mucosa, muscles, and oral mucosa.

It is important to maintain close approximation of the oral and nasal layers to avoid creating dead space between the mucoperiosteal flaps. In this dead space, blood can easily gather, creating a clot and thereby preventing normal healing. By implementing two-layer closure where both layers are in contact with each other through the entire length of the hard palate, repair is reinforced and has greater chances for success. When the amount of tissue on the oral and nasal sides seems inadequate to bridge the gap, such as in cases of complete wide clefts, a specially designed incision must be used to create mucoperiosteal flaps that will be sufficient enough to suture together without tension.

Another technique that may be employed when two-layer closure proves to be difficult involves the incorporation of the mucoperiosteal flaps from the vomer to create part of the layer on the nasal side. In many cases of unilateral complete cleft of the lip, alveolus, and palate, the vomer is attached to the palatal shelf on the noncleft side. The mucoperiosteal flap raised from the vomer is sutured to the raised mucoperiosteal flap on the nasal side of the smaller maxillary segment, thereby creating the nasal layer. In bilateral clefts, the mucoperiosteal flaps from the vomer help to create the nasal layer on both sides of the vomer, allowing for complete closure and successful healing.

To ensure complete closure of the hard palate, it is necessary to raise and approximate the mucoperiosteal flaps without tension along the entire palatal cleft. To relax the mucoperiosteal flaps on both the oral and nasal sides, flap incisions must be specially designed so that tissue can be borrowed from the oral layer and added to the nasal layer. This increases the width of the mucoperiosteal flaps on the nasal side while decreasing the width of the mucoperiosteal flaps on the oral side. The narrower flaps on the oral side can then be approximated and sutured together to close the palatal cleft.

The surgeon must pay special attention to completely close the cleft in the anterior portion of the palate, an area susceptible to the development of oronasal fistulae. This is probably the most difficult task of the operation. The mucoperiosteal flaps in the area immediately posterior to the hard palate must also be relaxed because excessive tension may impede healing and also cause dehiscence resulting in oronasal fistulae. In cases of bilateral cleft with a protruding premaxilla, oronasal fistulae are left open in the anterior portion of the palate to facilitate repositioning of the premaxilla at a later age. In each case our goal is to provide a sufficient amount of tissue for tension-free closure of nasal and oral layers in the hard palate and the entire soft palate to secure proper healing and avoid oronasal fistulae. This approach is typical for two-flap palatoplasty. At the same time, the surgeon must be careful not to leave large areas of bone exposed following the transposition of mucoperiosteal flaps for palatal closure.

Lengthening of the soft palate

Some surgical techniques aim to lengthen the soft palate, the reasoning being that a sufficiently long soft palate is fundamental to normal speech production. The Wardill-Kilner pushback technique of three or four-flap palatoplasty may be employed to achieve this effect. In this approach, the surgeon raises and repositions the mucoperiosteal flaps, leaving two triangular areas of bone exposed in the anterior portion of the palate (Fig. 7-6, A-D).

This technique is based on the assumption that the mere retropositioning of the mucoperiosteal flaps will permanently lengthen the soft palate. In reality, this lengthening is only effec-

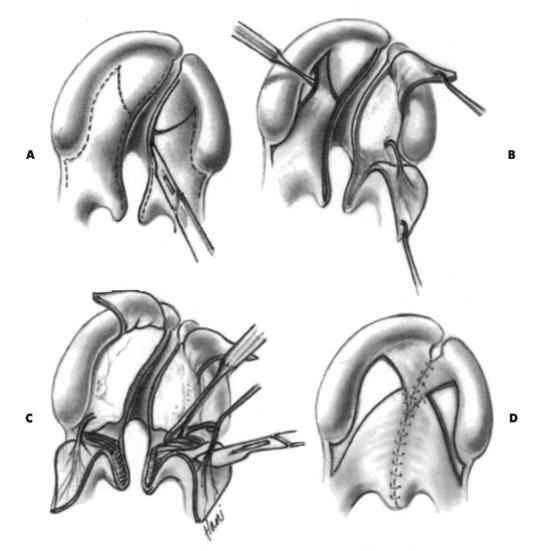

Fig. 7-6 Wardill-Kilner four-flap pushback palatoplasty. **A,** Design of the four flaps. **B,** Elevation of mucoperiosteal flaps. **C,** Releasing muscle attachments of the soft palate from the posterior edge of the hard palate. **D,** Closure of the palatal cleft with pushback of the posterior flaps. Note two large triangular areas of exposed bare bone. Closure of the anterior palate is incomplete.

tive for a short period of time. Because the nasal mucoperiosteum is not retropositioned to the same degree as on the oral side, postoperative contraction occurs over several weeks and returns the soft palate to its approximate length before surgery.

For this technique to be successful, the mucoperiosteum on the nasal side must also be dissected from the posterior edges of the hard palate so that both sides of the soft palate are retropositioned to the same degree. However, detaching the nasal mucoperiosteum from the posterior edge of the hard palate creates a diamond-shaped defect on the nasal side because there is not enough mucosa to cover the raw surface left by the transposed mucoperiosteal flaps. Although this raw area helps to lengthen the soft palate during surgery, it heals by secondary intention, causing scar contracture, which pulls the soft palate forward and shortens it again after some period of time. Simply put, the Wardill-Kilner technique does not adequately lengthen the soft palate as is expected by surgical design. By leaving areas of bone exposed in the anterior portion of the palate, this technique creates conditions for secondary scar contracture and the possibility of subsequent maxillary growth aberrations.

Another disadvantage of the Wardill-Kilner pushback technique is the creation of oronasal fistulae in the anterior portion of the palate and quite frequently, on the border between the hard and soft palate. Since the surface of the nasal layer is raw in this area, single layer closure employed in the Wardill-Kilner technique is not sufficient. Oronasal fistulae that cause distorted speech production require secondary closure, which may be difficult in the anterior portion of the palate. For this reason, techniques that attempt to lengthen the soft palate by repositioning the mucoperiosteal flaps on the oral side and in turn neglect the presence of the oronasal fistulae in the anterior palate do not contribute to speech rehabilitation nor to complete closure of the palatal cleft.

Furlow technique

In 1978 Furlow introduced a new technique for reconstruction of the soft palate with simultaneous lengthening. His double-opposing Z-plasty technique of soft palate repair lengthens the palate and reorients the muscles to produce a functional muscle sling. This is combined with minimal undermining of the hard palate mucoperiosteum, thus reducing the potential for detrimental effects of raising mucoperiosteal flaps on facial growth. Furlow performs this

operation without relaxing incisions. He undermines the medial edges of the mucoperiosteum on the hard palate to create less tension during closure. La Rossa, who modified this operation, indicates improved speech results and points out the following advantages of the Furlow procedure:

1. Lengthening of the soft palate without hard palate mucoperiosteal lengthening flaps
2. Reduced dissection and trauma to the palatal muscles by maintaining their attachment to the mucosa on at least one surface
3. Reorientation of the palatal musculature to a more anatomically correct position, thereby reconstructing the "levator sling"
4. Closure of the soft palate without a straight midline scar
5. Reduced chance of fistulae
6. Improved speech results

The potential disadvantages are as follows:
1. Probable increased operative time
2. Possible increase in scarring
3. Possible increased incidence of posterior crossbite

The use of Furlow double Z-plasty to lengthen the soft palate must be critically evaluated because this procedure, which definitely results in lengthening of the soft palate, also creates tension in the horizontal dimension resulting in narrowing of the posterior segments of the maxilla and subsequent posterior crossbite. This surgery is also technically more difficult than routine straightline closure of the soft palate. In our opinion, the percentage of fistulae remains high and speech results do not seem to be any better than those achieved with two-flap palatoplasty.

Alveolar bone grafting

In many cases of complete unilateral and bilateral cleft of the lip, alveolus, and palate, alveolar clefting presents an additional problem. The question arises whether to close the alveolar cleft at the time of primary lip repair or at the time of cleft palate repair. Surgeons and orthodontists also must decide whether or not to use alveolar bone grafting. I strongly discourage bone grafting at an early age because it locks the maxillary segments in positions that may inhibit further growth and development and disturb the occlusal relationship.

Alveolar bone grafting is an issue that must be understood by all professionals participating in the multidisciplinary management of cleft patients. This technique is used in cases of complete unilateral and bilateral cleft of the lip, alveolus, and palate. Indications for alveolar bone grafting in unilateral clefts include the presence of a gap and the indentation of the alveolus in the cleft area, as well as the presence of a canine dental follicle. Even if the tooth follicle is present, the tooth will not erupt without the presence of bone in the alveolar arch. For this reason, bone grafting is beneficial when performed between 7 to 9 years of age to facilitate the eruption of the canine.

Orthodontic treatment must precede bone grafting to properly form the alveolar arch and to ensure a proper occlusal relationship. In some cases of unilateral complete cleft, there may be no indication for alveolar bone grafting. There may be no gap between the teeth and cleft line, nor any indentation of the alveolus. Bone grafting is indicated more frequently in bilateral clefts than in unilateral clefts.

When the premaxilla protrudes, bilateral bone grafting is performed simultaneously with surgical retropositioning of the premaxilla and closure of the oronasal and nasolabial fistulas. This is usually performed at 6 to 8 years of age to secure the premaxilla within the alveolar arch and to allow the teeth to erupt into the bone grafts.

Exposure of the bare palatal bone

Another problem in cleft palate repair is related to the exposure of bare bone following the transposition of the mucoperiosteal flaps for closure of the palatal cleft. In very wide clefts, the transposition of the flaps may leave areas of bare bone on the palatal shelves. Depending on the surgical technique, it is possible to close this secondary defect as well as the primary cleft defect with the same mucoperiosteal flap. This can be achieved by changing the inclination of the mucoperiosteal flap from a sloping to a horizontal position, much like the lowering of a drawbridge. By applying this principle in two-flap palatoplasty and attending to the closure of the lateral defects, it is possible to avoid exposing bare bone in the majority of cases.

In other surgical techniques, bone is routinely exposed as a result of the surgical design. For example, the Wardill-Kilner pushback three- or four-flap palatoplasty technique exposes a triangular area of bone following the repositioning of the mucoperiosteal flaps on the oral side. Exposure of bare bone lateral to the mucoperiosteal flaps also occurs routinely in the von Langenbeck technique.

The guidelines of two-flap palatoplasty

The guidelines of two-flap palatoplasty are summarized here to facilitate an understanding of the principles that direct this surgical technique. These guidelines are not presented in the order of their importance.

1. In all types of cleft palate, palatoplasty is performed in one stage with the aim of achieving the following goals:
   A. Complete closure of the palatal cleft
   B. The creation of an adequately functioning soft palate
      An exception to guideline A occurs in cases of bilateral cleft of the lip, alveolus, and palate with a protruding premaxilla in which oronasal fistulas are left in the anterior portion of the palate to facilitate the surgical retropositioning of the premaxilla.
      One-stage, two-flap palatoplasty avoids a series of complications that may occur in two-stage cleft palate repair in which closure of the hard palate is delayed. The one-stage approach eliminates the need for a second operation to close the hard palate, avoids occasional difficulties that sometimes interfere with closure of the entire palate, and attempts to avoid retraction of the soft palate as a result of scar contracture and tension.

2. One-stage, two-flap palatoplasty described by Bardach in 1967 and 1984, and by Bardach and Salyer in 1987 and 1990, is designed as a compilation of maneuvers taken from a variety of surgical techniques. Some of the maneuvers described in these operations are newly developed. Maneuvers borrowed from other techniques include the raising of the mucoperiosteal flaps on the oral and nasal sides, two-layer closure of the hard palate, and three-layer closure of the soft palate.
   Original maneuvers include the following: the design of the mucoperiosteal flaps on the oral side; conservative elevation of the mucoperiosteal flaps in the area of the neurovascular bundles; complete dissection of the muscles of the soft palate from the posterior edge of the hard palate and from the periosteum on the nasal side; vertical mattress sutures to closely approximate the mucoperiosteal flaps on the oral and nasal sides, to avoid leaving dead space between the layers and to stabilize the oral layer in a desired

position; and precise closure of both layers in the anterior portion of the palate.

Another important innovation, contributed by Bardach and Nosal, is the geometric model, which explains the transposition of the mucoperiosteal flaps and the possibility of closing the palatal cleft while covering bare bone on the palatal shelves.

3. Cleft palate repair should be performed at 6 to 18 months of age with the aim of completely closing the palatal cleft and creating an adequately functioning soft palate. The choice of timing for closure of the palatal cleft depends on the type and severity of cleft. The mildest forms of cleft palate may be successfully operated on at 6 to 8 months of age. Cleft palate associated with cleft of the lip and alveolus, unilateral or bilateral, may be operated on at 9 to 18 months of age, depending on the severity of the cleft, the position of the maxillary segments, and the decision to use presurgical orthopedic treatment.

4. Special attention is required to close the cleft in the anterior portion of the palate. This is probably the most difficult maneuver in cleft palate repair. For this reason, the incisions creating the mucoperiosteal flaps must be carefully designed so that they provide an adequate amount of tissue for two-layer closure. The width of the cleft in the anterior portion of the palate and the inclination of the palatal shelves determine how much mucoperiosteum will need to be incorporated into the nasal layer. Often it is necessary to leave more mucoperiosteum at the edge of the cleft on the oral side so that it can be incorporated into the flap on the nasal side to allow for tension-free closure.

Precise and complete closure of the nasal layer in the area of the hard palate is essential to the success of the operation. In the majority of cases, the incision on the margin of the cleft in the anterior portion of the palate extends to the border between the oral and nasal mucosa, which is easily distinguished by its shade. Transposition of the mucoperiosteal flaps to close the palatal cleft always follows the freeing up of the flaps so that no tension is felt when they are sutured together at the midline.

5. Raising the mucoperiosteal flaps is not difficult in primary cleft palate repair. However, in secondary operations the procedure is more difficult and is usually accompanied by more bleeding. When raising the mucoperiosteal flaps in the primary operation, the surgeon should begin undermining the flap not at the tip but lateral to it, at approximately ⅓ of the distance from the tip. A periosteal elevator may be used to undermine the flap from the bone under the periosteum. By undermining the flap and moving the elevator forward, the tip of the flap is easily elevated. The remaining blunt dissection of the flap from the palatal shelf is done using a roll of gauze. This stage of the operation usually takes only a few minutes and causes little or no bleeding.

Caution must be exercised when lengthening the neurovascular bundle. By gently pulling the flap, the neurovascular bundle is easily exposed. Its length may then be extended by separating it from the mucoperiosteal flap at a distance necessary to avoid tension of the transposed flap. Sharp dissection of the neurovascular bundle must be performed with great caution to ensure its continued attachment to the anterior portion of the flap, which provides it with a sufficient blood supply.

6. When preparing the mucoperiosteal flaps on the oral and nasal sides, both layers must be sufficiently released and mobilized to avoid tension in any particular area. In most cases, the greatest tension occurs in the area between the hard and soft palate. In some surgical techniques, the hamulus is fractured to facilitate medial approximation of the mucoperiosteal flaps on the oral side. In two-flap palatoplasty, however, we do not fracture the hamulus nor enter the space next to it (Ernst's space). We see no advantage in performing this procedure because it does not release tension in the area between the hard and soft palate as is commonly believed. In our experience, we have achieved better relaxation by lengthening the neurovascular bundle since it is the primary cause of limited flap mobility.

Some surgeons sever the neurovascular bundle to avoid tension when approximating the mucoperiosteal flaps. This procedure impairs the blood supply to the flap, resulting in serious complications. The rate of partial necrosis of the mucoperiosteal flaps is much higher following this procedure than when the neurovascular bundle remains attached to the flap. Some surgeons release the tension of the neurovascular bundle by removing the posterior wall of the major palatine foramen. We find these procedures to be less advantageous than partial, sharp dissection of the neurovascular bundle from the mucoperiosteal flap.

Partial dissection of the neurovascular bundle from its attachment to the flap increases the mobility to the mucoperiostcal flap and also provides the flap with an adequate blood supply. Releasing the neurovascular bundle from the major palatine foramen by removing its posterior wall provides limited mobility to the flap and therefore does not result in tension-free closure of the palatal cleft.

7. It is necessary to close the cleft in two layers, making sure that the nasal and oral layers are approximated and sutured together without tension, which may jeopardize the healing process. Vertical mattress sutures enhance the two-flap palatoplasty technique. These sutures provide close approximation of both layers, stabilize the mucoperiosteal flaps on the oral side in the desired position, and avoid leaving dead space between the flaps.

If the oral and nasal layers are not closely approximated, two complications may hinder the healing process: blood may accumulate, forming a bloodclot in the empty space between the layers; and the unattached oral layer may loosen from the palatal shelves, resulting in large oronasal fistulas in the anterior portion of the palate.

To prevent the latter complication, some surgeons support the oral flaps with a special dressing to stabilize them in close approximation to the underlying palatal shelves. The use of an iodoform gauze dressing to secure the flaps has serious disadvantages due to the possibility of wound contamination and the exertion of excessive pressure on the mucoperiosteal flaps. The two-flap palatoplasty technique successfully prevents both developments due to the use of vertical mattress sutures, which closely approximate the oral and nasal layers of the mucoperiosteal flaps, thus stabilizing them in the desired position and eliminating empty space between them.

8. Creating mucoperiosteal flaps from the vomer greatly enhances tension-free closure of the nasal layer. In some cases of complete cleft palate only and complete unilateral and bilateral cleft lip, alveolus, and palate, mucoperiosteal flaps from the vomer can be used to create the nasal layer. In many cases of unilateral complete cleft of the lip, alveolus, and palate, the vomer is attached to the palatal shelf of the larger maxillary segment. This position of the vomer also facilitates the use of mucoperiosteal flaps, which can be raised from the vomer, turned over, and sutured to the mucoperiosteal flap raised from the palatal shelf on the nasal side.

Some surgeons use the vomer flap for one-layer closure of the anterior portion of the palate. This type of palatal closure does not ensure complete closure of the anterior portion, especially in the area next to the alveolar ridge. Whenever possible, we prefer two-layer closure of the palatal cleft using mucoperiosteal flaps from the vomer.

In complete cleft of the palate only and in complete bilateral palatal clefts, the vomer is usually located in the midline. This position allows the surgeon to use mucoperiosteal flaps raised from the vomer to be sutured together with mucoperiosteal flaps raised on the nasal surface of the palatal shelves. This approach facilitates tension-free closure of the nasal layer along the entire hard palate and partially into the soft palate. At the posterior edge of the hard palate, the vomer decreases in height. By suturing the mucoperiosteal flaps on the nasal side of the palatal shelves to the mucoperiosteal flaps on the posterior edge of the vomer, the soft palate is lifted, creating a better position of the soft palate to achieve velopharyngeal closure. This technique developed by Salyer often helps to achieve normal speech production.

9. Many surgeons and speech pathologists believe that lengthening the soft palate directly correlates with improved speech production. In some surgical techniques, lengthening the soft palate is a primary objective. Wardill-Kilner three- and four-flap palatoplasty is a pushback technique in which the soft palate is lengthened by retropositioning the mucoperiosteal flaps on the oral side and cutting through the nasal mucoperiosteum along the posterior edge of the hard palate. Although this approach substantially lengthens the

soft palate, subsequent healing of the raw area produces scar contracture on the nasal side.

Another surgical technique aimed at lengthening the soft palate is Furlow palatoplasty in which large Z-plasty is performed to lengthen the soft palate. Neither the von Langenbeck technique nor two-flap palatoplasty emphasize lengthening the soft palate, although some maneuvers in two-flap palatoplasty may contribute to a slight lengthening of the soft palate due to the careful detachment of the soft palate muscles from the nasal mucoperiosteum and from the posterior edge of the hard palate.

10. The soft palate is closed in three layers. The first layer consists of the nasal mucosa extending up to the tip of the uvula. The second layer consists of the muscles of the soft palate. At the time of surgical repair, these muscles are treated as a muscular complex that must be carefully and precisely detached from the posterior edge of the hard palate and returned to its normal horizontal position. This lowering of the muscle complex creates a palatal sling. Also, muscle fibers attached to the nasal periosteum must be released to allow for better repositioning of the muscles on both sides of the soft palate.

The muscle layer may be sutured separately from the mucosal layers or may be sutured jointly with the nasal and oral layers using horizontal and vertical mattress sutures. The advantage of suturing the muscle layer to the mucosal layer on the oral and nasal sides is that the sutures do not remain within the muscle layer which, on rare occasions, may complicate the healing process.

The third layer to be closed is the oral mucosa. It can be closed separately from the muscle layer or sutured together with the muscle layer using vertical mattress sutures. Closure of the soft palate must be performed without tension, especially in the area between the hard and soft palate. It is also important to remember to recreate the uvula, a structure that seems significant to the parents of the patient.

11. Speech production determines the success of any surgical technique used in cleft palate repair. In the vast majority of cases, if speech production is satisfactory, the technique is considered successful and acceptable. On the other hand, a high rate of speech problems following cleft palate repair indicates that a particular technique is less successful.

No matter how well-designed the surgical technique, the results will not be satisfactory if surgical repair is performed by an inexperienced surgeon. The results of cleft palate repair depend not only on surgical technique but also on the proficiency of the surgeon as well as all of the factors previously described.

The difficulty in evaluating surgical techniques causes widespread uncertainty among surgeons and speech pathologists as to which technique is best. However, an especially serious problem is the evaluation of surgical proficiency, because there are no objective tests to judge surgical performance other than short-term and long-term results. It would be interesting to examine the speech and surgical results in a series of patients who have been operated on by one surgeon, and then compare the results with another series of patients in whom the same technique was used by different surgeons. This type of comparative study would allow for a scientific evaluation of the advantages and disadvantages of surgical techniques, as well as assessment of surgical proficiency. At the present time, our assessment is based on very few well-designed and well-executed late results studies in addition to studies based on observations taken from clinical experience. Unfortunately, there are no well-designed prospective studies at this time.

12. Delayed closure of the hard palate is no longer justified since surgeons now work closely with orthodontists in the multidisciplinary treatment of cleft patients. The incorporation of orthodontic care in the treatment protocol allows the surgeon to close the soft and hard palate simultaneously without the risk of developing maxillofacial deformities. The two-stage technique is still applied by some surgeons and recommended by some orthodontists. The results from several advanced cleft centers indicate that one-stage cleft palate repair produces better speech results and more successful closure of the palate than the two-stage procedure.

13. The idea that cleft palate repair is detrimental to maxillofacial growth is based on

the assumption that each operation on the cleft palate results in the denudation of palatal bone lateral to the medially transposed mucoperiosteal flaps and that scarring in this area leads to maxillary growth aberrations.

Clinical observations and experimental studies do not justify this widespread belief for two main reasons: every cleft palate repair does not necessarily lead to the exposure of bare palatal bone; in addition, close cooperation with the orthodontist and combined surgical-orthodontic care successfully prevents secondary maxillofacial deformities. In the majority of cases that employ two-flap palatoplasty, it is possible to cover the laterally exposed bone simultaneously with closure of the palatal cleft. In wide palatal clefts, the bone lateral to the mucoperiosteal flaps on the oral side will usually be exposed because there is not enough tissue available to close both the palatal cleft and bare bone. However, covering the bone with Avatine at the time of surgery stimulates fast epithelialization, and scar contracture is prevented, thus avoiding growth aberrations of the maxilla.

14. Nosal's geometric analysis exposed the fallacy that cleft palate repair results in exposure of bare bone lateral to the medially transposed mucoperiosteal flaps. It also proved that many palatal clefts may be repaired without exposing any bare bone, depending on the width of the palatal cleft and the widths and inclination of the palatal shelves.

15. Unfortunately, cleft palate surgery is neither described nor discussed as explicitly as cleft lip surgery. This is because the results of lip surgery are highly visible, whereas the results of cleft palate repair are not, except when there are complications such as oronasal fistulas or hypernasality. Surgical techniques vary; no single technique is widely accepted as the operation of choice.

Cleft palate repair seems to be more difficult and causes more problems than cleft lip repair. This situation is related not only to less experienced surgeons but also to surgeons who perform a great number of cleft palate operations. Complications reported in the literature related to the high incidence of oronasal fistulae and hypernasality requiring a pharyngeal flap indicate that palatoplasty requires a high level of surgical skill and deep understanding of the surgical technique.

SURGICAL TECHNIQUE: TWO-FLAP PALATOPLASTY

The surgical technique described in this chapter is a one-stage, two-flap palatoplasty which, in our experience, leads to optimal speech and surgical results. It allows the surgeon to completely close the palatal cleft as well as create an adequately functioning soft palate. The details of the technique differ to some degree depending on the form of palatal cleft. To facilitate an understanding of these surgical procedures, the techniques as they are performed on the submucous cleft, cleft palate only, and unilateral and bilateral cleft of the lip, alveolus, and palate will be briefly described. The results of this procedure must be judged according to speech, maxillofacial growth, and the presence of oronasal fistulas.

Submucous cleft of the soft palate

Surgical repair of the submucous cleft depends on the extent of the cleft as well as the conditions and functioning of the soft palate and the lateral and posterior pharyngeal walls. The primary goal of this operation is to release the abnormal attachment of the muscles of the soft palate from the posterior edge of the hard palate, to reorient the muscles, and to suture them in their proper alignment. Tension caused by muscle approximation or the close attachment of the mucoperiosteum of the hard palate to the palatal shelves must also be released.

To achieve these goals, the M-shaped incision is carried through the mucoperiosteum on the oral side of the palate. The central tip of the "M" incision reaches the most anterior point of the palatal cleft. The lateral arms of the "M" incision curve around the posterior edge of the alveolus and extend into the pterygomandibular raphe. When mucoperiosteal flaps on the oral side are elevated, the neurovascular bundle is identified, and the posterior edge of the hard palate can be easily approached. The mucosal bridge that separates the two segments of the soft palate must then be removed to expose the muscles of the soft palate along the cleft. The muscle fibers are carefully detached from the posterior edge of the hard palate and from the nasal periosteum. The soft palate muscles are then reoriented in a horizontal position, resulting in the creation of a palatal sling, which improves the functioning of the soft palate. This procedure allows for some lengthening of the soft palate, which may be important in certain cases. The soft palate is sutured in three layers, beginning with the nasal mucosa and followed by the muscles and the oral mucosa. The mucoperiosteal flaps are returned to their beds and sutured in place.

Cleft palate only

Surgical repair of the cleft palate only depends on the form of the cleft. Closing the cleft of the soft palate only requires a different procedure than that employed in complete cleft of the soft and hard palate with the vomer positioned at the midline. Despite the differences in surgical procedures, the basic objectives are the same for both cleft forms: complete closure of the cleft and the creation of an adequately functioning soft palate.

Cleft of the soft palate

To close the soft palate, the surgeon begins by making incisions on the medial margins of the cleft, exposing the muscles on both sides. The incisions are carried forward the full length of the cleft, continuing into the hard palate if there is submucous clefting at the posterior edge of the hard palate. In some cases of cleft palate only, some surgeons may repair the palatal cleft by approximating the edges of the soft palate, following the incisions that expose the muscles on both sides of the cleft. On some occasions, this operation can be performed with almost no tension. However, the results are usually unsuccessful because the muscle attachments remain abnormal and the functioning of the soft palate remains impaired. Cleft palate without repositioning the muscles of the soft palate usually results in a short palate, which in turn leads to velopharyngeal incompetence. For this reason, I strongly discourage simple closure of the soft palate by approximation only without additional incisions to raise the mucoperiosteal flaps, detach the muscles of the soft palate, and create a muscle sling (Fig. 7-7, A-E).

When repairing the soft palate only, no matter how small the cleft, the mucoperiosteal flaps on the hard palate must be raised to expose the neurovascular bundle and the attachment of the muscles to the posterior edge of the hard palate. At this point, it is beneficial to extend the neurovascular bundle (even if there is only slight tension when approximating the mucoperiosteal flaps) since it adds to the mobility of the mucoperiosteal flaps and prevents retraction following the healing process. Accurate and

gentle detachment of the soft palate muscles from the posterior edge of the hard palate and sharp dissection of the muscle fibers from the nasal periosteum changes the position of the muscles from oblique to horizontal. They can then be sutured in their normal alignment. This step in the operation is important because it lengthens the soft palate to some degree and allows for better functioning.

Final closure of the palatal cleft begins with the suturing of the mucosa on the nasal side, followed by the muscle layer and the oral mucosa. The mucoperiosteal flaps on the oral side are transposed medially, approximated at the midline, and sutured in this position. Since no attempt is made to retroposition the mucoperiosteal flaps on the oral side, no bone is left exposed. In all cases of cleft palate, these guidelines should be followed to ensure optimal speech and surgical results.

Cleft of the hard and soft palate

Different approaches must be applied in cases involving cleft of the hard and soft palate. When the vomer is positioned at the midline of the cleft and on the same level as the edges of the palatal shelves, mucoperiosteal flaps from the vomer may be used to create the nasal layer for closure of the palatal cleft. Two technical aspects differentiate the combined closure of the hard and soft palate from closure of the soft palate only: the use of mucoperiosteal flaps from the vomer and the medial transposition of the mucoperiosteal flaps, which leaves an area of bone exposed lateral to them.

At the start of the operation, incisions are made at the margins of the cleft of the hard palate and carried into the soft palate. The extent of the incision in the hard palate depends on the width of the cleft and the position of the vomer, which may be at the level of or close to the level of the palatal shelves. In narrow or moderately wide clefts, the incision at the edge of the hard palatal cleft is carried through between the oral and nasal mucosa.

Another incision made along the lower edge of the vomer allows for the raising of two mucoperiosteal flaps on each side, which can then be approximated to the mucoperiosteal flaps raised on the nasal side of the palatal shelves. This approach ensures complete and secure closure of the nasal layer. It allows the mucoperiosteal flaps from the vomer to be sutured to the nasal layer with little or no tension.

Following the preparation of the mucoperi-

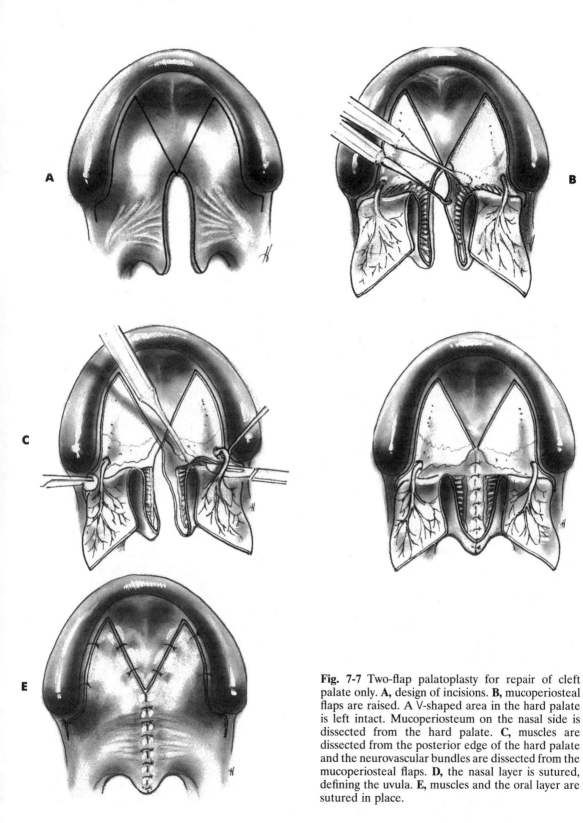

Fig. 7-7 Two-flap palatoplasty for repair of cleft palate only. **A,** design of incisions. **B,** mucoperiosteal flaps are raised. A ∨-shaped area in the hard palate is left intact. Mucoperiosteum on the nasal side is dissected from the hard palate. **C,** muscles are dissected from the posterior edge of the hard palate and the neurovascular bundles are dissected from the mucoperiosteal flaps. **D,** the nasal layer is sutured, defining the uvula. **E,** muscles and the oral layer are sutured in place.

osteal flaps for closure of the nasal side, the lateral incision is carried on to the oral side. This flap, raised from the underlying bone, exposes the neurovascular bundle, the foramen palatine major, and the posterior edge of the hard palate. At this point, the procedure follows the same steps as were described for soft palate closure. The muscles of the soft palate are released from their attachment to the posterior edge of the hard palate and repositioned into a horizontal alignment to ensure their proper functioning. It is important to sufficiently release the mucoperiosteal flaps on the oral side to avoid any tension when they are sutured together at the midline. Following closure of the mucosa and the muscles of the soft palate, the mucoperiosteal flaps from the oral side of the hard palate are sutured using vertical mattress sutures with the aim of approximating not only the flaps but also the oral and nasal layers, closing the empty space between them.

In cases when mucoperiosteal flaps from the vomer cannot be used to close the nasal layer due to the position of the vomer, a different surgical procedure is required. The incision along the margin of the palatal cleft must create sufficiently wide mucoperiosteal flaps to close the nasal layer without excessive tension. It should be carried on somewhat farther from the edge of the cleft on the oral side to allow for the incorporation of more mucoperiosteum into the flap on the nasal side. One must realize that leaving a wider strip of mucoperiosteum at the edge of the palatal cleft to be incorporated into the nasal layer will narrow the mucoperiosteal flaps on the oral side. In such cases, medial transposition of the mucoperiosteal flaps to close the palatal cleft will expose bare bone lateral to the flaps. I suggest covering the exposed bone with Avatine at the time of surgery to facilitate normal healing and to avoid scar contracture, which may lead to subsequent maxillary growth aberrations. The remaining steps of the operation are identical to those previously described and illustrated.

Unilateral complete cleft of the palate

Repair of the unilateral complete cleft of the palate requires a different approach than cases of cleft palate only since the cleft extends into the alveolus and the vomer is usually attached to the medial edge of the palatal shelf of the larger maxillary segment. In this form of cleft, the cleft palate divides the maxillary segments into larger and smaller portions. As was mentioned before, the palatal shelf of the larger maxillary segment may be attached to the vomer. However, if the vomer is positioned higher than the edge of

the palatal plate, it cannot be used to close the palatal cleft. If, on the other hand, the vomer is attached to the edge of the larger maxillary segment, the mucoperiosteal flap raised from the vomer may be easily sutured to the mucoperiosteal flap on the nasal side of the smaller maxillary segment, thus securing complete closure of the nasal layer. It is very important to extend the incisions on the cleft margins up to the alveolar cleft so that the mucoperiosteal flaps on the nasal side can be extended and sutured within the alveolar cleft and along the hard palate (Fig. 7-8, A-F).

I believe that insufficient attention is paid to closure of the anterior portion of the hard palate, and for this reason the highest rate of oronasal fistulae occur in this area. The mucoperiosteal flaps on the oral and nasal sides must be raised in a way that ensures medial flap transposition without tension when closing the palatal cleft in the anterior portion of the palate. The steps needed to achieve this are identical to those described for closure of the cleft palate only. They include deflecting the mucoperiosteal flaps, isolating and extending the neurovascular bundles, detaching the muscles of the soft palate from the posterior edge of the hard palate, and creating a muscle sling with the muscles joined in a horizontal position. The remaining steps do not differ from the previously described technique except when using vertical mattress sutures to approximate and extend the oral and nasal layers into the alveolar cleft.

Bilateral complete cleft of the palate

To close the bilateral palatal cleft, two-flap palatoplasty may vary depending on the positions of the premaxilla and the vomer. When the premaxilla protrudes, the anterior portion of the palatal cleft must not be closed until 6 or 7 years of age. At this time, surgical repair includes the surgical retropositioning of the protruding premaxilla, complete closure of the anterior portion of the palatal cleft and of both alveolar clefts, and bilateral alveolar bone grafting.

At the Iowa Cleft Palate Center, where this approach is favored, no presurgical orthopedics are used in cases of a protruding premaxilla. The protocol used by Olin and Bardach dictates unrestrained growth of the maxillary complex until 6 to 7 years of age when surgical repositioning of the premaxilla is performed. When the premaxilla is within the alveolar arches or slightly in front of them, primary palatoplasty may be performed to completely close the palatal cleft, including the alveolar cleft on the lingual side. Mucoperiosteal flaps from the

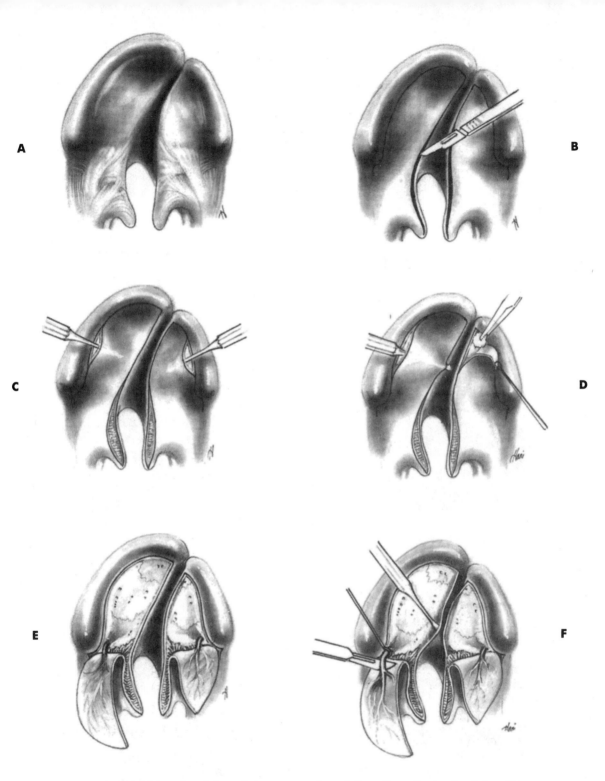

Fig. 7-8 A, initial undermining of the mucoperiosteal flaps from the hard palate with a Woodson elevator. **B,** a mucoperiosteal flap is raised from the vomer for closure of the nasal layer. On the cleft side, mucoperiosteum is widely dissected on the nasal side from the bone using a Padgett elevator. Dissection of the neurovascular bundle from the mucoperiosteal flap allows better mobilization of the flap. **C,** dissection of the muscles from the posterior edge of the bony palate on both sides. The muscle must be dissected from the entire posterior edge of the bony palate. The neurovascular bundle is dissected from the mucoperiosteal flap. **D,** nasal layer sutured in the area of the hard and soft palate. The 4-0 chromic sutures are tied with knots on the nasal side. Attention is directed to proper alignment of the soft palate. In the anterior portion, careful closure of the nasal layer is paramount. **E,** muscles of the soft palate are sutured together. **F,** mucoperiosteal flaps are sutured in place and the lateral incisions are closed. The explanation for closure of the lateral incisions is presented in the discussion on geometry of the two-flap palatoplasty.

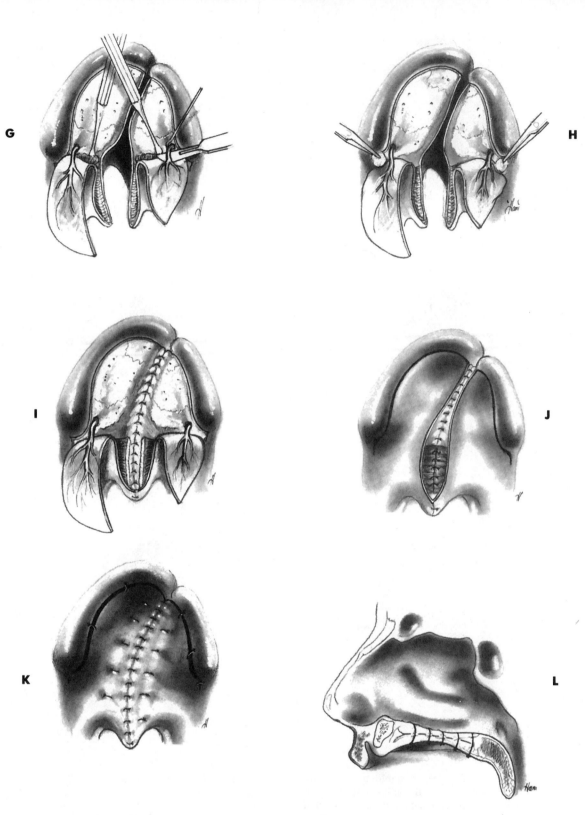

Fig. 7-8, cont. G, dissection of the muscles from the posterior edge of the bony palate on both sides. The muscle must be dissected from the entire posterior edge of the bony palate. The neurovascular bundle is dissected from the mucoperiosteal flap. **H,** gauze rolls are used to free the mucoperiosteal flaps behind the alveolar arch. **I,** nasal layer sutured in the area of the hard and soft palate. The 4-0 chromic sutures are tied with knots on the nasal side. Attention is directed to proper alignment of the soft palate. In the anterior portion, careful closure of the nasal layer is paramount. **J,** muscles of the soft palate are sutured together. **K,** mucoperiosteal flaps are sutured in place and the lateral incisions are closed. The explanation for closure of the lateral incisions is presented in the discussion on geometry of the two-flap palatoplasty. **L,** mucoperiosteal flaps in the area of the hard palate are sutured using vertical mattress sutures in the nasal layer, preventing dead space between layers.

vomer may help to secure complete closure of the nasal layer along the length of the hard palate (Fig. 7-9, A-F and Fig. 7-10, A, B).

To complete this procedure, the incision is carried along the lower edge of the vomer, raising mucoperiosteal flaps on either side of it. These flaps can be easily sutured together with the mucoperiosteal flaps raised on the nasal side of the palatal shelves. Raising the mucoperiosteal flaps on the oral side, isolating the neurovascular bundle, and extending its length by sharp, partial detachment from the mucoperiosteal flap increases the mobility of the flaps and minimizes tension. These steps reposition the muscles of the soft palate. Securing them in a horizontal position is identical to the procedure previously described.

RESULTS OF TWO-FLAP PALATOPLASTY WITH REGARD TO SPEECH PRODUCTION

The main goal of cleft palate repair, regardless of cleft form, is normal speech production. The morphology of the cleft palate, the proficiency of the surgeon, and the choice of surgical technique influence the outcome of surgical repair with regard to speech production. Late results studies performed at the Iowa Cleft Palate Center assess the effectiveness of two-flap palatoplasty in regard to speech production and residual oronasal fistulas.

The initial report presented by Morris and Van Demark in 1981 indicated that in 80% of patients with unilateral cleft lip, alveolus, and palate, velopharyngeal function was within normal limits. The late results of another study published in 1989 were based on the examination of 45 children with unilateral cleft lip, alveolus, and palate, who underwent two-flap palatoplasty. The results indicated that in 80% of patients, velopharyngeal function was within normal limits. The findings from this investigation indicate that as a primary palatoplasty technique, the two-flap method yields a velopharyngeal mechanism appropriate for normal speech in four of five patients. This success rate compares favorably with rates reported for other methods, which approximate 60 to 70%. In addition, this surgical technique resulted in a minimal percentage of oronasal fistulae (2% overall) as compared to two other techniques (Van Langenbeck and Wardill-Kilner) used at the Iowa Cleft Palate Center before 1973. The latter two techniques resulted in oronasal fistulae in 17% and 24% of patients, respectively.

Another late results study from the Iowa Cleft Palate Center, published in 1992, assesses speech results and the presence of oronasal fistulas following two-flap palatoplasty in patients with bilateral cleft lip, alveolus, and palate. According to these findings, 78% of the patients exhibited velopharyngeal competence within normal limits, while 22% underwent or needed secondary velopharyngeal surgery. Five patients out of 50 (10%) had an oronasal fistula in the anterior palate. These findings indicate that speech results in patients with unilateral and bilateral cleft palate following two-flap palatoplasty are superior to the speech results obtained using the same technique in patients with cleft palate only.

These studies provide a quantitative measure of the success rate of two-flap palatoplasty in regard to speech production. When this procedure is performed with care and technical skill, it results in complete closure of the palatal cleft, minimal frequency of oronasal fistulae, and the creation of an adequately functioning velopharyngeal mechanism.

TWO-STAGE PALATOPLASTY: PRIMARY VELOPLASTY

In two-stage palatoplasty, the cleft of the soft palate is closed during primary lip repair, but the cleft of the hard palate is left open. This procedure, originated by Schweckendiek in 1936, is based on the belief that closing the cleft of the soft palate at an early age fosters normal speech production, while delaying hard palate repair prevents secondary maxillofacial deformities caused by early surgical intervention on the hard palate.

Two-stage palatoplasty is a compromise between two opposing opinions related to the timing of palatoplasty and the iatrogenic effects of surgical repair of the cleft lip and palate. Some speech pathologists believe that early closure of the palatal cleft enhances normal speech. At the same time, many orthodontists believe that early cleft palate repair may hinder midfacial growth and development due to restrictions caused by cleft palate repair. The assumption that cleft palate repair is the main cause of secondary maxillofacial deformities is based on original studies by Herfert, later studies by Kremenak, and anecdotal data from unoperated adults with clefts. Their poorly substantiated conclusions indicate that cleft palate repair necessarily exposes bare bone, resulting in growth inhibition of the midfacial complex.

The intent with two-stage palatoplasty is to alleviate this problem by leaving the hard palate open for a long period of time. This supposedly allows for unrestrained growth of the maxillary segment, thereby preventing the development

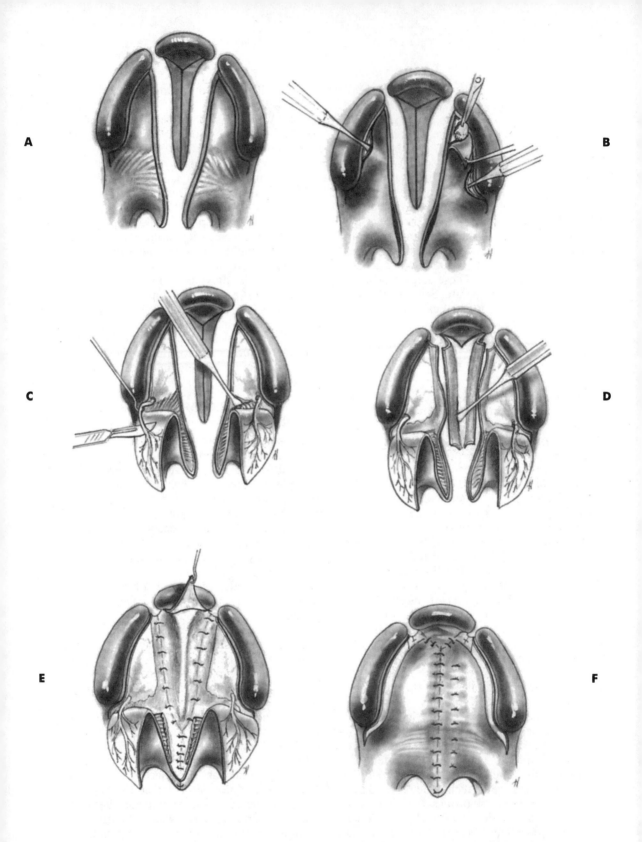

Fig. 7-9 Two-flap palatoplasty for bilateral cleft palate with a nonprotruding premaxilla. **A,** incision design on the palate, premaxilla, and lower edge of the septum. **B,** mucoperiosteal flaps are raised from the hard palate. **C,** mucoperiosteal flaps are raised. The muscles are freed from the posterior edge of the hard palate. The neurovascular bundles are partially dissected from the mucoperiosteal flaps. **D,** elevation of the mucoperiosteal flaps on both sides of the vomer and premaxilla, and dissection of the mucoperiosteal flaps on the nasal side of the hard palate. **E,** closure of the nasal layer. **F,** closure of the muscle and oral layers. In the area of the hard palate, vertical mattress sutures closely approximate the oral and nasal layers to prevent dead space. Later to the mucoperiosteal flaps, areas of bare bone remain exposed.

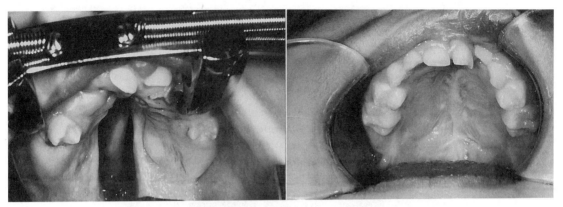

Fig. 7-10 A, Bilateral cleft of the palate. Note nasal septum in midline. Mucoperiosteal flaps from the nasal septum were used to create the nasal layer as demonstrated in Fig. 7-13. **B,** After one-stage two-flap palatoplasty.

of secondary maxillofacial deformities. This concept, quite popular in Europe, was adopted by some centers in this country and became popular in the 1970s. The positive and negative aspects of this approach, as with many other surgical techniques, makes it controversial.

Some clinicians considered early closure of the soft palate to be advantageous in that it may restore the normal functioning of the soft palate at an early age as well as narrow the cleft of the hard palate. However, this belief was not confirmed in a study conducted in Marburg, Germany by the Iowa Cleft Palate Team. All patients were operated on by Wolfram Schweckendiek (son of Herman Schweckendiek who introduced the two-stage palatoplasty technique).

This study revealed an unusually high incidence of velopharyngeal incompetence. We found poor speech results following delayed hard palate closure in patients operated on by this surgeon. These unsatisfactory speech results were also confirmed in a sample of patients with unilateral cleft lip, alveolus, and palate, operated on at the Iowa Cleft Palate Center. Our patients showed early signs of hypernasality and a compensatory articulation pattern. Poor speech results following two-stage palatoplasty were also reported by other surgeons and speech pathologists who observed that insufficient velopharyngeal closure leads to moderate to severe hypernasality.

Another observation related to two-stage palatoplasty is the occurrence of a short soft palate with limited mobility. Many patients in whom the hard palate was left open exhibited a narrowing of the palatal cleft after surgery over some period of time. It may be assumed that the

functioning of the soft palate contributes to the approximation of the palatal shelves, thus narrowing the palatal cleft. It was also observed that the palatal shelves within the hard palate change to an almost vertical position, making final closure technically difficult (Fig. 7-11, A-D).

On the other hand, the normal growth or almost normal growth and development of the maxillary complex in two-stage palatoplasty is undisputed. In the Marburg patients, we found that the maxilla grew undisturbed and that the cephalometric measurements matched the normal population. For this reason, Schweckendiek and many of his followers delay closure of the hard palate until 14 to 16 years of age.

Although it can be justifiably assumed that leaving the hard palate unrepaired contributes to better growth and development of the maxillary complex, it is no longer the only approach in which these ends are achieved. At the present time, close cooperation between surgeons and orthodontists makes it possible to enhance the results of surgical treatment because orthodontic management with constant monitoring successfully prevents the development of secondary maxillofacial deformities.

Currently, there are many variations of two-stage palatoplasty, few of which are justified from the viewpoint of speech development and maxillofacial growth. All these variations advocate closure of the soft palate before or simultaneously with cleft lip repair. These variations seem to be inconsequential in terms of the main objectives of two-stage palatoplasty. More clinical and comparative studies are necessary to assess the validity of two-stage palatoplasty in the multidisciplinary management of clefts.

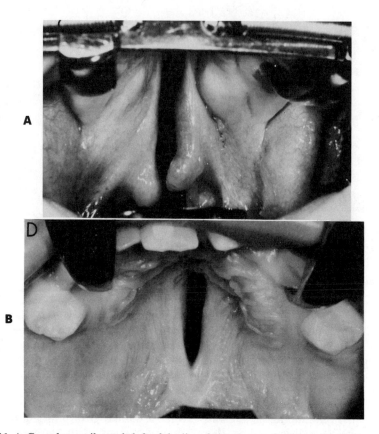

Fig. 7-11 A, Complete unilateral cleft of the lip, of alveolus, and palate; after primary lip repair
B, Soft palate is closed; cleft in the hard palate remains unrepaired.

As was indicated before, the sequence of surgical procedures in two-stage palatoplasty may differ among surgeons and centers. The original two-stage palatoplasty described by Schweckendiek and performed in some centers dictates that the cleft lip be repaired simultaneously with the soft palate. Schweckendiek performs this operation at 6 months of age, while many other surgeons perform the operation earlier, usually at 3 to 4 months of age. In the majority of cases, the soft palate is sutured together under tension because the mucoperiosteal flaps and the neurovascular bundles have not been released. This results in the shortening of the soft palate after surgery. In addition, this procedure leaves the muscles of the soft palate incorrectly attached to the posterior edge of the hard palate. Under these circumstances, the soft palate can hardly be expected to function normally.

However, the improved functioning of the soft palate after veloplasty contributes to the approximation of the maxillary segments and changes their position. Closure of the hard palate at a later age may be difficult because of the vertical positioning of the palatal shelves in the area of the hard palate. In the secondary operation, mucoperiosteal flaps are raised on the oral and nasal sides to close the hard palate in two layers. Detaching the muscles of the soft palate from the posterior edge of the hard palate may achieve some lengthening of the soft palate and create better mobility.

Two-stage palatoplasty is still accepted by some surgeons, orthodontists, and speech pathologists despite accumulated data indicating that speech is worse and maxillary growth is no better after this surgery than after one-stage palatal closure. Several clinical studies have proven that closure of the soft palate, usually performed at the time of primary cleft lip repair, may in fact adversely affect speech production. The large opening in the hard palate prevents normal speech development. Our experience has been similar to that of many other surgeons and speech pathologists. We have observed that

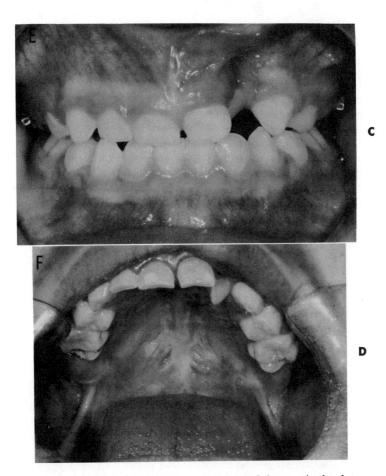

Fig. 7-11, cont. C and **D,** Occlusion and view of the repaired palate.

two-stage palatoplasty contributes to a variety of speech impairments at an early age. For this reason we have abandoned this approach.

COMPLICATIONS FOLLOWING PALATOPLASTY

Several complications may occur during or after cleft palate repair. During primary cleft palate repair, the use of proper local anesthetics and delicate surgical technique usually results in minimal bleeding (30 to 60 ml). However, if the palatine artery is severed, *excessive bleeding* will occur, requiring coagulation or ligation of the vessel. There is usually much more bleeding during secondary palatoplasty than during the primary operation because of scar tissue, which prevents smooth dissection of the mucoperiosteal flaps from the underlying palatal shelves. In secondary operations, special attention must be paid to controlling the bleeding by the use of local anesthetics with vasoconstrictors and careful, precise surgical technique.

Flap necrosis is a complication caused by inappropriate handling of tissue, the excessive use of vasoconstrictors, the creation of excessive tension when closing the palatal cleft, or poor stabilization of the mucoperiosteal flaps after the completion of cleft palate repair. To prevent flap necrosis, it is important not to apply excessive local anesthetics. It is also imperative to release the mucoperiosteal flaps on the oral and nasal sides so that they can be sutured together without tension. Avoiding tension, especially in the area on the border between the hard and soft palate where the width of the cleft is greatest, prevents dehiscence and necrosis of the flaps. In addition, proper stabilization of the mucoperiosteal flaps on the oral side, as is performed in two-flap palatoplasty using mattress sutures to join the oral and nasal layers, is essential in order to avoid loosening of the mucoperiosteal flaps and subsequent necrosis.

Oronasal fistula is the most common complication following palatoplasty. Oronasal fistulae are areas of communication between the oral and nasal cavities. They occur due to the failure of cleft palate repair, although on some occasions they are left open due to the design of the operation or an inability of the surgeon to achieve complete closure.

Generally, oronasal fistulae are located in the anterior portion of the hard palate or on the border between the hard and soft palate. Fistulae in the anterior portion may result from poorly designed surgical techniques that fail to close the most anterior portion of the hard palate. In cases of unilateral and bilateral complete clefts of the lip, alveolus, and palate, the von Langenbeck and Wardill-Kilner techniques may leave these kinds of fistulae. Depending on their size, oronasal fistulae may interfere with speech. On some occasions, soft tissue on the margins of the fistulae approximate closely enough so that speech is not affected. However, fluids and air leak through them.

The border between the hard and soft palate is the second most common location of oronasal fistulae. This is an area where surgeons encounter the greatest amount of tension when approximating and suturing the flaps to close the hard and soft palate. Oronasal fistulae located laterally to the palatal mucoperiosteal flaps may be more difficult to repair than those located at the midline of the palate. The most common and most difficult fistulas to repair are those located in the anterior portion of the palate and in the alveolus following bilateral cleft palate repair.

On many occasions, oronasal fistulae appear following maxillary expansion at the time of postsurgical orthodontic treatment. When these fistulas cause speech problems and leak air and fluids, surgical repair is necessary and must be performed as soon as possible. However, closure should be delayed at least 6 months after primary surgery until the tissue has established a normal blood supply. Various surgical procedures can be used to close oronasal fistulae depending on their location. We advocate the use of two-layer mucoperiosteal flaps to permanently close the fistula as opposed to obturators, which maintain the opening. Successful and permanent closure of oronasal fistulae is performed using a two-layer technique, which incorporates local and transposition flaps from the palate.

THE INFLUENCE OF CLEFT PALATE REPAIR ON MAXILLOFACIAL GROWTH

The majority of specialists involved in the multidisciplinary treatment of clefts falsely believe that early palatal surgery inhibits maxillofacial growth by injuring the periosteum of the bony palate and produces scarring following palatal repair. For many years (since the late 1940s and early 1950s) palatoplasty was considered to be the primary cause of maxillofacial growth aberrations. This opinion is still widespread, especially among orthodontists who advocate performing cleft palate repair at 18 to 36 months of age or later to avoid growth disturbances produced by early surgery. This opinion is not justified. Clinical and experimental data do not prove the detrimental effects of palatoplasty on maxillofacial growth. Experimental data by Herfert is poorly designed and lacks statistical analysis. Clinical data presented in published studies by Graber is also poorly designed and suffers from an inherent inability to isolate the effects of palatoplasty from other surgical and orthodontic procedures, which may influence maxillofacial growth.

It is important for all specialists conducting clinical and experimental cleft research to understand that it is impossible to design a clinical study in which a single surgical factor is isolated and studied apart from other factors that influence maxillofacial growth. For example, if a patient is born with a cleft lip, alveolus, and palate, and primary surgery is performed on the cleft lip at 3 months of age, and if prior to surgery presurgical orthodontic treatment was implemented, and following these procedures a year later the cleft palate is repaired followed by another orthodontic treatment, it becomes obvious that all of these procedures have a compound effect on maxillofacial growth and that it is impossible to isolate any single factor to study its effects.

Clinical studies that seemingly prove the influence of a particular surgical procedure on maxillofacial growth are inconclusive, and their validity is more than questionable. It is unfortunate that many surgeons and speech pathologists have adopted this unsubstantiated view and for this reason avoid early surgery, anticipating adverse effects on maxillofacial growth.

A series of studies from the Experimental Cleft Palate Surgical Laboratory at the University of Iowa supplements the data indicating that two-flap palatoplasty does not adversely effect maxillofacial growth. Although cleft palate surgery performed in rabbits and beagles results in various growth aberrations, it did not effect overall craniofacial growth. This observation, combined with the results of the experimental and clinical studies performed at the Iowa Cleft Palate Center, indicates that primary cleft lip repair is also responsible for maxillofacial growth disturbances due to the increased pressure of the repaired lip on the underlying maxillary skeleton. These findings lead us to formulate the hypothesis that both surgical procedures, cleft lip and palate repair, contribute to midfacial growth aberrations.

In addition to experimental research, some leading cleft surgeons have demonstrated that well-designed and delicately performed cleft palate repair has no adverse effect on maxillofacial growth (Salyer, Noordhoff, Jackson, Bardach). Early cleft palate repair, if used in conjunction with presurgical and postsurgical orthodontic treatment, maintains a normal occlusal relationship and fosters normal growth.

The belief that palatoplasty is detrimental to maxillofacial growth flourished at a time when surgical treatment was the dominant method of cleft habilitation, and multidisciplinary management was in its initial stages. Poor surgical techniques produced excessive tension which, without orthodontic treatment, led to severe secondary maxillofacial deformities. These deformities were caused by inhibited maxillary growth in the anteriorposterior direction. Malocclusion and severe prognathism due to the retarded growth of the maxilla were common. At the present time, greatly improved surgical techniques combined with thorough and careful orthodontic treatment nearly eliminate the possibility of developing severe growth aberrations and malocclusion. In our practice, only a minimal number of cases require prolonged orthodontic treatment or orthognatic surgery.

Currently, many leading surgeons advocate early cleft palate repair, operating without hesitation as early as 6 to 9 months of age. The great majority of surgeons operate at 12 to 18 months of age. Analyzing data from many cleft palate centers, we conclude that early cleft palate surgery, when performed by a highly skilled surgeon working in close cooperation with an experienced orthodontist, does not adversely effect maxillofacial growth.

Periodic examinations of the patient by all specialists involved in the treatment, especially by the surgeon and orthodontist, allow for timely orthodontic intervention, which is helpful in preventing growth aberrations and malocclusion. When orthodontists suggest delaying cleft palate repair due to the danger of inhibiting maxillary growth, speech pathologists do well to remember not only the fact that this danger is no more imminent than it was 25 years ago, but also the following idea most clearly expressed by Peet and Patterson: "The reason for operating

on cleft palates is to allow for the development of normal speech. This simple fact must never be forgotten despite a mass of literature of the harmful effects of early palate repair on the growth of the maxilla." Early versus late palatoplasty is not as acutely debated as it was in previous years when surgery was the dominant form of treatment and surgical technique and orthodontic care were not as advanced as they are now.

The choice of surgical technique for palate repair requires discussion. In many books and articles, surgeons and speech pathologists emphasize the relationship between surgical technique and speech results when determining the success or failure of surgical repair. Although this statement is partially correct, surgical technique must be evaluated in light of the skills of the surgeon who performs it. It is reasonable to assume that the same surgical technique performed by a highly skilled surgeon versus an inexperienced one will yield different results. Some surgical techniques seem to be, by design, more effective than others.

Some techniques have serious shortcomings and often lead to undesired complications. The von Langenbeck technique fails to completely close the most anterior portion of the hard palate in complete cleft of the lip, alveolus, and palate, resulting in oronasal fistulas in the anterior portion of the palate. In the Wardill-Kilner technique, the retropositioning of the mucoperiosteal flaps exposes large areas of bone on the palatal shelves. This contributes to maxillary growth aberrations due to scar contracture caused by the secondary healing of bare bone.

In contrast, the two-flap palatoplasty technique completely closes the palatal cleft, including the alveolar portion, and successfully prevents the development of oronasal fistulas. In this technique, a special effort is made to minimize the exposure of bare bone.

As was mentioned above, surgical techniques, no matter how well designed, will not guarantee success when performed by a surgeon with minimal experience and undeveloped skills. Much has been written about the advantages and disadvantages of various surgical techniques in cleft palate repair. However, minimal or no attention has been paid to the critical factor of the surgeon's proficiency. In analyzing the surgeon's proficiency and the importance of surgical technique, the success of the surgical treatment depends on the surgeon as well as the technique.

The success of cleft palate repair is determined primarily by speech development, maxillofacial growth, and the presence or absence of oronasal fistulae. Unquestionably, normal speech development is the major goal of palatoplasty. Cleft palate surgery cannot be considered successful if normal speech is not obtained, even when the cleft palate is completely closed and maxillofacial growth is undisturbed. Another measure is the development of growth aberrations of the maxillary complex. Periodic postsurgical evaluations allow the surgeon and orthodontist to decide if and when additional surgery or orthodontic intervention is necessary to prevent secondary growth disturbances.

A third factor helpful in evaluating the results of cleft palate repair is related to the anatomical conditions of the hard and soft palate. One must pay attention to the extent and quality of surgical repair on the palate. It is important to assess the presence or absence of oronasal fistulae and the length and mobility of the soft palate. In most cases, oronasal fistulas in the anterior portion of the hard palate or on the border between hard and soft palate are the result of inadequate surgical performance. Inadequate surgical repair may also be responsible for a short palate, although on many occasions the anatomical conditions before surgery determine the length of the soft palate. This may be especially true in cases of bilateral cleft of the lip and palate when, before surgery, the segments of the soft palate are short and the muscles are underdeveloped. Length of the soft palate is only one factor to consider when evaluating velopharyngeal closure, which is es-

sential for normal speech production; it must be evaluated within a complex framework of all structures of the velopharynx.

SUGGESTED READINGS

Bardach J: *Cleft palate repair: Two-flap palatoplasty, research, philosophy, technique, and results.* In Bardach J, Morris H, editors: Multidisciplinary management of cleft lip and palate, Philadelphia, 1990, WB Saunders.

Bardach J, Salyer K: Surgical techniques in cleft lip and palate, St. Louis, 1991, Mosby.

Bardach J, Salyer K: *Cleft palate repair.* In Bardach J, Salyer K, editors: Surgical techniques in cleft lip and palate, St. Louis, 1991, Mosby.

Bardach J, Salyer K: *Research in cleft lip and palate.* In Bardach J, Salyer K, editors: Surgical techniques in cleft lip and palate, St. Louis, 1991, Mosby.

Dorf D, Curtin J: *Early cleft palate repair and speech outcome: A ten-year experience.* In Bardach J, Morris H, editors: Multidisciplinary management of cleft lip and palate, Philadelphia, 1990, WB Saunders.

Kriens O: *Anatomy of the cleft palate.* In Bardach J, Morris H, editors: Multidisciplinary management of cleft lip and palate, Philadelphia, 1990, WB Saunders.

La Rossa D, Randall P, Cohen M, Cohen S: *The Furlow double reversing z-plasty for cleft palate repair: the first ten years of experience.* In Bardach J, Morris H, editors: Multidisciplinary management of cleft lip and palate. Philadelphia, 1990, WB Saunders.

Lindsay W, Witzel M: *Cleft palate repair: von Langenbeck technique.* In Bardach J, Morris H, editors: Multidisciplinary management of cleft lip and palate, Philadelphia, 1990, WB Saunders.

Perko M: *Two-stage palatoplasty.* In Bardach J, Morris H, editors: Multidisciplinary management of cleft lip and palate, Philadelphia, 1990, WB Saunders.

Schweckendiek W, Kruse E: *Two-stage palatoplasty: Schweckendiek technique.* In Bardach J, Morris H, editors: Multidisciplinary management of cleft lip and palate, Philadelphia, 1990, WB Saunders.

Skoog T: The use of periosteal flaps in the repair of the primary palate, *Cleft Palate J* 2:332 1965.

8 Communicative Impairment Associated with Clefting

Mary Anne Witzel

This chapter provides a framework for the student or clinician unfamiliar with patients with clefts to identify the communication impairments that may exist and to understand the possible causation of these problems, thus providing the patient with effective and efficient screening, assessment, treatment, and referral.

All children born with a cleft of the lip and/or palate or a syndrome associated with clefting are at risk for communication impairment. These problems can be minor or in some cases cause a significant communication handicap. Communication problems can be evident when the child begins to develop speech and language or can occur at various stages of maturation. In general, children who have a cleft lip and/or palate as part of a syndrome are at greater risk for more complex communication impairment than those with cleft lip and/or palate only. Identification of all phenotypic features and correct diagnosis of syndromes is crucial to understanding and identifying the communication problems that these children may have and selecting the most effective and efficient treatment.

Chapter 1 discusses the differences between the medical and behavioral models in the approach to patient care. It points out that the professions typically referred to as the behavioral sciences usually do not place great importance on the cause of a symptom from either the diagnostic or treatment perspective.

Speech-language pathologists, audiologists and, psychologists, however, should be prepared to approach the speech, language, hearing, and cognitive problems that individuals with clefting may exhibit from the medical model perspective. In the medical model the presenting problems are symptoms of a disease process. Once the disease is identified and its natural history and prognosis understood, the clinician is in a better position to recommend and conduct effective and efficient treatment for improvement or correction of communication impairment (Pollock et al., 1993).

Clinicians providing speech and language evaluation and treatment services as part of a cleft palate or craniofacial team should be well versed not only in the anatomy and function of the vocal tract but also in the implications that various phenotypic features, anomalies, or syndromes will have on all aspects of communication, including speech, language, hearing, and cognition.

Quality is doing things right the first time, for the right reasons. Quality of service depends on the correct diagnosis and selection of the most effective and efficient methods of treatment. Health care systems around the world can ill afford the costs associated with poor quality of service, and therefore the importance of careful differential diagnosis is significant.

Although the communication impairments that individuals with clefting may have are often related to abnormalities in the anatomy or function of various aspects of the vocal tract, all types of communication impairment can occur. Therefore the speech-language pathologist must be careful not to overlook impairments that may be less obvious in the initial assessment.

This chapter describes the types of communication impairment known to occur in cleft lip and/or palate and clefting conditions as well as the known causative factors. Although some clefting conditions and syndromes may have syndrome-specific communication impairments, these are not always well documented in the literature. Clinical researchers in the field of cleft palate and craniofacial disorders are accumulating and publishing data on the communicative phenotypes of many syndromes; however, much remains unknown. It is therefore important that clinicians approach each case with an open mind and consistently assess all aspects of communication to determine the types of impairment(s) that the patient has. Clinicians should also note any unusual phenotypic features that might contribute to the communication impairment or cause them to seek a genetic consultation (Pollock et al., 1993). It is also important that clinicians obtain knowledge of the existing literature when a specific syndrome diagnosis is made to understand the identified communication impairments that the patient is at risk for, as well as the natural history and prognosis for the condition.

It is beyond the scope of this chapter to review all the known communicative impairments associated with each clefting condition. Also, for many syndromes or conditions the complete communication phenotypes are not fully identified. In view of this, it is important that clinicians approach each patient with a consistent framework for evaluation so that all aspects of communication impairment can be identified and these important data can be accumulated (see Chapter 9).

SPEECH IMPAIRMENT

The formation of speech is a complex and coordinated task involving interaction of the structures of respiration and mastication, including the abdomen, diaphragm, chest wall, larynx, oropharynx, nasopharynx, hard palate, soft palate, nasal cavity, maxilla, mandible, lips, tongue, and teeth. To produce voice, these structures generate, shape, and direct the airstream through the vocal tract, which extends from the glottis to the anterior nares and lips. The flow of air through the vocal tract is altered by a series of valves (Fig. 8-1). These include the vocal cords, velopharyngeal (VP) sphincter, lips, and those made by contact or approximation of the tongue with the hard or soft palate, teeth, and lips. Thus, control of the airstream is possible at five sites: larynx, VP valve, nasal valve, tongue with hard palate, soft palate, and teeth, and lips together or with teeth (Witzel and Vallino, 1992).

Articulation

Formation of the sounds of speech is easily influenced by deviations in oral structure and function (Witzel et al., 1980; Vallino and Thomson, 1993) so that the risk of articulation problems is high in those with cleft lip and/or palate or other craniofacial abnormalities. Speech-language pathologists often classify speech sound errors as phonetic or phonologic. Phonetic errors or errors in the articulation or formation of the sounds of speech are related to abnormalities in anatomy, function, and/or motor control or specific problems in learning. Phonologic errors, however, indicate a difficulty in the child's organization, learning, and representation of the sound units and sound system of a

language. Since the anatomy and function of the vocal tract play such a large role in the articulation problems that these individuals exhibit, the most informative analysis of speech sound errors is usually the phonetic classification of voicing, manner of formation, and place of articulation. This allows easier identification of causation than the phonologic processes classification. However, phonetic or sound formation difficulties are thought to lead to persistent phonologic process simplifications (Chapman and Hardin, 1993) and should not be ignored.

Errors of voicing, manner of formation, or place of articulation can occur if the anatomy or function of any of the five valves of the vocal tract is affected. In general, the speech problems that these patients may exhibit are related

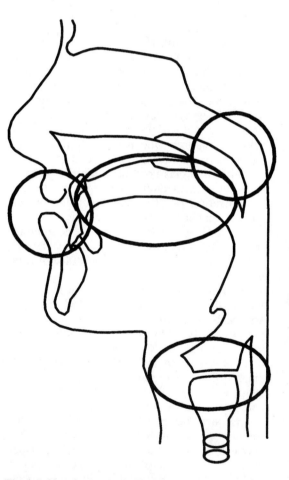

Fig. 8-1 Vocal tract, including sites where the airflow is modified to create speech sounds. (From Witzel MA, Vallino L: Speech problems in patients with dentofacial or craniofacial deformities. In Bell WH, editor: *Modern practice of orthognathic and reconstructive surgery,* vol 2, Philadelphia, 1992, WB Saunders.)

to (1) the anatomy and function of the vocal tract, including the larynx, VP valve, hard and soft palate, tongue, lips, teeth, jaws, and nose, (2) hearing, and (3) brain anatomy and function (Witzel and Vallino, 1992).

Speech begins with respiration. As the respiratory muscles contract, air is exhaled from the lungs and passes through the glottal opening of the larynx. At this level, the flow of air may or may not be interrupted by movement of the vocal cords. When the vocal cords approximate and vibrate during exhalation, voicing is produced. When the vocal cords abduct as air passes freely through the larynx, no voicing occurs. Sounds such as /b/, /d/, /z/, and /g/ are referred to as voiced sounds because they are produced by adduction and vibration of the vocal cords during exhalation of air, sending sound waves into the pharynx and oral cavity to be shaped by the tongue and lips. Voiceless sounds such as /p/, /t/, /s/, and /k/ result when the vocal cords abduct when the air passes through the larynx and is then stopped or narrowed by the tongue or lips. All vowels are voiced and are articulated with very little constriction in the vocal tract. They are created by variations in tongue height, tongue advancement, and lip rounding.

The unvoiced, or voiceless sounds (e.g., /s/) are often more difficult to produce than the voiced sounds (e.g., /z/). This may be influenced, however, by the adequacy of velopharyngeal closure, the type of consonant, and the age of the child.

Manner of formation refers to the degree of narrowing or constriction of the oral or pharyngeal cavities to impede or give frication to the airstream flowing through the vocal tract during articulation. It also refers to the direction of the airstream through the oral cavity over the tongue only or through the nasal and oral cavities simultaneously. For example, stop sounds (/p/, /b/, /t/, /d/, /k/, /g/) are formed when the lips or tongue block the airstream, causing a pressure buildup followed by a sudden release of air. The fricative sounds (/f/, /v/, /th/, /s/, /z/, /sh/, /zh/) are formed when the tongue or lips narrow the airstream to cause frication. The affricate sounds (/ch/, /j/) are formed when the tongue is first positioned as for a stop sound to impede the air and then the air is released through a constriction in the oral cavity that creates friction. The lateral sound (/l/) is produced when the tongue tip is held against the alveolar ridge and the air flows over the side of the tongue. The glides (/w/, /y/, /r/) are produced with gentle constriction of the lips or gentle

contact of the tongue against the palate, which requires minimal impedance of air. For the nasal consonants (/m/, /n/, /ng/) the lips and tongue are positioned for a stop sound, but the air is released through the nasal rather than the oral cavity by the opening of the VP valve (Witzel and Vallino, 1992).

In patients with velopharyngeal inadequacy (VPI), the airstream escapes into the nasal cavity and is not impeded orally to achieve the required air pressure for oral stop, fricative, affricate, lateral, and glide sounds. This phenomenon often results in weak production of pressure sounds. It has been found that most individuals with oral anomalies preserve the manner of formation of sounds but alter the place in the vocal tract where the sound is normally produced to achieve as much narrowing or constriction of the vocal tract as possible. When errors of manner do occur, oral pressure sounds such as /p/, /t/, /k/, /b/, /d/, and /g/ are perceived as weak due to the significant loss of oral pressure or as /m/ and /n/ substitutions. Errors of manner occur when there is a leak in the vocal tract either due to inadequate closure of the VP valve during production of oral sounds or a palatal fistula.

Place of formation refers to the location in the vocal tract where two articulators (e.g., tongue and palate) occlude, or narrow the vocal tract to form a sound. Bilabial sounds (/p/, /b/, /w/) are formed when the lips contact or approximate each other; labiodental sounds (/f/, /v/) are formed when the lower lip contacts the upper incisors. Lingual sounds (/th/, /t/, /d/, /l/, /s/, /z/, /sh/, /zh/, /ch/, /j/, /w/, /r/, /k/, /g/) occur when various parts of the tongue contact or approximate the incisor teeth, the alveolar ridge, the hard palate, or the soft palate. When errors of place occur, the result is usually the substitution of another sound for the consonant being produced. The individual may substitute a normal sound, such as /k/ for /t/ (kop for top) or a compensatory sound such as a pharyngeal stop (Witzel and Vallino, 1992).

A distinctive category of errors of place of articulation is commonly known as *compensatory articulation*. This term describes specific errors of place of articulation that may occur in patients who have inadequate closure of the VP valve or a cleft or fistula in the hard palate. They have been described by Morley (1967) as "compensatory adjustments" and by Bzoch (1979) as "laryngeal and pharyngeal gross substitution errors." The most detailed description has been provided by Trost (1981).

Compared with normal oral consonants,

these erroneous sounds, which are thought to occur in an attempt to shape the airstream below the VP valve, are produced more posterior and inferior in the vocal tract by posterior positioning of the tongue (pharyngeal stop, fricative, or affricate), associated true and false vocal fold adduction (glottal stop), or abnormal positioning of the arytenoid cartilage and epiglottis (laryngeal stop, fricative, or affricate) (Kawano et al., 1985). For example, the pharyngeal fricative, which may be substituted for fricative sounds, occurs when the dorsum of the posterior tongue approximates the posterior pharyngeal wall to give frication to the airstream. Because frication occurs below the VP valve, velopharyngeal closure is unnecessary to produce this compensatory sound (Hoch et al., 1986).

A common misconception about compensatory errors is that they are always the direct result of VP insufficiency or VP incompetence (Trost-Cardamone, 1989) and that patients who exhibit these errors require surgical or prosthetic management of VPI before these errors can be corrected by speech therapy (Hoch et al., 1986). Although compensatory articulation is sometimes a consequence of VPI, VPI may be a consequence of compensatory articulation because limited movements of the VP valve occur during production of these sounds. Hoch et al. (1986) have described increased movements of the components of the VP valve after speech therapy to improve compensatory articulation.

To date, 10 types of compensatory articulation substitutions have been identified in the literature (Trost, 1981; Kawano et al., 1985). These include sounds that are produced in a more posterior and lower place in the vocal tract than normal, such as the glottal stop, and those in which posterior or other abnormal positioning of the tongue is often implicated. In some cases, there is abnormal positioning and function of the larynx and the epiglottis. Warren (1986) proposes that compensatory articulation errors are produced in response to the individual's inability to direct the airflow normally through the vocal tract. This theory of regulation control is based on the premise that normal speech results from the flow and pressure of air, which are directed and controlled by the valves of the vocal tract (see Fig. 8-1). The flow and pressure of air through the oral cavity are reduced when the VP valve is inadequate or there is a fistula, causing problems with the formation of oral pressure sounds. In response to this inability to create sufficient airflow and pressure through the mouth or vocal tract, the individual may attempt to produce oral speech sounds by shaping the airflow in the lower vocal

tract, where sufficient airflow and pressure can be generated.

In addition to the ten types of compensatory articulation substitutions described above, this author has observed two additional substitutions (laryngeal stop and posterior nasal affricate).

Types of compensatory articulation errors

Glottal stop: The most well-known compensatory error is the glottal stop, a normal sound in many languages or dialects. In English it starts the production of vowel sounds when used in isolation or at the beginning of words. It becomes a compensatory error, however, when it is used as a substitution for stop consonant sounds. The glottal stop occurs when the vocal cords adduct and allow air pressure to build up below the glottis. When the glottal stop is used as a substitution for consonant stop sounds, the individual usually builds greater pressure below the glottis than is used for vowels, causing excessive tension in the lower vocal tract and more intense opening and closing of the vocal cords. When this pressure and tension are significant, nasopharyngoscopy shows the false vocal cords or ventricular folds to move medially and contact in the midline (Fig. 8-2). This finding may indi-

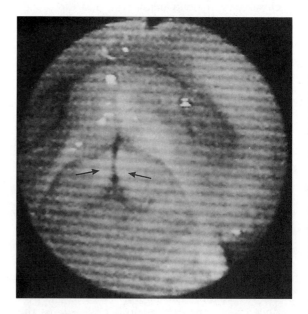

Fig. 8-2 Nasopharyngoscopic view of the larynx during production of a glottal stop substitution. Note the medial excursion of the false vocal folds so that they are meeting in the midline over the true vocal cords.

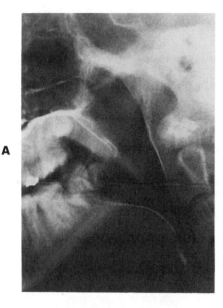

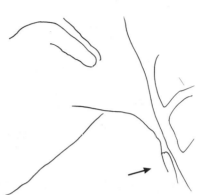

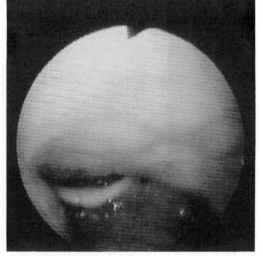

Fig. 8-3 A, Lateral still frame from a videofluoroscopy study showing posterior position of tongue and epiglottis to contact the pharynx for production of the laryngeal stop substitution. **B,** Nasopharyngoscopic view of base of tongue and epiglottis against the pharynx to produce the laryngeal stop substitution.

cate a more severe form of the glottal stop substitution whereby even greater subglottic pressure is involved.

Laryngeal stop: This is a substitution for stop sounds whereby the base of the tongue moves posteriorly toward the pharynx, causing the epiglottis to contact the pharynx, thereby momentarily blocking the airstream. It is also thought that the larynx moves in a superior direction during this activity to assist in temporarily stopping the airway (Fig. 8-3).

Laryngeal fricative: The laryngeal fricative is a substitution for fricative sounds whereby the base of the tongue moves posteriorly toward the pharynx, causing the epiglottis to approach the pharynx, thereby narrowing the airstream to create frication. It is also thought that the larynx moves superiorly during this activity to assist in the narrowing of the airstream (Fig. 8-4) (Kawano et al., 1985).

Laryngeal affricate: This is a substitution for affricate sounds whereby the base of the tongue moves posteriorly toward the pharynx, causing the epiglottis to briefly contact the pharynx and then constrict the airstream to create stopping and then frication. It is also thought that the larynx moves superiorly during this activity.

Pharyngeal stop: In this substitution for stop sounds the dorsum of the tongue moves posteriorly to contact the pharynx, causing a pressure buildup followed by a sudden release of air (Fig. 8-5) (Trost, 1981).

Pharyngeal fricative: A pharyngeal fricative is a substitution for fricative sounds whereby the dorsum of the tongue moves posteriorly toward the pharynx to constrict the airstream, causing frication (Fig. 8-6).

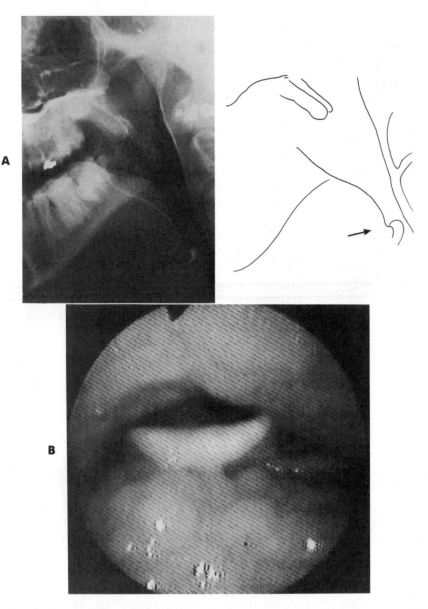

Fig. 8-4 A, Lateral still frame from a videofluoroscopy study showing posterior position of tongue and epiglottis to narrow the pharynx for production of the laryngeal fricative substitution. **B,** Nasopharyngoscopic view of base of tongue and epiglottis approaching the pharynx to produce the laryngeal fricative substitution.

Pharyngeal affricate: In this substitution for affricate sounds the dorsum of the tongue moves posteriorly, contacting the pharynx, and then constricting the airstream to create stopping and then frication (Fig. 8-7).

Posterior nasal fricative: This is a substitution for fricative sounds whereby the posterior dorsum of the tongue and soft palate are positioned to generate frication at the VP valve. The tongue and VP valve positions have been reported to be variable (Trost, 1981), but the error sound is always accompanied by audible nasal air emission. This error usually occurs without other compensatory errors (i.e., glottal stop) and is amenable to therapy. Once the child begins to articulate the fricative sounds using correct tongue placement, the nasal air

PHARYNGEAL STOP

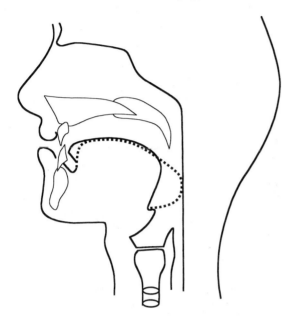

PHARYNGEAL AFFRICATE

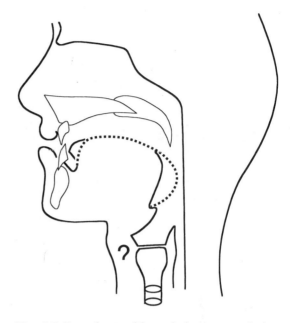

Fig. 8-5 Posterior position of the tongue during production of the pharyngeal stop substitution. (Modified from Trost JE: Articulatory additions to the classical description of the speech of persons with cleft palate, *Cleft Palate J* 18:193, 1981.)

Fig. 8-7 Posterior position of the tongue during production of the pharyngeal affricate substitution.

PHARYNGEAL FRICATIVE

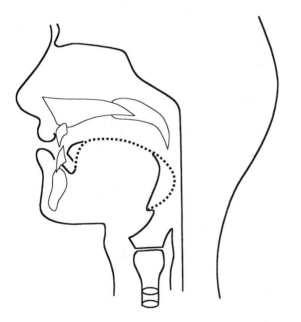

Fig. 8-6 Posterior position of the tongue during production of the pharyngeal fricative substitution.

emission is eliminated and VP closure occurs. This is often referred to as sound-specific VP inadequacy (Trost-Cardamone, 1986).

Posterior nasal affricate: In this substitution for affricate sounds the posterior dorsum of the tongue and soft palate are positioned to create both stopping and frication at the VP valve. This error sound is always accompanied by audible nasal air emission and usually occurs with the posterior nasal fricative but without other compensatory errors (i.e., glottal stop); is amenable to therapy. Once the child begins to articulate the affricate sounds using correct tongue placement, the nasal air emission is eliminated and VP closure occurs. This is often referred to as sound-specific VPI.

Middorsum palatal stop: This is a Substitution for stop sounds /t/, /d/, /k/, and /g/ made by the middorsum area of the tongue contacting the hard palate to create pressure buildup at the approximate place where the glide /j/ would be produced (Fig. 8-8). This error is often used when the patient has an open palatal fistula in an attempt to occlude the fistula while articulating stop sounds. It has also been noted, however, without a palatal fistula (Trost, 1981).

MID-DORSUM PALATAL STOP

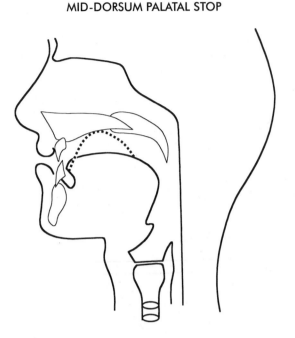

Fig. 8-8 Position of the tongue during production of the middorsum palatal stop substitution. (Modified from Trost JE: Articulatory additions to the classical description of the speech of persons with cleft palate, *Cleft Palate J* 18:197, 1981.)

Middorsum palatal fricative: In this substitution for fricative sounds the middorsum area of the tongue approaches the hard palate to create frication at the approximate place where the glide /j/ would be produced. Normal production of these fricative sounds occurs anterior to this with the tongue blade approaching the alveolar and prepalatal areas of the hard palate. This error is often used when the patient has an open palatal fistula in an attempt to occlude the fistula while articulating fricative sounds.

Middorsum palatal affricate: In this substitution for affricate sounds the middorsum area of the tongue contacts and approaches the hard palate to create pressure buildup and then frication at the approximate place where the glide /j/ would be produced. Normal production of the affricate sounds occurs anterior to this with the tongue blade approaching the prepalatal areas of the hard palate. This error is often used when the patient has an open palatal fistula in an attempt to occlude the fistula while articulating affricate sounds.

The middorsum palatal stop, fricative, and affricate are not the result of VPI, nor do they necessarily cause decreased function of the VP valve. They most often occur in response to an open palatal fistula.

Other errors of place include auditory or visual distortions of sounds produced in the anterior area of the mouth. The tongue may protrude through or between the teeth, causing distortion in the formation of linguo-alveolar and linguopalatal sounds (Fig. 8-9). Atypical lip movements caused by a repaired cleft lip, problems with cranial nerve innervation, or malocclusion may cause substitution or distortion of the bilabial, labiodental, tip dental, tip alveolar, blade alveolar, and blade prepalatal sounds.

Phonology

There are few reports in the literature of the phonologic abilities of children with clefting. The existing studies, however, indicate that the speech sound errors that many children with cleft lip and/or palate exhibit may not be purely phonetic and may also have a phonologic component (Lynch et al., 1983; Estrem and Broen, 1989; Powers et al, 1990; Chapman and Hardin, 1992; Chapman, 1993), suggesting a difficulty with the child's ability to organize and represent the sound units and system of language.

The most descriptive study to date of phonologic processes in preschool children with cleft palate (with or without cleft lip) (Chapman, 1993) indicated early delays in phonologic development particularly for the processes of deletion of final consonants, syllable reduction, and backing. However, these delays were less apparent by 4 to 5 years of age when the phonologic skills of the children with cleft palate were similar to noncleft counterparts.

To date, there are no published reports of phonologic abilities in specific syndromes associated with clefting. This information may provide the clinician with an additional framework for planning and conducting treatment of speech problems in these children.

Resonance

The resonance of voice (the amplification of sound waves produced by the vibrations of the vocal cords) is influenced by the size, shape, and surface of the infraglottal and supraglottal resonating structures and cavities. These resonators include the trachea, bronchial tube, lungs, rib cage, laryngeal ventricle, epiglottis, thyroid cartilage, aryepiglottic folds, pharynx,

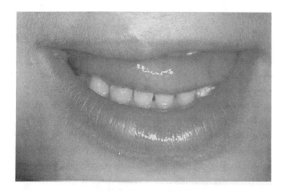

Fig. 8-9 Tongue protrusion through a space created by missing teeth at the site of a cleft during production of lingual alveolar sound /s/. (From Witzel MA, Vallino L: Speech problems in patients with dentofacial or craniofacial deformities. In Bell WH, editor: *Modern practice of orthognathic and reconstructive surgery,* vol 2, Philadelphia: 1992, WB Saunders.)

tongue, oral cavity, facial muscles, cheek muscles, mastication muscles, soft and hard palates, nasal cavity, and paranasal sinuses (Witzel and Vallino, 1992).

A sound wave is produced when a mechanical disturbance, such as the vibration of the vocal cords, creates a high-pressure area that moves through air. When this high-pressure area passes through an enclosed space, the waves are repeated and amplified, and a resonating cavity is created. The volume of the cavity determines the number of simultaneous sound waves. All surfaces have a natural frequency at which they begin to vibrate. If the frequency in a cavity surface is the same as that of the sound wave, the surface also vibrates, sending separate sound waves, called the sounding board effect (Gray, 1959). Each type of speech sound, which is categorized according to the manner and place of production, involves different resonating cavities and structures.

As the airstream enters the pharynx, it is directed through the oral or nasal cavity or both by the opening and closing of the VP valve. The degree of closure of the VP valve is related to the consonant and vowel sounds produced.

Several types of abnormal vocal resonance problems may exist or coexist in patients who have clefting or craniofacial abnormalities. Hypernasality is the speech problem most often associated with cleft palate and syndromes associated with clefting. This abnormality of resonance occurs when the sound waves emanating from the vocal folds enter both the oral and nasal cavities during speech, causing both cavity chambers to vibrate and enhance the sound

waves. The degree can range from mild to severe. It is perceived when vowels and consonants such as /l/ and vocalic /r/ are produced. In most cases, hypernasality results from inadequate closure of the VP valve during speech, but it may also be caused by the entrance of air into the nasal cavity through an open cleft palate or fistula in the hard or soft palate. Other subtle factors also need to be considered, such as tissue mass and elasticity, structural deviations in the nose, constriction or tension in the vocal tract, mouth opening, respiratory efforts, tongue movements, timing of VP closure in relation to laryngeal, lingual, and labial movements for speech, and nasal resistance (Witzel and Stringer, 1988).

The initiation of the coordinated movements of the speech mechanism may also be a factor in the hypernasality of such patients. Several investigators have shown that speakers with cleft palate may show differences in the timing of VP closure (Forner 1983; Folkins, 1985; Karnell et al., 1985). These differences are thought to be attempts to compensate for varying degrees of inadequate closure. Momentary hypernasality and/or nasal air emission at the outset of speech may result if VP closure is not completed before the sound waves are generated from the vocal cords, allowing some sound waves to enter the nasal cavity. Other individuals have difficulty sustaining VP closure during speech, resulting in intermittent hypernasality and nasal air emission.

Oral cavity constriction during speech may increase hypernasal resonance by forcing more sound waves into the nasal cavity. This constriction may be the result of restricting mouth opening during speech, posterior or superior positioning of the dorsum of the tongue during articulation of some sounds, or abnormal positioning or tension of the pharynx (Boone, 1983).

Other types of abnormal resonance include hyponasality, denasality, cul de sac, and muffled. Hyponasal resonance occurs when a partial blockage in the nose increases the airflow resistance, thereby reducing the sound wave vibration in the nasal cavity and altering the acoustic production of the nasal consonants (/m/, /n/, and /ng/).

Denasality occurs when the nose is completely blocked, preventing almost all vibration of sound waves in the nasal cavity. In this situation the nasal consonants approximate the oral consonants /b/, /d/, and /g/.

Partial or complete blockage of the nasal airway may be caused by collapse of the anterior nasal valve, a deviated nasal septum, enlarged nasal turbinates, nasal polyps, high palatal vault, choanal atresia, enlarged adenoid tissue, retro-displaced maxilla, or an obstructive pharyngeal flap. Patients with these conditions are usually mouth breathers.

Another resonance abnormality is known as cul-de-sac resonance. Its cause and perceptual quality are poorly understood and documented. McWilliams and colleagues (1990) believe that it results from an anterior rather than a posterior nasal obstruction and gives a muffled quality to nasal consonants. Without precise descriptions of the perceptual correlates of this phenomenon, these authors refer to it as a variation of hyponasality and denasality.

Hyponasality and denasality are not the opposites of hypernasality. These two forms of resonance can occur together in the same patient, unless there is total nasal obstruction that will obscure hypernasality. Some patients with VPI may also have partial or total obstruction on one side of the nasal airway. This sometimes occurs in those with unilateral cleft lip and palate. The effect of the obstruction on speech resonance may not be appreciated until after surgical or prosthetic treatment of VPI, when the listener's perception of it is heightened. Conversely, in patients with VPI, correcting nasal obstruction can increase the perception of hypernasality and nasal air emission.

Clinicians working with patients with craniofacial anomalies sometimes refer to muffled resonance. This term has been used to describe the unusual resonance in patients with Treacher Collins syndrome or Nager syndrome. These patients have a very shallow nasopharynx and oropharynx and bony deformities of the facial skeleton that limit their resonating cavity. The tongue often assumes a posterior position in the pharynx, further limiting resonance. Many also have VPI.

Nasal air emission

Nasal air emission, or nasal escape, is silent or audible airflow through the nose during production of sounds in which airflow should be directed through the mouth. It usually results from inadequate closure of the VP valve but can also be the result of a fistula in the hard or soft palate. Nasal air emission in the absence of a fistula indicates that the VP valve closes incompletely but not necessarily that it is inadequate. This emission, when audible, has been considered a separate speech characteristic, an error of articulation, and a secondary manifestation of VPI (Peterson-Falzone, 1986).

Nasal air emission and hypernasality are not synonymous, although they often coexist and are interrelated. Nasal air emission can occur without the perception of hypernasality, as in individuals who have sound-specific VPI. Conversely, hypernasality can occur without nasal air emission, as in the person with a submucous cleft palate who can achieve VP closure but whose soft palate is thin and hypoplastic, causing the air waves in the vocal tract to vibrate the soft palate enough to displace the air in the nasal cavity (McWilliams et al., 1990).

If nasal air emission is intense, it will often be audible to the listener and be perceived as a snorting sound. If it meets resistance in the nasal cavity due to a partial or complete blockage, turbulent noises will be perceived. This turbulence is most noticeable on sounds that require sustained closure of the VP valve, such as the fricative and affricate sounds.

The nasal alae and surrounding facial musculature will contract during speech in some patients with abnormal nasal air emission in an attempt to limit the emission. This grimacing may enhance the sound of nasal air emission and distract the listener-observer by affecting the esthetic appearance of the face during speech.

If partial or complete blockage of the nasal airway is present, normal occurring nasal air emission for nasal sounds will be reduced or absent, resulting in hyponasal or denasal speech.

Phonation

Problems of laryngeal voice, or phonation, in patients with clefting have not been well documented. There have been descriptions of problems such as hoarseness, breathiness, abnormal pitch, soft voice, and strangled voice (McWilliams et al., 1990). These problems may be functional or a direct response to abnormal anatomy or pathology.

Patients with borderline VP closure and cleft palate are thought to be at risk for hoarseness secondary to hyperfunctional use of the vocal cords, resulting in vocal cord edema, nodules, or other pathology. It is hypothesized that this occurs as the patient uses laryngeal hyperfunction to compensate for borderline VP valving (McWilliams et al., 1969). Vocal cord pathology may also be evident in patients who consistently use the glottal stop substitution with increased laryngeal hyperfunction.

Breathiness secondary to poor lubrication of the vocal cords has been reported in ectrodactyly - ectrodermal - dysplasia - clefting syndrome (Gorlin et al., 1990). Abnormal pitch has been documented in Apert syndrome (Witzel, 1983) and velo-cardio-facial syndrome (Shprintzen et al., 1978). Diplophonia may occur when there is abnormal innervation of the vagus nerve to the larynx, as found in some cases of hemifacial microsomia. Laryngeal stridor may occur in cases of laryngomalacia.

Use of a soft voice may be related to the individual's inability to create sufficient oral pressure during speech, or it may be an attempt to reduce the perception of hypernasality or nasal air emission. A strangled voice often results from insufficient mouth opening during articulation. This may also be an attempt by the speaker to reduce the perception of abnormal resonance and nasal air emission.

Intelligibility

Intelligibility is a general judgment of speech that refers to how well a listener understands it. Intelligibility of speech is influenced by many variables, including articulation, resonanace, nasal air emission, laryngeal phonation, rate and fluency of speech, stress, accent, and intonation. Intelligibility is decreased by both articulation and hypernasality. Of the two, articulation seems to have a more direct influence than hypernasality (Subtelny et al., 1972; Moore and Summers, 1973).

Intelligibility ratings offer only a global judgment of speech. They do not determine specific aspects of speech, such as articulation or nasal resonance, or specific consequences of surgery or prosthetic treatment. Ratings of intelligibility may be affected by the familiarity or ease with which the listener adapts to the speaker's errors, the conversation topic, and the length and complexity of the utterances.

Acceptability

Acceptability of speech is the subjective impression of the pleasingness of speech. It involves the perception and judgment of both the sound of speech and the appearance of the speaker (Witzel and Vallino, 1992).

Sound of speech. There are few reports of the reactions and judgments of listeners (including parents, peers, and laypersons) to the speech problems that individuals with clefting exhibit. Several authors have investigated the perceptual preferences of the listener for compensatory articulation or nasal air emission in children with repaired cleft palate; single words produced with compensatory articulation are more acceptable to both parents and other children than are single words produced with nasal air emission (Paynter and Kinard, 1979).

Appearance of speech. Speech quality and facial attractiveness are both powerful factors in determining interpersonal attitudes and behavior (Glass and Starr, 1979). The visual cues received by an observer while watching an individual speak may either enhance or detract from the intelligibility of the speaker's articulation (Wells, 1971). Abnormalities in the facial appearance during speech that may distract the listener-observer include atypical movements of the lips, jaws, and tongue during formation of bilabial, labiodental, and linguoalveolar sounds. Facial and occlusal anomalies combined with these abnormal movements may affect judgment of facial appearance, speech acceptability, and social acceptability (Klaiman et al., 1988).

LANGUAGE IMPAIRMENT
Receptive and expressive language

Clinicians often focus on the speech and hearing problems associated with clefting. Therefore, language delays and disorders have not received as much attention. In general, language development has been found to be delayed in children with cleft lip and palate and cleft palate only (Lynch, 1986; McWilliams et al., 1990). However, for many children, especially those with cleft lip and palate or cleft palate only without an identified syndrome, these delays improve with age (Shames and Rubin, 1971, Musgrave et al., 1975).

In the past decade, neurolinguistic deficits have been identified in many of the genetic syndromes associated with clefting. These neurolinguistic deficits often result in varying degrees of receptive and expressive language delay or disorders, reading disorders, or learning disabilities (Gilger, 1992; Schaefer et al., 1992). There is a great need for more research and data in the area of language development and proficiency, particularly for syndromes associated with clefting, so that early identification and appropriate treatment planning can occur.

The features of language

The five major features of language—phonology, semantics, syntax, morphology, and pragmatics—are closely related and intertwined. Clinical research on the abilities of children with cleft lip and palate, cleft palate only, and syndromes associated with clefting in these five areas of language is beginning to emerge, but at this time our level of knowledge is basic.

Expanding our knowledge base in the abilities and weaknesses in the features of language will provide the clinician with an additional framework for planning and conducting treatment of language problems in these children.

Phonology. There are few reports in the literature of the phonologic abilities of children with clefting. The existing studies, however, indicate that the speech sound errors that many children with cleft lip and/or palate exhibit may not be purely phonetic and may also have a phonologic component (Lynch et al., 1983; Estrem and Broen, 1989; Powers et al; 1990; Chapman and Hardin, 1992; Chapman, 1993), suggesting a difficulty with the child's ability to organize and represent the sound units and system of language.

The most descriptive study to date of phonologic processes in preschool children with cleft palate (with or without cleft lip) was by Chapman (1993), indicating early delays in phonologic development particularly for the processes of deletion of final consonants, syllable reduction, and backing. However, these delays were less apparent by 4 to 5 years of age, when the phonologic skills of the children with cleft palate were similar to noncleft counterparts. To date, there are no published reports of phonologic abilities in specific syndromes associated with clefting.

Semantics, syntax, morphology, and pragmatics. Information on these features in those with clefting or conditions associated with clefting is almost nonexistent. In the area of syntax, it has been reported that mean sentence length is shorter in those with clefts in comparison to noncleft peers (McWilliams et al., 1990).

Learning and reading disability

Language learning disability may occur in children with clefting if they have verbal deficits. Research by Richman (1980) and Richman and Eliason (1984) has indicated that children with cleft lip and palate are susceptible to verbal expressive deficits, whereas those with cleft palate only are more likely to demonstrate poor associative reasoning and pervasive language disability.

In some conditions associated with clefting, such as velo-cardio-facial syndrome, Prader-Willi syndrome, neurofibromatosis, and fetal alcohol syndrome, learning disability is a frequent phenotypic feature. It may be related to generalized cognitive deficits, central nervous system dysfunction, or specific components of language. Some have specific verbal expressive deficits and some have poor associative reasoning, indicating a general language learning disability. Neuropsychologic testing should be considered for any patient with a history of developmental delay, receptive or expressive language difficulties, or a syndrome known to have a high incidence of learning disabilities.

Reading disability has also been identified in both cleft lip and palate and cleft palate only groups of children (Richman et al., 1988), and the incidence is higher than in the general population (Richman and Eliason, 1986). Approximately one third of children with cleft lip and palate and one half of children with cleft palate only will experience difficulty in reading abilities. The studies by Richman and Eliason (1984) suggest that those with cleft palate only tend to make whole word gestalt-type errors, whereas those with cleft lip and palate are more likely to make phonetic errors.

Specific reading disability has not been reported in conditions associated with clefting; however, those with identified cognitive deficits or general language learning disability would be at high risk for reading disability.

Cognitive impairment

Numerous studies have been undertaken to examine the intellectual abilities of children with various types of clefting (Richman and Eliason, 1986; McWilliams et al., 1990). In general, the studies indicate that those with cleft lip and palate have intelligence quotients that fall within the average range. The risk for deficits in intelligence is increased in those with cleft palate only, especially when other congenital anomalies are present. Cognitive impairment can range from a specific language or learning disability to severe mental retardation. Children with clefting conditions should be followed closely during their developmental stages so that delays in development can be identified early and appropriate intervention strategies planned and administered.

Hearing impairment

All individuals with conditions associated with clefting are at risk for hearing loss, and any type of hearing loss can occur. Although conductive hearing loss is the most common, sensorineural and mixed losses also occur. These losses can be fluctuating, static, progressive, or have delayed onset. They can be acquired or congenital, unilateral or bilateral. The severity can range from mild to profound. It is therefore extremely important that all individuals with clefting or conditions associated with clefting have early and routine audiologic and otologic assessment, with follow-up and treatment as appropriate. Hearing loss, depending on the type, degree, configuration, and age of onset, can have variable effects on speech and language development, behavior, academic achievement, social interaction, and social acceptance.

Conductive hearing loss. Children with clefting are at high risk for fluctuating mild to moderate conductive hearing loss, since the incidence of otitis media (the accumulation of fluid in the middle ear space) has been reported as high as 100% (Paradise et al., 1969). With otologic care and routine audiologic follow-up the risk for hearing loss can be minimized. Children with fluctuating conductive hearing losses will receive inconsistent speech and language information. This is thought to contribute to early speech and language delays, which may ultimately affect academic performance. The most common cause of conductive hearing loss is abnormal anatomy and/or function of the eustachian tube. However, conductive hearing loss may also be the result of anatomic abnormality of the structures of the external (Fig. 8-10) or middle ear or the tympanic membrane, or it may be the result of abnormal function of any of these structures.

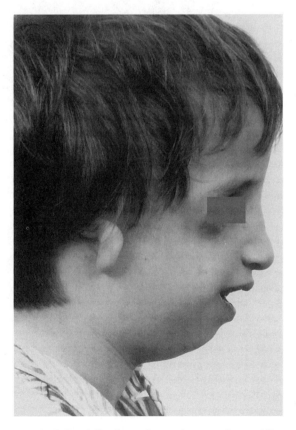

Fig. 8-10 Partially formed ear in a patient with Treacher Collins syndrome.

Sensorineural hearing loss. Sensorineural hearing loss, although not as common as conductive hearing loss, is also a finding in individuals with conditions associated with clefting. It is usually congenital and static due to structural malformation in the inner ear, the spiral ganglion and stria vascularis, the cochlear neurons, or the auditory nerve. It may be progressive in syndromes such as neurofibromatosis where tumorous growths impinge on the auditory nerve (Jung, 1989). The sensorineural hearing loss may be of any configuration (i.e., sloping or flat), any degree (i.e., mild to profound), and affect all or only some frequencies. This type of hearing loss affects the perception or clarity of the sound being heard, resulting in a distortion of sounds and difficulty in discriminating among the sounds of speech.

Mixed loss. A mixed loss occurs when there is both a conductive loss and a sensorineural loss. For example, a child with Treacher Collins syndrome may have a conductive loss due to atresia or microtia of the outer ear and a sensorineural loss due to a structural malformation in the inner ear (Pron et al., 1993).

Unilateral and bilateral loss. Unilateral hearing loss is a frequent finding in the oculo-auriculo-vertebral spectrum of the branchial arch disorders such as hemifacial microsomia. These losses are usually conductive but may also be sensorineural or mixed. The affect of unilateral hearing loss on speech and language development and proficiency is usually thought to be negligible; however, this is an area where more investigative research is needed.

Bilateral hearing loss, if significant enough to cause difficulty in the perception of speech and environmental sounds, can handicap speech, language, and social interaction. A hearing loss may become symptomatic at the 15 to 20 dB level for some children, particularly if the hearing loss occurs before speech and language development begins.

Tinnitus and vestibular dysfunction. Tinnitus and vestibular dysfunction can occur as the result of abnormalities in the anatomy or function of the cochlea or fibers of the auditory nerve. Tinnitus may also be secondary to infection of the middle or inner ear, intracranial lesions that affect the central auditory nervous system, or transmission of normal or abnormal vascular pulsations to the cochlea. These problems are difficult to assess in young children, and the incidence in craniofacial anomalies is unknown (Black and Lilly, 1990).

PHENOTYPIC FEATURES AFFECTING SPEECH

Nose

The nose may be abnormal in size and shape and there may be varying degrees of nasal obstruction. In those with cleft lip and palate the cross-sectional area of the nose is smaller than normal (Warren, 1984). Obstruction may be total or partial because of a deviated nasal septum, enlarged turbinates, mucosal swelling and inflammation, slumping of the nasal alae, and tissue remnants in the anterior portion of the nose after cleft lip repair. When the nose is small or there is obstruction, there may be increased nasal airway resistance during speech, contributing to hyponasality or denasality.

Lips

The lips may affect the articulation of bilabial and labiodental sounds if there is a repaired cleft lip, abnormal nerve innervation, or if the lips are in an abnormal position because of the position of the maxilla or mandible. Most clinicians disregard the potential effects of the cleft lip on speech because patients who have clefts of the lip only are usually reported to have normal articulation and resonance.

In general, complete bilateral clefts of the lip may have a more significant effect on speech than complete unilateral clefts of the lip. The movements and flexibility of the upper lip for formation of vowels and bilabial sounds are often reduced due to deficiency, tightness, or excessive scarring of the orbicularis oris muscle.

In patients who have cleft lip and palate and maxillary hypoplasia, the lower lip often assumes an everted or protruded position at rest (Fig. 8-11). During speech, as the patient attempts to position the lips for bilabial and labiodental sounds, excessive motion of the lower lip is observed, detracting from the facial appearance. When deformities of the jaws and malocclusion prevent easy closure of the lips, the bilabial sounds are affected (Fig. 8-12).

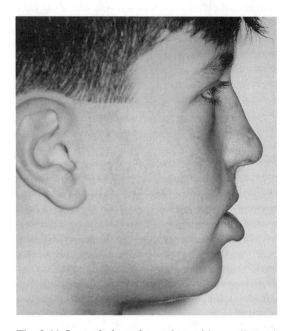

Fig. 8-11 Lateral view of a patient with a unilateral cleft lip and palate. Note the everted lower lip. (From Witzel MA, Vallino L: Speech problems in patients with dentofacial or craniofacial deformities. In Bell WH, editor: *Modern practice of orthognathic and reconstructive surgery,* vol 2, Philadelphia: 1992, WB Saunders.)

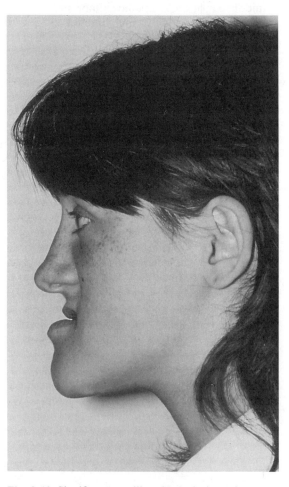

Fig. 8-12 Significant maxillary hypoplasia and negative overjet in a patient with cleft lip and palate showing difficulty in lip closure for bilabial sounds.

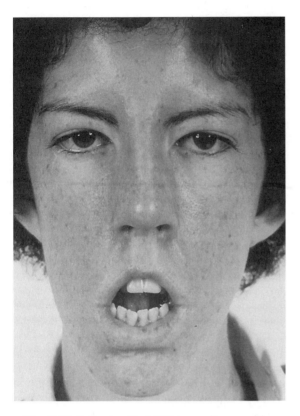

Fig. 8-13 Patient with Möbius syndrome with an inability to obtain lip closure due to bilateral seventh nerve paralysis. (From Witzel MA, Vallino L: Speech problems in patients with dentofacial or craniofacial deformities. In Bell WH, editor: *Modern practice of orthognathic and reconstructive surgery,* vol 2, Philadelphia: 1992, WB Saunders.)

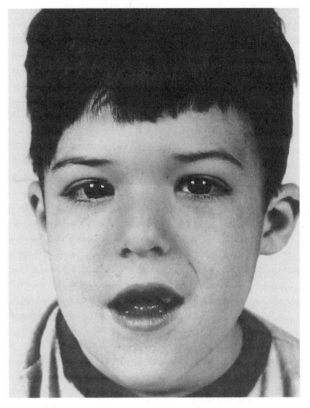

Fig. 8-14 Patient with velo-cardio-facial syndrome. Note the thin vermilion border of the upper lip.

Unilateral or bilateral underdevelopment or paralysis of the seventh cranial nerve, as found in hemifacial microsomia and Möbius syndrome, impede or prevent bilabial and labiodental sounds (Fig. 8-13).

Abnormalities in the anatomy of the upper or lower lip may be indications of syndromes of clefting and therefore be indirectly related to the presenting speech problems. For example, the vermilion of the upper lip may be abnormally thin in velo-cardio-facial syndrome (Fig. 8-14), and there are pits or mounds in the lower lip in Van der Woude syndrome (Fig. 8-15).

Teeth

Interdental spacing and missing teeth. Lingual-alveolar sounds, particularly /s/ and /z/, are affected by spaces in the anterior dental arch due to the cleft or by missing or rotated incisor teeth (Fig. 8-16). When the interdental space is large, the tongue moves forward into and often

through it during speech, distracting the listener-observer. Missing teeth or interdental spaces cause a central or lateral and in some cases bilateral lisp for the lingual-alveolar and lingual-palatal sounds. These errors are perceived both auditorily and visually, causing distortion of the speaker's appearance.

Occlusion. Occlusal defects often have a detrimental effect on the production of anterior speech sounds. Patients with protrusion of the maxillary incisors (positive overjet) can have difficulty approximating the lips for bilabial sounds (Fig. 8-17). If the airstream cannot be directed anteriorly, the sibilant-fricative sounds can become distorted. Patients with protrusion of the mandibular incisors (negative overjet) may incorrectly place the lower incisors against the upper lip to produce the labiodental /f/ and /v/ sounds, resulting in visual facial distortion (Fig. 8-18).

The lingual-aveolar sounds /s/ and /z/ are frequently distorted if the tongue is carried low, protruded, or if the frication within the oral port is impeded. The /r/ and /l/ sounds may also be affected if the tongue cannot retrude accurately and sufficiently for the correct production.

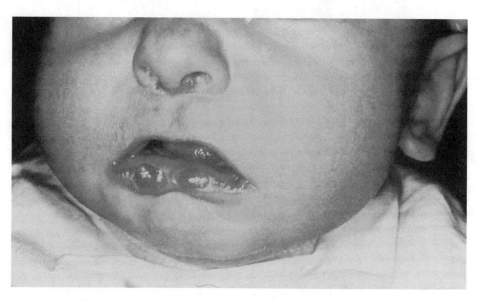

Fig. 8-15 Lip pits on the lower lip in a patient with Van der Woude syndrome.

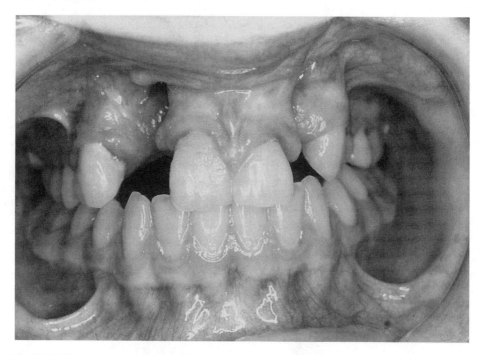

Fig. 8-16 Missing teeth and spaces in the anterior upper dental arch in a patient with bilateral cleft lip and palate. (From McWilliams BJ, Witzel MA: *Cleft palate in human communication disorders: an introduction,* New York, 1994, Macmillan.)

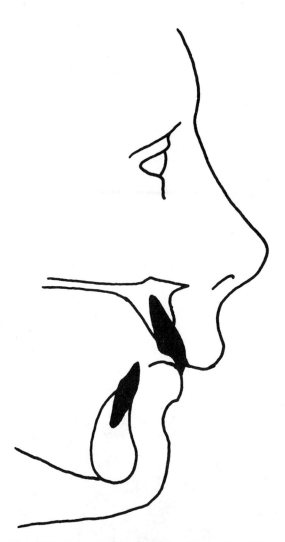 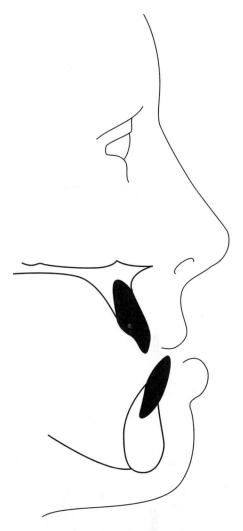

Fig. 8-17 Retrognathic facial profile and positive overjet malocclusion. (From Witzel MA: Speech Problems in craniofacial anomalies, *Communicative Disorders* 8(4):49, 1983.)

Fig. 8-18 Prognathic facial profile and negative overjet malocclusion. (From Witzel MA: Speech problems in craniofacial anomalies, *Communicative Disorders* 8(4):49, 1983.)

An open bite malocclusion (Fig. 8-19) can prevent the lips from approximating for the formation of the bilabial or labiodental sounds and cause facial distortions. There may also be speech and facial distortion during sibilant-fricative–blade alveolar and blade prepalatal sounds, if the patient has difficulty directing the required airstream or protrudes the tongue through the open bite.

Maxilla

The shape, size, and position of the maxilla can also affect speech sound production. Patients with unilateral cleft lip and palate may have

unilateral collapse of the maxillary arch, and those with bilateral cleft lip and palate may have bilateral collapse (Fig. 8-20). This abnormality often causes the required airstream for the blade alveolar and blade prepalatal sounds to be directed laterally or bilaterally resulting in distortion. The lingual-alveolar sounds may be substituted by the back velar sounds /k/ or /g/ or the middorsum palatal stop if the patient has difficulty achieving a comfortable site to produce these sounds.

Maxillary hypoplasia affects articulation when it is accompanied by negative overjet with or without open bite. In these cases, there may

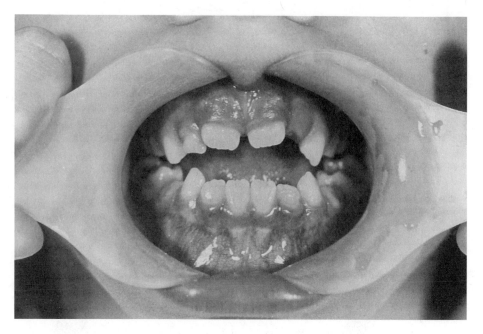

Fig. 8-19 Open bite malocclusion.

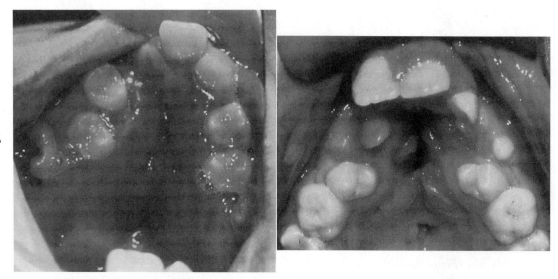

Fig. 8-20 A, Unilateral maxillary collapse. **B,** Bilateral maxillary collapse. (From Witzel MA, Vallino L: Speech problems in patients with dentofacial or craniofacial deformities. In Bell WH, editor: *Modern practice of orthognathic and reconstructive surgery,* vol 2, Philadelphia: 1992, WB Saunders.)

be abnormal production of the bilabial, lingual-dental, and lingual-alveolar sounds (see Fig. 8-12 and 8-18).

Hypoplasia of the maxilla may also contribute to the resonance of voice. When the maxilla and nasal airway are hypoplastic, they may limit the enhancement and vibrations of the sound waves generated by the vocal cords, causing a reduction in nasal resonance. Patients with Apert or Crouzon syndrome often have a retrodisplaced hypoplastic maxilla, shallow nasopharynx, and long thick soft palate, which contribute to their characteristic hyponasal resonance (Fig. 8-21).

Maxillary prognathia and positive overjet with

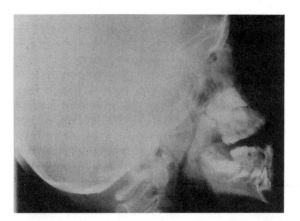

Fig. 8-21 Lateral x-ray of a patient with Apert syndrome showing a retrodisplaced maxilla, shallow nasopharynx, and long, thick soft palate. (From Witzel MA, Vallino L: Speech problems in patients with dentofacial or craniofacial deformities. In Bell WH, editor: *Modern practice of orthognathic and reconstructive surgery,* vol 2, Philadelphia: 1992, WB Saunders.)

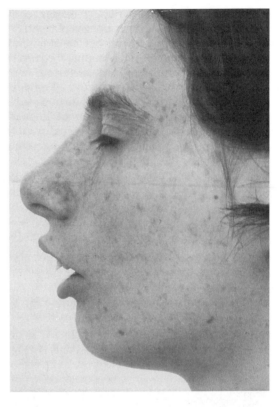

Fig. 8-22 Maxillary prognathia and positive overjet.

or without open bite may result in an abnormal facial appearance and abnormal production of bilabial sounds if there is difficulty with lip closure. The listener-observer may misperceive abnormal visual and auditory cues and the speaker's lingual-alveolar and lingual-dental sounds because of the difficulty in channeling a direct anterior airstream (Fig. 8-17 and 8-22).

Mandible

Retrognathia (see Fig. 8-17) and prognathia (see Fig. 8-18) of the mandible, when accompanied by significant positive or negative overjet with or without open bite, may also affect articulation. These problems contribute to abnormal production of bilabial, labiodental, lingual-alveolar, and lingual-palatal sounds and an unusual appearance of speech.

Tongue

The tongue is usually normal in size, shape, anatomy, and function in patients with clefting only. However, in some syndromes associated with clefting the tongue is abnormal, contributing to speech problems.

Macroglossia, or an abnormally large tongue, is associated with syndromes such as Down and Beckwith-Weidemann (Fig. 8-23). Not only does macroglossia affect the appearance when speaking and eating, but it also interferes with accurate production of lingual-dental, lingual-alveolar, and lingual-palatal sounds. In severe cases, the blade of the tongue contacts the upper lip

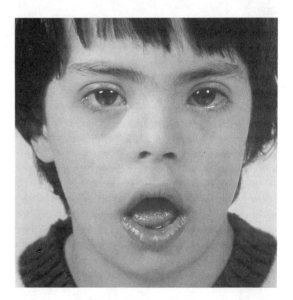

Fig. 8-23 Macroglossia, or enlarged tongue, in a child with Down syndrome. (From Witzel MA, Vallino L: Speech problems in patients with dentofacial or craniofacial deformities. In Bell WH, editor: *Modern practice of orthognathic and reconstructive surgery,* vol 2, Philadelphia: 1992, WB Saunders.)

for bilabial sounds and the upper incisor teeth for labiodental, tip dental, tip alveolar, blade alveolar, blade prepalatal, front palatal, and central palatal sounds. Lip rounding for vowels and the glides /w/ and /r/ may be distorted.

Microglossia, or an abnormally small tongue, as found in syndromes such as hypoglossia-hypodactyly also limit production of lingual-dental, lingual-alveolar, and lingual-palatal sounds when the tongue cannot contact the teeth, alveolus, and palate (Fig. 8-24).

Ankyloglossia, or tongue-tie, often occurs in children without any other abnormal phenotypic features. Although it is rarely mentioned in texts on oral and craniofacial syndromes as a specific phenotypic feature, it should always be investigated on oral exam. When it prevents tongue tip contact with the alveolar ridge, lingual-dental sounds may be affected. Ankyloglossia may also prevent the patient from adequately clearing food from the buccal sulcus area.

If the tongue is cleft or has lobules, as in oral-facial-digital syndrome types I and II (Fig.

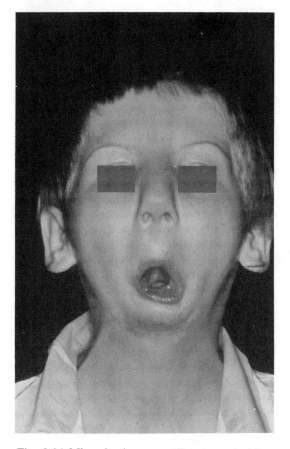

Fig. 8-24 Microglossia, or small tongue, in hypoglossia-hypodactyly.

8-25), or tumors as in neurofibromatosis, accurate placement for articulation of lingual-alveolar and lingual-palatal sounds is difficult.

Abnormal cranial nerve innervation of the tongue often occurs in syndromes such as hemifacial microsomia. In this syndrome, the cranial nerves are often unilaterally deficient and the tongue deviates to the affected side. This may result in difficulty for accurate tongue placement of all sounds requiring tongue posturing.

Accurate tongue placement is often difficult when there are missing incisor teeth or increased interdental spacing because the tongue frequently slides forward into gaps during speech, causing both auditory and visual distortions of the lingual-alveolar and lingual-palatal sounds.

When there is a significant negative overjet, the tongue may be visible during speech as the patient produces the lingual-alveolar sounds by contacting the alveolar area of the mandibular arch. Lingual-alveolar sounds may be further distorted if the tongue is humped to use the blade against the maxillary alveolus because of difficulty in retracting the tongue for accurate tongue tip placement.

Patients with inadequate closure of the VP valve during speech often have abnormal tongue placement. In some patients, the tongue is carried low and forward in the mouth; in others the tongue is abnormally elevated or retracted during articulation. For example, lingual-alveolar, lingual-pharyngeal, and lingual-epiglottic-pharyngeal contacts and approximations occur in those with compensatory articulation. Tongue humping and use of the middorsum area of the tongue may occur in those with an open fistula in the hard palate.

Hard palate

Abnormalities of the hard palate, including an unrepaired cleft, a fistula after palate repair (Fig. 8-26), maxillary collapse, or other abnormal configuration, affect tongue placement and posturing as well as airflow through the oral cavity. Compensatory errors such as the middorsum palatal stop, fricative, and affricate are thought to occur in response to an open palatal cleft or fistula or significant maxillary collapse that prevents adequate tongue placement for these sounds. If the oral airflow is directed through the fistula during production of oral pressure sounds, nasal air emission and hypernasality may result.

If the hard palate is abnormally low and flat, oral resonance may be altered and precise contact between the tongue and palate may be

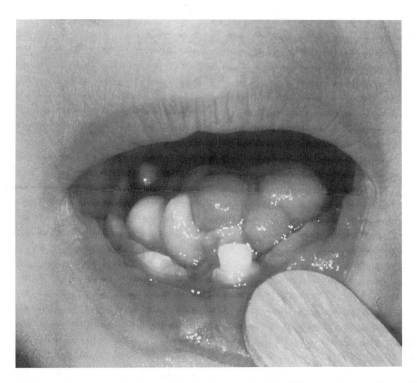

Fig. 8-25 Lobules in the tongue in a patient with oral-facial-digital syndrome. (From Witzel MA, Vallino L: Speech problems in patients with dentofacial or craniofacial deformities. In Bell WH, editor: *Modern practice of orthognathic and reconstructive surgery,* vol 2, Philadelphia: 1992, WB Saunders.)

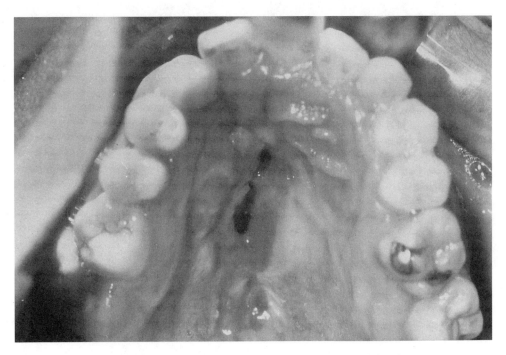

Fig. 8-26 Fistula in the hard palate in a patient with cleft palate.

compromised, causing distortion of the lingual-palatal sounds. The palate is rarely abnormally high in conditions associated with clefting; however, it may occur in patients with a long narrow face. The lingual-palatal sounds may be compromised if the patient is not able to achieve the tongue contact necessary for the production of lingual-palatal sounds. The hard palate often has hypertrophy of its lateral aspects with a deep midline fissure in patients with Apert syndrome (Fig. 8-27). This configuration can restrict the anterior flow of air through the oral cavity, distorting the lingual-palatal fricative sounds.

Soft palate

Deficiencies in the anatomy and function of the soft palate and surrounding musculature are common in conditions associated with clefting. When they occur, they usually result in VPI, which in turn leads to hypernasal resonance, abnormal nasal air emission, weak oral pressure sounds, or compensatory articulation errors. When a fistula in the soft palate persists after palate repair, hypernasality and nasal air emission may occur and there may be compensatory articulation patterns.

The most frequent causes of VPI are structural defects of the soft palate. These include overt or submucous cleft palate (Fig. 8-28), repaired cleft palate with a persistent structural or functional inadequacy, and an abnormally small or unusually shaped soft palate. Although many children with velo-cardio-facial syndrome have an overt or submucous cleft of the soft palate, some present with a short soft palate in relation to the size of the nasopharynx. In the Nager syndrome, the soft palate is abnormally small or hypoplastic (Jackson et al., 1989).

Cranial nerve impairment that results in unilateral or bilateral paresis or paralysis of the soft palate and/or pharyngeal musculature can result in VPI that involves one side of the VP valve only or the entire valve (Fig. 8-29). Unilateral VPI is usually seen in syndromes such as hemifacial microsomia. In these patients, the soft palate deviates to the unaffected or normal side during phonation.

Although clefting sometimes occurs in the syndromes of Apert and Crouzon, the soft palate is usually abnormally long and thick (Peterson-Falzone et al., 1981) (see Fig. 8-21), and this is believed to contribute to the hyponasality, mouth breathing, and forward posturing of the tongue within the oral cavity in these patients.

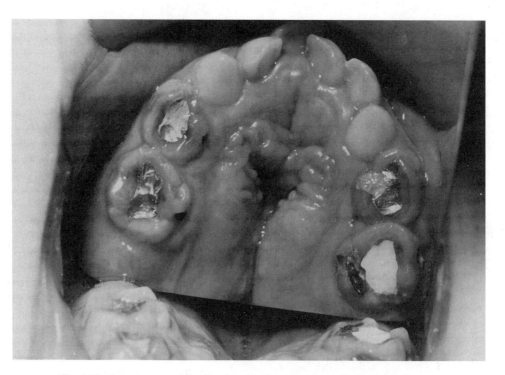

Fig. 8-27 Appearance of the hard palate in a patient with Apert syndrome.

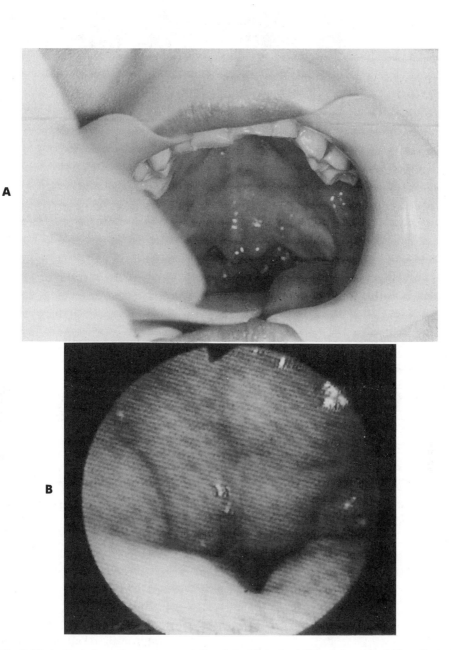

Fig. 8-28 A, Oral view of submucous cleft palate. Note the bifid uvula and midline diastasis. **B,** Nasopharyngoscopic view of submucous cleft palate. Note the midline notching of the soft palate.

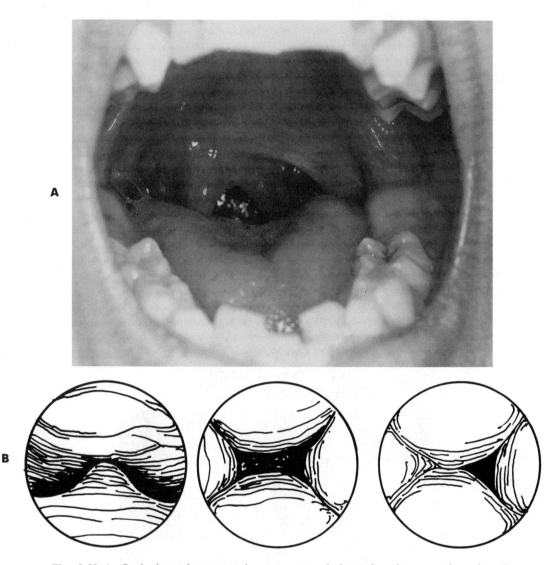

Fig. 8-29 A, Oral view of asymmetric movement of the soft palate on phonation. **B,** Nasopharyngoscopic view of asymmetric velopharyngeal insufficiency during speech. (From Witzel MA, Posnick JC: Patterns and location of velopharyngeal valving problems: atypical findings on video nasopharyngoscopy, *Cleft Palate J* 26:6, 1989.)

Pharynx

Abnormalities in the anatomy and function of the pharynx occur frequently in conditions associated with clefting. The pharynx may be enlarged relative to the size of other surrounding structures, particularly the soft palate. Terms such as deep or capacious pharynx have been used to describe this disproportion. VPI with its concomitant speech problems usually accompanies an enlarged pharynx.

The abnormally long and thick soft palate and the retrodisplaced maxilla in Apert and Crouzon syndromes result in a shallow nasopharynx (Peterson-Falzone et al., 1981) (see Fig. 8-21). Patients with Treacher Collins syndrome or Nager syndrome have a small pharynx with hypoplastic musculature (Shprintzen et al., 1979; Jackson et al., 1989). These abnormalities in the size and function of the pharynx are implicated in the hyponasal resonance that is often noted in Apert and Crouzon syndromes and the muffled resonance that is often found in Treacher Collins and Nager syndromes.

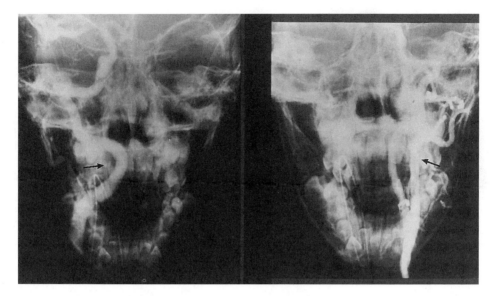

Fig. 8-30 Abnormal medial deviation of the carotid arteries in a patient with velocardiofacial syndrome. (From MacKenzie-Stepner K et al: Abnormal carotid arteries in velocardiofacial syndrome: a report of three cases, *Plast Reconstr Surg* 80:348, 1987.)

Pharyngeal hypotonia is frequently reported in velo-cardio-facial syndrome (Goldberg et al., 1993) and thought to contribute to the VPI that these patients exhibit. Some patients with velo-cardio-facial syndrome have medial displacement of one or both carotid arteries into the pharynx so that they lie just superficial to the pharyngeal musculature (MacKenzie-Stepner et al., 1987) (Fig. 8-30). Although this abnormal finding does not directly influence speech, it may complicate the treatment of VPI when these arteries are in the site of surgical treatment.

Hypertrophic adenoidal and tonsillar tissue causing partial or complete pharyngeal obstruction may cause hyponasal resonance and anterior tongue carriage during articulation, distorting the lingual-dental and lingual-alveolar sounds. Enlarged tonsils may reduce airflow into the nasal cavity during speech, particularly when they impinge on the VP ports in patients who have a pharyngeal flap. If the palatine tonsils are enlarged and positioned between the soft palate and the pharynx, they may impede the closure of the soft palate during speech, resulting in nasal escape and hypernasal resonance (MacKenzie-Stepner et al., 1987; Shprintzen et al., 1987).

When there is an irregular shape or vertical crevices in the adenoid tissue, air may escape through the VP valve during speech and cause hypernasality and nasal air emission, even though velar adenoidal contact is achieved during speech (Witzel and Posnick, 1989) (Fig. 8-31).

Tonsillectomy is not contraindicated on the basis of speech, even in those with cleft palate. However, adenoidectomy will cause or unmask VPI in many patients with cleft palate, submucous cleft palate, or congenital palatal insufficiency (Witzel et al., 1986).

Larynx

Abnormalities in the anatomy and function of the larynx and epiglottis have not been well documented in patients with clefting, since it is not usually part of the examination protocol for many clinicians. However, there may be abnormalities in the anatomy and function of the larynx that account for the voice problems sometimes noted.

The entire vocal tract including the larynx should always be visually assessed when problems with either resonance or laryngeal phonation are suspected. The congenital anomalies of the larynx that have been noted in conditions associated with clefting are often the result of underdevelopment of the laryngeal structures, and these problems may be unilateral or bilateral. For example, in ocular-genital-laryngeal syndrome (Opitz syndrome) the larynx is often small with short, thick cords resulting in an abnormally high-pitched voice (Fig. 8-32).

Other problems with anatomy that have been reported include laryngomalacia resulting in laryngeal stridor, laryngeal web, subglottic stenosis, and laryngotracheal cleft. These abnormalities usually cause problems in the quality and pitch of voice. There may also be unilateral or bilateral abnormalities in the

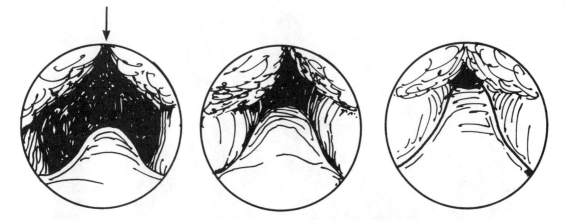

Fig. 8-31 Vertical crevices in adenoid resulting in leakage of air through the velopharyngeal port during speech. (From Witzel MA, Posnick JC: Patterns and location of velopharyngeal valving problems: atypical findings on video nasopharyngoscopy, *Cleft Palate J* 26:66, 1989.)

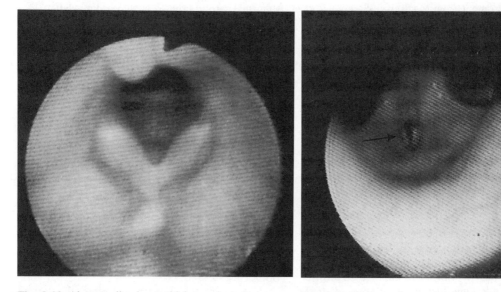

Fig. 8-32 Abnormally short, thick vocal cords in a patient with Opitz C syndrome.

Fig. 8-33 Unilateral paresis of the right vocal cord.

innervation of the larynx. Unilateral paresis of the branches of the vagus nerve has been observed in hemifacial microsomia (Fig. 8-33). This may result in a diplophonic voice quality.

Lesions on the vocal cords or other evidence of hyperfunctional use are also evident. It is not unusual to find edematous vocal cords or nodules (Fig. 8-34) in patients with borderline VP closure and hoarseness. Many patients with borderline or inadequate VP closure and/or compensatory articulation errors have also been

noted in our examinations to have enlarged or prominent ventricular folds suggestive of hyperfunctional use of these folds.

Other unusual findings that we have observed during examination of the larynx in patients with clefting conditions include a cleft epiglottis in a patient with Stickler syndrome (Fig. 8-35), a bifid epiglottis in velo-cardio-facial syndrome, and a protracted epiglottis in Treacher Collins and Nagar syndromes.

There is a definite need for more documen-

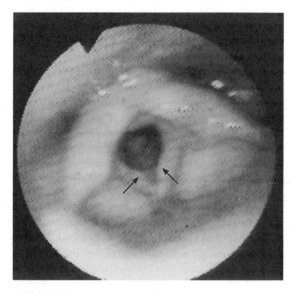

Fig. 8-34 Bilateral vocal cord nodules in a patient with velopharyngeal insufficiency.

tation of the anatomy and function of the structures of the lower vocal tract and the effect on laryngeal voice production in conditions associated with clefting.

PHENOTYPIC FEATURES AFFECTING LANGUAGE

Although there is little research to date on the language profiles of children with various types of clefting conditions, it is known that in some of these conditions there are specific problems with the anatomy and function of the brain and central nervous system, and these may certainly impair receptive and expressive language as well as learning and reading abilities.

Recent developments in diagnostic imaging techniques of the brain and central nervous system allow evaluation of the structural, metabolic, and electrophysiologic aspects (Schaefer et al., 1992). These assessment techniques in combination with neurobehavioral and neuro-

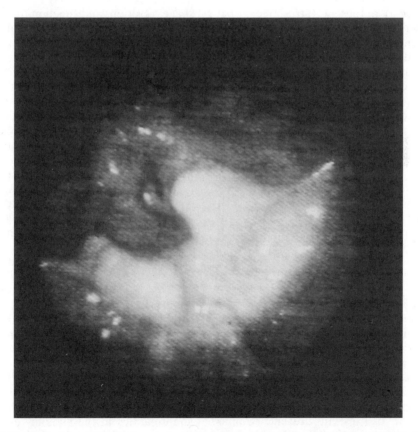

Fig. 8-35 Cleft of the epiglottis in a patient with Stickler syndrome. (From Witzel MA, Stringer DA: Methods of assessing velopharyngeal function. In Bardach J, Morris H, editors: *Multidisciplinary management of cleft lip and palate.* Philadelphia; 1990, WB Saunders.)

psychologic testing can provide much needed information on CNS anatomy and function in individuals with craniofacial anomalies.

Congenital problems of the brain that have been documented in various syndromes associated with clefting include microcephaly (an abnormally small brain), macrocephaly (an abnormally large brain), holoprosencephaly (impaired midline cleavage of the forebrain), agenesis or absence of the corpus callosum, Arnold-Chiari malformation, hydrocephaly, tumors, and encephaloceles. Some patients also have seizures and increased intracranial pressure.

PHENOTYPIC FEATURES AFFECTING HEARING

Structural and functional abnormalities of the outer, middle, and inner ear as well as the tympanic membrane and eustachian tube that result in hearing loss can impede speech production and development as well as receptive and expressive language, behavior, and learning abilities.

External ear and auditory canal

Small (microtia) or absent (atresia) external ears (Fig. 8-11) are often associated with small or absent auditory canals, which impede the flow of sound waves into the middle ear, resulting in a conductive hearing impairment. These problems are frequent findings in Treacher Collins syndrome, Nager syndrome, oral-facial-digital syndrome type II, and hemifacial microsomia (Sando et al., 1990).

Tympanic membrane

The tympanic membrane may be absent or hypoplastic, as in Apert or Crouzon syndrome; or there may be abnormalities in its shape or position, as found in Treacher Collins syndrome. These abnormalities and others, including replacement of the tympanic membrane by a bony plate or fibrous tissue, will result in a conductive impairment (Sando et al., 1990).

Middle ear and ossicular chain

Abnormalities of the middle ear and ossicular chain resulting in a conductive loss occur in many conditions associated with clefting. The middle ear cavity may be abnormally small, deformed (rectangular rather than oval), or in some cases missing. There may be absence, underdevelopment, abnormal development, or fixation of the ossicles. In Treacher Collins syndrome, for example, the middle ear cavity may be absent or abnormally small, and the ossicles may be absent, poorly developed,

and/or ankylosed (Pron et al., 1993). Congenital malformations of the incus have also been reported in Stickler and oral-facial-digital type II syndromes; discontinuity of the ossicular chain in Wildervanck syndrome; displaced or malformed ossicles in branchial-otic-renal (BOR) syndrome and thickened ossicles in oto-palatal-digital syndrome (Gorlin et al., 1990; Sando et al., 1990). The nerve supply that innervates the tympanic cavity and its structures may also be abnormal. The nerves may be absent, hypoplastic, or displaced. For example, in the oculoauriculovertebral spectrum the facial nerve may be hypoplastic and the chorda tympani nerve absent, and in Möbius syndrome the facial nerve may be absent (Sando et al., 1990).

The jugular vein may invade the middle ear cavity in some patients with Apert or Crouzon syndrome (Crysdale, 1986, personal communication), not only interfering with function of the ossicles but also increasing the surgical risk when inserting ventilating tubes.

Eustachian tubes

The eustachian tubes may be abnormal in size, shape, position, and function, thereby preventing normal aeration, pressure equalization, and fluid drainage of the middle ear and contributing to conductive hearing loss. Eustachian tube dysfunction resulting in otitis media is common in infants with cleft palate, reportedly as high as 100% (Paradise et al., 1969). The resultant hearing loss is conductive and usually fluctuating, whereas hearing loss caused by anatomic abnormalities is usually more permanent.

In patients with clefting, the eustachian tubes may not dilate effectively due to dysfunction or deficiency of the tensor veli palatini muscle, which is a muscle of the soft palate. In the infant and young child, the eustachian tube normally lies in a horizontal position. As the child grows, the angle of inclination becomes more vertical, allowing easier drainage of middle ear fluid. Some authors have also described such factors as hypercompliance of the eustachian tube, abnormal muscles, and adenoid hypertrophy as causative factors in eustachian tube dysfunction in patients with clefting (Bluestone, 1971; Rood and Stool, 1981).

Inner ear, cochlea, vestibular apparatus and auditory nerve

Sensorineural hearing loss will result from abnormalities in the anatomy and function of the inner ear, cochlea, vestibular apparatus, and auditory nerve. For example, in Wildervanck syndrome the semicircular canal may be abnormal and the labyrinth hypoplastic. In neurofibromatosis there may be tumors, known as acoustic neuromas, impinging on the auditory nerve. The Mondini deformity has been found associated with the Klippel-Feil anomaly (Gorlin et al., 1990).

SUMMARY

This chapter provides an overview of the types of communication problems that can occur in individuals with clefting and the possible causes of these problems. Although many phenotypic characteristics have been identified and reported in the literature for the various syndromes and conditions associated with clefting, the clinician should not assume that all have been delineated because many of these conditions are rare and the severity or degree of expression is often variable. The speech-language pathologist or audiologist should approach each patient with an open mind and carefully document all the communication impairments that the patient exhibits. The causative factors should also be determined; this often requires the input of other specialists on the cleft palate or craniofacial team. This information will help plan and deliver appropriate and effective interventions.

REFERENCES

Boone DR: *The voice and voice therapy,* ed 3, Englewood Cliffs NJ, 1983, Prentice Hall.

Black OF, Lilly DJ: Tinnitus in children. In Bluestone CD, Stool S, editors: *Pediatric otolaryngology,* ed 2, vol 1, Philadelphia, 1990, WB Saunders.

Bluestone CD: Eustachian tube obstruction in the infant with cleft palate, *Ann Otol Rhinol Laryngol* 80(suppl 2):1, 1971.

Bzoch KR: *Communication disorders related to cleft lip and palate,* Boston, 1979, Little, Brown.

Chapman KL: Phonologic processes in children with cleft palate, *Cleft Palate-Craniofacial J* 30:64, 1993.

Chapman KL, Hardin MA: Phonetic and phonologic skills of two year olds with cleft palate, *Cleft Palate-Craniofacial J* 29:433, 1992.

Estrem TL, Broen PA: Early speech production of children with cleft palate, *J Speech Hearing Res* 32:12, 1989.

Folkins JW: Issues in speech motor control and their relation to the speech of individuals with cleft palate, *Cleft Palate J* 22:106, 1985.

Forner LL: Speech segment durations produced by five and six year old speakers with and without cleft palates, *Cleft Palate J* 20:185, 1983.

Gilger JW: Genetics in disorders of language, *Clin Commun Disorders* 2:35, 1992.

Glass L, Starr CD: A study of relationships between judgments of speech and appearance of patients with orofacial clefts, *Cleft Palate J* 16:436, 1979.

Gorlin RJ, Cohen MM, Levin RS: *Syndromes of the head and neck,* ed 3, New York, 1990, Oxford University Press.

Gray GW, Wise CM: *The bases of speech,* New York, 1959, Harper and Brothers.

Hoch L, Golding-Kushner K, Seigal-Sadewitz VL, and Shprintzen RJ: Speech therapy, *Semin Speech Lang* 7:313, 1986.

Jackson IT, Bauer B, and Saleh J: A significant feature of Nagar's syndrome: palatal agenesis, *Plast Reconstr Surg* 84:219, 1989.

Jung HJ: *Genetic syndromes in communication disorders.* Boston, 1989, Little, Brown.

Karnell MP, Folkins JW, Morris HL: Relationships between the perception of nasalization and speech movements in speakers with cleft palate, *J Speech Hear Res* 28:63, 1985.

Kawano M, Isshiki N, Harita Y, and Tanokuchi F: Laryngeal fricative in cleft palate speech, *Acta otolaryngol* (suppl) 419:180, 1985.

Klaiman P, Witzel MA, Margar-Bacal F, and Munro IR: Changes in aesthetic appearance and intelligibility of speech after partial glossectomy in patients with Down syndrome, *Plast Reconstr Surg* 82:403, 1988.

Lynch JI: Language of cleft infants: lessening the risk of delay through programming. In McWilliams BJ, editor: *Seminars in speech and language,* York, 1986, Thieme.

Lynch JI, Fox DR, Brookshire BL: Phonological proficiency of two cleft palate toddlers with school age follow-up, *J Speech Hearing Disord* 48:274, 1983.

Mackenzie-Stepner K, Witzel MA, Stringer DA, Lindsay WK, Munro IR, and Hughes H: Abnormal carotid arteries in velocardiofacial syndrome: a report of three cases, *Plast Reconstr Surg* 80:347, 1987.

Mackenzie-Stepner K, Witzel MA, Stringer DA, and Laskin RL: Velopharyngeal insufficiency due to hypertrophic tonsils. A report of two cases, *Int J Pediatr Otorhinolaryngol* 14:57, 1987.

McWilliams BJ, Bluestone CD, Musgrave RH: Diagnostic implications of vocal cord nodules in children with cleft palate, *Laryngoscope* 79:2072, 1969.

McWilliams BJ, Morris HL, Shelton RL: *Cleft palate speech,* ed 2, Philadelphia, 1990, BC Decker.

Moore WH, Summers RK: Phonetic contexts: their effects of perceived nasality in cleft palate speakers, *Cleft Palate J* 10:72, 1973.

Morley ME: *Cleft palate and speech,* ed 6, Baltimore, 1967, Williams & Wilkins.

Musgrave RH, McWilliams BJ, Matthews HP: A review of the results of two different surgical procedures for the repair of clefts of the soft palate only, *Cleft Palate J* 12:281, 1975.

Paynter ET, Kinard MW: Perceptual preferences between compensatory articulation and nasal escape of air in children with velopharyngeal incompetence, *Cleft Palate J* 16:262, 1979.

Peterson-Falzone SJ. Speech characteristics: updating clinical decisions, *Semin Speech Lang* 7:269, 1986.

Pollock H, Ferketic M, Shprintzen RJ, and Witzel MA: *Delineation and diagnosis of craniofacial syndromes: effect on case management* (videotape), Rockville Pike, M, 1993, American Speech Language Hearing Association.

Powers G, Dunn C, Erikson C: Speech analysis of four children with repaired cleft palates, *J Speech Hear Disord* 55:542, 1990.

Pron G, Galloway C, Armstrong D, and Posnick J: Ear malformation and hearing loss in patients with Treacher Collins syndrome, *Cleft Palate-Craniofacial J* 30:97, 1993.

Richman LC, Eliason MJ: Development in children with cleft lip and/or palate: intellectual, cognitive personality and parental factors. In McWilliams BJ, editor: *Seminars in speech and language,* New York, 1986, Thieme.

Richman LC, Eliason MJ, Lindgren SD: Reading disability in children with clefts, *Cleft Palate J* 25:21, 1988.

Rood S R, Stool SE: Cleft palate related otopathologic disease, *Otolaryngol Clin North Am* 14:865, 1981.

Sando I, Shibahara Y, Wood RP: Congenital anomalies of the external and middle ear. In Bluestone CD, Stool S, editors: *Pediatric otolaryngology,* ed 2, vol 1, Philadelphia, 1990, WB Saunders.

Schaefer GB, Mathy-Laikko P, Bodensteiner JB: Neurogenetic aspects of communication disorders, *Clin Commun Disorders* 2:9, 1992.

Shprintzen RJ, Goldberg RB, Lewin ML, Sidoti EJ, Berkman MD, Argamoso RV, and Young D: A new syndrome involving cleft palate, cardiac anomalies, typical facies, and learning disabilities: velocardiofacial syndrome, *Cleft Palate J* 15:56, 1978.

Shprintzen RJ, Croft C, Berkman MD, and Rakoff SD: Pharyngeal hypoplasia in Treacher Collins syndrome, *Arch Otolaryngol* 105:127, 1979.

Shprintzen RJ, Sher AE, Croft CB: Hypernasal speech caused by tonsillar hypertrophy, *Int J Pediatr Otorhinolaryngol* 14:45, 1987.

Subtelny JD, Van Hattum RJ, Meyers BB: Ratings and measures of cleft palate speech, *Cleft Palate J* 9:18, 1972.

Trost JE: Articulatory additions to the classical description of the speech of persons with cleft palate, *Cleft Palate J* 18:193, 1981.

Trost-Cardamone JE: Effects of velopharyngeal incompetency on speech, *J Childhood Commun Disorders* 10:31, 1986.

Trost-Cardamone JE: Coming to terms with VPI: a response to Loney and Bloem, *Cleft Palate J* 26:68, 1989.

Vallino LD, Tompson B: Perceptual characteristics of consonant errors associated with malocclusion, *J Oral Maxillofac Surg* 51:850, 1993.

Warren DW: A quantitative technique for assessing nasal airway impairment, *Am J Orthod* 86:306, 1984.

Warren DW: Compensatory speech behaviors in cleft palate: a regulation control phenomenon? *Cleft Palate J* 23:251, 1986.

Wells CG: *Cleft palate and its associated speech disorders,* New York, 1971, McGraw Hill.

Witzel MA, Rich RH, Margar-Bacal F, and Cox C: Speech problems in craniofacial anomalies, *Commun Disorders* 8:45, 1983.

Witzel MA et al: Velopharyngeal insufficiency after adenoidectomy: an eight year review, *Int J Pediatr Otorhinolaryngol* 11:15, 1986.

Witzel MA, Posnick JC: Patterns and location of velopharyngeal valving problems: atypical findings on video nasopharyngoscopy, *Cleft Palate J* 26:63, 1989.

Witzel MA, Ross RB, Munro IR: Articulation before and after facial osteotomy, *J Maxillofac Surg* 8:195, 1980.

Witzel MA, Stringer DA: Methods of assessing velopharyngeal function. In Bardach J, Morris H, editors: *Multidisciplinary management of cleft lip and palate,* Philadelphia, 1990, WB Saunders.

Witzel MA, Vallino LD: Speech problems in patients with dentofacial or craniofacial deformities. In WH Bell, editor: *Modern practice of orthognathic and reconstructive surgery,* vol 2, Philadelphia, 1992, WB Saunders.

9 The Evaluation and Remediation of Language Impairment

Luigi Girolametto

NEED FOR LANGUAGE INTERVENTION

Language impairment is not a normal outcome for *all* children with cleft palate or cleft lip and palate. Although many past studies have revealed a high incidence of language-related deficits in this population compared with normally developing peers (e.g., Spriestersbach et al., 1958; Morris, 1962), some of these children learn communication and language skills at a rate comparable to their peers. A handful of recent studies report comparable or even superior performance in specific areas of communicative behavior, e.g., prelinguistic development (Pecyna et al., 1987), parental language input (Chapman and Hardin, 1991), and language comprehension (Long and Dalston, 1983). In light of the costly and time-consuming nature of language intervention, the clinician must therefore avoid the assumption that every child with cleft palate possesses a language delay.

Undeniably, however, there exists a subgroup, or several subgroups, of children with cleft palate and cleft lip and palate for whom the risk of a transitory or permanent impairment in receptive and expressive language functioning is a certain outcome (e.g., McWilliams et al., 1990; Dalston, 1990). This may be due, in part, to the concomitant presence of other handicapping conditions such as a hearing impairment, mental retardation, cognitive impairment, attentional/affective disorders, or various syndromes associated with clefting. We concur with Shames and Rubin (1979) that the cleft palate population is heterogeneous with respect to outcomes in developmental areas, especially language.

Some children with cleft palate appear to overcome early developmental difficulties to achieve age-appropriate expressive language skills (Morris, 1962), cognitive and learning skills (Musgrave et al., 1975), and pragmatic communication behaviors (Shames and Rubin, 1979) by early school age. Others appear to experience long-term language difficulties as evidenced by reports of morphosyntactic difficul-

ties (Shames and Rubin, 1979), pragmatic impairments (Warr-Leeper et al., 1988), and learning disabilities (e.g., Richman and Eliason, 1984; Richman, Eliason, and Lindgren, 1988; Shprintzen and Goldberg, 1985). These latter studies challenge the clinician to carefully monitor the development of language once an impairment is diagnosed and to be cautious about interpreting an apparent catch-up in language development. Early language impairments often result in learning and reading problems in the school-age years.

The necessity for language screening and assessment in the early years is underscored by McWilliams et al. (1990), who point out that "as clinicians, we should be aware of the possibility of language disabilities in children with clefts, understand the necessity for careful evaluation, and be prepared to intervene when it is appropriate to do so."

ASSESSMENT OF COMMUNICATION AND LANGUAGE IMPAIRMENT

Clearly, if the clinician wishes to assess the language abilities of infants and young children with clefts, additional time and effort are required beyond what might be routinely taken for an evaluation of speech and the oral-peripheral mechanism. (See Chapters 8 and 10 for a discussion of the assessment of speech development. This chapter focuses on the assessment and intervention of communication and language impairments in infants and young children with clefts.)

Infant/toddler assessment

The assessment of early communication skills and language development from birth to 18 months focuses on three major areas of communicative behavior: parent-child interaction, early social communication skills (e.g., social interaction, joint attention, behavior regulation, pragmatic functions), and receptive and expressive language skills (especially vocabulary acquisition).

Parent-child interaction

The assessment of parent-child interaction in the early years is predicated by theoretical explanations of early language development. Although the process of language acquisition is not known, most major theories of acquisition assume that language emerges from the early reciprocal interactions in which a parent's willingness to engage children in interaction and respond to their cues facilitates the emergence of early social-conversational skills. These skills (turn-taking, joint reference, topic initiation, and responsiveness), in turn, provide a structure that permits the development of intentionality and the extraction of meaning and linguistic rules from the adult's speech (Lieven, 1978; Snow, 1978; Kaye and Charney, 1981; Wells, 1986).

It may be hypothesized that some parents of infants with clefts have initial difficulties interacting in an optimal manner, particularly if their children are medically unstable, temperamentally difficult, do not vocalize, smile, or demonstrate reciprocal eye gaze, or have concomitant developmental difficulties that place them at risk for language delay (e.g., diagnosis of a clefting syndrome). Alternatively, as toddlers develop language, reduced intelligibility may make them difficult for parents to understand, thus resulting in a diminished feedback loop in which the child receives fewer contingent responses (expansions, expatiations) after his or her utterances. Routine screening of parent-child interaction is prohibitive. Only if the clinician suspects that the interaction may not be supportive of optimal communication development is measurement of the parent-child interaction system per se warranted.

Assessment instruments that profile the interactions between parents and their children rate various features of "motherese" (i.e., adaptations that adults make in their speech to young children), which are derived from the literature and are highly correlated with accelerated language acquisition in children who are not handicapped. These profiles focus on the assessment of three main clusters of facilitative motherese techniques: child-oriented techniques that establish episodes of joint attention and involvement (e.g., face-to-face contact, affective involvement, noticing and responding to the child's cues), interaction-promoting techniques that establish balanced turn-taking in interactions (e.g., waiting expectantly for a response, signaling for responses using voice and body language cues), and language-modeling techniques that help the child induce the relationships among language form, content, and use (e.g., labeling objects, use of short utterances, repeti-

tion). Some scales also rate child interaction behaviors such as turn-taking, joint attention, affect, and gaze aversion. Several published interaction rating scales are listed in Appendix A.

We have found that these scales are easy to understand and use in a clinical setting. We have found it necessary, however, to make several observations of parent-child interaction and routinely interview parents about the representativeness of the interaction to ensure accuracy of interpretation. A major disadvantage of all rating scales is the absence of specific profiles of adequate versus inadequate parental input. We do not yet know what levels of parental responsiveness and interaction are necessary to promote optimal communicative development (Tannock and Girolametto, 1992).

Early social-communication abilities and vocabulary acquisition

The major focus of assessment in infants and young children below 18 months with developmental abilities is the child's ability to negotiate conversation (initiate, maintain, and respond) for the purposes of social interaction, joint attention, and behavior regulation. The child's ability to express communicative functions such as requesting and commenting in a nonverbal, vocal, or gestural mode is presumed to be a precursor to language content and form (Bruner, 1983; Schaffer, 1989). At this early level the child develops receptive and expressive vocabulary, as well as comprehension of simple commands and questions.

It can be assumed that some children with clefts have difficulty acquiring early communicative competency, particularly if the cleft is concomitant with other handicapping conditions. There is conflicting evidence about the long-term effects of a delay at this early stage in development. Whereas Shames and Rubin (1979) found that children with clefts acquired communicative functions later than their peers but caught up by their fourth year, Warr-Leeper et al. (1988) found the opposite, namely that pragmatic difficulties with peers emerged once children with clefts reached school age.

Screening for early communicative impairment is facilitated by the recent explosion of measurement instruments that are parent administered, obtained through parent interview, or through direct observation of the child. It is no longer viable to wait for the child to have acquired some language before estimating a delay in acquisition. Given the enormous variability in development and the recent emergence of assessment batteries, standardized instruments are preferred over those which are nonstandardized. Appendix B lists only those that are standardized and norm-referenced.

Preschool language assessment

The assessment of receptive and expressive language abilities for children who have some measureable language skills is an area familiar to most clinicians. Typically, measurement includes the areas of receptive and expressive vocabulary, comprehension of utterances differing in length, structural complexity, and conceptual information, appropriate expressive use of morphology and syntax, and age-appropriate discourse and conversational skills.

Assessment instruments have been available for some time, including screening instruments of overall receptive and expressive language functioning. As measures of receptive language, we routinely use the Receptive Scale of the Reynell Developmental Language Scales-U.S. Edition (Reynell and Gruber, 1990), the Peabody Picture Vocabulary Test-Revised (Dunn and Dunn, 1981), and the Test of Auditory Comprehension of Language-Revised (Carrow-Woolfolk, 1985). Production measures used include the Structured Photographic Expressive Language Test (Werner and Kreshek, 1983) for screening purposes, the Expressive One-Word Picture Vocabulary Test-Revised (Gardner, 1990), and informal language sampling. Although standardized tests assessing the pragmatics of conversation are available, we have relied primarily on teacher reports and informal observation.

INTERVENTION FOR COMMUNICATION AND LANGUAGE IMPAIRMENT
Intervention approaches

The importance of early language intervention is underscored by the finding that language impairment in young children is also a major risk factor for later educational and mental health problems (Prizant et al., 1990; Rescorla, 1991). Once a diagnosis of language impairment is made, the need to provide early language intervention in the most effective and efficient manner possible is crucial to the mental, social, and academic well-being of children with clefts.

Language intervention approaches vary along a continuum from highly structured didactic programs that use behaviorally-based teaching procedures (e.g., elicited imitation, reinforcement, shaping, chaining) to child-centered, interactive approaches that facilitate communication through repeated exposure to language in naturalistic, conversational contexts (Fey, 1986). These approaches are derived from philosophically distinct theories of how children acquire language (Tannock and Girolametto, 1992). In the middle of the continuum are hybrid models of intervention that incorporate aspects of didactic approaches but apply them in naturalistic contexts.

Traditionally, didactic approaches have been considered most appropriate for preverbal or minimally verbal children (Friedman and Friedman, 1980; Cole and Dale, 1986; Fey, 1986; Carrow-Woolfolk, 1988), whereas interactive models of intervention are considered more suitable for children who are using short phrases. Unfortunately, there is a paucity of empirical research to support this assertion, and we do not yet know which programs work for which children, nor can we assume that one approach will work for all children irrespective of their stage of development or communicative profile (Fey and Cleave, 1990; Wilcox, Kouri, and Caswell, 1991). Faced with a wide range of intervention approaches, the clinician must assess the relative value of each and select the one that best addresses the needs of individual children.

Language intervention may take many forms: parent-focused programs, preschool treatment nurseries, individual one-on-one therapy, or small group therapy. We focus on parent-focused intervention and small group therapy as viable means of providing service to the child with cleft lip and palate.

Parent-focused intervention

From a practical perspective, parents of infants and toddlers are in an ideal position to assume a pivotal role in the stimulation of communication development because they have frequent and extensive contacts with their children, can provide intervention at various intervals throughout the day, and are generally motivated to help their children. Parental involvement in intervention is also consistent with the empowerment of parents advocated by the Education of the Handicapped Act Amendments of 1986 (P.L. 99-457, Part H). Parent involvement may take many different forms from general parent education programs, commitment to completing homework assignments or monitoring progress, to assuming responsibility as the major change agent (Fey, 1986). The extent of parental involvement may vary in households in which both parents are working, or in which extenuating family circumstances such as poor health, lack of employment, or marital discord are present (Dunst, Leet, and Tivette, 1988).

Parent education programs that aim to give parents general information about normal development and possible outcomes is desirable for **all** families of children with clefting disorders. The agenda for a parent education session may focus on the normal development of speech and language, typical speech and language difficulties of children with clefts, general principles of speech and language stimulation, and specific activities for stimulating speech and language development. Information may be shared individually with parents or in small parent groups before or after surgery for closure of the cleft palate (6 to 18 months of age). The clinician's desire to provide information must be coupled with sensitivity to the parents' needs and their readiness to accept their child's disability.

Parent education programs are appropriate as preventive programs, but unfortunately they do not meet the specific needs of the child with a language impairment, in which case more direct parent-focused intervention is desirable. Intensive, parent-focused intervention, in which the parent accepts responsibility as the primary change agent, may be necessary for parents of some children with clefts who have a confirmed delay in communication skills or who are at risk of communication delay (e.g., a clefting syndrome). A popular form of parent training focuses on increasing the use of child-oriented, interaction-promoting, and language-modeling techniques (Norris and Hoffman, 1990; Tannock and Girolametto, 1992). Numerous models of this **interactive** language intervention have been developed for parents of infants (e.g., Klein et al., 1988; Girolametto and Ushycky, 1989), toddlers (e.g., Manolson, 1992; Mahoney and Powell, 1986), and preschool children (e.g., Weistuch et al., 1991; MacDonald, 1989). Inclusion in such a program must be preceded by screening the child's communication to determine if this type of intervention is warranted. A brief description of several interactive program packages is presented in Appendix C.

Small group therapy

Children with language impairment who have concomitant developmental and cognitive delays (e.g., clefting syndrome) should receive language treatment within a multidisciplinary setting such as a preschool treatment program or nursery. For children who present with a primary impairment in speech and language, we advocate group language intervention as opposed to individual treatment. Regardless of the theoretical orientation (didactic versus interactive teaching), language content, form, and use are best taught in group settings that are naturalistic and promote peer interaction. Naturalistic therapy is facilitated by themes or scripted events such as going on a picnic, visiting a farm, or going shopping. Both articulation/ phonology targets and language goals may be

incorporated into these themes. Advocates of nonspeech sound practice may include nonspeech targets as well. A sample agenda for a young preschool group is included in Appendix D. In this sample agenda up to four preschoolers participate in a session of 1.5 hours in which the theme reflects the real-life experience of one of the group members — taking an airplane trip to visit grandparents. In this example, practice of nonspeech sounds or phonology/ articulation targets occurs at the beginning of the group session as a separate activity. The target sounds and words are then integrated into activities that include these targets with high frequency, and also teach the vocabulary, semantic relations, or morphosyntactic goals of the session. The target sound in this activity is /sh/, which is practiced once in a didactic manner, at the beginning of the session, and twice incidentally, during the packing activity and the craft activity. Language goals for these children are two-word utterances (three morphemes) of the type agent + object (e.g., boy walking) and three-word utterances of the type agent + action + object (e.g., "I want X" or "I see X"). In this example group homogeneity permits the same goals to be targeted for all children, but it is also possible to target individualized phonology or articulation goals during the same session so that children pack different objects into their suitcases. Similarly, language targets may vary, depending on the receptive and expressive levels of the children in the group.

We recommend that parental involvement continue to be an important adjunct to direct therapy. In this sample agenda time is reserved at the end of therapy for the clinician to discuss specific home practice activities. Alternatively, parents may participate in selected group sessions as volunteers. In this case they may observe an activity, assume the therapist's role with their own and other children, and receive feedback on their performance. For example, during phonology practice a parent may ask the children choice questions ("Do you want a shoe or a shirt?") and expect a one-word response with the target sound.

As mentioned earlier in this chapter, language intervention is a long-term venture for most children with language impairment. As children approach school age, conventional speech and language goals must be supplemented by the discourse skills necessary for classroom success and exposure to early literacy through print (Constable and Van Kleeck, 1985; Hughes, 1989). In this way we create a bridge between preschool language therapy and the classroom setting to address the child's future academic needs.

Appendix A

Rating Scales for Parent-Child Interaction

Observation of Communicative Interaction (Klein and Briggs, 1987) is an informal assessment guide designed for rating the interaction of parents with infants up to 12 months; it is available in English and Spanish. Although applicable to all parent-infant dyads, it was originally developed to examine interactions of infants and mothers who are socially disadvantaged. The 10-item scale rates maternal interaction techniques along a 4-point continuum of frequency (1 = rarely/never; 2 = sometimes; 3 = often; 4 = optimally). It does not rate infant interactive or communicative behavior. Items include child-oriented techniques (responsiveness, provides tactile and kinesthetic stimulation, smiles contingently, facilitates eye contact), interaction-promoting techniques (varies prosody, encourages conversation) and language-modeling techniques (interprets, recasts, labels, imitates).

The *Interaction Rating Scales* (Clarke and Seifer, 1985) include three items that rate child or dyadic behavior (e.g., child gaze aversion, child social referencing, dyadic reciprocity) and seven items that rate parent behaviors representative of child-oriented techniques (acknowledging, direction of gaze, affect), interaction-promoting techniques (forcing, overriding) and language-modeling techniques (imitating, expanding). Items are evaluated using a 5-point scale reflecting judgments of the appropriateness of use (1 = poor; 3 = moderate; 5 = excellent).

The *ECO Scales* (MacDonald, 1989) consists of five rating scales that assess competencies in the areas of social play, reciprocal interactions, preverbal communication, language, and pragmatics of conversation. Both child and parent behaviors are rated. Competencies span the continuum from early prelinguistic interactions to mature conversational behavior. Specific child behaviors and parent techniques are subjectively rated using a 9-point scale that captures the frequency of occurrence (e.g., 1 = never; 5 = occasionally; 9 = frequently) or agreement (e.g., 1 = strongly disagree; 9 = strongly agree). The scales include a large number of items and can be used in their entirety, or the clinician may select a particular scale to use based on the age and abilities of the child.

You and Your Baby: Building Communication (Girolametto and Ushycky, 1989) is a two-pronged evaluation procedure that includes an observation form for summarizing the infant's and toddler's interaction, play, and communication behavior and a scale for evaluating specific parental techniques using binary ratings of "Satisfactory" or "Needs Improvement." Designed as a parental self-assessment, this scale has been widely used by clinicians and is available in English and French. Items include child-oriented techniques (stay at child's level to encourage eye contact, respond, share activities), interaction-promoting techniques (wait, signal for turns, play turn-taking games, be animated), and language-modeling techniques (imitate, label, expand, and talk about what is happening).

Appendix B

Assessment Instruments for Early Communicative Behavior

The *MacArthur Communicative Development Inventories* (Fenson et al., 1993) are parent-administered assessments of communication behaviors in infants and toddlers. The *words and gestures* form is designed for ages 8 to 16 months and focuses on emerging receptive and expressive vocabulary, play, and communicative gestures. The separate *words and sentences* form is designed for children between 16 and 30 months and assesses expressive vocabulary, morphosyntactic development, and use of multiword utterances. A manual accompanies the test forms and provides extensive information on reliability, validity, and scoring procedures. We have found that this scale is easy to administer before or between clinic visits and is easily scored. Experimental editions are available in several languages including Spanish, Cantonese, and Japanese. Unfortunately, the results are only as valid as the accuracy of parental report.

Assessing Linguistic Behaviours (ABL) (Olswang et al., 1987) is designed to profile the abilities of infants and toddlers in the developmental range of birth to 2 years. It includes five separate clinician-administered scales for the comprehensive assessment of early communicative development: cognitive precursors to language, play, communicative intentions, receptive language, and language production. The scales may be administered and scored separately, since an overall profile is not obtained. A training tape accompanies the manual. The assessment procedures rely heavily on videotaped observations and coding and may be prohibitive in terms of the time required. We have found the Communicative Intention Scale and the Language Comprehension Scales to be particularly useful.

The *Rossetti Infant-Toddler Language Scale (ITLS)* (Rossetti, 1990) is a comprehensive, criterion-referenced instrument that judges the child's mastery of behaviors in six separate scales from birth to 3 years: interaction-attachment, pragmatics, gesture, play, language comprehension, and language expression. Scale items may be scored as present or absent by one of three means: spontaneous observation, direct elicitation, or parent report. The interaction-attachment scale includes items reflecting both infant and parent interactive behaviors and is an alternative to the parent-child interaction rating scales listed above.

The *Communication and Symbolic Behavior Scales (CSBS)* (Wetherby and Prizant, 1991) measures the development of early communication skills from 8 months to 2 years in seven different areas: communicative functions, communicative means (gestures, vocalizations), reciprocity, social/affective signaling, verbal symbolic behavior, and play. Similar to the ABL, administration relies on videotaped communication sampling and subsequent coding, which may be time consuming. In addition to sampling, a caregiver questionnaire and structured eliciting contexts (i.e., communicative temptations) are used. The child's performance is rated on 20 five-point rating scales reflecting the frequency of occurrence, which varies for each specific behavior (e.g., for Gestural Means, 1 = none; 3 = three different conventional gestures; 5 = at least five different conventional gestures).

Appendix C

Interactive Parent-focused Programs

Mother-Infant Communication Project (Klein, Briggs, and Huffman, 1988)
The major focus is on communicative interaction strategies, especially child-oriented and interaction-promoting strategies. Service delivery components include a newborn phase, conducted in the hospital neonatal intensive care unit, and a follow-up phase, conducted through home visits, a center-based program, and small parent groups.
    Mother-Infant Communication Project
    California State University, Los Angeles
    Childhood Special Education
    5151 State University Drive
    Los Angeles, CA 90032

You and Your Baby: Building Communication (Girolametto and Ushycky, 1989)
Techniques from all three clusters of techniques — child-oriented, interaction-promoting, and language-modeling — are taught. Service delivery components include a 6-week center-based program for groups of parents and their infants, and individual consultations with videotaping.
    The Hanen Centre
    Suite 3-390, 252 Bloor St. West
    Toronto, Ontario M5S 1V6

Ecological Communication Organization (MacDonald, 1989)
This program is suitable for children of any age and is particularly appropriate for parents of children who are prelinguistic and minimally interactive. Techniques are taught individually or in parent groups, through a center-based program with home activities. The program has been applied to other caregivers as well.
    James D. MacDonald, PhD
    Parent-Child Communication Project

Nisonger Center for Developmental
    Disabilities
Ohio State University
1581 Dodd Drive
Columbus, OH 43210

Transactional Intervention Program: Teacher's Guide (Mahoney and Powell, 1986)
This program was designed to promote a responsive style of interaction with children from birth to age 3 years. The emphasis is on child-oriented and interaction-promoting techniques.
    Pediatric Research Training Center
    University of Connecticut Health Center
    Farmington, CT 06032

The Hanen Program for Parents (Manolson, 1992)
This program is designed to be implemented in a 12-week group program for parents. Three home visits provide individual consultation for the family. Techniques include child-oriented, interaction-promoting, and language-modeling techniques. A parent manual, "It Takes Two to Talk" and teaching video tapes are available.
    The Hanen Centre
    Suite 3-330, 252 Bloor St. West
    Toronto, Ontario M5S 1V6

Language Interaction Intervention (Weistuch et al., 1991)
This program was designed for parents of children with expressive language delays and focuses primarily on language-modeling techniques.
    Lucille Weistuch, PhD
    Department of Communication Disorders
    Montclair State College
    Upper Montclair, NJ 07743

Appendix D

Sample Agenda for a Preschool Language Group

Theme:	Taking an airplane ride
Phonology Target:	Stridents [sh]
Language Target:	Agent + Action + Object (I want *X;* I see *X*) Agent + Action (boy walk*ing*)

The clinician may introduce this session's theme using a book about airplanes or free play with an airport play set. In this way, the children's experiential knowledge is activated.

1. Phonology practice   15 minutes
Children make a list of things they would pack in a suitcase. Clinician prints the list in large letters on a wall board and draws a picture beside the corresponding word. Clinician integrates the target sound using the following words: shoe, shirt, shampoo, shorts, shower cap.

2. Activity 1   15 minutes
Each child gets an empty paper suitcase. Pictured objects are displayed on a wall board beside the printed word and include phonology targets as well as distractors (pictures of a refrigerator, stove, slide) that cannot be packed.

Clinician goes first and models "I want *X.*" Children take turns packing five pictured objects each.

3. Activity 2   15 minutes
Clinician and children pretend to be on an airplane. Clinician (or volunteer) places picture cards on the floor. Clinician goes first, pretends to look out the airplane window and models "I see *X.*" Children take five turns each looking out the window.

4. Snack   15 minutes
Clinician (or volunteer) pretends to be flight attendant. Clinician asks each child "Can I get you something to drink?" Expected response is "I want *X.*"

5. Craft   15 minutes
Children choose pictures to paste onto their airport scene. Pictures depict Agent + Object scenarios. Phonology words may be incorporated.

6. Parent session   15 minutes
Parents are given feedback on their children's achievements in the session, as well as ideas for stimulating speech and language goals at home.

REFERENCES

Bruner J: *Child's talk: learning to use language.* Oxford, 1983, Oxford University Press.

Carrow-Woolfolk E: *Theory, assessment and intervention in language disorders,* Philadelphia, 1988, Grune & Stratton.

Carrow-Woolfolk E: *Test for auditory comprehension of language-Revised,* Allan, Texas, 1985, DLM Teaching Resources.

Chapman K, Hardin M: Language input of mothers interacting with their young children with cleft lip and palate. *Cleft Palate-Craniofacial J* 28:78, 1991.

Cole K, Dale P: Direct language instruction and interactive language instruction with language delayed preschool children: a comparison study. *Speech Hearing Res* 29:206, 1986.

Dalston R: Communication skills of children with cleft lip and palate: a status report. In Bardach J, Morris H, editors: *Multidisciplinary management of cleft lip and palate,* Philadelphia, 1990, WB Saunders.

Dunn L, Dunn L: *Peabody picture vocabulary test-Revised,* Circle Pines, Minn, 1981, American Guidance Service.

Dunst C, Leet H, Trivette C: Family resources, personal well-being, and early intervention, *J Spec Educ* 22:108, 1988.

Fenson L, Dale P, Reznick S, Thal D, Bates E, Hartung J, Pethick S, Reilly J: *The MacArthur communicative development inventory.* San Diego, 1993, Singular Publishing Group, Inc.

Fey M: *Language intervention with young children,* Austin, Texas, 1986, Pro-Ed.

Fey M, Cleave P: Early language intervention, *Semin Speech Language* 11:165, 1990.

Friedman P, Friedman K: Accounting for individual differences when comparing the effectiveness of remedial language teaching methods, *Appl Psycholing* 1:151, 1980.

Girolametto L, Ushycky I: *You and your baby: building communication,* Toronto, 1989, Hanen Centre.

Gardner M: *Expressive one-word picture vocabulary test-Revised,* Novato, Calif, 1990, Academic Therapy Publications.

Kaye K, Charney R: Conversational asymmetry between mothers and children, *Child Language* 8:35, 1981.

Klein D, Briggs M, Huffman P: *Mother-infant communication project: facilitating caregiver-infant interaction,* Los Angeles, 1988, California State University, Division of Special Education.

Lieven E: Conversations between mothers and young children: individual differences and their possible implications for the study of language learning. In Snow C, Waterson N, editors: *The development of communication,* New York, 1978, Wiley & Sons.

Long N, Dalston R: Comprehension abilities of one-year-old infants with cleft lip and palate. *Cleft Palate J* 20: 303, 1983.

Mahoney G, Powell A: *Transactional intervention program: teacher's guide.* Farmington, Conn, 1986, Pediatric Research and Training Center, University of Connecticut Health Center.

Manolson A: *It takes two to talk,* Toronto, 1992, Hanen Centre.

MacDonald J: *Becoming partners with children,* San Antonio, Texas, 1989, Special Press.

McWilliams B, Morris H, Shelton R: *Cleft palate speech,* Philadelphia, 1990, B.C. Decker.

Morris H: Communication skills of children with cleft lip and palate, *Speech Hearing Res* 5:79, 1962.

Musgrave R, McWilliams B, Matthews H: A review of the results of two different surgical approaches for the repair of clefts of the soft palate only, *Cleft Palate J* 12:281, 1975.

Norris J, Hoffman P: Language intervention within naturalistic environments, *Language, Speech and Hearing Services in the Schools* 21:72, 1990.

Olswang L, Stoel-Gammon C, Coggins T, Carpenter R: *Assessing linguistic behaviors.* Seattle, 1987, University of Washington Press.

Pecyna P, Feeny-Giacoma M, Neiman G: Development of the object permanence concept in cleft lip and palate and noncleft lip and palate infants. *J Commun Disord* 20:233, 1987.

Prizant B, Audet L, Burke G, Hummel L, Maher S, Theodore G: Communication disorders and emotional/behavioural disorders in children and adolescents, *Speech Hearing Dis* 55:179, 1990.

Rescorla L: Identifying expressive language delay at age two, *Topics in Language Disorders* 11:14, 1991.

Reynell J, Gruber C: *Reynell developmental language scales-U.S. Edition.* Los Angeles, 1990, Western Psychological Services.

Richman L, Eliason M: Type of reading disability related to cleft type and neuropsychological patterns, *Cleft Palate J* 21:1, 1984.

Richman L, Eliason M, Lindgren S: Reading disability in children with clefts, *Cleft Palate J* 25:21, 1988.

Rosetti L: *Infant-toddler language scale.* East Moline, Ill, 1990, LinguiSystems.

Scarborough H, Dobrich W: Development of children with early language delay, *J Speech Hearing Res* 33:70, 1990.

Schaffer H: Language development in context. In von Tetzchner S, Siegel L, Smith L, editors: *The social and cognitive aspects of normal and atypical language development,* New York, 1989, Springer-Verlag.

Shames G, Rubin H: Psycholinguistic measures of language and speech. In Bzoch K, editor: *Communicative disorders related to cleft lip and palate,* Boston, 1979, Little, Brown.

Snow C: The conversational context of language acquisition. In Campbell R, Smith P, editors: *Recent advances in the psychology of language,* New York, 1978, Plenum Press.

Spriestersbach D, Darley F, Morris H: Language skills in children with cleft palate, *J Speech Hearing Res* 1:279, 1958.

Shprintzen RJ, Goldberg R: *Multiple anomaly syndromes and learning disabilities.* In Smith S, editor: *Genetics and learning disabilities,* San Diego, 1985, College Hill Press, pp 153-174.

Tannock R, Girolametto L: Reassessing parent-focused language intervention programs. In Warren S, Reichle J, editors: *Causes and effects in communication and language intervention,* Baltimore, 1992, Paul Brookes.

Warr-Leeper G et al: A comparison of the performance of preschool children with cleft lip and/or palate on the test of pragmatic skills. Paper presented at the Annual Meeting of the American Cleft Palate-Craniofacial Association, Williamsburg, Virginia, 1988.

Weistuch L, Lewis M, Sullivan M: Use of a language interaction intervention in the preschools. *J Early Intervention* 15:278, 1991.

Wetherby A, Prizant B: *Communication and symbolic behavior scales.* San Antonio, 1991, Special Press, Inc.

Wells G: Language, learning and teaching: helping children to make knowledge their own. In Lowenthal F, Vandamme F, editors: *Pragmatics and education,* New York, 1986, Plenum Press.

Werner E, Kresheck J: *Structured photographic expressive language test,* Sandwich, Ill, 1983, Janelle Publications.

Wilcox J, Kouri T, Caswell S: Early language intervention: a comparison of classroom and individual treatment, *Am J Speech-Language Pathol* 1:49, 1991.

10 The Evaluation of Speech Disorders Associated with Clefting

Linda L. D'Antonio and Nancy J. Scherer

This chapter is written for the speech-language pathologist who may be confronted for the first time with the challenge of evaluating the communication skills of an individual with a cleft palate or other craniofacial disorder. You may be a student or a newly trained speech pathologist unfamiliar with evaluation of patients in a medical setting. You may be an experienced clinician who has never worked with this population, confronted with your first cleft client. Or you may have found yourself challenged with the seemingly overwhelming task of providing speech-language pathology services for a cleft palate/craniofacial team. What do you do? Where do you begin? Where do you go for advice?

First you must realize that you are not alone. Most training programs provide little if any exposure to the area of cleft palate/craniofacial disorders. This chapter is not an attempt (nor is it possible) to make you an expert in cleft palate or to give you all of the training you would need to serve as an independent member of a cleft palate/craniofacial team. Rather it is a tool to guide you in the *content areas* that generally are of concern for patients with cleft palate. It is essential that the reader of this chapter understand that the information provided here is not intended to be a substitute for training and experience. Nor is it a substitute for more thorough discussions of communication impairment associated with cleft palate.

This chapter discusses (1) the role of the speech and language pathologist in assessing speech (particularly on a cleft palate/craniofacial team), (2) the differences between screening and evaluation, (3) the critical information you need to obtain from your patients, (4) difficult patient populations you are likely to encounter, (5) suggestions for eliciting the necessary information, and (6) how to report your findings and recommendations along with your role in making management recommendations to the cleft palate team and to community care providers.

A NOTE ON TERMINOLOGY

Although the title of this Chapter is "The evaluation of speech disorders associated with clefting," the role of the speech-language pathologist is to assess overall communication skills in patients with cleft palate and often other craniofacial anomalies. Therefore, although we continue to use the term *speech evaluation* within this chapter, it should be recognized that we are referring to the more comprehensive communication process. Additionally, the term *evaluation* may be a misnomer. In most cleft palate team settings in the United States the speech pathologist is not afforded the luxury of spending the amount of time with each patient necessary to conduct comprehensive evaluations of speech and language. Almost all teams perform an in-depth speech and language evaluation at some point in a child's development or receive reports of comprehensive evaluations conducted elsewhere. However, typically, a basic speech and/or speech and language screening is conducted on a more routine basis during team visits. Therefore this chapter focuses on the areas of development and communication that should be screened in a brief team visit. Obviously, all areas of development, speech, and language that we discuss in this chapter cannot be evaluated or screened in detail. However, the speech pathologist can use information obtained during a brief screening to select areas of concern for further screening or to identify the children who require further in-depth assessments. The content areas discussed within the screening process are the same areas to be addressed in a full speech and language evaluation, but in greater depth.

THE ROLE OF THE SPEECH-LANGUAGE PATHOLOGIST

The speech-language pathologist should be involved with a child with cleft palate from early infancy throughout growth and development. Over time the objectives of the speech-language consult and involvement with the family and patient will change. For example, Philips (1990) advocates three types of speech-language programs between birth and age 3. She suggests that at ages 3 to 12 months the focus should be parent education. From 12 to 30 months the clinician should develop and monitor a speech and language stimulation program "to support and promote the child's phonologic and linguistic development," to help avoid compensatory speech patterns, and to begin assessment of velopharyngeal (VP) function. From 30 months on the speech-language pathologist begins direct remediation.

Similarly, O'Gara and Logemann (1990) suggest that early referral and longitudinal involvement of the speech-language pathologist are necessary to instruct parents in the active daily role they play in their child's communication development. Specifically, they indicate that parents need information regarding the following:

1. The role that the normal noncleft hard and soft palates play in normal speech sound acquisition
2. The restrictions imposed by the unrepaired cleft hard or soft palate on the variety of consonant phones produced by their child during babbling and perhaps first word productions
3. The avoidance of positive reinforcement of consonant constrictions that involve backed glottal and pharyngeal place features

Additionally, during the early stages of development the speech-language pathologist should educate and remind parents and other professionals of the potential deleterious role of conductive hearing loss on communication development.

After the age of 36 months, the attention of the speech-language pathologist begins to focus more on speech production, particularly articulation, phonology, VP function, and overall intelligibility. Most texts and chapters that describe the evaluation of speech disorders associated with clefting focus on issues related to resonance, VP function, and articulation. For example, Morris (1990) writes:

The speech-language pathologist in contemporary practice is prepared to deal with aspects of communication that relate to speech production, language, and voice. Since cleft lip and palate and related disorders are primarily structural defects that affect the articulators and the mechanisms for controlling oronasal resonance, speech production and voice are of prime concern. Of the two, it frequently is more expedient and efficient to focus on speech production.

The burden of conducting assessments that may lead to critical management decisions such as surgical intervention can cause the speech pathologist to focus almost exclusively on aspects of speech production, particularly VP function. However, it is important to understand that speech production is only one part of the communication process that may be associated with palatal clefting. A large percentage of children who present with cleft palate also may be affected by another more complex craniofacial anomaly or by a multiple malformation syndrome (Pashayan, 1983; Jones, 1988). Siegel-Sadewitz and Shprintzen (1982) have shown that most syndromes associated with clefting have a variety of identifiable communication disorders that may be far more involved than impairments in speech production alone. Therefore the speech-language pathologist must screen all aspects of communication and be aware of the diversity of impairments that could be found in this population. In our clinical experience it is particularly important to monitor language and other developmental skills in addition to the more obvious speech production skills at least into the middle school years. For example, information pertaining to language skills can be very important for identifying children who should be monitored more closely for later reading and academic problems (Eliason and Richman, 1990).

RATIONALE FOR A PHYSIOLOGIC/ DEVELOPMENTAL APPROACH

As discussed previously, there is great pressure in some settings for the speech pathologist to focus primarily or even exclusively on resonance and VP function with respect to surgical success or secondary management. However, the velopharynx is only one part of a complex, interrelated series of structures that form the human vocal tract. Therefore even a simple speech evaluation must take into consideration the structures and processes of the entire speech production mechanism. Fig. 10-1 shows a schematic representation of the vocal tract as proposed by Netsell et al. (1989) for structuring clinical speech physiology evaluations and assessing vocal tract function. In this representation the vocal tract comprises 10 functional components. A functional component is defined as a vocal tract structure or structures used to generate or valve the speech airstream. These components must function in a highly coordinated and temporally constrained manner. There is evidence that impairment in one vocal tract component may cause or be associated with impairment in other components. For

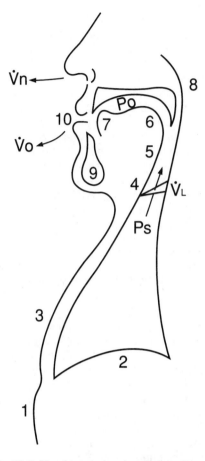

STRUCTURES

1 – Abdominal muscles
2 – Diaphragm
3 – Rib cage
4 – Larynx
5 – Tongue/pharynx
6 – Posterior tongue
7 – Anterior tongue
8 – Velopharynx
9 – Jaw
10 – Lips

AERODYNAMICS

Ps – Subglottal air pressure
Po – Intraoral air pressure
$\dot{V}_L$ – Laryngeal air flow
$\dot{V}o$ – Oral air flow
$\dot{V}n$ – Nasal air flow

Fig. 10-1 Vocal tract, showing designation of 10 functional components that generate or valve the speech airstream and the aerodynamic variables that can be measured. (Reprinted with permission from Netsell R, Lotz W, Barlow S: A speech physiology examination for individuals with dysarthria. In Yorkston K, Beukelman D, editors: *Recent advances in clinical dysarthria,* Boston, 1989, College-Hill.)

example, Warren (1986) suggests that impairment of the VP valve alone can lead to alterations in function along the entire vocal tract. Similarly, Dalston et al (1992) suggest that nasal cavity function can affect articulation patterns. Therefore the speech-language pathologist should be certain to consider the entire vocal tract when evaluating a patient with cleft palate and thereby avoid the common mistake of focusing exclusively or primarily on the cleft and VP function.

We have stated our view that it is essential to evaluate speech production as part of the greater communication process and that a speech evaluation should address the entire vocal tract. Additionally, in our clinical experience it is valuable (if not essential) to assess speech production within the context of motor speech development. Although this concept may seem foreign initially, speech-language pathologists use some motor speech development data routinely. For example, in assessing the speech production of a 3-year-old, the experienced clinician would not be alarmed at the absence or distortion of the /s/ sound for which the young child does not have the necessary motor skills to produce accurately or consistently. However, Netsell (1981) hypothesizes that the development of each vocal tract component can be assessed independently (Fig. 10-2). This approach has particular appeal and advantages for assessment of prespeech and early speech activity in the cleft population. For example, one could expect delays and impairment in the VP mechanism and tongue positioning due to the early presence of a cleft and possible velopharyngeal incompetence (VPI). However, delays in the other components de-

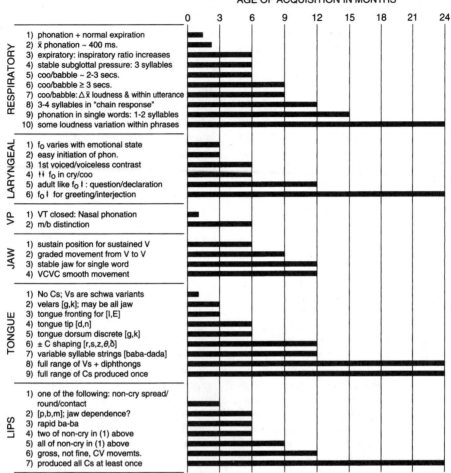

AGE OF ACQUISITION IN MONTHS

RESPIRATORY
1) phonation + normal expiration
2) x̄ phonation ~ 400 ms.
3) expiratory: inspiratory ratio increases
4) stable subglottal pressure: 3 syllables
5) coo/babble ~ 2-3 secs.
6) coo/babble ≥ 3 secs.
7) coo/babble: Δ x̄ loudness & within utterance
8) 3-4 syllables in "chain response"
9) phonation in single words: 1-2 syllables
10) some loudness variation within phrases

LARYNGEAL
1) f_0 varies with emotional state
2) easy initiation of phon.
3) 1st voiced/voiceless contrast
4) ↑↓ f_0 in cry/coo
5) adult like f_0 ↑ : question/declaration
6) f_0 ↑ for greeting/interjection

VP
1) VT closed: Nasal phonation
2) m/b distinction

JAW
1) sustain position for sustained V
2) graded movement from V to V
3) stable jaw for single word
4) VCVC smooth movement

TONGUE
1) No Cs; Vs are schwa variants
2) velars [g,k]; may be all jaw
3) tongue fronting for [I,E]
4) tongue tip [d,n]
5) tongue dorsum discrete [g,k]
6) ± C shaping [r,s,z,θ,ð]
7) variable syllable strings [baba-dada]
8) full range of Vs + diphthongs
9) full range of Cs produced once

LIPS
1) one of the following: non-cry spread/round/contact
2) [p,b,m]; jaw dependence?
3) rapid ba-ba
4) two of non-cry in (1) above
5) all of non-cry in (1) above
6) gross, not fine, CV movemts.
7) produced all Cs at least once

Fig. 10-2 Hypothesized speech motor milestones in the first 2 years. Selected speech behaviors listed for each of the functional components of the speech mechanism were selected to show increasing control of each component. These behaviors were drawn from the existing literature and are based predominantly on data obtained from phonetic transcription. The termination of the horizontal bar associated with each behavior represents the approximate age at which the speech act might be expected to be established in the child's speech production capabilities. (Modified from Netsell R: The acquisition of speech motor control: a perspective with directions for research. In R Stark, editor: *Language behavior in infancy and early childhood,* New York, 1981, Elsevier Science Publishing.)

scribed in Fig. 10-2 may be related to the presence of the cleft in a compensatory manner or may be an early warning signal of a more involved speech motor control disorder.

Appendix A provides a clinical protocol for observations and elicitation tasks for assessing the components of the vocal tract with the minimum age at which success for each task might be expected. This protocol was prepared by Miller et al (1979) according to the physiologic developmental approach described in Fig. 10-2.

We have discussed the importance of assessing speech production as one part of the complete vocal tract and as a developmental motor control process. It also is important to assess speech as part of a more global developmental communication process. As we have seen, children with cleft palate are at risk for a variety of communication impairments. Generally, children with cleft palate are followed by a cleft palate team from birth to late adolescence or adulthood. Therefore it is important to use an assessment model that addresses the important milestones at each stage of development. Inherent in the developmental approach is the understanding that a child progresses through a sequence or hierarchy of stages which are not necessarily linked to chronologic age for many children with congenital anomalies.

Information regarding a child's development is an essential component of a communication evaluation. For instance, in the cleft population early assessment of developmental processes in speech, language, motor development, and cognitive functioning may provide early predictors of a later communication delay or disorder or of a more serious global impairment. In addition to differentiating between a communication impairment and a more global impairment, a developmental approach to screening and evaluation also may be beneficial in differentiating among subtypes of speech/language impairment. For example, understanding a child's developmental profile should allow the clinician to differentiate between a phonologic process error and a developmental articulation error. In another situation a developmental approach can differentiate between an expressive language disorder, which one might expect in a child with an impaired speech production mechanism, and a receptive-expressive delay/disorder, which would be of more concern and may point to a more complex impairment. Finally, a physiologic/developmental model naturally lends itself to the transition from assessment to intervention by suggesting where a child "should be" and "what comes next." The combined physiologic/developmental model can be seen at work in the following screening protocols.

THE SCREENING PROCESS: THE NECESSARY INFORMATION TO BE OBTAINED

As mentioned previously, cleft care provided within a team approach usually is carried out over a patient's first 18 years of life. Therefore important information to obtain in a speech and language screening differs significantly over time depending on the patient's age and the information needed by other team members to determine readiness for various physical management procedures.

Many speech-language pathologists are tied to a single screening tool or screening protocol regardless of age and must adapt the existing forms as they conduct their screening. This rapid adaptation often is difficult, especially under tight time constraints or when screening numerous patients of differing ages in a single clinic. Therefore for some time we have advocated the use of developmental stage screening forms, which serve to remind the clinician to address the relevant content areas for that general age range. Sample screening forms are shown and discussed with respect to the important information for four developmental groups: infant, toddler/preschool, school age, and teen/adult.

The infant screening

The box that appears on p. 181 shows a sample infant screening form. Typically we use the term *infant* to refer to the age range from birth to 18 months of age. However, this form, like the others, should be used in a flexible manner based on estimated maturational age rather than actual chronologic age. During this stage the speech-language pathologist makes first contact with the parents and child. It is also during this time that lip repair is completed (when a cleft lip is present) and the stage during which primary palate repair usually is performed.

As suggested earlier, the speech-language pathologist should be involved with the family and patient from the first visit to the cleft palate/craniofacial team. During the earliest interactions the focus generally is on parent education. However, even in the most early stages of infancy there are opportunities for the trained interviewer and observer to screen oral structure and function, hearing responsiveness, socialization, and parent-child interaction, which may provide important information regarding later communication and general development. At this stage good interviewing and observation skills are critical, since more formal evaluation procedures are not possible. Additionally, strong counseling skills are advantageous to gain insight into family concerns and interactions that may be important to the child's long-term care.

History, parent report, and observation. The focus of the parent report section is to gather information regarding the child's feeding, airway, motor and communication development. Keep in mind that developmental information is only as good as the source. Information obtained from parent report is the parents' perception of the child's development, and thus the accuracy of the information may be influenced by the parents' understanding of development and the value the family places on the child's development. Good interviewing technique and astute behavioral observation are invaluable. Even with the potential problems of using parent report, the benefits still outweigh the potential problems if the interview is facilitated properly by the speech-language pathologist.

CRANIOFACIAL SPEECH-LANGUAGE SCREENING: INFANT

Name:

DOB:

Age:

Diagnosis:

Funding:

Date of Screening:

HISTORY/PARENT REPORT

Feeding:

Airway:

Motor Milestones:

_____ Diminished head lag (2 to 4 mo)

_____ Control of torso sitting supported (2 to 4 mo)

_____ Rhythmic movement of legs and arms (2 to 4 mo)

_____ Sits unassisted (4 to 8 mo)

_____ Reaches for objects (0 to 5 mo)

_____ Walks unassisted (13 to 18 mo)

COMMUNICATION DEVELOPMENT

_____ Alertness:

_____ Social Smile:

_____ Sound:

_____ Visual:

_____ Tracking:

_____ Orienting to Sound:

Prelinguistic Skills

_____ Vowels (cooing)

_____ Babbling CV   CVC   CVCV

_____ Gesture-requests by pointing

_____ Understands person or object names

_____ Understands action words: jump, drink, kiss

_____ Inhibits to "no"

_____ True words

_____ Compensatory articulations

OROMOTOR/SPEECH MECHANISM

Structure:

Function:

PHONATION

_____ No apparent concern

_____ Suspect

Quality:

_____ Harsh

_____ Breathy

_____ Strained

_____ Volume/loudness

_____ Pitch

_____ Other _____

_____

SUMMARY/IMPRESSIONS:

RECOMMENDATIONS:

_____ Audiological evaluation

_____ Additional speech/language evaluation

_____ Developmental assessment

_____ Developmental programming

_____ Follow with team

_____ Rescreen recommended _____

_____ Other _____

Seen and examined by: _____

Speech-Language Pathologist   License #

Feeding. Assessment of feeding for nutritional purposes is critical and usually is carried out by the pediatrician or nurse. However, some information about the feeding process is important to the speech-language pathologist because it provides a means for assessing the structure and function of the speech mechanism during a complex motor task. Infants who show a significant lack of coordination during feeding or evidence of aspiration may be referred for a thorough swallowing/feeding evaluation. Although early feeding problems may or may not predict later motor speech problems, they certainly suggest a child who is at risk for speech impairment and who should be followed closely. Morris and Klein (1987) provide an excellent resource for the evaluation of early feeding skills with some discussion of the relationship between general and speech development. They provide detailed information regarding assessment and treatment with a section specifically focused on infants with cleft palate.

Feeding problems also may result from causes other than motor or structural deficits. Particularly in the cleft population, the success of early parent-child bonding may influence feeding. Feeding then becomes a window into aspects of parent-child interaction that may influence speech and language development later.

Airway. Information regarding airway function is essential because it may indicate a potentially life-threatening problem that warrants immediate intervention. Generally, the assessment of airway concerns is the responsibility of the pediatrician or otolaryngologist. However, the speech pathologist should be sensitive to signs and symptoms of airway impairment in infants and young children. Airway obstruction may be caused by deformities of the nose, midface, oral cavity, mandible, oropharynx, hypopharynx, skullbase, larynx, and trachea. The infant is an obligate nose breather for approximately the first 6 weeks of life. With growth, the larynx descends in the neck, which allows for more adult-like respiratory patterns through the nose and mouth. In infancy, observable or reported signs of airway obstruction may include obstruction of the nose or nasopharynx, which is characterized by snoring or snorting sounds or laryngeal and subglottic obstruction characterized by stridor a higher frequency sound. Snoring generally is considered a sign of partial airway obstruction, whereas overt sleep apnea is a complete cessation of breathing during sleep (Handler, 1985).

Airway obstruction may be mild or severe. It can have potentially life-threatening or devel-opmental consequences (Gray, 1990). Persistent airway impairment can affect later speech quality in a variety of ways. Most commonly hyper-trophied adenoids and tonsils or nasal obstruction can create hyponasal resonance or cause the child to become a chronic mouth breather, in which case articulation can be affected. Additionally, laryngeal abnormalities such as persistent laryngomalacia (collapse of redundant supraglottic tissue into the glottis during respiration) can result in impaired breath support for speech and abnormal laryngeal voice quality. Although this condition is reported to resolve in normal children by 18 months of age, it is not uncommon for it to persist in children with craniofacial anomalies (Gray, 1990). As with feeding problems, parent report or a history of airway impairment also may suggest the presence of a more complex craniofacial anomaly or a multiple malformation syndrome and thus can be an early finding to identify children who should be referred for additional evaluations or be followed closely by the team. Additionally, some children with cleft palate also have conditions that require tracheostomy. In these instances it is the speech pathologist's responsibility to ascertain whether the family is aware of the risk for communication impairment in children with tracheostomies and to determine whether adequate parent education, communication stimulation, or therapy is being provided.

Motor development. It is well known that motor milestones are an indicator of general development and relate to speech and language acquisition. It is particularly important to screen motor development in the infant, since it is one of the first indicators to be observed and monitored. There are several well-known developmental screening tests that outline fine and gross motor development. Popular examples are The Denver Developmental Screening Test (1969) and The Bayley Scales of Infant Development (1969). However, for purposes of screening motor development in the infant with cleft palate, it is effective and sufficient to monitor a few selected motor milestones routinely and refer for full developmental evaluation when motor development is suspect or obviously delayed. There are three primary reasons for vigilance in such monitoring. Observed delays or impairment in motor function may be (1) an indication of a specific motor impairment such as cerebral palsy or other neurologic conditions, (2) an indicator of a more global developmental delay or multiple malformation syndrome, and (3) predictive of later speech and language delay or impairment. In the cleft palate population Kemp-Fincham et al (1990) make a case for careful monitoring of early motor milestones before 6 months of age as it relates specifically to the onset of babbling and development and expansion of phoneme repertoire before the onset of word production. They use information regarding motor development to suggest that initial palatoplasty should be timed with or occur between 4 and 6 months of age to correspond with this period of rapid increase in motor control and phonemic expansion.

Communication development. The focus of the communication screening during the infant stage is to identify early precursors of later receptive and expressive language and speech function. A variety of communication processes are developing simultaneously between birth and 18 months of age. Although all or even most aspects of communication development cannot be observed during this period, some processes are particularly good windows into development and thus make them good screening items. Fig. 10-3 shows critical age ranges for various speech and language processes taken from a number of screening tools (Assessing Linguistic Behaviors, 1989; MacArthur Communication Development Inventory, 1989; Rossetti Infant-Toddler Language Scale, 1990).

It is important for screening items to sample aspects of comprehension, play, communicative gesture, phoneme repertoire, syllable structure, and word use, since these communicative behaviors provide early evidence of possible speech and language disorders. This profile of performance may permit early differential diagnosis between specific impairments (e.g., articulation and expressive language delay/disorders) as shown by phoneme repertoire, syllable structure, and word use versus more global impairments (e.g., developmental delay or receptive-expressive language disorder). Information regarding parent-child interaction also may be useful in this differential diagnosis.

The communication areas screened during infancy warrant further discussion. Comprehension and play items are important to assess because they provide an indication of the child's language abilities that do not rely on intact speech production skills. The benefits of such an approach are obvious in the cleft palate population where the possibility of poor speech production skills and reduced intelligibility may make traditional language testing difficult to interpret. Comprehension of language is an essential process to screen but is difficult to assess reliably. Young children in a busy clinic setting often do not respond to comprehension questions, whereas they do respond at home in a familiar setting. When comprehension screening is not successful, screening of developmental play milestones can help the speech and language pathologist identify elements of play that correspond to language comprehension milestones (Thal and Bates, 1988; Thal et al, 1991). Also, screening of play in combination with communicative gestures (e.g., pointing to indicate requests) gives an indication of the child's nonverbal skills that relate to overall cognitive level.

Early articulation performance can be assessed in babbling and words through description of the child's phoneme repertoire and syllable structure. Traditionally, most non-speech pathologists think articulation can be assessed only with the onset of word production. However, current data suggest that there is a continuity between sound repertoire and syllable structure in babbling and later speech articulation Kemp-Fincham et al, 1990; O'Gara and Logemann, 1990; Trost-Cardamone, 1990). Therefore, when assessing the communication skills of the infant with cleft palate, a valuable window to later articulation development may be found in the sounds present in the child's babbling. O'Gara and Logemann (1990) suggest that precursors to compensatory articulation errors can be found in the infant's early phoneme repertoire and can therefore be targeted for early monitoring and intervention, thus avoiding a firm establishment of such errors in the child's later phonemic repertoire and phonologic system. Trost-Cardamone (1990) suggests "it is possible that onset and practice of compensatory valving placements could begin with babbling." However, she reports there are no strong data to support this notion in her sample of eight babies. Despite the lack of hard data establishing that compensatory articulation and valving patterns may have their origins in babbling, it is wise for the speech pathologist to monitor the infant's early phoneme repertoire and educate the parents regarding the significance of abnormal sound development.

Onset and variety of word use is the first reliable indicator of speech and language performance. As with language comprehension assessment, screening of word use in a clinic setting can be unpredictable at this age level. Parent questionnaires such as the MacArthur Communicative Development Inventory (1989) and the Rossetti Infant-Toddler Language

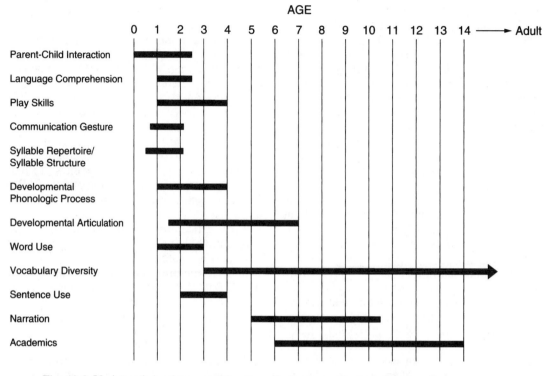

Fig. 10-3 Variety of developmental language behaviors with the corresponding age range during which these behaviors are particularly sensitive indicators of general language development.

Scale (1990) are two published, normed screening tools that can augment clinical observation and elicitation during screening. Parents may complete the questionnaires while they are waiting during the clinic visits, and the questionnaires can be scored and interpreted by the speech and language pathologist.

Oromotor/speech mechanism. The primary purpose of assessing the oromotor/speech mechanism is to differentiate the role of true structural restrictions from impairments of speech function. In infancy it is possible to identify motor concerns that place the child at risk for later motor speech problems, but complete assessment is not possible until the child is older. Since assessment of motor speech performance is difficult, information regarding oromotor function is critical. As mentioned previously, feeding may be the first opportunity to assess the functional abilities of the oromotor mechanism. For nonverbal children, feeding may be the only opportunity to assess oromotor function. However, for children who are beginning to talk, both nonspeech and speech tasks should be assessed. Most standard speech mechanism exams incorporate nonspeech tasks.

However, infants cannot perform most structured, voluntary oromotor tasks outside of a meaningful context. Nevertheless, some function may be observed during spontaneous movements or from elicited actions. For example, pursing lips may be observed when the child kisses a parent or blows bubbles. Range of tongue motion may be observed when licking a sweet solution from outside of the lips, elevating the tongue to reach peanut butter placed on the alveolar ridge, or locating cereal placed between the teeth and cheek.

Information regarding syllable structure is important but again should be elicited in meaningful contexts. For the infant, nonmeaningful syllable repetition such as "pah-tah-kah" usually cannot be obtained. However, the use of word imitation may provide the desired information by varying the length and complexity of the utterance. For example, the clinician may begin with consonant-vowel combinations such as "boo" and expand to consonant-vowel-consonant combinations such as "boot" and consonant - vowel - consonant - vowel sequences such as "booboo" or "peek-a-boo." Also, for older infants repetition of "patty-cake" is a useful target stimulus for rapid syllable repetition. The clinician should be certain to use simple words that young children would know and early developing phonemes that are appropriate for the child's developmental age.

Phonation. As seen in Fig. 10-2, rapid development of laryngeal/voice function takes place in the first 12 months of life. From birth to 3 months fundamental frequency (pitch) varies with emotional state, and there should be easy onset of phonation. From birth to 6 months the first voiced/voiceless contrasts should appear in babbling and there should be an increase or decrease in fundamental frequency during crying and cooing. Between birth and 12 months the infant begins to vary pitch for question versus declaration. Additionally, as stated earlier, abnormal laryngeal voice quality may be a sign of airway obstruction or airway dysfunction and in some cases may point to a more complex craniofacial disorder or a more involved syndrome than identified previously. Therefore it is important for the speech-language pathologist to be sensitive to phonatory function and quality even at this early stage of development.

The toddler/preschool screening

The box on pp. 186-187 shows a sample toddler/preschool screening form. It is during this stage of development that overt speech and language skills become accessible to direct observation and evaluation. Receptive and expressive language, articulation, resonance, and phonation are developed enough that they can be assessed separately. Additionally, the predictive value of screening results increases as the child matures. During the toddler/preschool stage speech and language function may begin to predict later specific speech and language impairment and academic strengths and weaknesses.

History, parent report, and observation. History, parent report, and clinician observation continue to be important sources of information during the toddler/preschool stage. However, in most situations the clinician has more opportunities to observe the child and verify information provided by the parents. As with the infant, the content areas to be reviewed and discussed with the family include feeding, now subdivided into chewing and swallowing; signs or symptoms of airway dysfunction, including snoring, allergies, and asthma; and continued monitoring of fine and gross motor skills. As with the infant, the speech-language pathologist should continue to emphasize the importance of aggressive monitoring of conductive hearing loss and educate parents of the relationship between fluctuating

hearing loss and delays or disorders of language development. Additionally, it is important at this stage of development to obtain detailed information from the parents regarding any educational programing, speech and language stimulation, or direct speech and language therapy the child may be receiving. The services available for children in this age group vary widely from state to state. Therefore the speech-language pathologist working with the cleft population should be familiar with the local resources available for preschool children with special needs. This is crucial for appropriate parent counseling and patient referral.

Language. It is essential that receptive and expressive language be assessed at this developmental level. The rapid expansion of language development in noncleft children during the toddler years highlights the importance of an extended screening or thorough evaluation between 2 and 3 years of age. Figure 10-3 on p. 184 shows a variety of language development behaviors with the corresponding age range during which these behaviors are particularly sensitive screening areas for general language development. It is important to recognize that the age range associated with each language behavior on this chart is not meant to show the total developmental range of the behavior; rather, the age ranges are considered to be the time period during which the corresponding behavior has been shown to be most predictive of overall language development. The language behaviors and corresponding screening ages were taken from several recently developed screening tools and developmental tests, including Assessing Linguistic Behaviors (1989), MacArthur Communication Development Inventory (1989), the Rossetti Infant-Toddler Language Scale (1990), Miller (1984), and Lahey (1988).

In addition to the familiar early indicators of language development such as parent-child interaction, language comprehension, and communication gestures, the assessment of play skills is incorporated in the list of screening behaviors. Recent literature has shown that developmental play skills often may be an indicator or predictor of language development (Thal and Bates, 1988; Thal and others, 1991). The assessment of play skills does not require speech production capabilities. Therefore, for the child with limited speech production proficiency or compromised intelligibility (as often occurs in children with cleft palate) the use of play assessment may be particularly valuable because it provides an estimate of the child's

CRANIOFACIAL SPEECH-LANGUAGE SCREENING: TODDLER/PRESCHOOL

Name: Diagnosis:
DOB: Funding:
Age: Date of Screening:

HISTORY/PARENT REPORT/OBSERVATION   PRIMARY LANGUAGE_____

Feeding: Chewing   Swallowing
Airway: Snoring   Allergies   Asthma   Trach_____

Motor Milestones:
_____ Use spoon to feed self (12-17 mo)
_____ Runs (19-24 mo)
_____ Builds a block tower (3 blocks/19-24 mo, 8 blocks/25-30 mo)
_____ Copies vertical and circular pattern (19-24 mo)
_____ Kicks/throws ball (25-30 mo)
_____ Walks up stairs (assisted 19-24 mo, unassisted 25-36 mo)
_____ Rides tricycle using pedals (31-36 mo)
_____ Draws vertical and horizontal strokes (25-30 mo), circles (31-36 mo)
_____ Cuts with scissors (31-36 mo)
_____ Heel-to-toe walk (4-5 yr)
_____ Draws a person, 3 parts (4-5 yr)

Hearing:_____

School: _____

Educational Program: _____   Special Services: _____

Speech Therapy at: _____

   Frequency: _____   Goals: _____

EVALUATION SUMMARY

Language:	Receptive:	No Concerns	Suspect	Delay/Disorder
	Expressive:	No Concerns	Suspect	Delay/Disorder

Oromotor/Speech Mechanism

Lip Closure:	Adequate	Inadequate	Asymmetric

Tongue:_____

Hard Palate: _____   Soft Palate: _____

   Fistula: Not Observed   Size _____   Location _____

Diadochokinetics _____

Articulation:

Developmental errors/Phonological processes: _____

Compensatory articulation: _____

Dental distortions: _____

Other:	Dialect	Rate	Reduced Excurions	Deterioration in conversation

Resonance	WNL				
	Hypernasal	NA	MILD	MODERATE	SEVERE
	Hyponasal	NA	MILD	MODERATE	SEVERE
	Mixed	NA	MILD	MODERATE	SEVERE
	Audible Nasal Emission	NA	MILD	MODERATE	SEVERE

Phonation	WNL	Hoarse	Breathy	Soft	Phonation Breaks	Vocal Abuse

NAME _____ DATE _____

SPEECH INTELLIGIBILITY RATING

	Clinician	Parent
1. Intelligible	_____	_____
2. Listener Attention Needed	_____	_____
3. Occasional Repetition of Words Required	_____	_____
4. Repetitions/Rephrasing Necessary	_____	_____
5. Isolated Words Understood	_____	_____
6. Occasionally Understood by Adult	_____	_____
7. Unintelligible	_____	_____

OVERALL SEVERITY OF COMMUNICATION IMPAIRMENT

_____ No concern
_____ Mild
_____ Moderate
_____ Severe

RECOMMENDATIONS:

_____ Audiological evaluation

_____ Complete speech/language evaluation at: _____

_____ "Bedside Swallow" eval: _____

_____ Nasendoscopy/aerodynamics

_____ Cognitive/academic/behavioral assessment at: _____

_____ Request School Reports/IEP/Speech Eval/Progress Report

_____ Rescreen recommended: _____

_____ Follow with team

_____ Other: _____

Speech-language therapy recommended at: _____

Frequency: _____

Intensity: Group   Individual   Both

Duration: _____

Goals: _____

_____

Other: _____

Seen and examined by: _____
                                Speech-Language Pathologist   License #

developmental level and language skills, independent of speech production.

A sample language worksheet is provided in Appendix B, which describes specific tasks and information that can be obtained during a clinic visit from parent report or observation. It should be noted that the worksheet attempts to extend language information typically obtained in a screening but does not replace a complete speech and language evaluation should the screening show areas of possible deficit. The worksheet contains suggested items for screening play, language comprehension, and expression for the 18 to 36-month range and the 3 to

4-year age range. The chronologic age levels indicate suggested screening ages rather than norms for the items. Play items have been selected based on the work of Thal and Bates (1988) and Thal et al (1991), who found that two play milestones were predictive of later language expression. The first play item on the worksheet—single functional toy play, or the appropriate use of toys (e.g., cup for drinking, car for pushing)—predicted later single word use. The second item—combines functional play, or the use of toys to create imaginative play (e.g., puts bib on doll, feeds doll, puts doll to bed)—predicted later sentence use. A third item was added for the older preschool age child—role play (e.g., takes the role of favorite characters in stories)—a task that requires integration of pragmatic, language comprehension, and production skills similar to those used in conversation and narration.

Language comprehension items were taken from The Rossetti Infant-Toddler Language Scale (1990) and Assessing Linguistic Behaviors (1989). The critical items included in the worksheet sample vocabulary categories in single-word and two- to three-word sentences. Vocabulary sampling is important because it is an indicator of global language comprehension. Additionally, vocabulary proficiency has been identified as a predictor of later reading problems (Eliason and Richman, 1990). The Peabody Picture Vocabulary Test (1981) is a quick, readily accessible test that can be administered in a screening if deficient language comprehension is suspected; other standardized comprehension measures are too time consuming for screening purposes.

Although comprehension of more complex language is expected by 3 years of age, screening of complex language requires more time than usually is available in a clinic visit. If there are concerns for language comprehension, a referral for a thorough speech and language evaluation should be made. It is essential to rule out the possibility of a language comprehension impairment, since this aspect of communication performance is particularly important for later academic success.

Expressive language can be sampled during a screening session. The speech pathologist should not rely exclusively on parent report of the child's language use at this age level because parents frequently fill in or correct the child's actual sentences inadvertently, thus eliminating crucial morphologic and syntactic errors that may have clinical relevance. Items suggested for screening expressive language during a brief clinic visit are presented in the language worksheet and were taken from the Rossetti Infant-Toddler Language Scale (1990), Assessing Linguistic Behaviors (1989), and The Preschool Language Scale—Revised (1992). The expressive language parameters of language use, overall sentence complexity, as indicated by mean length of utterance (MLU), expressive vocabulary, and narration are included as means for screening expressive language development.

Language and phonology represent rule-based processes. When language delay is noted, phonologic delay should be suspected. A standard sampling of phonologic processes might be included in the screening when a phonologic impairment is noted.

Oromotor/speech mechanism. Information on oromotor structure and speech motor function should be assessed thoroughly for all children. However, a careful intraoral examination and motor speech evaluation are particularly important during the toddler/preschool age range, since it usually is the first opportunity to evaluate oromotor function during speech activity. As with the infant, the oromotor exam must assess both structure and function.

Children with cleft palate or a suspected cleft usually will have received many intraoral examinations from medical and dental specialists. In most cases, by the time the speech pathologist evaluates the child, oral structure will have been well documented. Therefore the intraoral exam should be brief and the speech pathologist should assess those structures which are likely to affect speech production. For example, the lips should be assessed for any restrictions that would prevent lip closure or other movements necessary for correct articulation. Likewise, the tongue should be evaluated for its potential to reach articulatory targets. The diagnosis of tongue-tie (i.e., a short lingual frenulum) is commonly suggested by many parents and health care professionals. This diagnosis should be made only if the child cannot achieve the maximum range of lingual movements needed for correct articulatory placement. Dentition should be inspected for malocclusion and missing teeth, which might restrict or affect articulation. Additionally, the presence of any dental appliances such as maxillary expansion devices or palatal obturators should be noted and assessed, since they might affect articulatory precision and speech quality. The oral cavity should be inspected for hypertrophic tonsils or any structural deviations that might interfere with the full range of articulatory motion. The hard and soft palates should be examined for the presence of palatal fistulae. If a fistula is present, the patient and parent should be questioned regarding the patency of the fistula and its effects on eating, drinking, and speech. It is not uncommon for a child to present with a palatal fistula of which the parent and surgeon have no awareness. Skillful observation and patient questioning are useful in establishing the presence of a patent, symptomatic fistula. (The role of palatal fistulae on speech production and issues pertaining to the evaluation of fistulae are discussed in the section on resonance).

The soft palate should be examined carefully. In our experience it is not uncommon for a child with a repaired cleft to present with a dehisced soft palate, which may have been ignored by other professionals. However, in many cases thorough evaluation, particularly endoscopic visualization, will later prove the defect to have a significant detrimental effect on speech. Careful examination of the soft palate is particularly important in the patient with hypernasality with no diagnosis of clefting. The most posterior portion of the soft palate should be examined carefully to aid in the possible diagnosis of submucous cleft palate. This diagnosis is often missed in children who have no obvious symptoms of clefting other than hypernasality or speech production impairment related to VP dysfunction. If a vertical line is seen in the uvula, the examiner should use a tongue depressor to lift the uvula to determine if there is an actual split in the tissue. Often mucus will hold the two halves of the uvula together, and the diagnosis will be overlooked or more tentative than when an actual split is observed.

A note of caution should be mentioned concerning intraoral examinations. Many speech pathologists and medical specialists perform an intraoral examination to assess velar length and movement. Most commonly soft palate motion is observed during sustained or repeated production of the vowel "ah." Although this practice may provide some useful information (especially whether the hard and soft palates are intact and the size and position of the tonsils relative to the soft palate), it is imperative that the speech pathologist understand that an intraoral view of soft palate length and function is not an adequate (nor often accurate) description of velar function. Additionally, velar movement during sustained or repeated vowel production is not predictive of velar function during dynamic speech activity. Furthermore, intraoral view reveals little information regarding the pattern of VP closure (i.e., the contribution of the

lateral and posterior walls), the level at which closure is achieved, and the size and role of the adenoids in VP closure.

During a brief screening the assessment of the motor speech mechanism often is accomplished simultaneously with assessment of speech production tasks. Useful information can be elicited during repetitive syllable production, production of modeled words, and spontaneous use of words. If a speech motor planning disorder is suspected, further assessment is warranted. Imitation of words and phrases controlled for length and complexity are critical. An oromotor exam developed for children 2 years 6 months to 6 years 11 months that includes these critical elements and is standardized is the Clinical Assessment of Oropharyngeal Motor Development in Young Children (Robbins & Klee, 1987). A more detailed but informal protocol for speech motor evaluation has been discussed and is presented in Appendix A.

When significant motor speech impairment is seen to affect speech production and intelligibility, it is essential to consider the use of an alternative communication system in addition to the child's verbal attempts. This is particularly important for the toddler or preschool child who is attempting to develop receptive and expressive language skills with a severely impaired speech production mechanism. The alternative system such as signing or a communication board usually is a temporary communication system that will facilitate functional communication until the speech motor function improves and the child is capable of intelligible speech production. In cases of severe motor speech impairment, as with some patients with cerebral palsy or other neurologic conditions, the augmentative system may become the child's principal means of communication.

Speech production. Palatal clefting may affect speech production in a number of ways, including hypernasal resonance, nasal substitutions, compensatory articulation, sibilant distortion, and increased risk for disorders of phonation. The box on p. 190 presents definitions of several speech symptoms associated with cleft palate and VP dysfunction. In addition to these definitions another topic related to terminology is discussed by McWilliams and others (1990), who point out that individuals with VP incompetence typically are described as displaying hypernasal voice quality. However, the term *voice* more accurately refers to problems associated with phonation. Therefore, they suggest the use of the term ***phonation disorders*** to refer to problems that occur at the level of the larynx and

RESONANCE, ARTICULATION, AND PHONATION DISORDERS FREQUENTLY ASSOCIATED WITH CLEFT PALATE AND/OR VELOPHARYNGEAL DYSFUNCTION

Hypernasality

The perception of inordinate nasal resonance during the production of *vowels*. This results from inappropriate coupling of the oral and nasal cavities. (The term *inordinate* is used because low vowels and vowels in nasal consonant contexts are normally somewhat nasalized).

Nasal emission

Nasal air escape associated with production of *consonants* requiring high oral pressure. It occurs when air is forced through an incompletely closed velopharyngeal port. Nasal emission may be audible or not.
Note: Hypernasality and *nasal emission* are not synonymous, although they often occur together and are both symptoms of velopharyngeal dysfunction.

Hyponasality

A reduction in normal nasal resonance usually resulting from blockage or partial blockage of the nasal airway by any number of causes, including upper respiratory tract infection, hypertrophied turbinate, and a wide, obstructing pharyngeal flap.

Hyper-hyponasality

The simultaneous occurrence of hypernasality and hyponasality in the same speaker usually as the result of incomplete velopharyngeal closure in the presence of high nasal resistance that is not sufficient to block nasal resonance completely.

Cul-de-sac resonance

A variation of hyponasality usually associated with tight anterior nasal constriction often resulting in a muffled quality.

Nasal substitution

The articulators are placed appropriately for an intended oral consonant. However, incomplete velopharyngeal closure causes the sound to be produced as a nasal consonant. For example, b becomes m and d becomes n. Such substitutions frequently are called homorganic nasals.

Compensatory articulation

The articulators are placed inappropriately so as to enable creation of the plosive or fricative characteristics of the sounds they replace. For example, if a patient cannot build up oral pressure for the fricatives (e.g., s) or plosives (e.g., p) because of velopharyngeal dysfunction, they may create those pressures below the level of the velopharyngeal port. Such substitutions include glottal stops, pharyngeal stops, and pharyngeal fricatives among others.

Sibilant distortion

Inappropriate tongue placement for the sounds /s/ and /z/.

Laryngeal/voice symptoms

A variety of phonation disorders may accompany velopharyngeal dysfunction, including hoarseness, low speaking volume, strained or strangled voice quality, and unusual pitch alterations. The most recent theory for the cooccurrence of velopharyngeal and laryngeal symptoms is that speakers with velopharyngeal dysfunction may attempt to compensate for the inability to achieve complete closure and maintain adequate speech pressures by compensatory activity at the level of the larynx.

---

the term *resonance disorders* to refer to hypernasality and other disturbances that occur supraglottally. This use of clearly defined, physiologically based terminology leads to a more accurate and precise nomenclature and facilitates interdisciplinary communication. It is used in our discussion of speech production.

The following sections present a general discussion of articulation, resonance, VP function, and phonation. The theoretical and clinical issues discussed regarding these areas of speech production apply to all age groups from toddler to adult. Obviously, the toddler or preschool child will demonstrate less speech production than the school-age child and the adult. Addi-

tionally, the toddler/preschool speech production system is in a period of rapid expansion, so greater variability is expected. Nevertheless, the principals regarding speech production presented within the toddler/preschool section of this chapter apply throughout the later developmental stages. Even though all of the areas of speech production remain important throughout the child's development, screenings and evaluations will shift in focus based on the information needed by the other professionals to develop an appropriate management plan for the child.

Articulation. Articulation, resonance, and VP function are inextricably linked. Although we discuss these processes separately, it should be understood they are highly interrelated and should be evaluated with this interrelationship in mind. Several contributors may impair articulation development or articulation skills. These factors include past or present VP dysfunction, timing of palate repair, palatal fistulae, abnormalities in the skeletal relationship between the maxilla and mandible, dental abnormalities, and nasal airway deviations.

It is essential that the speech-language pathologist be aware that not all children with cleft lip and palate necessarily develop articulation disorders. This is important information that often is not relayed to parents of children with cleft palate. Additionally, children with palatal clefts should be expected to demonstrate developmental articulation errors just as those observed for children without cleft palate. Therefore, especially during the toddler/preschool age range, information about normal articulation development is an essential component of parent counseling and often will relieve much parental anxiety.

ARTICULATION TESTING. The speech-language pathologist should assess articulation skills routinely. The type of testing will depend on the information the speech pathologist desires from the testing process. For example, articulation testing for children with cleft palate may be used for determining whether the child has an articulation or phonologic disorder or whether the pattern of articulation errors suggests the presence of VPI or both. Another primary goal of the articulation test is to determine whether the child is consistent or inconsistent in the errors noted and whether he or she is stimulable for correct or improved articulatory productions.

Most speech pathologists are familiar with a number of articulation tests and frequently are most comfortable with one or two specific tests. Any articulation test can be utilized for testing the child with cleft palate; however, two tests have been developed specifically for the cleft palate population. The Iowa Pressure Articulation Test (Morris et al, 1961) is composed of 43 plosives, fricatives, and affricatives likely to be misarticulated in the presence of incomplete VP closure. This articulation test is focused primarily on the identification of VPI. A second test developed specifically for individuals with cleft palate is the Bzoch Error Pattern Diagnostic Articulation Tests (Bzoch, 1979). Like the Iowa Pressure Articulation Test, this test samples plosives, fricatives, and affricates. Articulation errors are placed into five categories: nasal emission, distortion, simple substitution, gross substitution, and omission.

In some time-limited clinical screening situations formal articulation testing is not possible. In these situations repetition of modeled words and sentences with a representative sample of sounds should be used to elicit a sample of the child's articulation skills. However, it should always be understood that production of modeled stimulus items does not provide an accurate estimate of the child's articulation skills. Regardless of the test or procedure used, most experienced clinicians agree the important information to be obtained from the assessment of articulation is an analysis of error patterns. It is not sufficient to note the number of errors or simply the sounds that are in error, and whether they are omissions, distortions, or substitutions. At a minimum, articulation errors should be identified by place and manner of articulation and the presence of nasal emission. The clinician also should note any relevant visual descriptions regarding sound production such as incomplete, inconsistent, or asymmetric lip closure, tongue placement with respect to dentition or tongue position along an anterior-posterior continuum.

Results of the articulation test or articulation sample can be analyzed in a variety of ways. The most common error pattern analyses include place-manner-voice, distinctive feature, and phonologic process analyses. Regardless of the system used, it is important to document the consistency of articulation patterns. That is, sounds should be identified as to whether they are consistently produced correctly, inconsistently produced correctly, or consistently misarticulated.

Morris (1990) discusses the importance of analyzing error patterns:

Specifically, the examiner must indicate in the scoring procedure whether speech production errors are oral or nasal in character. The distinction is important in regard to the apparent etiology of the error patterns: Errors that are nasalized raise questions about velopharyngeal function; errors that are oral indicate that velopharyngeal function is within normal limits but articulation placement is not. Obviously, cleft palate patients frequently show both error types on the same sound production, and the scoring procedure must be sufficiently flexible to reflect that as well.

The scoring procedure also must reflect use of "unusual" speech sound substitutions. Two examples are the glottal stop and the pharyngeal fricative. . . . Trost has suggested others as well: the pharyngeal stop, the mid-dorsum palatal stop and the posterior nasal fricative.

In addition to testing articulation in single words and short phrases, it is essential to observe articulation skills and error patterns in conversational speech. It is not uncommon for children to demonstrate excellent articulation placement for single words and show a significant deterioration in connected speech. When this occurs, further probing should be conducted. Once again, it is important to note the pattern of errors. The clinician should attempt to determine if the cause of the deterioration is a reduction in articulatory precision, a decrease in the range of articulatory motion, a consistent pattern of sound omission or distortion (perhaps related to a particular location such as word final position or cluster reduction), or if the errors are inconsistent and apparently random. In many cases an inconsistent deterioration in articulation skills with increased length and complexity of utterance is indicative of a speech motor planning disorder such as dyspraxia. If this is suspected, further evaluation should be conducted using some of the suggestions described in this chapter for assessing the dyspraxic child presented in the section entitled Unexpected but common populations.

COMPENSATORY ARTICULATION. This consists of articulation errors thought to be articulatory gestures that the child adopts during speech development to compensate for inadequate VP closure. In general, for most children with cleft palate, when articulation errors are present, tongue placement is shifted posteriorly (backed) in an attempt to valve the airstream before it escapes or is diminished through an open VP port or through an open cleft. Most commonly the correct place of articulation is sacrificed while the correct manner of articulation is preserved (Trost, 1981). The most commonly described compensatory articulations are the glottal stop, which is a common replacement for /t/ and /d/, and the pharyngeal fricative often used as a replacement for sibilants and affricates. Morris (1990) discusses the nature of such compensatory articulation patterns:

> The presumption is that these substitutions are adopted because of deficits of the oral structures. Specifically, the suggestion is that the glottal stop and the pharyngeal fricative compensate for velopharyngeal dysfunction because the plosiveness or fricativeness can be obtained by a buildup of air pressure "posterior" (in this case, below) to the velopharyngeal mechanism. Because these sound substitutions are learned behavior, they may persist after the physical deficit (velopharyngeal dysfunction) has been resolved. For that reason, the occurrence of substitutions like the glottal stop does not always yield useful information about velopharyngeal function during speech. Speech therapy is clearly required to teach more "anterior" articulation patterns.

The presence of compensatory articulation errors makes both diagnosis and management decisions more complex for the speech pathologist. Fortunately, a recent study by Peterson-Falzone (1990) suggests that there may be a much lower occurrence of compensatory articulation errors in the cleft population than has been suggested previously. In a retrospective analysis of 240 children from three cleft palate treatment centers, she found that 87.5% of the children studied showed noncompensatory (i.e., developmental, dialectal, and/or structural) articulation errors, and only 21.7% of the children demonstrated compensatory errors. Furthermore, when the less severe error, the middorsum palatal stop, was removed from the more severe compensatory articulations, the percentage of children demonstrating compensatory articulation errors was reduced to 12.5%. Therefore, although the new clinician should be familiar with identifying compensatory articulation errors and the principles of origin and treatment, the actual frequency of occurrence may not be as high as some authors have suggested. Their presence and frequency should be noted in the assessment of articulation and they should be targeted for immediate remediation.

ARTICULATION AND VELOPHARYNGEAL FUNCTION. Although most clinicians would agree that many of the misarticulation patterns found in the speech of individuals with cleft palate probably are the result of past or present VP dysfunction, there is a lack of research data to confirm such a causal relationship. Peterson-Falzone (1986) sums up the controversy:

> The relationship between velopharyngeal closure and speech is rarely as clear-cut as both the clinician and the research worker would like. Studies relating specific speech problems (and the severity of those problems) to measurements of velopharyngeal closure have often yielded contradictory and confusing results because of problems in measuring both speech output and the function of the velopharyngeal system.

The controversy concerning the relationship between articulation and VP function carries over into issues relating to diagnosis and management. There is no disagreement that articulation errors present in the speech of individuals with cleft palate should be addressed in speech therapy. However, there are several opinions regarding the timing of articulation therapy in general and in particular its value (if any) in managing VP dysfunction.

The most conservative view is that there are few experimental data to support a causal relationship between the use of articulation therapy and improvement in VP function. McWilliams et al. (1990) state that without experimental data "articulation therapy should be employed where needed to change articulation. However, its use as a procedure for influencing velopharyngeal function is not warranted."

No one would argue that articulation therapy cannot eliminate a large VP gap due to the absence of adequate tissue. However, Van Demark and Harden (1990) cite several studies that show decreased perception of hypernasality and audible nasal emission (i.e., symptoms of VP dysfunction) in some children following intensive articulation therapy. They suggest that "this improvement, along with concomitant improvement in articulation, may facilitate speech intelligibility for select children and minimize the need for surgical management."

Hoch et al. (1986) point out that traditionally it was believed that articulation therapy for children with documented VPI should be deferred until physical management of the VP mechanism was accomplished. One argument for this approach is that inappropriate therapy (especially for young children) may lead to posterior tongue posturing to facilitate VP closure, which can then result in undesirable compensatory articulation patterns that may be difficult to remediate after surgery. Hoch and her coauthors suggest that articulation therapy can improve VP function before physical management. The authors assert that the changes in VP function associated with the improved articulation may alter subsequent surgical planning. Based on their experience with articulation therapy before surgical intervention, the authors recommend the following:

To summarize, when VPI is observed in association with compensatory articulation errors (most specifically glottal stop substitutions), we believe that surgical correction of the VPI should be deferred. This approach is contrary to the widely accepted practice of first physically managing the VPI. We suggest that it is more appropriate to eliminate the compensatory articulation errors first with a well-planned speech-therapy program. The rationale is that improvement of oral articulation may have the benefit of improving the valving of the velopharyngeal sphincter. Furthermore, in at least a small percentage of cases, correction of the oral articulation disorder will eliminate the need for surgery altogether (Shprintzen, 1990). In addition, when oral articulation has been normalized the effects of surgery can be immediately appreciated and assessed.

The preceding discussion concerning the relationship between articulation and VP function is included in this section to alert the unfamiliar speech pathologist to the controversy and its impact on clinical practice. It is common for the speech pathologist to be asked to choose between two management alternatives for a patient, i.e., further speech therapy or physical management. An awareness of the different opinions regarding the use and timing of articulation therapy will help prepare the speech pathologist for making such decisions and provide a rationale for the selected course of action. Additionally, it should alert the team speech pathologist to the need to make very specific recommendations regarding the type of therapy needed when referring a child elsewhere for "speech therapy".

Resonance. During the preschool years the speech pathologist can begin to assess resonance and VP function with some accuracy. As the child's phonemic repertoire, articulatory skills, and expressive language expand, there are more opportunities to evaluate whether VP valving is adequate for speech production. Generally, the more developed the child's speech production skills are, the more accurately resonance and VP function can be assessed. Before discussing clinical assessment it is important to consider some issues related to terminology and to discuss the goals of the evaluation of resonance and VP function.

TERMINOLOGY. Traditionally, when symptoms suggest that the velopharynx is not functioning correctly, we have referred to the problem as velopharyngeal incompetence (VPI). However, hearing hypernasality or nasal emission (i.e., symptoms associated with VPI) does not indicate necessarily that the velopharynx cannot work. These symptoms merely indicate that the velopharynx is not functioning correctly at that time. Wendell Johnson, one of the fathers of modern speech pathology and a semanticist, explored the relationship between language and science. He wrote: "The language of science is the better part of the method of science...it must be used meaningfully...." He taught us that **the way we talk about a topic influences the way we think about it** (Johnson, 1946). Therefore, when a clinician hears hypernasality or nasal emission, i.e. symptoms of VPI, and in turn makes a diagnosis of VPI the semantic label he or she has used can have far-reaching implications. For example, the diagnosis of VPI suggests to many clinicians that the VP mechanism cannot achieve closure and that only physical management (either surgical or prosthetic) will correct the problem. Additionally, such a label may bias the inexperienced speech pathologist to discontinue speech therapy on the grounds that additional therapy will be of no value until physical management is completed. Furthermore, if the diagnosis is incorrect, surgical or prosthetic attempts to manage the problem often will be of little value. In this instance the clinician has used imprecise language, which can unintentionally lead to erroneous assumptions and inappropriate actions.

Previous authors have made recommendations for standardizing the nomenclature. For example, Loney and Bloem (1987) reviewed the literature and found no consensus or precise definitions of the terms *velopharyngeal incompetence, velopharyngeal inadequacy,* and *velopharyngeal insufficiency.* They found that authors frequently use all three terms interchangeably or one term to describe all types of VP malfunction. They suggest that "inconsistencies in terminology present an obstacle to communication among members of multidisciplinary teams concerned with rehabilitation of patients with velopharyngeal problems." They recommended adoption of a standardized nomenclature. Trost-Cardamone (1989) proposes a taxonomy for VP disorders based on etiology. She states:

Impaired velopharyngeal closure for speech can result from a variety of etiologies. Moreover, there are perceptual speech characteristics that are pathognomonic of velopharyngeal impairment and that can distinguish among certain subtypes of velopharyngeal function problems. In both diagnosis and treatment, it is necessary for the clinician to have a taxonomic system for reference, which should serve to relate etiology to deviant velopharyngeal and speech production patterns. This is especially important because the nature of the velopharyngeal function disorder allows for certain treatment alternatives and excludes others.

Trost-Cardamone suggests the following taxonomy:

Velopharyngeal inadequacy is the generic term used to denote any type of abnormal velopharyngeal function....Within the broad group of inadequacies, there are subgroups of structural, neurogenic, and mislearning or functional origins.

Under the broad classification of velopharyngeal inadequacy she delineates three etiologic categories: velopharyngeal insufficiency, velopharyngeal incompetence, and velopharyngeal mislearning. Each of these are defined as follows:

Velopharyngeal insufficiency includes any structural defect of the velum or pharyngeal wall at the level of the nasopharynx; there is not enough tissue to accomplish closure, or there is some type of mechanical interference to closure. Most often these problems are congenital.

Velopharyngeal incompetence includes neurogenic etiologies that result in impaired motor control or impaired motor programming of the velopharynx-....Motor control disorders can cause partial or total paresis of the soft palate and pharyngeal walls. Depending upon the nature, level and locus of the nervous system lesion, velopharyngeal incompetence often disturbs velopharyngeal closure for protective and reflexive acts of gagging and swallowing, as well as for speech.

Velopharyngeal mislearning includes etiologies that are not caused by structural defects or by neuromotor pathologies of the velopharyngeal complex.

In this latter category of VP mislearning, Trost-Cardamone includes phone specific nasal emission and velopharyngeal symptoms associated with deafness or hearing impairment. She concludes:

This classification extends the proposal of Loney and Bloem by offering professionals an etiologically based system that can be applied in research and treatment. It uses diagnostic categories that are clinically meaningful and can be expanded or reorganized as new findings occur. For these reasons, it has potential for unravelling the terminological confusions regarding "VPI."

The use of clearly defined nomenclature is a critical factor in clinical practice where unclear terminology may lead to inappropriate assumptions and inappropriate management. However, in clinical practice the delineation proposed by Trost-Cardamone may be too cumbersome for daily use and may not accomplish the goal of improved interprofessional communication.

Therefore, a more simple and direct approach for routine, clinical practice is to use the generic and all-encompassing term *velopharyngeal dysfunction.* This term does not assume or rule out any possible cause of the perceived speech symptoms or management approach. As described by Netsell (1988), VP dysfunction during speech may be the result of structural deficits, neurologic disorders, faulty learning, or a combination of sources. Dalston (1991) uses the term velopharyngeal dysfunction and defines it as follows:

...any impairment of the velopharyngeal complex. It may result from a lack of sufficient tissue to enable contact to be effected between the soft palate and the posterior pharyngeal wall ("velopharyngeal insufficiency"), a lack of neuromuscular competency in moving velopharyngeal structures into contact with one another ("velopharyngeal incompetency" or both. Finally, it may be due to maladaptive articulatory habits that do not reflect physical or neuromuscular impairment (e.g., phoneme specific nasal emission).

By not implying the source of the symptoms, the term *dysfunction* acknowledges that some features of the VP valving mechanism are not functioning appropriately, but no cause or treatment approach is implied or suggested until appropriate diagnostic testing can be conducted. Once an etiology is established clearly, the taxonomy proposed by Trost-Cardamone is quite appropriate and meaningful.

This discussion of terminology may seem academic and of little relevance for routine clinical practice. However, it is included here to illustrate for the unfamiliar clinician the potential impact terminology can have in the diagnosis and management of patients with resonance or velopharyngeal disorders. Regardless of the terminology you choose to use in practice, it is important to be aware of the risks involved when diagnostic terminology is not defined clearly.

DIFFERENTIAL DIAGNOSIS. One of the most important determinations made by the speech pathologist in assessing the speech of patients with cleft palate is whether VP function is adequate for speech production and whether behavioral management can improve this function or if physical management is indicated. Shprintzen and Golding-Kushner (1989) suggest that this is one of the most critical roles a speech-language pathologist can have because it is one of the few situations in which the speech pathologist's evaluation and recommendations may lead to surgery.

In the evaluation of resonance, the speech pathologist must be aware that speech symptoms often attributed to VPI may come from a variety of sources or combination of sources. As mentioned previously, hypernasality and/or nasal emission may be the result of the lack of sufficient tissue to allow closure of the VP port; neuromotor impairment involving innervation of muscles of the VP port as in many congenital anomalies, neurologic diseases, or head injury; mislearning or other behavioral factors as in instances of phoneme-specific nasal emission or lack of oral/nasal discrimination; or from other structural involvement such as a palatal fistulae, which may allow nasal air escape or enlarged tonsils, shown to result in impaired VP function in some instances.

The process of differential diagnosis can be quite difficult, since speech symptoms that may appear to be quite similar and indistinct to the casual listener or inexperienced observer (or in some instances even the experienced listener) may in fact be quite diverse in both etiology and therefore appropriate management. For example, in the cleft population it is not uncommon to observe hypernasality and nasal emission in a patient with a repaired cleft and a residual oronasal fistula. Casual perceptual

observation cannot determine the source of these symptoms. Therefore, it would be inappropriate to label the phenomenon VPI without investigating the symptoms further. In some instances the symptoms may be solely attributable to air escape through the fistula. In this case the diagnosis would be hypernasality and nasal emission due to a patent oronasal fistula and may be unrelated to the VP mechanism. The appropriate management would be repair or obturation of the fistula. In other cases the symptoms may appear to be attributable to a lack of proper VP function or to a combination of the two. In these cases diagnosis and management planning become far more complicated, especially if attempted by listener evaluation alone.

Another illustration of the need for differential diagnosis is the phenomenon of phoneme-specific velopharyngeal inadequacy (Trost, 1981) or phoneme-specific nasal emission (Peterson-Falzone and Graham, 1990). This is the perception of nasal emission isolated to specific pressure consonants such as /s/ and /z/, as opposed to the consistent nasal emission generally seen when the VP valve is incapable of closure. The inexperienced clinician (and until recent years, even some experienced clinicians) have mistaken this articulation-based error for true VPI. Many patients have been referred for or have received inappropriate physical management for what is basically an articulation error requiring behavioral therapy for effective remediation.

As these examples illustrate quite clearly, the evaluation of VP function for speech must be carried out by a speech pathologist with expertise in this area. Although some cases may be straightforward, most are not. A detailed description of symptoms, their frequency and severity, and their response to behavioral probes help to define the problem and lead to appropriate management suggestions. In many instances the process of accurate differential diagnosis is difficult or impossible to make without the help of instrumental evaluation methods.

CLINICAL ASSESSMENT. In routine clinical practice and especially in screening patients with cleft palate, the primary tool of the speech pathologist is the auditory perceptual or listener evaluation of speech. The speech pathologist must make clinical judgments to determine whether there is a deviation in resonance, the nature of that deviation, and the severity. Ultimately, despite any structural deviations or the results of instrumental testing, it is how the speech sounds to the unfamiliar listener that determines whether there is a resonance disorder. As described in the box on p. 190, several resonance disorders may accompany clefting. The speech pathologist must determine whether a deviation in resonance exists and if so to what degree it deviates from normal.

A common criticism of perceptual ratings is that, although they have high face validity, frequently they are limited by poor reliability. Therefore it is useful to use some form of standard rating scale for judgments of the presence and severity of hypernasality, hyponasality, mixed resonance, and cul-de-sac resonance. A variety of rating scales are presented and discussed in McWilliams et al (1990). It should be noted that some scales suggest that hypernasality and hyponasality be rated on the same continuum. These two resonance disorders are reflections of quite different abnormalities and therefore should be rated on distinctly separate scales.

In addition to the use of a numerical rating scale it is essential that the speech pathologist address the issues of intrarater and interrater reliability. It is important for the clinician to establish agreement with other clinicians. This can be done informally with colleagues who conduct similar evaluations. Or it can be done more formally using a published series of rating tapes produced by McWilliams and Philips (1979). Just as interrater reliability is important, so is intrarater reliability. This is a measure of how often a clinician agrees with his or her own rating of the same variable. This is relatively easy for the practicing clinician to establish and should be done periodically either formally or informally.

To elicit an adequate speech sample, most clinicians use a standard list of words and sentences developed specifically to assess resonance and VP function. Examples are the Pittsburgh Sentences described by McWilliams and Philips (1979). There are many similar sentences and phrases used by cleft palate teams and speech pathologists. The actual sentence or phrase is not important. What is important is the phonetic makeup of each utterance and the diagnostic information that can be obtained from its production. Philips (1986) described the Pittsburgh Sentences and explained the rationale for their use as a tool for assessing resonance and velopharyngeal function.

1. Mama made lemon jam.
2. Put the baby in the buggy.
3. Kindly give Kate the cake.
4. Go get the wagon for the girl.
5. Sissy sees the sun in the sky.
6. The ship goes in shallow water.
7. Jim and Charlie chew gum.
8. Please tie the stamps with string.

The first sentence will assist in distinguishing between hyponasal and hypernasal resonance, a differentiation that confuses parents, teachers, and some clinicians. Frequently, children are described as "talking through the nose" or sounding "nasal" when in fact, there is a lack of nasal resonance, hyponasality, caused by an abnormal reduction in nasal airflow. In such cases, the /m/s in *Mama m*ade, lemon, and j*am* will sound more like /b/, and the /n/ in lem*on* will approach a /d/. When hyponasality is present without other speech characteristics suggestive of VPI the clinician may consider the appropriateness of referral to an otolaryngologist. However, when speech characteristics indicative of VPI are observed on the other sentences with or without hyponasality, further speech evaluation to assess velopharyngeal function is indicated.

The remaining sentences are loaded with what are known as the pressure consonants, that is, sounds that demand velopharyngeal closure. These are the plosives...and the fricatives and affricates....Their placement in sentences that also contain consonant clusters and the nasal consonants...creates relatively difficult contexts for a speaker with VPI. Evidence of hypernasal resonance (even when it is in combination with hyponasality), reduced oral pressure on consonant sounds, audible nasal air escape, nasal air turbulence, or compensatory articulation is reason to suspect the possibility of VPI with or without cleft palate. Further information about the velopharyngeal valve is required regardless of the consistency or severity of the manifestations.

As noted in the definitions provided in the box on p. 190, hypernasality and nasal emission are not synonymous although they often occur together. They are both symptoms of VP dysfunction; however, the observation of one of these symptoms does not necessarily predict the presence of the other. Although nasal emission is not technically a disorder of resonance, it is included in this section as a disorder of the VP valving mechanism. Its presence may signal a true VPI or it may be the result of disordered articulation.

The assessment of nasal emission should include information regarding its presence, frequency, and severity in addition to patterns of facial movement, including nares constriction, nasal grimacing, and other facial constrictions. It is particularly important to note the pattern of nasal emission. For example, does it occur consistently for all oral consonants or for only some consonants? If it occurs for only some sounds, is there a pattern to the occurrence? That is, is it more likely to occur for sounds from a particular place or manner of articulation? Or, does nasal emission occur more often for consonants in a particular position within a word, e.g., word initial or word final positions. This analysis of the pattern of nasal emission is valuable for both diagnostic purposes and for planning management.

Some young children, especially in the toddler/preschool age range, may demonstrate inconsistent nasal emission that appears to be related to a failure to have achieved the correct manner distinction between oral and nasal sounds. That is, they may not have acquired the oral/nasal contrast. In many instances the very young or delayed child may not discriminate between oral and nasal contrasts in his or her own productions or in the models of the speech pathologist. In these cases determining the child's discrimination capabilities is the first step in determining production capabilities. Many young children who present with inconsistent nasal emission are stimulable for correct production of oral consonants once they recognize and understand the difference between oral and nasal airflow.

When assessing nasal emission is it particularly important to differentiate between nasal emission due to an incompetent VP valve and nasal emission that is the result of an articulation-based error. For example, audible nasal air escape may be heard with the posterior nasal fricative. In this case the source of the nasal frication is linguovelar contact with airflow directed through the open VP port (Trost, 1981). The observed nasal emission is the result of a compensatory articulation. Audible nasal emission also may be isolated to specific consonants (especially /s,z/) and referred to as phoneme-specific VPI (Trost, 1981) or phoneme-specific nasal emission (Peterson-Falzone and Graham, 1990). Trost (1981) defines this pattern of nasal emission as

the occurrence of nasal air emission and audible posterior nasal frication on certain pressure consonants only. That is, this abnormal pattern of airflow occurs in the absence of any hypernasal resonance, and the remainder of the pressure consonants are produced with adequate closure.

We know that hypernasality is the result of incomplete closure of the VP port. Audible nasal emission may be attributed to inadequacy of the port or to articulatory errors. However, both symptoms also may result from a patent oronasal fistula (with or without VPI). Significant controversy exists concerning accurate identification of a symptomatic fistula, the extent of the effects on speech, and decisions regarding surgical repair. There are many opinions expressed in the surgical literature. There is a common misconception that there is a relationship between the size and location of a palatal fistula and its effects on speech (Randall, 1986). A more conservative view is that the functional significance of a palatal fistula must be determined for each patient individually. D'Antonio et al (1992) showed a significant improvement in perceptual judgments of hypernasality, frequency of nasal emission, perceived oral pressure, and speech quality when comparing speech ratings with fistulae unoccluded and temporarily occluded with chewing gum. However, there was no consistent relationship between the improvement in speech characteristics between the unoccluded and occluded conditions based on size and location of the fistulae. Results of the same study suggested that an important factor influencing changes in speech and aerodynamic characteristics when a palatal fistula is obturated is the individual's nasal cavity resistance (i.e., the degree to which the nose resists the flow of air through it). Additionally, Isberg and Henningsson (1987) showed a relationship between temporary obturation of a patent oronasal fistula and concomitant improvement in VP valving. They suggest that occlusion of a palatal fistula regardless of size or location was associated with improvement in lateral wall motion of the VP port. Results from these studies concerning palatal fistulae are presented here to emphasize that a number of factors are likely to contribute to the effects of palatal fistulae on speech. Therefore, when a palatal fistula is observed, no statement concerning its effect on hypernasality, nasal emission, or speech quality can be made without comparing speech characteristics with the fistula unoccluded and occluded. For most children this can be done quite easily with chewing gum or with a nontoxic self-adhesive material described by Reisberg et al (1985).

In addition to a true VPI, articulation-based errors, and palatal fistulae, there is one other important, yet little discussed, cause shown to result in hypernasality and nasal emission. In some cases hypertrophic tonsils can prevent complete VP closure, resulting in hypernasality, nasal emission, or both (Shprintzen et al 1987; Mackenzie-Stepner et al, 1987). It should be emphasized that the determination that the tonsils were the likely cause of the resonance and VP symptoms was based on perceptual, endoscopic, and multiview video-fluoroscopic studies. The speech pathologist should be aware that enlarged tonsils can be detrimental to resonance and VP function. However, the decision to remove tonsils in a patient with VP symptoms should be made only after instrumental assessment and not based on listener judgments alone.

Finally, as shown in the box on p. 190, individuals with cleft palate also may demonstrate hyponasal resonance, mixed hyperhyponasal resonance, or cul-de-sac resonance. Patients with repaired cleft palate frequently have structural deviations of the nasal airway that can result in a resistance to nasal airflow. Additionally, individuals with cleft palate are subject to the same sources of anterior airway obstruction as noncleft patients. When hyponasality is present, the speech pathologist should question the patient and parents to determine whether the symptoms are transitory (as with a cold or upper respiratory tract infection) or if they are chronic and persistent. Traditionally, the anterior nasal airway has been overlooked in most speech evaluations. However, recent research has suggested that the nasal cavity is an important factor affecting not only resonance but articulation and VP function as well (Warren, 1986; Dalston et al, 1992). Therefore a comprehensive screening or evaluation of resonance should include a thorough assessment of the contributions of the nasal cavity. If chronic hyponasality, mixed resonance, or cul--de-sac resonance is observed, further evaluation is indicated and referral for otolaryngologic evaluation should be considered.

STIMULABILITY TESTING. When VP function is variable, as it often is, particularly in young children with cleft palate, an important source of diagnostic information is stimulability testing (Morris, 1990). A cornerstone of modern speech therapy is that a child's ability to be stimulated for improved speech production through auditory, visual, and in some instances tactile cues is a good prognostic indicator of potential for long-term improvement. Such stimulability testing is particularly useful in the child with variable VP function. It can provide valuable information about whether behavioral management is likely to remediate the velopharyngeal symptoms or if such amelioration of symptoms appears unlikely.

Morris (1984) suggests there are two major subgroups of patients with marginal VP dysfunction and proposes that the two groups can be distinguished by the response to short-term therapeutic intervention.

The first group is the **almost-but-not-quite (ABNQ) subgroup.** This group tends to present with mild and consistent nasalization of speech that is highly consistent among and within tasks. Morris suggests:

Speech training is not successful with the ABNQ group for the purpose of improving velopharyngeal function. That is because the patient apparently has already extended the mechanism to the physiologic limits and does so consistently. If trial training for that purpose is provided to confirm the diagnosis of ABNQ marginal incompetence, it should be discontinued after 6 hours of treatment if no improvement in velopharyngeal function is observed.

In this case the lack of response to highly focused therapy suggests that physical management is the treatment of choice if the impairment is significant enough to warrant intervention.

The second diagnostic group of marginal VP function described by Morris is the **sometimes-but-not-always (SBNA) subgroup.** Patients in this group generally show marked inconsistency in VP function. Morris indicates that some patients in this category will show improvement with training and some will not. He believes that the major diagnostic determinant in this group is the lack of positive response to directed speech therapy focused on improving VP function. Morris suggests that patients in this group usually demonstrate that they are capable of increasing oral productions within their speech repertoire at the single sound or single word level. However, they often are unable to generalize this pattern into connected, conversational speech. Morris explains the importance of diagnostic therapy in this group.

Diagnosis of these patients is frequently controversial. Inexperienced speech pathologists fail to interpret correctly the lack of improvement from training. Parents are falsely optimistic about the outcome because they observe the variance in speech production that is typical of the group. Surgeons and dentists who work often with cleft patients overinterpret the observation that the SBNA patient can perform well on single word tasks or highly specific speech activities. As a consequence, it is vital that observations about response to speech training (or rather, lack of it) be included as part of the diagnostic findings for these patients.

Morris suggests that a child in the SBNA subgroup who will be capable of achieving complete, consistent VP closure should do so after approximately 10 hours of intensive, focused training. On the other hand, he believes that if no improvement is observed in connected speech within 10 to 20 hours of training, the diagnosis of SBNA should be made.

Unfortunately, patients with inconsistent velopharyngeal function usually represent the greatest dilemma for the speech pathologist and other team members in attempting to establish an appropriate management plan. Often these patients' inability to achieve consistent closure is a complex, interrelated problem with several contributing variables. For instance, it is likely that many of these patients demonstrate poor timing of VP movements and poor coordination with other articulators and vocal tract components, which may result in the observed variability. Since inconsistencies in VP function can be quite complex in origin and manifestation, it is not uncommon for the patient with variable function to show limited improvement following physical management. Therefore, decisions regarding management of these patients should be undertaken with great caution after in-depth and thoughtful assessment. Detailed counseling of the patient and the patient's family concerning realistic expectations from physical intervention should be a high priority.

INSTRUMENTAL ASSESSMENT. The foregoing discussion of the evaluation of resonance and VP function has focused on the listener evaluation of the perceptual characteristics of speech. For most clinical speech pathologists this is the primary tool available for assessing resonance and VP function. As mentioned previously, the perceptual characteristics of speech determine whether there is a deviation from normal. The human auditory perceptual system is the best judge of this subjective impression. However, in cases where diagnosis is complex or when physical management is under consideration, instrumental assessment, particularly direct visualization of the VP mechanism should be undertaken. Two methods of direct visualization of the velopharynx during dynamic speech activity are multiview videofluoroscopy and flexible fiberoptic nasendoscopy. These methods are discussed in Chapter 11. However, it is important for the clinician to realize that there are a number of instrumental methods available for assessing VP function for speech. They vary from one another in the information they provide, clinical practicality, validity, and reliability and whether they allow direct or indirect observation. If the reader desires further information concerning various methods available for assessing VP function for speech, the following references will serve as excellent resources for further study of the topic (Dalston and Warren, 1985; Folkins and Moon, 1990; Karnell and Seaver, 1990; D'Antonio, 1992).

ISSUES RELATED TO MANAGEMENT. The final result of the clinical assessment of speech production should be a rating or judgment of the child's overall intelligibility and a rating of the severity of the communication impairment. Information from the assessment and the ratings of intelligibility and severity are used with data from the overall screening to make recommendations and develop a management plan. The three broad categories of management for VP dysfunction are speech therapy, prosthetic management, and surgical intervention. Once a diagnosis has been established, attention turns toward the question of whether management of any kind is indicated. McWilliams et al (1990) stress the importance of the speech pathologist's role on a cleft palate team in making treatment recommendations:

We want to emphasize our conviction that it is the role of the speech pathologist to judge the adequacy of velopharyngeal function for speech production. This is done in collaboration with other professionals who also provide valuable information about the mechanism and its function and suggest alternatives for management. If physical management is chosen as the preferred method of treatment the surgeon or the dentist is legally and ethically accountable to the patient and family for proper treatment and must always have the last word about whether or not to perform the surgery or construct the prosthesis. However, it is the speech pathologist who decides whether or not the proposed physical management is indicated for speech improvement.

No form of management is without its own costs. Although surgical management may be the most permanent and carry the most physical risks, prosthetic management and speech therapy also require significant compliance, time commitment, and often emotional commitment. Therefore no management alternative should be undertaken casually.

All three of these management categories are familiar to clinicians involved in cleft care. Most team members have personal biases about the particular effectiveness and value of each method. However, in reality the new or unfamiliar speech pathologist should be aware that there has been little prospective research on treatment outcome for any of these methods. Much of what clinicians believe to be true about each method's effectiveness usually is based on personal experience and training. Therefore decisions regarding the appropriateness of a given intervention method necessarily will vary among teams and individual providers depending not only on the differential diagnosis for a particular patient, but also on operational variables such as the availability of services, expertise and experience of care providers, compliance of patients and families, and many other practical considerations.

It is incumbent on the speech pathologist to interpret the available evaluation data and to determine whether management of any form will improve **speech intelligibility, speech quality, or quality of life.** Unfortunately there is no formula for making such decisions easily. For example, in one instance a patient may present with a significant communication impairment of which VP dysfunction is only a small source of the overall decreased communication competence. In such a case a cost-benefit analysis might lead to the decision not to offer physical management, especially surgical management. Another patient might present with mild VP dysfunction with no other communication impairment. Although the symptoms may be slight, the patient or the family may feel that even a small observable stigma will result in detrimental effects and reduced life options. Again a cost-benefit analysis may suggest that physical management is likely to result in only a minimal improvement in speech quality. However, in this case even a small improvement may be enough to translate into significant improvements in quality of life. In this situation it may be appropriate to offer physical management, even surgical management.

Despite our ability to collect detailed scientific data concerning the source and magnitude of VP symptoms, in the final analysis decisions regarding management are part of the **art of cleft care.**

Phonation. Individuals with cleft palate or VPI are at risk for laryngeal/voice disorders. The relationship between VP and laryngeal dysfunction may be congenital or behavioral (D'Antonio et al., 1988). For example, as mentioned previously, palatal clefting may be associated with a number of multiple malformation syndromes for which resonance and phonation disorders frequently cooccur. Also, as we have discussed previously, the vocal tract is a series of interrelated valves. An impairment in one valve may lead to compensatory activity or impairment in another valve. Specifically, speakers with impaired VP valving may use increased respiratory effort or abnormal laryngeal valving, both of which are potentially damaging to the larynx and may result in observable laryngeal pathology or voice symptoms or both. D'Antonio et al. (1988) reported 41% of 85 patients with symptoms of VP dysfunction had abnormal voice characteristics, or observable laryngeal abnormalities, or both. This occurrence of laryngeal/voice disorders is substantially greater than would be expected in an unaffected population of children.

McWilliams et al (1969) reported on 43 children with cleft palate and hoarseness. Laryngoscopy and lateral view videofluoroscopy were performed on 32 children who were described as chronically hoarse. Of the children who received instrumental evaluations, 84% had some vocal fold pathology and 59% had borderline VP closure. In a follow-up study McWilliams et al (1973) showed that alteration of the VP valving in these children often resulted in improvement in voice symptoms. These data suggest a relationship between borderline VP function and laryngeal pathology. The authors further suggest that some children compensate for minimal VPI by increased laryngeal valving. They speculated there is a relationship between faulty valving, hoarseness and speech therapy. They suggest that children with VPI and hoarseness should not receive speech therapy focused on elimination of the VP dysfunction, since such therapy may result in compensatory laryngeal valving, which in turn can result in vocal fold pathology. Results from these studies suggest that all patients with cleft palate and/or VPI should be evaluated routinely for the presence of a voice disorder.

McWilliams et al (1990) describe a protocol for assessment of phonation in patients with cleft palate. They suggest the first step is to listen to voice characteristics and determine if a disorder is present. If it is, then a thorough perceptual voice evaluation should be conducted. This should include a history that attempts to determine whether the voice symptoms are recent or chronic. It also is important to determine whether the voice heard at the time of the screening is typical for the child or atypical. If the symptoms are atypical and can be related to a cause such as a cold or recent (but not chronic) vocal abuse, then the symptoms should be noted, reported, and monitored closely over time. However, if they are reported or observed to be chronic, then further evaluation should be recommended.

A careful interview should suggest whether the voice symptoms originate from a behavioral cause, a physical cause, or the potential of both. For example, disorders such as excessive loudness, reduced loudness, or abnormal use of pitch range often are behavioral variables that usually are not indicative of vocal fold pathology. However, disorders such as harshness, breathiness, and phonation breaks may have behavioral origins but also are signs of vocal fold pathology such as vocal fold nodules, thickening, and edema. Patients with these voice symptoms should be referred for evaluation by an oto-laryngologist.

Whether vocal fold pathology is present or not, recommendation should be made for close monitoring of voice symptoms. If the symptoms are significant enough to draw attention to the child, to detract from what the child is attempting to communicate, or if there is the potential for the causative behaviors to result in further laryngeal/voice impairment, then intervention should be recommended. There is a common belief that preschool and early school-age children cannot benefit from voice therapy. This may be true if the therapy follows a cognitive approach to voice education. However, most voice disorders among children have a significant behavioral component, which can be targeted and altered with behavior modification techniques. Therefore, for children with phonation disorders it is appropriate to recommend direct behavioral intervention combined with parent/family education with goals and strategies for modification of voice use and elimination of vocally abusive behaviors.

Fluency. In addition to articulation, resonance, and phonation, an area of speech production that should be considered, especially at this age, is fluency. There is no higher occurrence of dysfluency in the cleft palate population than in the noncleft population. In fact, it has been hypothesized that there may be a lower occurrence of stuttering in patients with structural impairments of the VP mechanism (Dalston et al 1987). However, as we know, many preschool children display normal dysfluency. For parents with a child who is experiencing other communication impairment or is at risk for these deficits, the presence of these normal dysfluencies may cause significant concern. It is important to educate and reassure the family and to report and monitor any evidence of dysfluency in this population just as you would in other children who manifest such behaviors.

The school-age screening

Evaluation of the school-age child is similar in content areas to the screening of the toddler/preschool child. The box on pp. 202-203 shows a sample school-age screening form. As with earlier developmental stages, information concerning feeding is relevant. A child of this age who continues to present with chewing and swallowing difficulties should be referred for more thorough evaluations and should be evaluated for neurologic impairment. Similarly, signs and symptoms of airway concerns continue to be

relevant. Once again an unremitting history of airway symptoms or newly identified symptoms should be of significant concern at this age and should be evaluated thoroughly and managed aggressively by the cleft palate team. At this stage the speech pathologist should be particularly aware of the link between chronic hypoxia (as seen in children with overt sleep apnea) and symptoms of chronic fatigue, irritability, and lack of attention, all of which can affect academic performance, behavior, and social interaction. For the school-age child, monitoring of motor milestones becomes less important except in children with severe developmental delay or physical impairments. However, it is important for the speech-language pathologist to know that adultlike speech motor control is not achieved until approximately age 11 or 12 (Kent, 1976) and should therefore continue to be monitored in the early and middle school years. The screening of the school-age child should include detailed information about current educational programing, speech and language services, and other special services as well as information concerning academic strengths and weaknesses. At this age the clinician may obtain much information directly from the child rather than depend solely on parent report. The child may provide important information about his or her own views of appearance and speech quality and intelligibility. Persistent articulation disorders should be targeted for aggressive management. If resonance and VP symptoms persist, it is critical to establish an aggressive monitoring or management plan to normalize the child's speech quality as soon as possible to avoid social and psychologic concerns. An especially important issue during the school-age years is the child's attitude regarding special programing, especially speech and language services. Additionally, observations of parent-child interactions and differences in parent and child reports can provide invaluable information regarding family dynamics and other important psychosocial issues.

We have discussed the importance of monitoring language development in the cleft palate population. Typically, children with moderate to severe language impairment have been identified by school age, but children with subtle language and learning problems may not be identified until they are engaged in formal education. These children with subtle language comprehension or expression deficits may be identified by their teachers with complaints of poor attention, poor social and pragmatic skills, reading and spelling problems, and written

CRANIOFACIAL SPEECH-LANGUAGE SCREENING: SCHOOL AGE

Name: Diagnosis:
DOB: Funding:
Age: Date of Screening:

HISTORY/PARENT REPORT   PRIMARY LANGUAGE _____

Feeding: Chewing   Swallowing
Airway: Snoring   Allergies   Asthma   Trach_____

Motor Milestones: No concerns _____   Suspect _____   Delayed _____

Hearing:_____

School: _____

Educational Program: _____   Special Services: _____

Speech Therapy at: _____
        Frequency: _____   Goals: _____
_____

EVALUATION SUMMARY
  Language: Receptive: No Concerns   Suspect   Delay/Disorder
             Expressive: No Concerns   Suspect   Delay/Disorder
Oromotor/Speech Mechanism

  Lip Closure: Adequate   Inadequate   Asymmetric
  Tongue:_____
  Hard Palate: _____   Soft Palate: _____
    Fistula: Not Observed   Size _____   Location _____
  Diadochokinetics _____
Articulation:
  Developmental errors: _____
  Compensatory articulation: _____
  Dental distortions: _____
  Other: Dialect   Rate   Reduced Excurions   Deterioration in conversation

Resonance	WNL				
	Hypernasal	NA	MILD	MODERATE	SEVERE
	Hyponasal	NA	MILD	MODERATE	SEVERE
	Mixed	NA	MILD	MODERATE	SEVERE
	Audible Nasal Emission	NA	MILD	MODERATE	SEVERE

Phonation	WNL	Hoarse	Breathy	Soft	Phonation Breaks	Vocal Abuse

language deficits. In particular, children with subtle language impairments often show difficulty with language comprehension of abstract vocabulary, complex sentence structure (e.g., The boy, who forgot his money, went home.), and passage or paragraph comprehension. Expressive language impairments often appear as word finding and formulation problems such as "He wanted to a a a. He went up there. You know, he wanted to...." These problems can restrict the child's ability to respond in classroom settings and interact in social conversation.

Identification of children with these subtle language deficits presents a difficult task for the cleft palate team's speech and language pathologist. A screening of language processes often is ineffective in identifying these elusive deficits. However, information regarding academic and social interactions can provide im-

NAME _____   DATE _____

SPEECH INTELLIGIBILITY RATING

	Clinician	Parent
1. Intelligible	_____	_____
2. Listener Attention Needed	_____	_____
3. Occasional Repetition of Words Required	_____	_____
4. Repetitions/Rephrasing Necessary	_____	_____
5. Isolated Words Understood	_____	_____
6. Occasionally Understood by Adult	_____	_____
7. Unintelligible	_____	_____

OVERALL SEVERITY OF COMMUNICATION IMPAIRMENT

_____ No concern
_____ Mild
_____ Moderate
_____ Severe

RECOMMENDATIONS:

_____ Audiological evaluation
_____ Complete speech/language evaluation at: _____
_____ "Bedside Swallow" eval: _____
_____ Nasendoscopy/aerodynamics
_____ Cognitive/academic/behavioral assessment at: _____
_____ Request School Reports/IEP/Speech Eval/Progress Report
_____ Rescreen recommended: _____
_____ Follow with team
_____ Other: _____

Speech-language therapy recommended at: _____

Frequency: _____

Intensity: Group   Individual   Both

Duration: _____

Goals: _____
_____

Other: _____

Seen and examined by: _____
                          Speech-Language Pathologist   License #

portant indicators of possible subtle language impairments. During the clinic visit the speech-language pathologist can obtain information from a discussion regarding grades, teacher comments, standardized achievement test results, homework assignments, and individual educational plans (IEPs). Teacher reports of poor academic performance may, in themselves, be an adequate reason to refer for a complete language evaluation. Although academic performance may be influenced by many motivational and learning variables, a language assessment is essential in differentiating the possible etiology of learning problems. In addition to reviewing educational performance, it is important for the speech-language pathologist to engage the child in conversation that requires organization of information in expressive language. Suggestions for eliciting a language and narrative sample are provided in the section entitled How to elicit important information.

The teen/adult screening

The teen/adult screening differs little from the school-age screening. However, in most instances patients in this age range scheduled for team visits, which include speech and language assessment usually present with persistent, long-standing speech production concerns that have been resistant to treatment. Or these patients may be returning to the cleft team for further surgical procedures that may affect speech. For example, many patients in the teen years are considered candidates for orthognathic surgery such as maxillary advancement. In these cases the speech pathologist must evaluate speech production, particularly VP function, and counsel the patient and other team members regarding the possibility of a deterioration in resonance and speech quality following advancement of the maxilla.

For this age group it is critical for the speech-language pathologist to determine the patient's wishes regarding speech quality and intelligibility and the desire for further management. It is not uncommon to find patients in the teen years who present with moderate to severe speech impairments (and in some instances language impairments) who refuse to consider any further treatment. It is important in these cases for the speech pathologist to present treatment recommendations as options the patient may choose to accept or reject. In our clinical experience, by the time patients with cleft palate reach the teen years and continue to present with an articulation or resonance impairment they usually are most interested in a surgical alternative and have "burned out" on speech therapy.

On the other hand, adults who present to cleft palate/craniofacial teams for evaluation and management of persistent speech production disorders often come to the evaluation process with significant motivation and expectations for improvement. For these patients a frank and honest interview should be conducted to determine the patient's perception of speech quality and intelligibility and the perceived effect it will

have in the patient's life. It is especially important to counsel these patients on the *realistic* potential for improvement in speech with further management.

HOW TO ELICIT IMPORTANT INFORMATION

It is not uncommon to hear the inexperienced speech pathologist express frustration at not being able to obtain adequate information during screening clinics regarding a child's speech and language skills. There are a number of methods for eliciting representative information regarding speech and language during a brief screening. Therefore we have listed some suggestions for maximizing the information that can be obtained even in a brief visit. Obviously, all of the following methods will not be necessary or practical for all children or for all clinical settings but are presented as options for expanding the clinician's strategies for obtaining desired information.

Parent questionnaires

Parent report is a time-efficient way of obtaining speech and language information, especially when it is obtained in a standard format such as a parent questionnaire. Good examples of parent questionnaires include The Vineland Adaptive Behavior Scales (1984), MacArthur Communication Development Inventory (1989), and the Rossetti Infant/Toddler Language Scale (1990). These questionnaires can be completed by the parents while they are waiting in the clinic rooms and reviewed by the speech-language pathologist during the visit or at a later time. Questionnaires are particularly valuable as a basis for beginning the parent interview and assessing parent reliability as an informant.

The speech-language screening kit

Generally, the speech-language screening is carried out in a medical clinic setting and the child understands that this is a medical appointment. This is taxing for the speech pathologist who may be most comfortable and effective at evaluation in a child-oriented environment. In our clinical experience (and particularly in training new clinicians) it is invaluable to prepare and have available a speech-language screening kit. Having a set of toys prepared in a kit facilitates communication and is of great assistance to the clinician in eliciting a speech-language sample, particularly in young children. A suggested list of toys and stimulus items is provided in Appendix C.

Elicitation tasks

A standard articulation test or word list should be available in the screening kit along with a list of words and sentences for assessing resonance and VP function. The speech pathologist should be prepared to elicit words in response to picture identification or imitation. In the young child this may require use of rewards or reinforcers such as pegs in a pegboard, blocks in a container, or food. Once again, the speech pathologist should be prepared with stimulus materials and reinforcers.

Language sample

Spontaneous language sampling provides invaluable information particularly for children who are suspect for language delays but present with subtle symptoms that may be overlooked in standardized language tests. Although this method can provide exceptionally valuable information, it is time consuming and is not familiar to many speech pathologists. Nevertheless, its use is warranted especially in complex cases when a diagnosis of language impairment is suspected but has not been confirmed by more traditional means. Several available texts describe language sample collection and analysis procedures in detail (Miller, 1984; Stickler, 1987). Some suggestions for general collection procedures are discussed briefly here. Language samples typically are collected during conversation or storytelling or narration. Approximately 25 utterances or sentences produced by the child are transcribed and analyzed for vocabulary, grammar, and pragmatic use. It is important to allow the child to initiate and lead the conversation as much as possible. Frequent questions from the clinician can restrict the child's participation and distort the semantic and syntactic complexity of the sample. The availability of a selection of age-appropriate toys is the best approach for facilitating spontaneous language use from the child. Spontaneously imitated utterances should be analyzed separately from truly spontaneous utterances. Inclusion of imitations may inflate the estimate of semantic and syntactic complexity.

Narrative sample

For the school-age child it is important to observe conversation and narration or storytelling. The narrative sample provides information regarding the child's ability to remember, organize, and formulate language not necessarily required in conversation. As with the language sample, how the narrative sample is collected influences the information obtained. Lahey (1989) suggests collecting narrative samples in more than one way. For example, have the child retell a recently viewed television show, formulate a story from a wordless picture book, and tell how to make a peanut butter sandwich. The obvious time constraints of the clinic screening limit narrative sampling, but the clinician should have several options available. We suggest that the speech pathologist may wish to use the story from the Goldman-Fristoe Test of Articulation (1969) and have one wordless picture book available in the speech and language screening kit for rapid access. This is particularly useful for obtaining a language sample and sample of connected speech in the child who is reluctant to produce spontaneous speech and language samples of adequate length.

UNEXPECTED (BUT COMMON) POPULATIONS

The speech-language pathologist who serves on a cleft palate/craniofacial team frequently will be asked to evaluate patients with complex multifactorial speech production disorders that may or may not be related to an overt cleft of the hard and/or soft palate. As we have discussed, palatal clefting is often associated with other physical and cognitive impairments. In these cases the speech and language pathologist must address all the potential contribution sources to the communication impairment. Second, cleft palate/craniofacial teams often serve as a regional resource for complicated patients with known or suspected physical impairments of the speech production mechanism, even in the absence of a cleft palate. It is not uncommon for such teams to have a relatively large number of patients referred primarily for evaluation of speech to rule out a cleft palate or VPI. In most of these instances the patient presents with other physical, motor, and/or cognitive impairments that make differential diagnosis difficult. In our clinical experience there are several groups of patients which the speech pathologist may not expect to encounter in working with a cleft palate team but which are frequently referred for evaluation. Among the most common of these unexpected populations are the "nonoral" child, the severely cognitively impaired patient, the severely motorically impaired patient, the dysarthric patient, and the dyspraxic child. Obviously, these diagnostic categories are not mutually exclusive. One or more of these diagnoses can occur in the same patient, with or without a cleft palate. The speech and language pathologist must be prepared for these patients with complex, multifactorial speech production impairments.

Perhaps the most interesting and most problematic of these patients is the nonoral child. This can be a young child in the toddler/preschool age or early school-age range who uses no obvious, recognizable, meaningful speech productions and has no hearing loss to account for the lack of speech production. They may present with little or extensive vocalization but a severely limited phoneme repertoire. When these children do appear to have speech production, their speech is characterized predominantly by vowels and the early developing nasal consonants /m/ and /n/. This pattern results in nasal sounding speech and stimulates concerns that the child has a physical oromotor deficit such as a submucous cleft palate accompanied by VPI. These children may have some generalized developmental delay or physical impairment, but often these impairments are not commensurate with the severe speech production disorder. Most often these children have received numerous evaluations and consultations and are referred to the cleft palate/craniofacial team to determine if there is a structural, oromotor basis for their impairment. In our experience the referring speech pathologist often is hopeful that a structural abnormality that is at the root of or a significant contributor to such an impairment can be identified. In fact, it is not uncommon for the parents and referring speech pathologist to suggest that the child has normal receptive language skills and normal expressive language (independent of speech production). However, careful language screening usually shows subtle or obvious deficits in both receptive and expressive language. In our experience these children have a more global impairment that often manifests itself more overtly as the child develops. It is not likely that the presence of an overt cleft palate, a submucous cleft, or even severe VP incompetence would be the sole cause of such a disorder. In these cases the child should receive a thorough evaluation including medical testing for neurologic impairment, and developmental/psychologic testing. The speech-language evaluation should include a thorough developmental history, a detailed description of the child's current system for making needs and wants known, including gesturing and word approximations, a reliable history of therapeutic and educational programing, language comprehension and expression testing that do not rely on speech production, and stimulability testing for improved oromotor function including production or approximation of early developing phonemes and words. Trial teaching can be used with augmentative communication systems to provide invaluable diagnostic and prognostic information. Additionally, as we have discussed previously, assessment of play competence can be used to provide an indication of nonverbal skills that correlate with language capabilities and cognitive function. Although these children present early with a profound communication impairment, they often respond quite well to an appropriate, intensive speech and language intervention program that includes oromotor programing, direct speech articulation therapy, and language therapy that focuses on the child's areas of weakness. Once some meaningful speech production has been established, it then becomes possible to assess the role of structural deficits. In some cases there may be true VPI. However, such a diagnosis should not be made until the child has had an adequate, appropriate course of therapy and has developed correct articulatory *placement* for at least three or four early developing oral consonants such as /p,b,d,f/. Once correct articulatory placement can be elicited, VP function can be evaluated and its contribution to the speech production impairment can be established.

A similar patient population includes the child with dyspraxia or a motor speech planning disorder. These children may present with persistent and severe speech production impairments including articulation disorders and inconsistent VP function that have been resistant to therapeutic interventions. Generally, these children can produce many or most phonemes in isolation but produce errors (often inconsistent errors) when attempting to combine these sounds in words or speech of increasing length. As with the nonoral child these children often are referred to cleft palate teams (whether a cleft is present or not) by community speech pathologists or pediatricians who cannot account for the poor progress in therapy.

Once again a thorough history, cognitive testing, and speech and language evaluation, not dependent on speech production, should be conducted. A comprehensive motor speech evaluation should be conducted that includes production of single phonemes, words, short sentences, and conversational speech. The articulation errors should be noted at each level, and the level at which the child's production capabilities deteriorate should be noted with respect to place and manner of articulation, length of utterance, and semantic-syntactic complexity.

One of the most important diagnostic indicators for this population is the child's performance during stimulability testing when the phonemic context is controlled and auditory, visual, and tactile cues are used. For most dyspraxic children articulation will improve significantly when asked to build on phonemes that are firmly established in the repertoire. Expansion from these correctly produced sounds should move only one feature or degree of complexity at a time. If the child responds positively to such an approach during diagnostic therapy, then a motor-based speech therapy plan should be followed with intensive therapy including an aggressive home program and, if possible, incorporation with his or her core curriculum in the classroom. For these children a phonologic approach, especially a therapy plan in which phoneme classes are cycled, should be avoided because they do not allow for the development of the motor programs needed by these children. It is important for the speech-language pathologist who evaluates these children to be aware that most children with dyspraxic speech characteristics often have associated overt or subtle impairments in receptive and/or expressive language and often require special academic placement to meet their communication needs and particularly to facilitate their therapy program, which should be intensive and comprehensive. Additionally, such children may often present with other motor impairments or delays that require or would benefit from therapeutic intervention, such as physical therapy or adaptive physical education. As mentioned previously, many of these children present with mild or severe VP dysfunction. Many times, diagnostic therapy shows that these children are unaware of manner distinctions between oral and nasal consonants. For example, even when given models in the clinician's speech productions they are unable to properly discriminate between nasal consonants (nose sounds) and oral consonants (mouth sounds). Often actively teaching this discrimination facilitates improved VP function. In these cases the symptoms of VP dysfunction are related to the motor planning and articulation disorder rather than to a true structural VP incompetence.

Another complex but common patient population often encountered by cleft palate/craniofacial teams is the child with velo-cardio-facial syndrome (Shprintzen et al., 1978; Gorlin, et al., 1990). Other specific syndromes have not been singled out in this chapter. However, our clinical experience suggests that the constellation of problems encountered in this patient population warrants inclusion in this section. This syndrome is associated with a number of findings, including overt or submucous cleft of the secondary palate, hypernasal speech, cardiac defects, specific learning disabilities, poor muscle coordination, hypotonia in infancy, retruded mandible, flat midface, long vertical face with a large fleshy nose, and broad nasal bridge (Shprintzen et al., 1978). The expression of the syndrome can be quite variable and in many cases geneticists and other professionals must rely on what Williams et al. (1985) refer to as "a *gestalt* type of approach to its diagnosis."

In our experience with many cleft palate teams and community care providers this diagnosis often is overlooked, sometimes in even the most obvious expressions of the syndrome. The reason for this is unclear but may be related to the relative newness of the syndrome and lack of exposure on the part of many geneticists, pediatricians, and other health care providers. Frequently children affected with this syndrome come to the speech and language pathologist or to a cleft palate/craniofacial team with a primary complaint of hypernasal speech and articulation disorder. Often these children have undergone numerous medical and developmental consults that have not resulted in a definitive diagnosis. However, to the clinician familiar with velo-cardio-facial syndrome the diagnosis may seem obvious.

We believe that the speech-language pathologist should be particularly aware of this syndrome and the possibility of associated speech, language, learning, and psychologic deficits in affected patients. Previous reports describe some of the communication and developmental impairments associated with this diagnosis (Shprintzen et al., 1978; Siegel-Sadewitz and Shprintzen, 1982; Golding-Kushner et al., 1985). However, more research and descriptions of clinical populations are needed concerning the communication skills of these children. We would like to emphasize that many children with this syndrome present with specific speech production impairments that are unusual, compared with the nonsyndromic cleft palate population and that frequently are unusually resistant to traditional speech therapy.

In addition to symptoms of VP dysfunction, they often present with symptoms similar to those described above for the dyspraxic child. They often show significant inconsistency in place and manner of articulation and in many cases poor stimulability and poor carryover skills to connected speech. Therefore, whereas these children present as difficult diagnostic dilemmas for the cleft palate team, they present a particular challenge for the speech-language pathologist both in diagnosis and treatment planning (Mackenzie-Stepner et al., 1987; D'Antonio and Marsh, 1987).

A final and little discussed population that should be mentioned in this chapter is the immigrant (or child of recent immigrants) who presents to the cleft palate/craniofacial team with an unrepaired or partially repaired cleft and is either a non-English speaker or speaker of English as a second language. These patients are a special challenge for the entire cleft palate team but particularly for the speech-language pathologist. It often is difficult to obtain a good health and developmental history from most of these patients due to fragmentation in health care and obvious language barriers. Additionally, cultural differences often make it difficult to obtain valid speech, language, and developmental data in the same manner that the clinician is used to approaching the standard screening or evaluation process. It is difficult for the speech pathologist to be prepared for all possible populations. However, if the clinician has a particularly large number of patients from a given culture or language group, it would be important to obtain some information regarding the phonemic inventory of the language, a simple core vocabulary, and information regarding child rearing practices.

REPORTING RESULTS AND MAKING TREATMENT RECOMMENDATIONS

Dalston (1991) has suggested that the result of the speech and language assessment of patients with cleft palate should result in an individualized care plan (ICP), which includes statements regarding the following:

- Medical diagnosis/diagnoses
- Historical information regarding previous evaluations and treatment
- Identification of speech impairments
- Identification of language impairments
- Identification of patient/family concerns and expectations
- Statement of short-term goals and estimated dates of attainment
- Statement of long-term goals
- Implementation plan, including identification of the therapist or facility responsible for providing treatment, if known, or a statement of efforts to be made in helping the family acquire needed services; this plan also should include recommendations concerning the frequency of intervention and

the name of the team speech-language pathologist who is available to interact with a therapist providing treatment elsewhere
- Statement of speech-language reevaluation date and areas that need particular attention at that time, if any; such reevaluations may or may not coincide with regularly scheduled team evaluations.

Reports to the cleft palate team

Report of the speech and language screening may take many forms, depending on the practices of the individual cleft palate team. Results may be reported verbally to the team and summarized by another team member (who usually is not a speech-language pathologist). A check form or computer data sheet may be used with or without a summary statement. Or the speech pathologist may write or dictate a summary or formal report at the time of the clinic visit or at a latter time. Whichever format is used, it is essential to remember that the speech and language screening is only as good as the final report (i.e., the information obtained must be reported in a useful manner to other professionals who rely on this information to make management decisions). A common mistake among most speech-language pathologists is that the results of their evaluations often are presented using technical terms and professional jargon that is not understood by other medical specialists. On the other hand they may use specialized medical terminology that is unfamiliar to the community-based speech-language pathologist who will be working with the child. Therefore, it is incumbent on the team speech pathologist to learn to communicate the results of the speech and language screening in a manner that can be understood by all of the professionals involved.

Verbal and written reports also are a valuable opportunity to educate other team members and other medical specialists regarding important aspects of speech, language and communication. As depicted in Fig. 10-4, there is a surprising lack of understanding in the medical community regarding aspects of communication apart from the readily observable speech production process. There is an overwhelming misunderstanding that speech production is synonymous with language comprehension and expression.

Reports are most useful for future reference if results are presented in a consistent, standard format. In this way other professionals and the speech pathologist can find information rapidly regarding the precise area of interest without

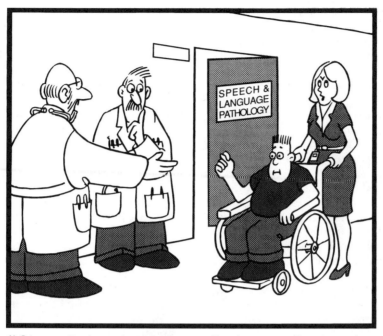

"Oh well, he doesn't talk–he won't need a speech evaluation"

Fig. 10-4 Common lack of understanding regarding "speech," "language," and "communication." (Reprinted with permission from D'Antonio L: Evaluation and management of velopharyngeal dysfunction: a speech pathologist's viewpoint. In Lehman J, editor: *Problems in plastic and reconstructive surgery,* Philadelphia, 1992, JP Lippincott.)

the necessity of reading through a full report. Additionally, because these reports usually become part of the child's permanent medical record (which may be quite voluminous in many cases) and searches through previous speech and language evaluations are often necessary, it is important to provide a concise but thorough summary paragraph that succinctly lists findings, impressions, and recommendations.

Reports to the community-based speech-language pathologist

Most cleft palate teams do not have the resources to provide the in-depth evaluation and ongoing speech therapy needed by many children with communication disorders associated with palatal clefting. Therefore it is the role of the team speech pathologist to make recommendations for further evaluation and treatment of communication impairment found during the team screening.

Recommendations for therapy should include frequency of therapy, duration of sessions, whether sessions should be group or individual, and therapy goals. In some situations recommendations should include suggestions for the actual therapy approach that is most appropriate for a given child. For example, in the case of the dyspraxic child who has shown little improvement in a traditional phonologic or phonemic articulation program the team speech pathologist might suggest a motor-based therapy plan such as that described in the section Unexpected (but common) populations. Similarly, the team speech pathologist might suggest the need for additional community services such as placement in a communication handicapped classroom, occupational/physical therapy, cognitive testing, or the development of a home-based therapy program.

The cleft palate team and the team speech-language pathologist usually have little control over the accessibility of services for their patients. The type and availability of services for handicapped children and adults vary dramatically from state to state and county to county within a state. While the team speech pathologist should be familiar with the resources available, the limitation of services should not influence the recommendations. That is, it is our opinion that the cleft palate team and the team speech pathologist should serve as an advocate for the child with cleft palate. Therefore the optimal therapy plan should be developed and presented to the family and community-based speech-language pathologists even though these services may be difficult to obtain.

Public law now mandates special services for handicapped children up to age 3. Unfortunately, although some services are available, there is no guarantee that they are appropriate or adequate for the child with cleft palate. Therefore an important role of the team speech pathologist, when time allows, is to monitor the community-based therapy of the team's patients. Economic constraints often dictate that fewer services are available than are needed by the child with communication impairment associated with palatal clefting. However, if the team speech pathologist serves as an advocate for the child and pursues the ideal therapeutic services needed, it is more likely that the child will get adequate services than without this advocacy. Just as the speech pathology report and recommendations can serve to educate other members of the cleft palate team, the report and the therapy suggestions in that report provide a valuable opportunity to assist and educate community-based speech pathologists regarding the communication needs of children with cleft palate.

SUMMARY

This chapter provides practical information to assist speech-language pathologists in screening and evaluating the communication skills of patients with cleft palate. Topics include the role of the speech-language pathologist on a cleft palate/craniofacial team, the differences between screening and evaluation, suggestions for the critical areas of information that should be obtained in either a screening or thorough evaluation, suggestions for how to elicit important information in an efficient manner, a discussion of unexpected populations you are likely to encounter, and suggestions regarding effective reporting of results to the cleft palate team and community care providers.

Our goal in presenting this information is to provide a practical, useful clinical resource for clinicians. However, if you are to be involved with a cleft population on a regular, ongoing basis there is no substitute for experience under the supervision of a veteran speech and language pathologist who has practiced with this population for a number of years. If you expect to participate on a team and find yourself unprepared or ill prepared, you may wish to contact experienced clinicians to act as advisors or optimally to find such a clinician to serve as a mentor.

ACKNOWLEDGMENT

We wish to acknowledge Helen Sharp, M.S., for comments on an early draft of this chapter and for contributions to the Screening Forms. We also wish to thank Ms. Debbie Lennox for assistance in manuscript preparation and Loma Linda University Media Services for assistance in preparation of illustrations and figures.

Appendix A

Observations and Elicitation Tasks in Informal Assessment of the Speech Production Mechanism

Miller J, Rosen P, Netsell R: Differentiating productive language deficits and speech motor control problems in children. Paper presented at the Wisconsin Speech and Hearing Association meeting, April 29, 1979.

The following section lists observations that can be made and elicitation tasks that can be used to determine the adequacy of the speech production mechanism. The techniques are presented in a manner such that one may make decisions related to the (1) lips, (2) teeth, (3) tongue, (4) jaw, (5) velopharynx and hard palate, (6) larynx, and (7) respiratory system. Although the systems involved in producing speech have been divided so that independent decisions can be made about each part of the system, this is *not* to suggest that these systems function independently.

The ideas presented are in no way meant to be exhaustive. Each clinician must vary the suggested techniques to meet the needs of the individual child and to make the suggestions comfortable for his or her clinical style. As one becomes familiar with the proposed framework, it will also become clear how one observed or elicited behavior can aid in decision making across systems (e.g., *puppy* gives information related to lip, tongue, jaw, velopharyngeal, laryngeal, and respiratory functioning).

A minimum age has been associated with some of the elicitation tasks to help ensure success for both child and clinician. The selected age range for each task is based on what a child would be expected to understand and/or imitate at that level of development.

The source material utilized in compiling the observation and elicitation tasks is drawn from unpublished papers, clinical protocols, and published work. (See the boxes on pp. 212-216 and Fig. A-1.)

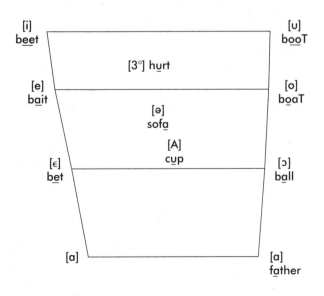

OBSERVATION AND ELICITATION TASKS: LIPS

Observe
1. Presence or absence of scarring
2. Smile (bilateral retraction)
3. Symmetric smile
4. Lip posture (open or closed)
5. Upper lip length (normal or short)
6. Protrude (kiss, /w/)
7. Round (/u/, food; /o/, boat)
8. Production of sounds or word with bilabials (list sounds during parent-child interaction that include /p/, /b/, or /m/).
9. Jaw dependence in production of bilabials
10. Drooling
11. Snack
    a. Lip closure in chewing
    b. Lip closure around straw
    c. Use of lips to clean away food

Elicit
1. *Nonspeech tasks*
   a. Smile (tickle child)
   b. Kiss baby,
      kiss mommy
   c. Blow a kiss
2. *Speech tasks*
   a. "oh, oh" (knock toy over)
   b. "mm" (while eating)
   c. Set out toys that can be acted upon with bilabial sounds, syllables, or words (consider sounds reported as within the child's sound repertoire)
   d. "Where's mama? Call mama."
   e. Ask name of toys.
   f. Bubbles—imitate *pop pop* as bubbles disappear.
   g. Use xylophone: sing bilabial sound or word up and down scale.
   h. Ask the child to imitate the words, *baby, mama, puppy.*

Minimum age to expect success with the elicitation task
1. *Nonspeech tasks*
   a. 7 months
   b. 8-12 months (demonstrated);
      16 months (verbal direction)
   c. 8-12 months
2. *Speech tasks*
   a. 12-18 months
   b. 12-18 months
   c. 12-18 months
   d. 12-18 months
   e. 18-24 months
   f. 18-24 months
   g. 18-24 months
   h. 18-24 months

OBSERVATION AND ELICITATION TASKS: TEETH

Observe
1. Occlusion
   a. Normal bite
   b. Overbite
   c. Underbite
2. Vertical relation to incisors
   a. Normal
   b. Open bite
3. Continuity of cutting edge of incisors and cuspids
   a. Normal
   b. Rotated, jumbled
   c. Missing teeth
   d. Supernumerary teeth
4. Caries/cavities (degree of problem)
5. Braces/retainer

Elicit
If the child has a problem with dentition, determine if there is a possible relationship to speech problem by using certain words and sounds (e.g., /f/, /sh/, /th/).

OBSERVATION AND ELICITATION TASKS: TONGUE

Observe
1. Structure
   a. Tongue at rest
   b. Size in relation to dental arches
   c. Symmetry (atrophy?)
2. Function
   a. List all vowels and consonants to determine the tongue's function in production of the sounds:
      (1) /t/, /d/, /n/ (tongue tip)
      (2) /g/, /k/ (tongue dorsum)
      (3) vowel production (see chart): *ba ga da* or words *buttercup, pattycake*)
   b. Observe use of jaw movement for tongue sounds (a bite block will help determine dependence)
   c. Observe spontaneous tongue movements:
      (1) Tongue thrust in swallowing
      (2) Tongue protrusion in play
      (3) Licking lips
      (4) Tongue movement while eating

Elicit
1. *Nonspeech tasks*
   a. Sucker: allow the child a taste, then hold the sucker in front of the lips to elicit tongue protrusion; next hold in the corners of the mouth to elicit tongue lateralization (hold child's head forward)

Continued.

OBSERVATION AND ELICITATION TASKS: TONGUE — cont'd

   b. Peanut butter on tongue depressor (same procedure as for sucker)
   c. Give the "raspberries"
   d. Use models (clinician, puppet, doll, parent) to demonstrate tongue protrusion and lateralization; use mirror play
   e. Quiet, *sh*
   f. Freddie Frog toy: tongue protrudes out of mouth to catch the fly (motivate older children)
   g. Use of the tongue as a make believe broom to sweep the "dirt" out of the house (mouth)
   h. "Simon Says" game
   i. "Pretend to be naughty and stick your tongue out at me."

Speech tasks
   a. If the child will repeat or imitate sounds, syllables, or words:
     (1) Tongue tip sounds /t/, /d/, /n/: *no, daddy, dog;* start with sounds or words within the child's repertoire
     (2) Dorsum of tongue /k/, /g/: *go, cake, key*
     (3) Range of vowels *pi, pe, pa, pu*
   b. Use bite block to determine jaw dependence
   c. Diadochokinetic rates
     (1) Model performance
     (2) Use visual markers
     (3) Count number of times /p/, /t/, /k/ produced per second
     (4) Have child produce words rapidly (e.g., *buttercup* or *pattycake*)

Minimum age to expect success with the elicitation task

1. *Nonspeech tasks*
   a. 12-18 months
   b. 12-18 months
   c. 12 months
   d. 12-18 months with a human model and 2 years for imitation of nonhuman object
   e. 18-24 months
   f. 2 years +
   g. 3½-4 years
   h. 3½-4 years
   i. 3½-4 years
2. *Speech tasks*
   a. (1) Within repertoire 12-18 months; not in repertoire 18-24 months
     (2) Same as (1)
     (3) Same as (1)
   b. 2 years
   c. 2 years

OBSERVATION AND ELICITATION TASKS: JAW

Observe
1. *Structure*
   a. Facial symmetry
   b. Mandible
     (1) Micrognathia
     (2) Macrognathia
     (3) Profile
2. *Function*
   a. Mobility of jaw
     (1) During speech
     (2) Nonspeech movements
     (3) Eating
   b. Is jaw thrust present?
   c. Grading of jaw
     (1) Smooth movement from vowel to vowel
     (2) Smooth movement from consonant to vowel: (CV) to CV
   d. Stability of jaw
     (1) For sustained vowel
     (2) For single word production

Elicit
1. Chatter teeth: "Brr, cold." How many times can upper and lower incisors be clenched together?
2. To help determine the child's dependence of jaw movement for production of bilabial and lingual sounds, a bite block can be used to stabilize the jaw and eliminate its contribution to the sound production. For children under 2 years of age, the use of a bite block is difficult. For use with any child, make certain that you can retrieve the bite block easily by holding on to it or attaching a string to it.

OBSERVATION AND ELICITATION TASKS: VELOPHARYNX AND HARD PALATE

Observe

1. *Structure*
   a. Hard palate
      (1) Normal
      (2) Repaired cleft (scarring)
      (3) Unrepaired cleft
      (4) Flat contour
      (5) Deep and normal contour
      (6) Fistulas
   b. Soft palate
      (1) Intactness
         (a) Normal
         (b) Repaired
         (c) Unrepaired
         (d) Symmetric
         (e) Asymmetric
      (2) Length
         (a) Satisfactory
         (b) Short
      (3) Uvula
         (a) Normal
         (b) Bifid
         (c) Deviates from midline
         (d) Absent
         (e) Long
2. *Function*
   a. Hypernasality (does the voice sound nasal?)
      (1) Vowels *ah* – prolonged
               ah – repeated
      (2) Nasal and nonnasal contrasts in words/ sentences: *mama, no no, m/b* distinction
   b. Nasal emission
      (1) Note fricative productions (e.g., kiss, fish)
      (2) Note any nasal flutter
   c. Is nasality continuous or intermittent? In what contexts – effort level, intensity, wide oral cavity, tongue position?
3. Presence of grimace

Elicit

1. Imitated isolated vowels
2. Words containing nasals/nonnasals; if child will imitate or look at picture book say:
   a. *mama*
   b. *puppy*
   c. *papa*
   d. *baby*
   e. *pumpkin*

3. While mouth is open, get child to say *ah-ah* (demonstrate on yourself; show them how that "little thing" (uvula) jumps up and down; use a mirror; watch for pharyngeal wall movement and symmetry
4. Sentences with and without nasals
   a. *Nonnasals*
      (1) Sue said hi.
      (2) The cat ate food.
   b. *Nasals*
      (1) Ten men came in.
      (2) My name is Tim.
      (3) I don't know.
      (4) Popcorn, please.
5. Vary contexts/facilitation techniques: "Let's see how many ways we can call mama." Whisper, loud, low pitch, high pitch, floppy (exaggerate mouth opening)
6. Gag reflex: use fingercot or tongue depressor, palpate at midline for cleft, move finger or blade back to gag
   a. Normal
   b. Hyperactive
   c. Hypoactive
   (Elicit gag reflex at the end of the assessment or check with the physician to see if this was done during the medical examination.)
7. Additional methods to measure nasal emission:
   a. Place finger under child's nose
   b. Nasal olive
   c. Small mirror
   d. Feather or tissue
   e. Rotometer – plastic tubing from nose allows flow of air to raise ball in a graduated cylinder
8. *Pui* (something smells bad); hold nose
9. "Make a sound. See if the sound stops when I hold your nose." Watch (demo) nasal vs. nonnasal.

Minimum age to expect success with the elicitation task

1. 12-18 months
2. If the word is within the child's repertoire, 12-18 months; if the words are new, 18-24 months
3. At least 2 years
4. At least 2 years
5. At least 2 years

OBSERVATION AND ELICITATION TASKS: LARYNX

Observe

Without a direct or indirect laryngeal examination by an ENT, all directions are based on perceptual characteristics of voice quality, pitch, and loudness.

1. Does the child's voice quality sound deviant?
2. Voice onset time: Is there a time lag between lip or tongue/palate release and the initiation of voicing?
3. Phonation time: amount of time voicing is sustained
4. Voiced/voiceless contrasts (e.g., *p*uppy vs. *b*aby, or *pa* vs. *ba*.
5. Intermittent voicing
6. Abrupt or gradual onset
7. Intonation patterns
8. Pitch variations in non-speech tasks (crying, laughing, sighing, coughing)
9. Pitch variations in speech tasks
10. Can the child whisper?

Elicit

1. Choose sounds or words within the child's repertoire which contain a voiced/voiceless contrast.
2. Variation in pitch
   a. Model the sound *ah* on a sliding scale.

   ah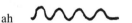

   ah

   b. Use visual cues (hands or paper cues) to demonstrate rising and falling pitch contours.
   c. Imitate a fire siren (Fisher-Price Village has a siren).

d. Use a xylophone to sing a musical scale.
e. Sing simple songs or nursery rhymes. Ask the child's parents which songs the child may know.
f. Role play with Fisher-Price people or puppets and use a low "daddy's voice" and a high "baby's voice."

3. Demonstrate phonation of a vowel *a* (count number of seconds sustained for respiration also). Listen for voice onset and phonation time.
   a. If child imitates, have child repeat the contrasting sounds or words, e.g., Sue, zoo; do, to.
   b. If child will not imitate, arrange environment to encourage the labeling of toys with voiced/voiceless contrasts.
   c. If child does not produce words, have toys available which the clinician can act upon and produce sounds to stimulate production.
4. Ask the child to talk softly because the baby is sleeping. "Sh, baby is sleeping" (model the quiet voice).
5. Ask the child to whisper a secret.

Minimum age to expect success with the elicitation task

1. Sounds or words within repertoire, 12-18 months; sounds or words are not within repertoire, 18-24 months
2. At least 2 years
3. At least 2 years
4. At least 2 years
5. 3½ to 4 years

OBSERVATION AND ELICITATION TASKS: RESPIRATION

Observe

1. During crying, babbling, or other speech behavior, use stop watch to time number of seconds child sustains respiration on one breath (maximum inhalation).
2. Present child with bubbles, balloons, whistles; encourage child to blow as long as possible (time exhalation).
3. Loudness changes in vocalization.

Elicit

(Minimum age to expect success with respiration elicitation tasks is at least 2 years.)

1. Hold airplane in front of child. Get child to phonate *ah* as the plane attempts to get to the airport. If child stops phonating, the plane crashes.
2. If child can count, attempt to have child count to 10 in one breath.
3. Water manometers
   a. U-tube manometers can be used with food coloring so that the water displacement is more visible to the child.
   b. Hold a toy animal at the level to which (5 cm) you want the child to displace the water. Tell the child that by blowing through the tube he or she can feed the animal.
   c. Use a beaker manometer with the straw immersed by 5 cm. Encourage the child to blow into the straw for 5 seconds.
4. Use bubbles, candles, or pinwheels to encourage the child to blow as you vary the distance of the object from their mouth.
5. Visual displays are beneficial in encouraging the child to sustain phonation.
   a. Let the child watch the stopwatch's hands move on the dial.
   b. Start the child phonating and lift the hands above the child's head while phonating.
   c. Use your hands and show the child that you want him or her to stretch the sound out as you move your hands apart.
   d. Use your fingers as counters; as the child phonates, drop one finger at a time and encourage phonation until all 10 fingers are down.
6. To determine if the child can make rapid changes in air volume:
   a. Attempt signs through nose.
   b. Have the child sniff or pant.
7. Variation in loudness
   a. Give child the model of how to vary vocal loudness by producing sounds, words, or singing a simple song.
   b. Whisper a secret.
   c. *Sh*, quiet, the baby is sleeping."
   d. "Let's call to mom in the next room" (demonstrate calling *mama* loudly).
   e. Hit a xylophone or drum softly and produce a quiet sound/word; hit the instrument hard and produce a loud sound/word.

Appendix B

Language Worksheet

	18-36 Months	3-4 Years

Play

1. Plays with two objects in a functional manner. For example, puts cup with saucer; puts spoon in cup; puts baby to bed; puts doll in car. — X
2. Combines functional play. For example, pours in cup, then drinks from cup, then washes cup; feeds doll, then kisses doll, then puts doll to bed. — X
3. Role play. For example, child takes the role of a character in a favorite story such as "The Three Bears." — (3-4 Years) X

Receptive language

1. Demonstrates understanding of commands with agents, objects, action, possession, descriptive attributes, and location by manipulating objects. For example, mommy eat; baby ride, mommy kiss daddy, baby's chair, red ball, baby in cup. — X
2. Peabody Picture Vocabulary Test—Revised. — (3-4 Years) X

	18-36 Months	3-4 Years

Expressive language

1. Uses language in play and communication during clinic visit. — X
2. Mean length of utterance for three longest utterances used during screening and by parent report (MacArthur Communication Development Inventory). — X
3. Vocabulary from parent report (MacArthur Communication Development Inventory). — X
   Number of words _____
   Percentile for age _____
4. Storytelling as observed in role play of favorite story (e.g., feltboard stories or wordless story books). — (3-4 Years) X

Phonology

1. Phonologic processes observed during clinic visit. — X   X
   Fronting _____
   Backing _____
   Stopping _____
   Reduplication _____
   Initial/final consonant delete _____
   Assimilation _____
   Cluster reduction _____
2. Assessment of phonologic processes—preschool Screening (Hodson, 1986). — (3-4 Years) X
   Pass   Fail

Appendix C

Suggested Materials for Speech-Language Screening Kit

1. Sesame Street character or other familiar doll or puppet with identifiable body parts and facial features
2. A few items of play food, plate, spoon, fork, cup
3. Small wind-up toys
4. Noisemakers (e.g., rattle, whistle, horn)
5. Five to eight blocks of different colors
6. Durable picture book for toddlers
7. Wordless picture book for school-age children
8. Feltboard story
9. Small remote-controlled car
10. Big-small contrasts
11. Toy vehicles, e.g. car, boat
12. People dolls and familiar toy objects (e.g., chair, table, bed)
13. Jar of bubbles and bubble wand
14. Stickers
15. Pegs and small pegboard
16. Food reinforcers (e.g., cereals, raisins)
17. Copy of story from Goldman-Fristoe Test of Articulation

REFERENCES

Bayley N: *Bayley scales of infant development,* San Antonio, 1969, The Psychological Corporation.

Bzoch KR: Communication disorders related to cleft lip and palate. Boston, 1979, Little, Brown.

Dalston RM: Standards of care for patients with craniofacial anomalies. Paper presented at the American Cleft Palate Craniofacial Association Consensus Conference, Pittsburgh, May 2-5, 1991.

Dalston RM, Martinkosky SJ, Hinton VA: Stuttering prevalence among patients at risk for velopharyngeal inadequacy: a preliminary investigation, *Cleft Palate J* 24:233, 1987.

Dalston RM, Warren DW: The diagnosis of velopharyngeal inadequacy, *Clin Plast Surg* 12:685, 1985.

Dalston RM, Warren DW, Dalston ET: A preliminary study of nasal airway patency and its potential effect on speech performance, *Cleft Palate J* 2:330, 1992.

Dantonio LL: Evaluation and management of velopharyngeal dysfunction: a speech pathologist's viewpoint. In Lehman J, editor: *Problems in plastic and reconstructive surgery,* Philadelphia, 1992, JB Lippincott.

Dantonio LL, Barlow SM, Warren DW: Studies of oronasal fistulae: implications for speech motor control. Paper presented at the Annual Meeting of the American Speech-Language Hearing Association, San Antonio, Nov 20-23, 1992.

Dantonio LL, Marsh J: Abnormal carotid arteries in the velocardiofacial syndrome: a report of two cases, *Plast Reconstr Surg* 80:471, 1987 (letter).

Dantonio LL, Muntz H, Province M, and Marsh J: Laryngeal-voice findings in patients with velopharyngeal dysfunction, *Laryngoscope* 98:432, 1988.

Dunn LM, Dunn LM: Peabody picture vocabulary test — Revised, Circle Pines, 1981, American Guidance Service.

Eliason MJ, Richman LC: Language development in preschool children with cleft, *Dev Neuropsychol* 6:173, 1990.

Folkins JW, Moon JB: Approaches to the study of speech production. In Bardach J, Morris HL, editors: *Multidisciplinary management of cleft lip and palate,* Philadelphia, 1990, WB Saunders.

Frankenburg WK, Dodds JB: *Denver developmental screening test,* Denver, 1969, University of Colorado Medical Center.

Golding-Kushner KJ, Weller G, Shprintzen RJ: Velocardio-facial syndrome: language and psychological profiles, *J Craniofac Genet Dev Biol* 5:259, 1985.

Goldman R, Fristoe M: *Goldman-Fristoe test of articulation,* Circle Pines, 1969, American Guidance Service.

Gorlin RJ, Cohen MM, Levin LS: *Syndromes of the head and neck,* ed 3, New York, 1990, Oxford University Press.

Gray S: Airway obstruction and apnea in cleft palate patients. In Bardach J, Morris HL, editors: *Multidisciplinary management of cleft lip and palate,* Philadelphia, 1990, WB Saunders.

Handler HD: Upper airway obstruction in craniofacial anomalies: diagnosis and management, *Birth Defects* 21:15, 1985.

Hoch L, Golding-Kushner K, Siegel-Sadewitz VL, and Shprintzen RJ: Speech therapy, *Semin Speech Language* 7:313, 1986.

Hodson BW: *The assessment of phonological processes — revised,* Austin, 1986, PRO-ED.

Isberg A, Henningsson G: Influence of palatal fistulas on velopharyngeal movements: a cineradiographic study, *Plast Reconstr Surg* 79:525, 1987.

Johnson W: *People in quandaries,* New York, 1946, Harper & Brothers.

Jones MC: Etiology of facial clefts: prospective evaluation of 428 patients, *Cleft Palate J* 25:16, 1988.

Karnell MP, Seaver EJ: Measurement problems in estimating velopharyngeal function. In Bardach J, Morris HL, editors: *Multidisciplinary management of cleft lip and palate,* Philadelphia, 1990, WB Saunders.

Kemp-Fincham SI, Kuehn DP, Trost-Cardamone JE: Speech development and the timing of primary palatoplasty. In Bardach J, Morris HL, editors: *Multidisciplinary management of cleft lip and palate,* Philadelphia, 1990, WB Saunders.

Kent RD: Anatomical and neuromuscular maturation of the speech mechanism: evidence from acoustic studies, *J Speech Hearing Dis* 19:421, 1976.

Lahey M: *Language disorders and language development,* New York, 1988, MacMillan.

Loney RW, Bloem TJ: Velopharyngeal dysfunction: recommendations for use of nomenclature, *Cleft Palate J* 24:334, 1987.

Macarthur: *The MacArthur Communicative Development Inventory,* San Diego, 1989, Development Psychology Lab, San Diego State University.

Mackenzie-Stepner K, Witzel MA, Stringer DA, and Laskin R: Velopharyngeal insufficiency due to hypertrophic tonsils. A report of two cases. *Int J Pediatr Otorhinolaryngol* 14:57, 1987.

Mackenzie-Stepner K, Witzel MA, Stringer DA, Lindsay WK, and Munro IR: Abnormal carotid arteries in the velocardiofacial syndrome: a report of three cases, *Plast Reconstr Surg* 80:347, 1987.

Mcwilliams BJ, Bluestone CD, Musgrave RH: Diagnostic implications of vocal cord nodules in children with cleft palate, *Laryngoscope* 79:2072, 1969.

Mcwilliams BJ, Lavorato AS, Bluestone CD: Vocal cord abnormalities in children with velopharyngeal valving problems, *Laryngoscope* 83:1745, 1973.

Mcwilliams BJ, Morris HL, Shelton RL: *Cleft palate speech,* ed 2, Toronto, 1990, BC Decker.

Mcwilliams BJ, Philips BJ: *Audio seminars in speech pathology: velopharyngeal incompetence,* Philadelphia, 1979, WB Saunders.

Miller J: *Assessing language production in children,* Oceanside, Calif, 1984, Academic Communication Associates.

Miller J, Rosen P, Netsell, R: Differentiating productive language deficits and speech motor control problems in children. Paper presented at the Wisconsin Speech and Hearing Association meeting, April 29, 1979.

Morris HL: Types of velopharyngeal incompetence. In Winitz H, editor: *Treating articulation disorders: for clinicians by clinicians,* Baltimore, 1984, University Park Press.

Morris HL: Clinical assessment by the speech pathologist. In Bardach J, Morris HL, editors: *Multidisciplinary management of cleft lip and palate,* Philadelphia, 1990, WB Saunders.

Morris HL, Spriestersbach DC, Darley FL: An articulation test for assessing competency of velopharyngeal closure, *J Speech Hearing Res* 4:48, 1961.

Morris S, Klein M: *Prefeeding skills: a comprehensive resource for feeding development,* Tucson, 1987, Communication Skill Builders.

Netsell R: The acquisition of speech motor control: a perspective with directions for research. In Stark R, editor: *Language behavior in infancy and early childhood,* New York, 1981, Elsevier Science Publishing.

Netsell R: Velopharyngeal dysfunction. In Yoder DE, Kent RD, editors: *Decision making in speech language pathology,* Toronto, 1988, BC Decker.

Netsell R, Daniel B: A physiologic approach to rehabilitation for adults with dysarthria, *Arch Phys Med Rehabil* 60:502, 1979.

O'Gara MM, Logemann JA: Early speech development in cleft palate babies. In Bardach J, Morris HL, editors: *Multidisciplinary management of cleft lip and palate,* Philadelphia, 1990, WB Saunders.

Olswang LB, Stoel-Gammon C, Coggins T, and Carpenter R: *Assessing linguistic behaviors.* Seattle, 1989, University of Washington Press.

Pashayan HM: What else to look for in a child born with a cleft of the lip and/or palate, *Cleft Palate J* 20:54, 1983.

Peterson SJ: A cross-sectional analysis of speech results following palatal closure. In Bardach J, Morris HL, editors: *Multidisciplinary management of cleft lip and palate,* Philadelphia, 1990, WB Saunders.

Peterson-Falzone SJ: Speech characteristics: updating clinical decisions, *Semin Speech Language* 7:269, 1986.

Peterson-Falzone SJ, Graham MS: Phoneme-specific nasal emission in children with and without physical anomalies of the velopharyngeal mechanism, *J Speech Hearing Dis* 55:132, 1990.

Philips BJ: Speech assessment, *Semin Speech Language* 7:297, 1986.

Philips BJ: Early speech management. In Bardach J, Morris HL, editors: Multidisciplinary management of cleft lip and palate, Philadelphia, 1990, WB Saunders.

Randall P: A commentary on management and timing of cleft palate fistula repair, *Plast Reconstr Surg* 78:746, 1986.

Reisberg DJ, Gold HO, Dorf DS: A technique for obturating palatal fistulas, *Cleft Palate J* 22:286, 1985.

Robbins J, Klee T: Clinical assessment of oropharyngeal motor development in young children, *J Speech Hearing Dis* 52:271, 1987.

Rossetti L: *The Rossetti infant-toddler language scale,* East Moline, 1990, Lingui Systems.

Shprintzen RJ: Surgery for speech: the planning of operations for velopharyngeal insufficiency with emphasis on the preoperative assessment of both pharyngeal physiology and articulation. In Huddart AG, Ferguson MWJ, editors: *Cleft lip and palate: long term results and future prospects,* vol 1, New York, 1990, Manchester University Press.

Shprintzen RJ, Goldberg RB, Lewin ML, Sidoti EJ, Berkman MD, Argamaso RV, and Young D: A new syndrome involving cleft palate, cardiac anomalies, typical facies, and learning disabilities: velo-cardio-facial syndrome, *Cleft Palate J* 5:56, 1978.

Shprintzen RJ, Golding-Kushner KJ: Evaluation of velopharyngeal insufficiency, *Otolaryngol Clin North Am* 22:519, 1989.

Shprintzen RJ, Sher AE, Croft CB: Hypernasal speech caused by tonsillar hypertrophy, *Int J Pediatr Otorhinolaryngol* 14:45, 1987.

Siegel-Sadewitz VL, Shprintzen RJ: The relationship of communication disorders to syndrome identification, *J Speech Hearing Dis* 47:338, 1982.

Sparrow S, Balla D, Cicchetti D: *Vineland adaptive behavior scales,* Circle Pines, 1984, American Guidance Service.

Stickler KR: *Guide to analysis of language transcripts,* Eau Claire, Wisc, 1987, Thinking Publications.

Thal D, Bates E: Language and gesture in late talkers, *J Speech Hearing Res* 31:115, 1988.

Thal D, Tobias S, Morrison D: Language and gesture in late talkers: a 1-year follow-up, *J Speech Hearing Res* 34:604, 1991.

Trost JE: Articulatory additions to the classical description of the speech of persons with cleft palate, *Cleft Palate J* 18:193, 1981.

Trost-Cardamone JE: Coming to terms with VPI: a response to Loney and Bloem, *Cleft Palate J* 26:68, 1989.

Trost-Cardamone JE: Speech in the first year of life: a perspective on early acquisition. In Kernahan DA, Rosenstein SW, editors: *Cleft lip and palate, a system of management,* Baltimore, 1990, Williams & Wilkins.

Van Demark DR, Hardin MA: Speech therapy for the child with cleft lip and palate. In Bardach J, Morris HL, editors: *Multidisciplinary management of cleft lip and palate,* Philadelphia, 1990, WB Saunders.

Warren DW: Compensatory speech behaviors in individuals with cleft palate: a regulation/control phenomenon? *Cleft Palate J* 23:251, 1986.

Williams MA, Shprintzen RJ, Goldberg RB: Male-to-male transmission of the velo-cardio-facial syndrome: a case report and review of 60 cases, *J Craniofac Genet Dev Biol* 5:175, 1985.

11 Instrumental Assessment of Velopharyngeal Valving

Robert J. Shprintzen

The instrumental assessment of velopharyngeal valving has occupied a substantial amount of space in the scientific literature for the past half century. A large number of devices have come and gone in the battery of tools used to study the process of velopharyngeal closure. The overwhelming majority of devices and procedures have long since disappeared from legitimate use in most "state-of-the-art" facilities. Only a handful of practical devices have remained, but the search continues for new procedures. In part, the continuous search for new instrumentation is driven by technology, especially in the area of imaging. The search for new procedures is also fueled by the fact that each individual procedure currently in use has some type of drawback leading to some degree of examiner dissatisfaction. In this chapter, procedures utilized to study velopharyngeal valving will be critically discussed. The majority of the chapter, however, will be devoted to an in-depth discussion of the current state-of-the-art procedures for the assessment of velopharyngeal valving problems.

TYPES OF ASSESSMENT PROCEDURES

The majority of clinicians would agree that procedures used to assess velopharyngeal valving disorders can be divided into two general categories: direct and indirect. In reality, these categories refer to the ability to actually see the velopharyngeal valve (i.e., direct visualization) versus studying some type of artifact or byproduct of velopharyngeal function (indirect). Indirect, or nonvisualizing procedures have been easier to apply because they are nonmedical in nature and can be implemented by nearly anyone, in or out of a medical facility. Procedures requiring direct visualization typically require some medical expertise and equipment, which can usually only be found within a hospital or medical environment. Though it might be argued that direct visualization procedures are too bothersome or expensive to be widely applied, especially within the confines of a speech

pathology clinic, one must consider if the information obtained from indirect procedures is sufficient for the recommendation of treatment. Indirect procedures include assessments of resonance (such as nasometry), air flow (such as pressure-flow, rhinometry, and manometry), and studies of muscle function (such as electromyography). Such studies have very limited value once direct assessments have provided a thorough observation of the VP valve. The only indirect measure of critical importance is listener judgment of resonance. The listener's assessment of resonance is the prime determiner of normal versus abnormal "nasality." The decision to treat a resonance disorder is wholly dependent on a judgment of abnormality.

The earliest report of direct observation of velopharyngeal closure is probably that of Hilton (1836), who observed the movements of the velum and lateral pharyngeal walls through a facial defect left by the spontaneous extrusion of a facial tumor in an adult. The first radiographic observations of the velopharyngeal structures came later that same century after the introduction of roentgenography and were reported as early as 1909 (Scheier, 1909). For the next 60 years, the lateral view radiograph (Fig. 11-1) became the standard procedure for the study of velopharyngeal closure, using both still cephalographs (Subtelny, 1964) and cineradiography (Moll, 1960). It was not until 1969 that two new procedures for the direct observation of the velopharyngeal valve were introduced, which would completely revise the scientific community's concept of velopharyngeal closure.

DIRECT PROCEDURES

Today, the "gold standard" for the assessment of velopharyngeal valving consists of two direct visualization procedures; multi-view videofluoroscopy and nasopharyngoscopy (Shprintzen and Golding-Kushner, 1989; Golding-Kushner et al., 1990). Both of these procedures were introduced in 1969 (Pigott, 1969; Skolnick, 1969) and have been followed by large numbers

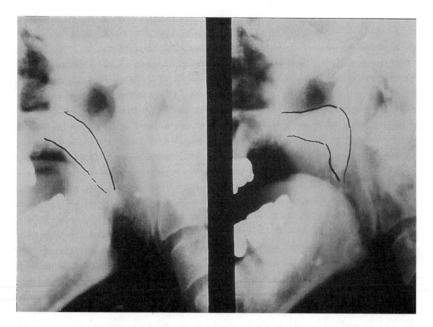

Fig. 11-1 Lateral view radiograph (from cineradiography) showing velum at rest (left) and during speech (right).

of publications reporting the results and efficacy of the techniques. These procedures will be described in detail first to serve as a base of comparison for other procedures which, in this author's opinion, have limited usefulness in the management of disorders related to velopharyngeal disorders. Because many patients will ultimately have some type of physical management of their velopharyngeal insufficiency (VPI), a direct observation of the movements and structure of the velopharyngeal valve is essential to successfully resolve the problem.

WHY NASOPHARYNGOSCOPIC AND MULTI-VIEW VIDEOFLUOROSCOPIC PROCEDURES?
New concepts in velopharyngeal valving

In his landmark investigations, Skolnick (1969, 1970, 1973) pointed out that velopharyngeal closure does not involve only the movement of the soft palate (velum) to the posterior pharyngeal wall. Since the advent of radiographs to study velopharyngeal closure nearly 100 years ago, lateral view studies have demonstrated that the palate moves posterosuperiorly to contact the adenoid in young children (Shprintzen and Golding-Kushner, 1989) and posterior pharyngeal wall in older children and adults (Fig. 11-2). However, a transverse (axial) perspective on the velopharyngeal valve shows that the velum does not fill the entire pharyngeal volume (Fig. 11-3). The pharyngeal walls extend laterally beyond

the outermost edges of the velum so that some degree of lateral pharyngeal wall motion is necessary if the velopharyngeal valve is to be closed completely. In other words, even if the velum were to contact the posterior aspect of the pharynx, if the lateral pharyngeal walls did not move, an insufficiency would occur (Fig. 11-4). This scenario is not at all unique and has been seen quite often. If only a lateral view videofluoroscopy were used to assess velopharyngeal function, the insufficiency could not be seen or diagnosed because the lateral pharyngeal walls cannot be seen in lateral view. Therefore, it is possible for a lateral view radiograph to show what appears to be velopharyngeal closure even though velopharyngeal insufficiency is occurring.

Though there has been some argument regarding the muscles that contribute to velopharyngeal valving, it is generally accepted that the levator veli palatini (levator) is responsible for the posterosuperior movement of the velum and that the superior constrictor is the major contributor to lateral pharyngeal wall motion. The musculus uvulae is also active during speech. These concepts of velopharyngeal function will be discussed in more detail later.

Another important concept relative to velopharyngeal valving was that of volumetric versus planar function of the mechanism (Shprintzen, 1983, 1989, 1992, Siegel-Sadewitz and Shprintzen, 1986). Many investigators discuss velopha-

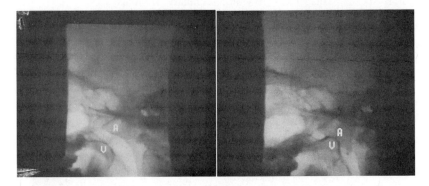

Fig. 11-2 Lateral view showing the velum (V) approximating to adenoid (A), beginning at rest (left) and during speech (right).

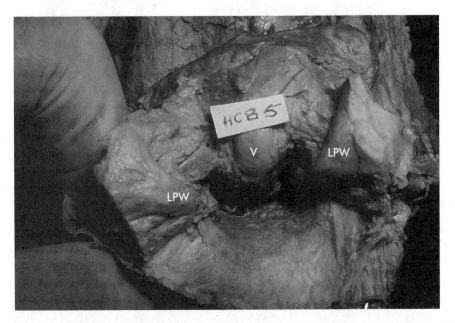

Fig. 11-3 Cadaver sections showing that the lateral pharyngeal walls (LPW) extend beyond the lateral edges of the velum (V), thus necessitating lateral pharyngeal wall motion to achieve velopharyngeal closure.

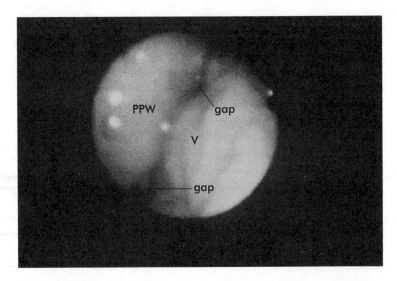

Fig. 11-4 Endoscopic view of an individual in whom the velum (V) approximates the posterior pharyngeal wall (PPW), but the lateral walls do not move medially leaving bilateral small gaps resulting in velopharyngeal insufficiency.

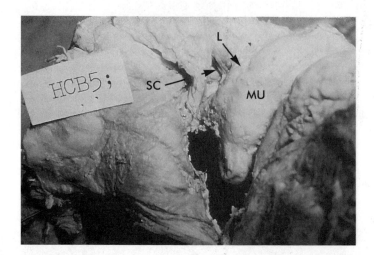

Fig. 11-5 Cadaver section demonstrating the course of the superior constrictor (SC) below the insertion of the levator veli palatini (LVP) in the velum below the musculus uvulae (MU).

ryngeal closure as if it occurs at a discrete two dimensional plane. For example, pressure flow studies calculate the area of a velopharyngeal gap (Warren, 1964; Warren, 1975). However, it has been pointed out that velopharyngeal closure does not occur at a discrete, flat plane, but rather in the coordinated movements of a volumetric tube with not only width and length, but also height (Shprintzen, 1983, 1989, 1992, Siegel-Sadewitz and Shprintzen, 1986). The cadaver specimen in Fig. 11-5 illustrates this point.

The levator enters the velum through the lateral pharyngeal wall at a slightly downward course. Because a thick portion of the levator is in the lateral pharyngeal wall, when it contracts, the portion of the lateral pharyngeal wall that contains it will move medially, carried by the sling-like constriction of the muscle. This movement of the lateral pharyngeal wall occurs at essentially the same level as the elevating velum, just beneath the torus tubarius (the nasopharyngeal orifice of the cartilage of the Eustachian tube), but is not the only level of motion that occurs in the lateral pharyngeal walls and is not the level of motion that contributes to velopharyngeal closure. The lateral pharyngeal wall motion essential to velopharyngeal closure comes from the uppermost fibers of the superior constrictor (Shprintzen et al., 1975). As is seen in Fig. 11-5, the uppermost fibers of the superior constrictor enter into the velum beneath the levator insertion. The course of the superior constrictor fibers begins along the midline of the posterior pharyngeal wall and then runs bilaterally toward the velum through the lateral

pharyngeal walls, underneath the salpingopharyngeal folds, in a slightly upward direction. These fibers form an incomplete sphincter with the anteriormost portion being the component that is in the velum intermingled with the other muscles in the palate. The only intrinsic muscle in the velum, the musculus uvulae, sits on top of all the other muscles and is often the largest muscle mass in the palate.

Contraction of the superior constrictor will move the lateral pharyngeal wall medially, but slightly below the plane of palatal elevation, thus making velopharyngeal closure a process that occurs over a vertical height of the pharynx as well as a horizontal level. It is therefore important that a diagnostic procedure be able to assess movement at all vertical levels of the pharynx.

Skolnick and colleagues (1973) introduced another concept that has become of major importance in both diagnosis and treatment of VPI. Skolnick and colleagues found that there is marked variability in the function of the velopharyngeal valve from person to person. Skolnick and colleagues reported that in their analysis of a number of normal and abnormal cases there were multiple patterns of movement in the velum, lateral pharyngeal walls, and posterior pharyngeal wall. They categorized their observations into four patterns of movement based on the anatomical plane in which the closure was oriented (Fig. 11-6):

Coronal — In the coronal pattern, the velum contacts the posterior pharyngeal wall broadly with the lateral pharyngeal walls moving medially just enough to contact the lateral edges. The majority of closure in anteroposterior.

Sagittal — In the sagittal pattern, the lateral pharyngeal walls move medially and touch in the midline. Because the lateral pharyngeal walls abut behind the velum, the soft palate never contacts the posterior pharyngeal wall.

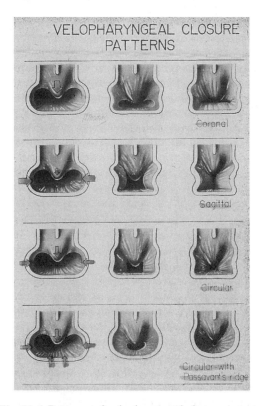

Fig. 11-6 Patterns of velopharyngeal closure as categorized by Skolnick et al (1973) seen in an axial view of the velopharyngeal sphincter. From Siegel-Sadewitz VL, Shprintzen RJ, Cleft Palate J 19, 196, 1982.

Circular — In the circular pattern, there is essentially equal movement in the velum and lateral pharyngeal walls. This pattern resembles a sphincteric configuration except for the absence of movement in the posterior pharyngeal wall.

Passavant's Ridge — Passavant's ridge refers to a forward movement of the posterior pharyngeal wall (Fig. 11-7), named after the first observer of this phenomenon, Gustav Passavant, a nineteenth century surgeon. In the Passavant's ridge pattern, the appearance is one of a true sphincter with all structures moving toward the midline.

The observations of Skolnick et al (1973) were subsequently confirmed in a larger series of cases of both normal individuals and individuals with cleft palate (Croft et al., 1981b). The importance of this finding cannot be stated strongly enough. The concept of variable motion in each component of velopharyngeal valving means that it is extremely important to evaluate every case with state-of-the-art visualization procedures because the symptomatic presentation of hypernasality does not predict a particular pattern of abnormal movement. If there are multiple patterns of movement, then it must require multiple types of treatment to address them. Clinicians must utilize diagnostic procedures that have high sensitivity and specificity for detecting these variations. Because physical management, surgery in particular, may depend on the diagnostic information obtained, false positives and false negatives should not be tolerated. Is there a single diagnostic procedure that will detect all problems without yielding potentially false results? No. We recommend the combined use of two procedures.

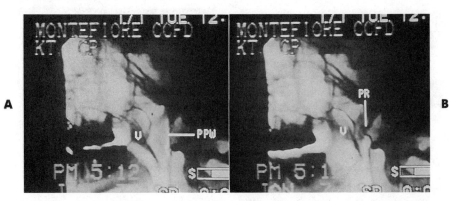

Fig. 11-7 Lateral view videofluoroscopy showing the velopharyngeal valve at rest (left) and during speech (right) with a Passavant's ridge in the posterior pharyngeal wall. The velum is labelled V, the posterior pharyngeal wall is PPW, and the Passavant's ridge is PR.

NASOPHARYNGOSCOPY

Nasopharyngoscopy was first described for the assessment of velopharyngeal function by Pigott (1969). The intent of nasopharyngoscopy is to provide a direct view of the velopharyngeal valve from above by passing a telescope through the nose that will not interfere with the normal production of speech. When the concept for endoscopy of the velopharyngeal valve was developed, the best instruments available for the procedure were rigid instruments, which were slender enough to be introduced into the nose (Fig. 11-8). The lens at the tip of the instrument allowed the examiner to look downward at a fixed angle. Pigott and Makepeace (1982) have recommended the use of a 70° downward-looking endoscope for the majority of cases.

Because the rigid endoscopes are not flexible, once they are introduced there is very little room for maneuverability of the instrument, and the examiner must look from above at the angle dictated by the lens system. The optical quality of the images is excellent and the area visible in the examination is quite wide, but the examiner remains bound to seeing only what the instrument will let him or her see. If there is a need to look at a different angle, it is necessary to have a completely different instrument.

Another problem with rigid instruments is the amount of discomfort experienced by the patient. Both the instrument and the internal structures of the nose are solid and firm. The nasal septum, turbinates, and nasal bones have little yield so that any pressure on them will result in significant pain. As a result, it is extremely difficult to get compliance from very young children (e.g., 4 and 5-year-olds) who are candidates for surgery, such as pharyngeal flap.

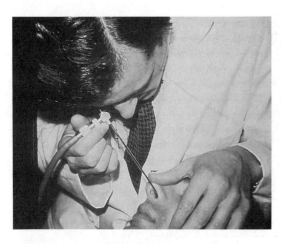

Fig. 11-8 Use of the rigid nasopharyngoscope.

In our early use of a rigid endoscope, we had very few compliant patients below the age of 6, and only slightly better than 50% compliance from children over 8 years of age. This is not acceptable for a technique that should be applied to all patients.

In the mid 1970s, the use of a slender fiber optic instrument was introduced by Japanese researchers from Osaka (Matsuya et al., 1974, Miyazaki et al., 1975). This instrument was a side-viewing endoscope that allowed a painless examination, but it was used essentially like a rigid endoscope because of its side-viewing construction. In other words, once the instrument was maneuvered into the postnasal space, it had to be positioned in the same manner as a rigid instrument and could not be passed further into the upper airway. However, it must be acknowledged that the Japanese report opened the door to applying a new generation of fiber optic technology to the study of speech disorders associated with cleft palate.

Shortly after the Japanese reports, the first slender end-viewing endoscopes were introduced to the American market. After obtaining our first 4 mm diameter endoscope in 1974 (a Machida ENT-4, or 4L), a series of reports began to appear in the scientific literature describing the use of the instrument (Shprintzen et al, 1978, 1979a, 1979b; Croft et al, 1978). Since that time, the overwhelming majority of instruments used for nasopharyngoscopy (and reported in the literature) have been end-viewing fiber optic endoscopes, and advances made in instrumentation have been related to improved optics and thinner devices.

Instrumentation

All fiber optic endoscopes have several things in common (Fig. 11-9). They are comprised of the portion that is inserted into the nose, a viewing end, and a light guide. The portion inserted into the nose is usually about 30 cm in length and covered in a black vinyl material. At the tip, there are two portions; a lens for gathering in the image, and a light conducting apparatus, which illuminates the pharynx (Fig. 11-9). The nasal portion of the instrument is extremely flexible and can be bent and twisted in any direction without altering the image seen through it. The body of the instrument (the portion held in the hand) has an eyepiece with a focus adjustment and a control apparatus (a lever or wheel) that flexes the distal end of the instrument through an arc of approximately 180° (Fig. 11-9). The light guide is a long vinyl coated cable, which inserts into a light source

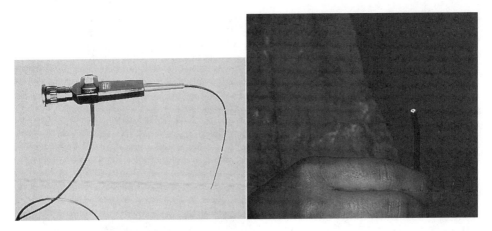

Fig. 11-9 Flexible nasopharyngolaryngoscope showing the body of the instrument with the control wheel and the illuminated tip.

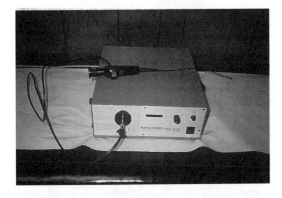

Fig. 11-10 Light source for a nasopharyngoscope with the light guide plugged into it.

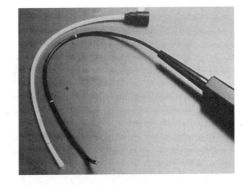

Fig. 11-11 Endosheath® device which keeps the nasopharyngoscope sterile.

(Fig. 11-10). The light source emits a high intensity light that is conducted through the light guide to the tip of the endoscope to illuminate the inside of the body. The light emitted from the tip of the endoscope does not generate heat and is therefore called a "cold light" because all of the heat is generated by the bulb that is contained in the light source.

At present, there are two types of end-viewing instruments in use categorized according to the ability to sterilize them. There are several instruments made by a number of manufacturers (Machida, Olympus, and Pentax) that have diameters ranging from 3.0 to 3.7 mm and can easily be rendered sterile for each examination with a new device called the Endosheath (Fig. 11-11). All of these instruments have excellent optics and maneuverability. The Endosheath is a sterile latex rubber sheath that is applied to the instrument for each use. At the tip of the Endosheath is a clear plastic lens covering,

which assures a fully sterile instrument. The endosheath adds only a fraction of a millimeter to the total thickness of the instrument. The Endosheath has been greeted with universal praise by patients because of their concern with infectious diseases being transmitted by medical instruments that are used repeatedly on many patients. Until the use of the Endosheath, it was necessary to first wash and then gas sterilize the endoscope after each use. Because gas sterilization takes time and is usually done at a different site in the hospital, the endoscope could not be used more than once or twice per day, which is unacceptable for busy centers. Cold sterilization using gluteraldehyde or some similar disinfectant is no longer considered to be a safe method for sterilizing endoscopes and immersion of endoscopes in caustic substances eventually damages the instrument.

The instruments that cannot be easily sterilized (i.e., they require gas sterilization) are the

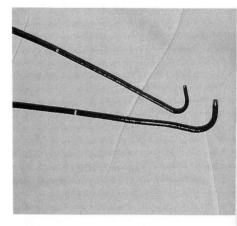

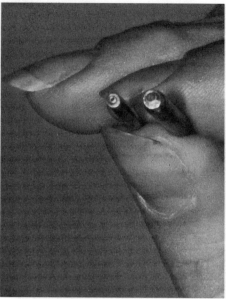

Fig. 11-12 Comparison of 2 mm and 3 mm naso-pharyngoscopes (Machida ENT-2 and Machida ENT-3) showing differences in thickness and surface area of the tip.

new generation of very thin nasopharyngo-scopes. The Machida ENT-2 is a very slender instrument, approximately 2 mm in diameter, with excellent optics that is easily passed into the noses of even very young children with no pain or discomfort. One might wonder why 1 mm thickness would make very much difference in compliance with examination. The answer is that the diameter is less an indicator of endo-scope size than is the surface area (Fig. 11-12). The entire tip of the endoscope is inserted into the nose so that the space occupied by the instrument in the nasal passage is more closely calculated by the surface area of the circular tip, or even more accurately by the volume of the instrument (the volume of a cylinder). Using surface area as an indicator, Table 11-1 com-pares the surface areas of four instruments as measured using the same electronic calipers (rounded to the nearest tenth of a millimeter): the Machida ENT-2, Machida ENT-3, Pentax FNL-10S, and Olympus ENF-P. The surface area of the instrument is computed by calculat-ing the area of a circle, πr^2. Thus, an instrument with a 2 mm diameter has a radius of 1 mm, and the surface area of the tip would be computed as the radius squared, (i.e., 1×1) multiplied by π, or 3.14159. Therefore, even though a 2 mm diameter instrument has a width two thirds that of a 3 mm instrument, its surface area is less than half. Similarly, compared to a 3.7 mm diameter instrument, a 2 mm instrument has a surface area less than a third that of the thicker instrument.

Table 11-1 Comparison of the diameter and total surface area of four currently available fiber optic nasopharyngoscopes

Instrument	Diameter	Surface area
Machida ENT-2	2.0mm	3.1mm^2
Machida ENT-3	3.0mm	7.1mm^2
Pentax FNL-10S	3.4mm	9.1mm^2
Olympus ENF-P	3.7mm	10.8mm^2

We have found a dramatically improved compliance rate with the 2 mm endoscope. In order to determine the value of individual instruments in terms of compliance, an experi-ment was conducted comparing the outcome of 200 consecutive examinations with each of the four instruments (a total of 800 examinations) listed in Table 11-1. The results were assessed according to age. In patients over the age of 12, there was no statistically significant difference between the rates of compliance with each instrument. However, in children 12 years of age or less, the 2 mm endoscope had a significantly better compliance rate than the other three instruments. The results were even more strik-ing in children under the age of 7 years. An analysis was also made of complaints of pain or discomfort. There were very few complaints of discomfort with the 2 mm endoscope (less than 5%), but a 30% to 60% rate of complaints with the other three instruments, the most being registered for the Olympus instrument, the least for the Machida 3L.

At present, there is no Endosheath available for the 2 mm instrument, which leaves clinicians in a quandary. The thicker instruments offer completely sterile examinations with the ability to use the endoscope as often as necessary on as many patients as necessary in a short time span, but with less than optimal compliance. The 2 mm instrument allows almost perfect compliance for even very young patients (4 and 5-year-olds), but the endoscope must be gas sterilized after each use, meaning that it is inaccessible for long periods of time. Our strategy has been to use both instruments. The 3 mm instrument is used routinely in order to maintain sterility; the 2 mm instrument is reserved for the youngest patients, or those patients where compliance may be questioned. Compliance is an extremely important factor in assessing a pediatric population. Because the data gathered from endoscopy are so critical to treatment planning, a successful examination should be of primary importance to the examiner. Some researchers have emphasized the importance of good optics for nasopharyngoscopy (Pigott and Makepeace, 1982). Though good optics is of importance, even the best optics are useless if an examination cannot be completed successfully.

Video recording

The majority of facilities or offices utilizing nasopharyngoscopy do not record the results of the examination. This is problematic because there is not as yet a standard or uniform method for reporting the results of endoscopic studies of the velopharyngeal valve. The person performing the endoscopic examination is usually not the same person who will be performing surgery. There is no way of knowing if the description of the endoscopic study made by the examiner is recreated mentally in an accurate manner by the surgeon. No study has ever been performed to assess the ability of written descriptions to convey a mental image of a visual endoscopic event. It is therefore important to record the results of endoscopic examinations on videotape so that as many clinicians as possible, including surgeons, can see the study. In a study of the reliability of endoscopic studies, D'Antonio et al. (1989) found that group judgments from videotaped studies were reliable sources of information for individual patients.

Videotaping of examinations is not at all difficult and, in some ways makes the entire examination procedure easier. There are two types of cameras that can be used for videotaping studies: small "chip cameras" and standard consumer electronics camcorders. Our preference is for the latter. Chip cameras (Fig. 11-13) are small, hand-held cameras that attach directly onto the eyepiece of the endoscope. They have no lens system and the video image is registered directly onto a video chip with the image being processed in a small electronic box attached to the camera portion by a cable. They are so light that they add little significant weight to the instrument so that examinations can be conducted in the same manner as they would without the camera except that the examiner must be watching a television screen rather than the image in the eyepiece. It should be pointed out that the image on the television screen appears much larger to the examiner. Camcorders must be tripod mounted because the camera is too heavy to hold while still controlling the endoscope (Fig. 11-14). Using a standard adaptor available from the endoscope manufacturer, cameras can be easily adapted to the nasopharyngoscope.

Our preference for a tripod mounted consumer video system is based on the following factors: price, light sensitivity, electronic features, and "hands free examination." Cost is a major factor. A standard "top of the line" camcorder (VHS or 8 mm) will cost less than a third the price of the least expensive endoscopic chip camera. Light sensitivity is also superior in the camcorder, often as low as 1 lux. Camcorders also offer a wide range of electronic features such as date and time generators, titlers, zoom, fade, and other enhancements to video imaging. Most important, by mounting the camera on a tripod, the examiner does not have to hold the instrument during the examination, leaving his or her hands free to hold the patient's head, point something out, or move the patient into a

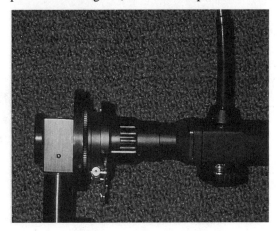

Fig. 11-13 Chip camera attached to nasopharyngoscope.

more favorable position. Using a tripod, only one hand is needed to keep the endoscope in position. The instrument can be advanced by swinging the tripod toward the patient and moved from side to side by rotating the endoscope clockwise or counterclockwise (Fig. 11-15).

EXAMINATION PROCEDURE

The first step in the examination process is gaining patient compliance. It is obviously helpful to have a natural rapport with children. The examiner should not be intimidating. It is always helpful to state at the very beginning that "I am not going to hurt you." This will be a true statement in nearly all cases if the patient is compliant, unfrightened, and proper topical anesthesia is administered.

Topical anesthesia

Using the 2 mm endoscope, it is usually sufficient to use only a light spray of Pontocaine (tetracaine hydrochloride, aqueous, 2%) into

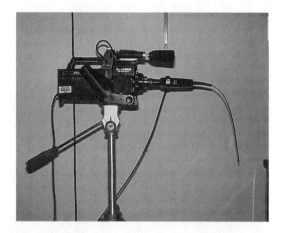

Fig. 11-14 Camcorder mounted nasopharyngoscope.

one nostril. Using the larger scopes, it is also suggested to use cotton packing soaked in Pontocaine inserted in the nose and left for approximately 5 minutes. We prefer Pontocaine because it acts quickly, has few side effects, and has a very mild odor, which is not at all noxious. In addition, Pontocaine is not astringent, as are many other local anesthetics, such as xylocaine or lidocaine. We prefer to spray the anesthetic into the nose with an atomizer rather than the pneumatic pump on the ENT cart, which is loud and tends to frighten young children. The best side of the nose is chosen by occluding each nostril and having the patient sniff in. The higher the pitch of the sound of the inhalation, the narrower the nasal passage. The larger passage is chosen and sprayed several times. We use strips of Webril cotton orthopedic bandage for nasal packing, cutting it into 3 mm wide strips, twirling it, dousing it with Pontocaine, and sliding it into the nose with small bayonet forceps (Fig. 11-16). This is left for 5 minutes and then removed before the examination.

It is important to explain in exact detail the entire process. The following excerpt is an actual transcription of a tape recorded endoscopic session between the author and a five-year-old patient:

Let me tell you exactly what I'm going to do, Michael. First, I'm not going to hurt you. Have you ever been on TV? Well, first I'm going to put your face on TV, and after that I'm going to put a picture of the inside of your nose on TV. Isn't that silly? Has the inside of your nose ever been on TV before? Well, let me tell you how I'm going to do that. You see that long piece of black spaghetti? [The examiner shows the patient the endoscope hanging from the camcorder] *Well, it's very thin and it will fit into the front of your nose very easily and it's attached to the TV camera so we can see inside your nose while you're talking to me. Now, if I just put this in your nose, you would probably sneeze because it would tickle you, so I'm going to*

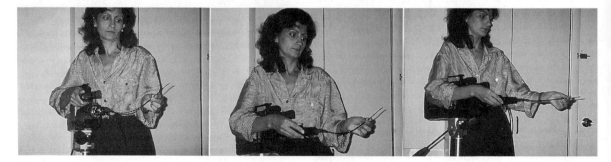

Fig. 11-15 Method of moving a camcorder mounted endoscope. As the tripod mounted camera is swiveled, the tip moves forward.

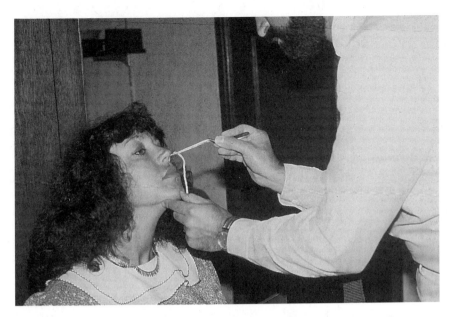

Fig. 11-16 Administration of nasal topical anesthesia on cotton packing.

put a little medicine into your nose that will make it so you won't sneeze. Let me show you the medicine. [The examiner shows the child an atomizer with some blue Pontocaine in it] *See? It looks like a perfume bottle. Does mommy have one like this?* [The examiner squirts a little Pontocaine in the air] *I'm going to squirt some of this blue medicine in your nose. It doesn't sting and it doesn't smell bad. Then I'm going to take a soft piece of cotton* [The examiner shows the child a small piece of cotton packing and rubs it against his hand to show him how soft it is] *and put some of the same medicine on it and put it into your nose with a pair of tweezers.* [The examiner shows the child a pair of small bayonet forceps and touches it to his hand to show him it won't hurt him] *I won't touch you with the tweezers, but I need to use them to put the cotton in your nose because my fingers are too big. OK, first let me spray your nose.* [The examiner sprays very lightly first so that there are no frightening jolts of spray or excessively loud noises] *OK, now I'll do it a few more times, just a little harder.* [The examiner gives the forceps to the child to hold] *Here, you be my assistant. Hold these tweezers for a second.* [The examiner places the cotton packing doused in Pontocaine in the patient's nose and takes the forceps back] *This looks like blue spaghetti, doesn't it? As this goes in your nose, you may feel a slight tickle, kind of like you have to sneeze, but it will stop right away.* [After the cotton is inserted into the nose, the examiner lets the child go into the waiting room to play for 5 minutes and calls him back in for the endoscopic examination] *Let me take the cotton out...you didn't swallow my blue spaghetti, did you? If you did, I'll have to charge you extra. Now we put your nose on TV. I'll tell you what to say. You can watch the whole thing right here on the television. If you feel anything you don't like, just tell me and I'll stop, OK? Remember, I won't hurt you. You may feel like there is something in your nose, but it won't hurt.* [The examination proceeds]

Endoscopic technique

The endoscope is inserted into the larger side of the nose under direct vision. Once the tip of the instrument is in the nostril, the examiner performs the rest of the insertion from the television screen. Basically, maneuvering the endoscope into the nose is like steering a car through a tortuous tunnel with hills, bumps, turns, and narrow passages. The idea is to steer clear of any obstacles and not hit them. The examiner's steering wheel is the control mechanism on the body of the endoscope, and the side-to-side movements are controlled by rotating the body of the scope. The examiner must take special care not to hit the turbinates or nasal septum, because these are the most sensitive areas of the nose.

The most advantageous viewing angle is obtained by passing the endoscope through the middle meatus of the nose (Fig. 11-17). If the endoscope is passed through the inferior meatus, the instrument enters the postnasal space sitting on top of the velum (Fig. 11-18). As the velum elevates, the endoscope will be lifted by

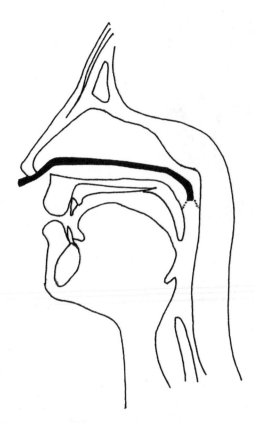

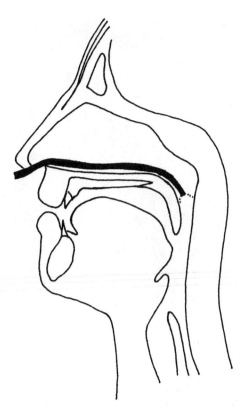

Fig. 11-17 Passing the endoscope through the middle meatus so that the instrument does not rest on the velum and is not moved by the velum during speech.

Fig. 11-18 Passing the endoscope through the inferior meatus so that the instrument is moved during speech as the velum elevates.

the soft palate. The examiner will not notice the movement, but it will be impossible to view the full movements of the velopharyngeal valve as a result. If the endoscope is in the middle meatus, it will be well above the plane of velar motion, and the tip can be flexed downward easily without interfering with the movements of velopharyngeal closure.

Though this superior level of viewing is advantageous, the major advantage of the fiber optic end-viewing nasopharyngoscope is its maneuverability and flexibility. This relates in particular to the previous discussion of velopharyngeal valving as a volumetric phenomenon. When the nasopharyngoscope traverses the choanae and enters the postnasal space, the velum and posterior wall of the nasopharynx can be seen (Fig. 11-19). By rotating the endoscope from side to side, the Eustachian tube orifices can be seen (Fig. 11-20). During speech, the palate will be seen to elevate towards the posterior pharyngeal wall and the lateral pharyngeal walls at the junction of the pharynx and palate will be seen to move medially in many patients. The lateral wall movement at this level represents contractions of the levator. Many examiners make a serious mistake at this point.

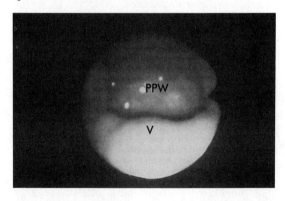

Fig. 11-19 Nasopharynx as viewed by endoscope showing the posterior pharyngeal wall (PPW) and velum (V).

Because they have seen something, they assume they have seen everything. What occurs at this superior level may not fully or accurately represent everything that is occurring in the velopharyngeal valve. As discussed earlier in this chapter, the movements of the velopharyngeal valve occur over a considerable height in the pharynx. If the endoscope is sitting high in the nasopharynx, the full extent of lateral pharyngeal wall motion and/or posterior pha-

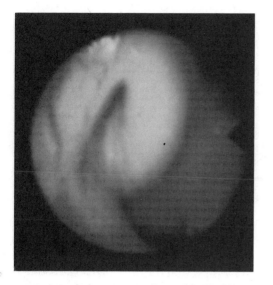

Fig. 11-20 Endoscopic view of a normal Eustachian tube orifice.

ryngeal wall motion may not be seen. This is especially true if there is good motion in the velum. If the velum moves well towards the posterior pharyngeal wall, the movement of the lateral pharyngeal walls and posterior pharyngeal wall (if there is a Passavant's ridge) related to superior constrictor contraction will occur at a point below the narrowing between the soft palate and pharynx. Of course, if there is little or no movement in the velopharyngeal valve during speech, the entire vertical height of the pharynx can be seen if the endoscope is positioned directly above the velopharynx.

In order to utilize an end-viewing flexible endoscope properly, the examiner must maneuver the instrument frequently. In order to see the entire vertical height of the pharynx, the endoscope must be moved in and out of the pharynx to visualize every structure, from the roof of the nasopharynx to the larynx. The instrument must also be moved from side to side if the entire circumference of the pharynx cannot be seen in the field of the endoscope. Figure 11-21 demonstrates the importance of

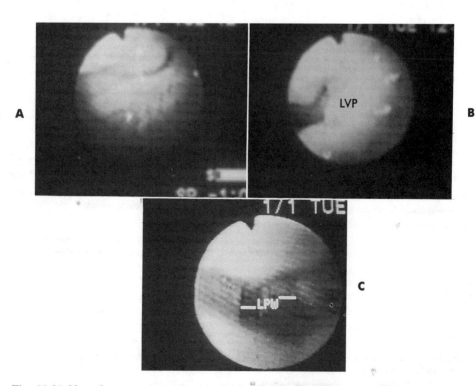

Fig. 11-21 Nasopharyngoscopy of an individual with submucous cleft palate showing two different levels of lateral pharyngeal wall motion. (A) View of the lateral pharyngeal wall at the level above the velum at rest, and (B) during speech showing medial movement of the levator sling (LVP). (C) Lower level of the pharynx beneath the adenoid and levator sling during speech, showing medial motion of the lateral walls (LPW), representing the contraction of the superior constrictor.

this type of maneuverability of the endoscope. This patient was referred for hypernasality with a previously undetected submucous cleft palate. The endoscope was positioned in the nasopharynx after passing through the middle meatus. Focusing on the palate and posterior pharyngeal wall, fair motion can be seen in the lateral pharyngeal walls (Fig. 11-21), which represents the belly of the levator as it enters the velum from the lateral pharyngeal walls (refer back to Fig. 11-5 for the anatomical relationship). The gap appears quite large from this perspective. As the endoscope is passed deeper into the pharynx, a second, more vigorous level of lateral wall motion is seen, which is caused by superior constrictor activity (Fig. 11-21). If the endoscope had not been passed deeper into the pharynx, this more active level of motion would not have been detected. Again, the examiner might have made the mistake of assuming that seeing the movement in the nasopharynx represented everything there was to see. Because many patients with clefts or hypernasality may also have voice disorders (see Chapters 9 and 14), it is important to look at the larynx for pathology. Flexible endoscopy is the ideal opportunity for observing the entire upper airway including the larynx.

The amount of the pharynx seen in the field of view of the endoscope depends in part on how close the tip of the endoscope is to the objective. If the endoscope is far away from the object being observed, more of that object will be seen. However, because a flexible endoscope can be moved easily from place to place in the pharynx, it is less critical to see the entire pharynx in one field of view.

Tonsils and adenoids

It is also extremely important to carefully observe the status of the presence and size of the lymphoid tissue. Though adenoids and tonsils are semantically both lymphoid masses, they are not in the same position and play very different roles in human speech. The adenoids are normally tucked into the posterior corner of the nasopharynx, a centimeter or more behind the posterior border of the nasal septum (vomer), which represents the choanal passage from the nose to the pharynx. The adenoids are an important anatomical feature for the development of normal speech. Several studies have pointed out that the adenoids are the primary site of contact for the velum in essentially all young children (Croft et al., 1981a; Siegel-Sadewitz and Shprintzen, 1986; Williams et al., 1987; Gereau and Shprintzen, 1988) and as such may be an important, if not essential structure

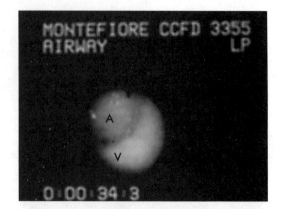

Fig. 11-22 Endoscopic view of adenoids (A) obstructing the choanae above the velum (V).

for learning normal speech. If hypertrophic, the adenoids may extend anteriorly to fill the choanae (Fig. 11-22) and cause denasality during speech. Hyponasality caused by adenoid hypertrophy is easily diagnosed by direct endoscopic observation of the choanae. If the adenoids are obstructing more than 50% of the choanae, the recommendation should be for adenoidectomy. In cases where the adenoids occupy the choanae, speech therapy will have no beneficial effect on decreasing hyponasal resonance.

Tonsils play no role in the development of normal speech. The normal position of the tonsils places them between the faucial pillars, which are in the oral cavity and not the pharyngeal airway (see Fig. 5-6). They are far below the level of velopharyngeal closure. In some cases, the tonsils may intrude into the pharynx if they are excessively large or positioned posterior to their normal placement. In this position, one or more of the following speech symptoms may occur. None are mutually exclusive:

1. Abnormal oral resonance, often referred to as "potato-in-the-mouth" speech pattern. This symptom is caused by a distortion of oral resonance by tonsils sitting in the pharynx, which can dampen the sound that would normally resonate in a larger cavity. This type of pattern may also be called "muffled."

2. Hypernasality and/or nasal emission of air. If the tonsils interfere with any of the component movements of the velopharyngeal valve, VPI will occur. Hypernasality related to tonsillar hypertrophy is often intermittent and variable, and may in part be phonemically influenced because of varying tongue position and varying pha-

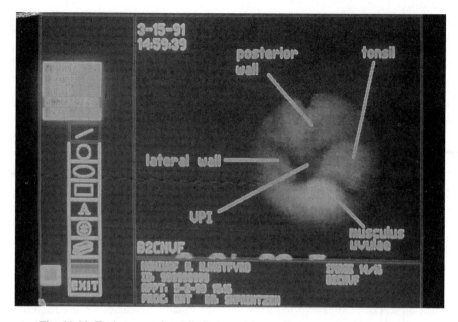

Fig. 11-23 Endoscopy of tonsils intruding abnormally into the nasopharynx.

ryngeal height changes related to resonance change.

3. Hyponasality. As stated above, this is not mutually exclusive of any of the other symptoms. The tonsils may physically obstruct nasal resonance by blocking the postnasal space (Fig. 11-23) yet still cause nasal escape or intermittent hypernasality by interfering with velopharyngeal closure. Mixed hypernasality and hyponasality is not an uncommon finding even in individuals with clefts who have VPI yet also have nasal obstruction secondary to septal deviations.

4. Vowel distortions. Vowel distortions are an unusual speech abnormality and are usually seen in children with dysarthria or other central nervous system impairments. Because vowels rely heavily on oral resonance without the stopping or frication of sound as found in consonants, the tendency for tonsillar hypertrophy to alter oral resonance will affect vowel phonation.

5. Consonant distortions. Individuals with cleft palate have articulatory errors related to tongue backing. In patients with tonsillar hypertrophy, the opposite is seen. Tongue protrusion is often seen in individuals with tonsillar hypertrophy as a maneuver for protecting the airway. In individuals with airway obstruction related to lymphoid tissue hypertrophy, the tongue is usually positioned anteroinferiorly in the mouth to maintain as patent an airway as possible posteriorly.

Nonspeech symptoms such as snoring, obstructive apnea, noisy respiration, stridor, decreased vitality, chronic pharyngitis, chronic postnasal drip, middle ear disease, and difficulty with deglutition (especially swallowing large pieces of difficult-to-chew food) are also common in patients with hypertrophic tonsils.

Though tonsils have been noted to cause velopharyngeal insufficiency (Shprintzen et al., 1987) when they interfere with lateral pharyngeal wall motion or velar elevation (see Fig. 5-8) many clinicians mistakenly warn patients that tonsillectomy will run the risk of prompting hypernasality, especially in individuals with palatal cleft. This is simply an erroneous association between tonsils and adenoids. It is true that adenoidectomy can induce hypernasality in some individuals (Croft et al., 1982), but tonsillectomy does not have the same risk. Tonsillectomy can be done with impunity with regard to speech (assuming an absence of surgical complications), even in individuals with clefts. Adenoids are almost always an asset to normal speech production and are only a liability when they are so large that they occlude the choanae and cause hyponasality. Tonsils are never an asset to normal speech production and are often a liability if hypertrophic, causing abnormal oral resonance or abnormal nasal resonance. Therefore, it is important to observe the placement and size of the tonsils endoscopically. If the symptoms presented by the patient are consistent with tonsillar hypertrophy and endoscopic examination shows tonsils sitting anywhere in the region of velopharyngeal closure, then tonsillectomy is indicated. Tonsillectomy may resolve the resonance and articulation problems caused by hypertrophic tonsils (Shprintzen et al., 1987; MacKenzie-Stepner et al., 1987a).

WHAT ELSE IS SEEN ON ENDOSCOPIC EXAMINATION?

The major advantage of nasopharyngoscopy over other diagnostic techniques is the ability to see internal anatomy directly. This should be of particular importance to surgeons who would want to see their operative field before reconstructive surgery. Therefore, even though the endoscopist is primarily concerned with observing the movements of the velopharyngeal valve during speech, extra care should be taken to notice structural anomalies or variations that could affect diagnosis or treatment.

Palatal morphology

In order to fully appreciate abnormalities of the palate, an understanding of normal endoscopic morphology is important to review. The normal palate is convex with a slight bulge in the midline, which becomes more prominent during speech. The convexity and bulge is caused by the midline mass of the musculus uvulae (Fig. 11-24). The musculus uvulae was once thought to be a vestigial structure in humans, but recent investigations have found it to be an important muscle in speech (Croft et al, 1978, 1981b;

Shprintzen, 1979; Lewin et al., 1980; Shprintzen, 1982; Siegel-Sadewitz and Shprintzen, 1982; Shprintzen et al., 1985). The musculus uvulae has a firm attachment only at its proximal end where it is firmly anchored to the palatal aponeurosis or to the posterior border of the hard palate. Its distal end hangs freely into the tip of the uvula. The musculus uvulae lies over all the other palatal muscles. During speech, the musculus uvulae contracts. Because it has a free end, contraction shortens the length of the muscle, causing it to thicken (Lewin et al., 1980; Croft et al., 1981a). The thickest portion of the muscle lies directly over the levator sling so that as the palate moves posterosuperiorly toward the posterior pharynx, it actually thickens (Croft et al., 1981a), which when seen in lateral view radiographs (Fig. 11-25) looks like a "knee" (sometimes referred to as a genu). This "knee" is labelled by some as the "levator eminence" presumably because the direction of movement follows the vector of the levator pull. However, the eminence on the velum is, in reality, the eminence of the musculus uvulae as it thickens on the nasal surface of the soft palate. Endoscopically, the musculus uvulae is an identifiable landmark, which indicates that the palate is morphologically normal.

Cleft palate, submucous cleft palate, and occult submucous cleft palate

Individuals with clefts of the palate have no identifiable musculus uvulae. As a midline palatal structure, the musculus uvulae is absent in individuals with midline palatal clefts. Individuals with repaired clefts tend to have a concavity or notch in the midline of the palate because of deficient muscle tissue, absence of the musculus uvulae, and contraction along the scar of the repair line (Fig. 11-26). It is common in individuals with repaired clefts to see small

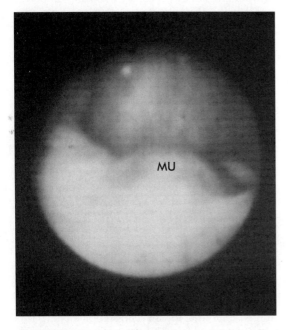

Fig. 11-24 Normal velar endoscopy with musculus uvulae (MU) seen as a convex bulge in the center of the velum.

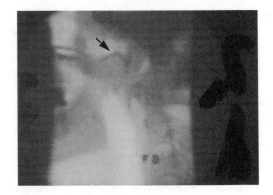

Fig. 11-25 Lateral view fluoroscopic view of the "levator eminence" *(arrow).*

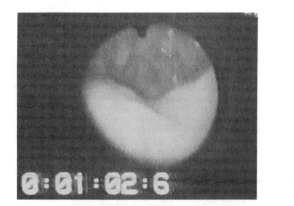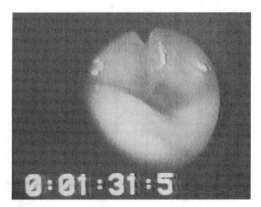

Fig. 11-26 Endoscopic appearance of the concave appearance of a repaired cleft at rest (left) and during speech (right).

midline gaps in the velopharyngeal valve corresponding to the midline deficiency of muscle (Fig. 11-26).

Submucous cleft palate represents a milder expression of overt palatal clefting. The malformation is, in essence, the same as overt clefting, but not as severe. Individuals with submucous cleft palate (see Chapter 1) have midline muscle deficiencies ranging from a complete absence of midline muscle (Fig. 11-27) where a zona pellucida is seen, to a minimally bifid uvula with some degree of midline muscle.

Endoscopic views of submucous cleft palate are quite similar to those seen in individuals with repaired palatal clefts. Rather than the midline convexity seen in normals, there is some degree of midline concavity or notching (Fig. 11-28). With palatal elevation during speech, this notch or concavity may deepen and cause a midline gap in the velopharyngeal valve. Individuals with large adenoids would not have the same risk for VPI even with a submucous cleft because the midline deficiency in the velum could be filled with adenoid tissue after the palate approximated to the adenoid pad (Fig. 11-29). It has been found that the great majority of individuals with submucous cleft palate (which is a very common anomaly in humans) have normal speech and only a slightly increased prevalence of middle ear disease (Schwartz et al., 1985).

Some individuals have hypernasal speech of mysterious origin. They have no obvious stigmata of cleft palate or submucous cleft palate, and no evidence of neurologic or neuromuscular disease. The hypernasality is consistent and does not appear to be a learned error, such as phoneme specific hypernasality. Are there "idiopathic" cases of VPI, or is our ability to detect all etiologies limited? The latter is more likely the case. As more vigorous diagnostic procedures are applied, more "mysterious" cases become clarified and explained. An example of this type of mystery is the *occult submucous cleft palate*. In 1975, Kaplan reported on a number of patients who had hypernasality of unexplained origin. During pharyngeal flap surgery, Kaplan dissected the velum and found that the muscle insertions were abnormal, similar to the type of abnormality found in cleft palate and submucous cleft palate. He labelled this anomaly *occult submucous cleft palate* because it was "mysterious" and because the only way to diagnose it, in his opinion, was palatal dissection at surgery. However, subsequent investigators have reported that individuals with occult submucous cleft have abnormalities on nasopharyngoscopic examination (Croft et al., 1978; Shprintzen, 1979; Lewin et al., 1980; Shprintzen, 1982). It was found that individuals with occult submucous clefts have endoscopic examinations that resemble those seen in individuals with submucous cleft palate (Fig. 11-30). The nasal surface of the velum was found to have a midline concavity, notch, or to be flat with no evidence of a musculus uvulae bulge. Therefore, simply stated, an occult submucous cleft palate is a palate that shows no evidence of abnormality on the oral surface (i.e., no bifid uvula, zona pellucida, muscle separation, or notching of the posterior border of the hard palate), but has anomalies of muscle presence and placement on its nasal surface that can be detected endoscopically. It has been suggested that this anomaly represents the mildest form of clefting (Shprintzen, 1982). The incidence and prevalence of occult submucous cleft palate is unknown because the only cases likely to be detected are those that are symptomatic. Unsymptomatic cases have no detectable anomalies that would lead to further examination.

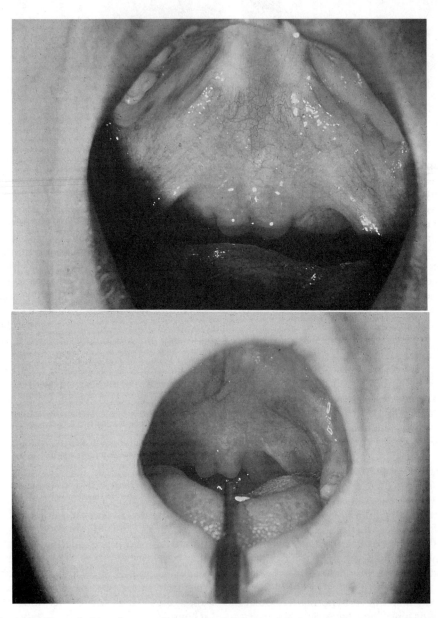

Fig. 11-27 Peroral view of severe (top) and mild (bottom) forms of submucous cleft palate.

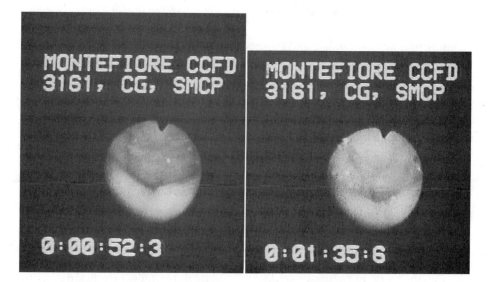

Fig. 11-28 Endoscopic view of submucous cleft palate at rest (left) showing a midline depression in the velum, and during speech (right) showing a small central gap.

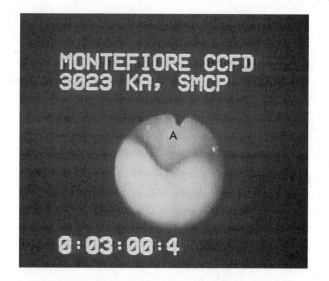

Fig. 11-29 Nasopharyngoscopic view of velopharyngeal closure against the adenoid (A) in an individual with submucous cleft palate.

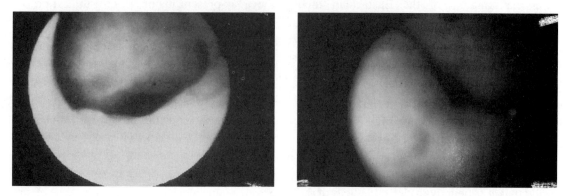

Fig. 11-30 Nasopharyngoscopic view of an occult submucous cleft palate at rest (left) and during speech (right). Note the midline concavity in the velum resulting in a small central gap.

Eustachian tube anomalies and middle ear disease

The association between cleft palate and middle ear disease is a well established one. There is some argument regarding the exact prevalence of middle ear disease in clefting. The publication of a landmark article in 1967 (Stool and Randall, 1967) cited a 94% prevalence of middle ear pathology in infants with clefts (cleft type or distribution was not reported). Paradise et al (1969) found that otitis media was universal in infants with clefts. In another landmark and often cited study, Bluestone (1971) concluded that Eustachian tube dysfunction was responsible for the high frequency of middle ear disease in infants with clefts. Bluestone utilized radiographic studies to determine that obstruction at the nasopharyngeal end of the Eustachian tube was the cause of failure to ventilate the middle ear. Bluestone related this finding to the early study of Rich (1920) who reported that the primary dilator of the Eustachian tube orifice was the tensor veli palatini. Bluestone therefore inferred that the obstruction he observed at the nasopharyngeal lumen of the Eustachian tube was caused by tensor dysfunction related to the cleft disrupting the tensor muscles. However, as pointed out in subsequent investigations (Shprintzen and Croft, 1981; Gereau et al., 1988), Rich's study was a functional anatomy study of dogs, not humans. There are differences in Eustachian tube function between humans and dogs. In any event, because the human tensor does not come into close approximation to the orifice of the Eustachian tube (it comes in contact with the tube closer to the isthmus), obstruction or constriction of the nasopharyngeal lumen of the tube could not be caused by tensor anomalies (Shprintzen and Croft, 1981; Shprintzen, 1982; Gereau et al., 1988). Some investigators have related Eustachian orifice obstruction to structural malformation of the Eustachian tube nasopharyngeal cartilage (Dickson and Dickson, 1972; Dickson, 1976; Maue-Dickson et al, 1976; Shprintzen and Croft, 1981; Shprintzen, 1982; Gereau et al., 1988). Those who cite structural malformation as being responsible for chronic middle ear disease have found reduced size of the nasopharyngeal lumen (Dickson and Dickson, 1972; Dickson, 1976; Maue-Dickson et al, 1976; Shprintzen and Croft, 1981; Shprintzen, 1982) and abnormal position of the orifice and levator muscle (Gereau et al., 1988). In a nasopharyngoscopic study, Gereau et al. (1988) found that in patients with clefts, the belly of the levator muscle elevated to fill the Eustachian orifice, completely blocking it in over 75% of the patients during both speech and swallowing. This phenomenon was not observed in the age and sex-matched normal controls. They concluded that nasopharyngoscopic assessment of Eustachian tube function may provide evidence of obstruction in individuals with clefts.

Recent investigations have also failed to reveal the universal nature of middle ear disease in patients with clefts as cited by Paradise et al. (1969). Gereau et al. (1988) found that middle ear disease was found in less than 80% of individuals with clefts and that there was some variation according to cleft type and syndromic diagnosis. A higher frequency of middle ear disease was found in more severe clefts. This observation is supported by data reported by Schwartz et al. (1985) who found a prevalence of acute otitis media in individuals with submucous cleft palate to be 64%, which was only slightly higher than the 49% frequency found in normal controls. These data reinforce the notion that submucous cleft palate represents a less severe form of the cleft anomaly, including both the prevalence of speech disorders and middle ear disease.

In summary, structural anomalies of the Eustachian tube have been discovered because of the application of nasopharyngoscopy to individuals with clefts. The connection between these structural anomalies and chronic middle ear disease in individuals with clefts is probable and points out the conventional wisdom of treating chronic middle ear disease aggressively with myringotomy and tube drainage, because ventilation by the normal Eustachian tube mechanism is problematic because of malformation.

Vascular anomalies

Recent studies have shown anomalies of the pharyngeal vasculature and have concluded that they may present major risks to surgical procedures for speech improvement. MacKenzie-Stepner et al. (1987b) reported on medial displacement and ectopic position of the internal carotid arteries in patients with velo-cardio-facial syndrome. Pulsations in the posterior pharyngeal wall were first noticed during nasopharyngoscopic examination of patients with velo-cardio-facial syndrome, which led the authors to perform angiography and CT angiography. They found internal carotid arteries in several patients that could have been in the operative field for pharyngeal flap surgery. Severing an internal carotid artery, one of the major vessels supplying blood to the brain, should obviously be avoided. In a subsequent study reviewing a larger number of patients with velo-cardio-facial syndrome with magnetic resonance angiography, Mitnick et al. (1995) found other anomalies of the pharyngeal vasculature, including anomalous vertebral arteries, hypoplastic arteries, and supernumerary arteries. As in the study of MacKenzie et al. (1987b), it was the endoscopic observation of pulsations of the posterior pharyngeal wall that led to the identification of the possibility of vascular anomalies in this group of patients. Similar pulsations have not yet been reported in conditions other than velo-cardio-facial syndrome, but clinical observation at this author's center has shown the same phenomenon in a small number of patients with clefts. Because the finding may not be syndrome specific, it is important for clinicians to endoscope every patient being considered for pharyngeal surgery to avoid the potentially disastrous complication of injuring major neck vessels.

MULTI-VIEW VIDEOFLUOROSCOPY

The use of motion pictures to study the movements of the velopharyngeal valve were first reported in 1930, initially as a method of studying swallowing (Barclay, 1930). The procedure was subsequently applied to speech during the next decade (Harrington, 1944). These studies were limited to the lateral view (midsagittal). In cineradiography, usually 16 to 24 frames of motion picture film are exposed every second. This procedure requires high doses of radiation, and the accuracy of the exposures cannot be monitored during the procedure. If studies are either overexposed or underexposed, it will not be known until after the film is developed. The procedure eventually changed so that rather than exposing individual film frames as separate radiographic pictures, the patient was fluoroscoped using an image intensifier and motion picture film that was shot from the fluoroscopic screen, hence the name cinefluoroscopy. Though cinefluoroscopy involved much less radiation than cineradiography, the dose was still high in comparison to other radiographic procedures. Furthermore, if the film were improperly exposed or processed, the image could not be retrieved.

With the advent of reliable and inexpensive videotape equipment, videofluoroscopy became the technique of choice for recording motion pictures. Videotape requires much less intensity of the fluoroscopic image for an adequate recording so that the total radiation would be much less than with filmed procedures (Isberg

et al, 1989). The low dosage offered by videofluoroscopy became even more pertinent when multiple views for studying velopharyngeal valving were introduced (Astley, 1958; Skolnick, 1969, 1970). Instant playback is an important and useful component of video recordings, as is freeze-frame, slow motion, frame-by-frame review, and 60 scan (the equivalent of frames) per second speed, which is far superior to motion picture film. Because the videotape recorder captures the image directly from the fluoroscopic table's television system, whatever is seen at the time of the study is being recorded in exactly that manner on the videotape.

In order to fully assess all components of velopharyngeal closure, Skolnick described the use of serial multiple radiographic views including the lateral, frontal, and base projections (Skolnick, 1969, 1970; Skolnick et al, 1973). Other views have been recommended since Skolnick's original papers, including the Towne's view, submentovertical, and oblique views. Though each individual view shows a different aspect of velopharyngeal function, the length of the fluoroscopic examination must be kept short in order to limit radiation exposure (Isberg et al, 1989). An International Working Group meeting in New York in 1989 recommended the use of at least two views for all cases: frontal and lateral. An "en face" view (base or Towne) may be added along with oblique projections in cases of asymmetry. The technique, advantages, and disadvantages of each projection are discussed later.

Who should be examined?

Because fluoroscopic assessment involves the use of ionizing radiation, it is recommended that any single patient not have more than one fluoroscopic examination unless repeat studies are absolutely critical to treatment planning. Nasopharyngoscopy can and should be used to supplement and enhance the data gathered from radiographic studies, especially when repeated examinations are necessary. However, as will be shown below and in Chapter 12, videofluoroscopic study in multiple views is absolutely essential to gathering information critical to making decisions about treatment. Because it is important to limit radiation exposure yet critical to perform multi-view videofluoroscopy, one must carefully consider the ideal time to schedule the examination and who should be examined. Parameters to be considered include the consistency of VPI, the status of articulation, the patient's age, and the timing of proposed treatments.

Consistency of VPI. As discussed in other chapters in this text (see Chapters 8, 10, 12, 16, and 17), not all dysfunction in the velopharyngeal valve implies an anatomical or physiological disorder that requires physical management. There are instances of inconsistent dysfunction (such as sound-specific VPI), which may be learned or tied to specific types of articulatory errors and are amenable to resolution with speech therapy. These types of problems should be easily recognized by a thorough clinical examination by the speech pathologist. If there is any question of the consistency of the VPI, nasopharyngoscopy should be scheduled before multi-view videofluoroscopy. If nasopharyngoscopy shows inconsistent velopharyngeal closure, then speech therapy should be scheduled immediately and videofluoroscopy deferred. After an appropriate period of therapy, nasopharyngoscopy should be repeated. Fluoroscopic examination should be reserved for patients who are not succeeding in therapy if an anatomical or physiological abnormality is suspected. If nasopharyngoscopy shows inconsistency in velopharyngeal valving, but no closure, multi-view videofluoroscopy may prove useful in determining the physiological nature of the variation and be useful in recommending treatment (especially if some type of physical management is being considered).

Status of articulation. There is a direct correlation between articulation and velopharyngeal valving. The correlation represents a bidirectional cause-and-effect relationship (see Chapters 8, 9, and 14). In one direction, individuals with velopharyngeal insufficiency, especially related to cleft palate, develop glottal stops and other "compensatory" articulation substitutions in an attempt to make intelligible consonant sounds. In the other direction, it has been shown that children with glottal stop substitutions develop gross VPI. Because articulation occurs at the glottis, which is below the level of the velopharyngeal valve, there is no reason for the VP valve to move. Therefore, the palate and lateral pharyngeal walls cease to function during speech. It has also been shown that in children who have some normal articulation and some glottal stop substitutions, the velopharyngeal valve functions well during normal placement and production, but is grossly incompetent during glottal stop substitutions (Henningson and Isberg, 1987; Hoch et al., 1987). Because of the nearly 1:1 correlation of glottal stops and gross VPI, it makes little sense to expose patients to radiation to observe an already predictable outcome. Also, it is not recom-

mended that patients with severely abnormal articulation have surgery to resolve their VPI. Because speech therapy (with or without speech bulb reduction as outlined in Chapter 16) may initiate marked movement in the velopharyngeal valve, which is not present during glottal articulation, it is important to resolve the articulatory status first to activate the valve and reduce the severity of VPI (see Chapter 14).

Age. Though some centers will perform pharyngoplasty at the first possible sign that there is VPI (Reath et al., 1987), it is strongly recommended that such surgery be deferred until language acquisition is complete and articulatory skills are more mature (at approximately 4.5 years of age). We have found marked improvement in velopharyngeal valving when VPI and articulatory errors are identified early and treated directly with speech therapy (see Chapter 14). Therefore, videofluoroscopic exposure should be deferred until surgery is either imminent or the patient is over 4 years of age (if articulation is not severely impaired). Fluoroscopic examinations performed earlier than this will probably not be successful in obtaining an indicative speech sample from the child, and early velopharyngeal valving efforts may not reflect the true physiologic capacity of the child.

Timing of treatments. If physical management of VPI is going to be deferred, it is recommended that videofluoroscopic examination be held off until treatment is imminent in order to minimize radiation exposure. The information provided by multi-view videofluoroscopy is considered critical to the successful management of VPI. Therefore, the information obtained from the study should be as relevant and close in time as possible to the actual treatment. Surgeons should not have to rely on one- or two-year-old studies to plan a surgical procedure.

FLUORSCOPIC TECHNIQUE

Videofluoroscopy can be performed in any fluoroscopic unit equipped with a television system. The only other necessary equipment is some barium contrast and a dropper (pipette). Because the fluoroscopic procedure is designed to assess the movements of the soft tissues of the pharynx, which are not clearly visible under radiographic assessment, it is necessary to coat the pharynx with barium, which is opaque to ionizing radiation.

Barium coating of the pharynx

In his original publication, Skolnick recommended instilling barium into the nose using a syringe tipped with a rubber catheter, which was passed deeply into the nose past the turbinates. A barium suspension mixed to the consistency of cream was injected through the catheter, which then coated the lateral pharyngeal walls and the nasal surface of the velum.

At our center, we have found that it is easier and less traumatic to the patient to utilize a simple dropper or pipette to administer the barium. We prefer to use flavored barium sulfate powder mixed with warm tap water to the consistency of cream (in other words, a thick, but easy flowing liquid). We use a dosage dropper, such as that used to administer medicine to young children or infants. This dropper is fairly large. The tip is rounded and fits snugly in most nostrils. Using the dropper, approximately 1 ml of barium is squirted into each nostril with the patient in a supine position (Fig. 11-31). In the past, we had recommended telling the child ahead of the procedure exactly what was going to be done. If there were an adverse reaction to the explanation, we would send a dropper home with the parents and instruct them how to behaviorally desensitize their child. After doing this for a year, we actually found our compliance rate getting poorer. It is probable that the child thought that if we were taking so much time to explain this procedure that it must be pretty awful. We therefore ceased telling the patients anything until the procedure was being done. At that time, all would be explained just before the procedure. The patient is simply instructed to lie down on the fluoroscopic table, and the barium is put in the nose as quickly as possible. Though some young children may cry initially, when they realize it did not hurt and that the barium has a pleasant taste, they stop. In the past 20 years, having done thousands of studies in this manner, there has been only one noncompliant patient (a 4-year-old who simply would not talk).

Fluoroscopic views

The number of possible angles that can be utilized to observe the velopharyngeal valve is literally infinite depending on the angle and direction from which the x-ray beam is directed. In order to determine which views should be used in any particular case, the clinicians must determine what type of information is necessary in order to fully diagnose and treat the patient. In general, at least the following basic types of information are important to obtain in the study:

Lateral pharyngeal wall movement and position
— The success or failure of both pharyngoplasty and speech bulb placement is most dependent on the amount of movement in the lateral pharyngeal walls. There is also diagnostic significance to both the amount

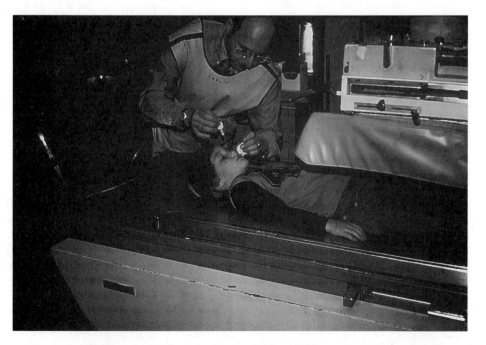

Fig. 11-31 Instilling barium into the nose prior to videofluoroscopy using a dropper.

of movement and the symmetry of movement. For example, absent movement indicative of a hypotonic pharynx is very common in velo-cardio-facial syndrome. Asymmetric motion is common in oculo-auriculo-vertebral dysplasia (hemifacial microsomia). The position of the lateral pharyngeal walls is also important with respect to the distance between them at rest. There are some disorders associated with an extremely narrow pharynx, which may be at high risk for the development of postoperative apnea following pharyngoplasty (Shprintzen, 1985).

Velar movement and structure — The amount of elevation and posterior movement of the soft palate is of obvious importance to understanding the function of the velopharyngeal valve. The vector of movement may point toward abnormality of muscle position. The amount of movement relative to the posterior pharyngeal wall can indicate if there are any restrictions on palatal mobility from previous operations or congenital disorders. The length of the palate relative to the depth of the nasopharynx should also be assessed. Structurally, the thickness of the palate at rest compared to its thickness during speech should be assessed. The presence of a normal musculus uvulae will result in increased thickness of the velum during phonation. Individuals with repaired palatal clefts or submucous clefts will not show an increase in thickness of the velum during speech.

Posterior pharyngeal wall movement and structure — The presence or absence of a Passavant's ridge should be assessed. Structurally, the relative size and position of the adenoid mass, especially in relation to the movement of the velum, must be noted.

Tongue movement and position — Many individuals with VPI attempt to valve the velopharyngeal port by thrusting the back of the tongue against the velum and lifting it into the nasopharynx (Fig. 11-32). This compensatory movement cannot be seen during nasopharyngoscopic examination because the tongue is below the palate and hidden by it from the view of the endoscope. The movement of the tongue during articulated sounds can be correlated to the process of velopharyngeal valving to determine if there are any relationships between oral articulation and velopharyngeal function. The position of the tongue during individual sounds will reveal the occurrence of tongue backing (see Chapter 14), which can result in acoustical alterations of consonant production.

In order to observe lateral pharyngeal wall motion, velar motion, posterior wall motion, and tongue position and movement, only two views would be necessary: frontal (P-A) and lateral. Other radiographic views would not provide information regarding the four basic requirements of videofluoroscopy and should therefore be used only to supplement the frontal and lateral views and not in their stead.

The currently used radiographic views and their relative value are detailed in the following section. It is recommended that any fluoroscopic examination be limited to two minutes or less and that a set speech sample be utilized, which will cover as many phonemic contexts as possible.

Starting the examination

The first step is, as in nasopharyngoscopy, to assure the patient that the examination will not hurt. Explain the equipment briefly to the patient so they understand that it cannot hurt

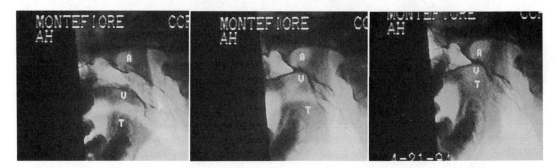

Fig. 11-32 Lateral view fluoroscopy showing the tongue pushing palate upward during speech.

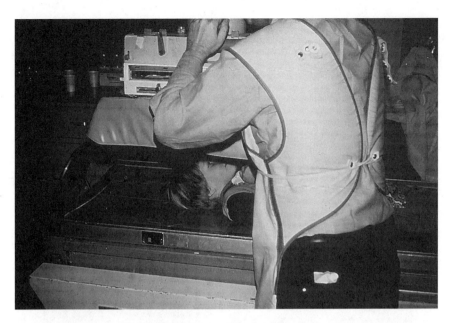

Fig. 11-33 Patient supine for frontal view.

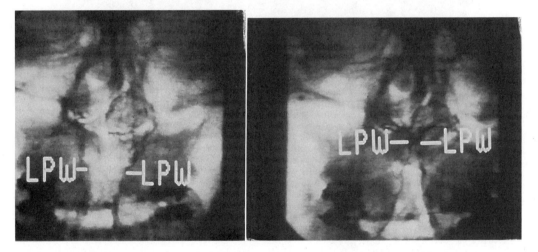

Fig. 11-34 Frontal view fluoroscopy, at rest (left) and during speech (right).

them. Put the patient on the horizontal fluoroscopic table and apply the proper shielding (Isberg et al., 1989). Review the speech sample and practice it, especially with very young children. It would be unacceptable to keep a patient under radiation exposure without obtaining an adequate speech sample for analysis. Therefore, it is important to let the patient know exactly what he or she should say when given the prompt. After rehearsing the speech sample, the barium should be instilled through both nostrils as described above with the patient supine.

Frontal view

Leaving the patient supine, the image intensifier can be passed directly over the patient's face (Fig. 11-33), which will provide the frontal view (also known as the P-A, or postero-anterior view). The X-ray beam comes up from the table and is registered by the image intensifier above the patient's face. It is preferable to leave the patient supine because the barium instilled into the patient's nose will remain pooled in the pharynx, thus providing the best possible coat. No difference has been found in lateral wall motion when patients are supine versus standing. With a good barium coat on the lateral walls, the medial movement of the lateral walls can be easily visualized (Fig. 11-34). The field of exposure should be kept wide enough to view both lateral pharyngeal walls, but well confined enough to prevent exposure of the entire neck.

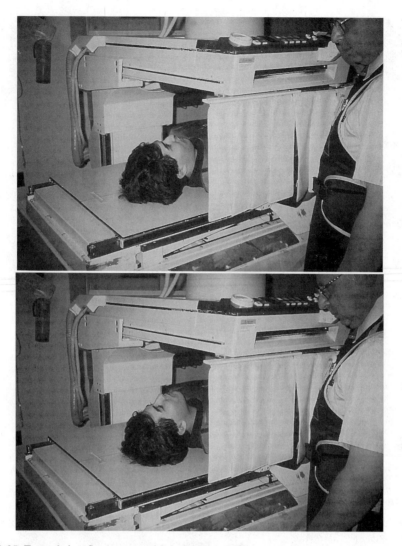

Fig. 11-35 Frontal view fluoroscopy with head horizontal so that the lateral walls are obscured by the palate (top), versus having the chin elevated (bottom) which makes the lateral walls easier to see.

If the barium coat is thick, it is often possible to see the superior surface of the velum elevating between the lateral pharyngeal walls. Also, if the tonsils are positioned posteriorly in the pharynx, barium will coat the posterior aspect of the tonsils and permit them to be seen in the fluoroscopic field. If the tonsils are visualized in frontal view fluoroscopy, it is likely that they are excessively large or abnormally positioned and require tonsillectomy.

Depending on the width of the pharynx, it may be necessary to tilt the head slightly in order to get an adequate frontal view (Fig. 11-35). When the lateral pharyngeal walls are widely spaced and the palate is parallel to the x-ray beam, they may be hidden by the tuberosities of the maxilla, which are densely radio-opaque. By tilting the head up (lifting the chin), the angle of the x-ray beam will be obliquely oriented in relation to the lateral walls and maxilla so that the pharynx will not be obscured.

Lateral view

The fluoroscopic table is then positioned vertically and the patient stands or sits with the midsagittal plane perpendicular to the x-ray beam (Fig. 11-36). The same speech sample is repeated. The field of exposure should avoid the thyroid gland, but it should be extended forward to see the tongue, teeth, and lips. In the lateral

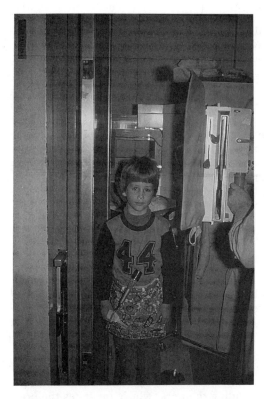

Fig. 11-36 Patient position for lateral view.

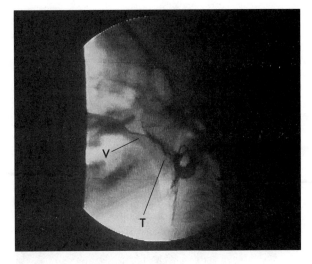

Fig. 11-37 Tonsils (T) posteriorly positioned in the pharynx posterior to the velum (V) as seen in lateral view fluoroscopy during speech.

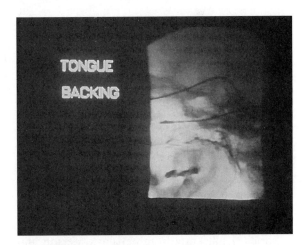

Fig. 11-38 Lateral view fluoroscopy showing "tongue backing" behind a fistula.

view, the velum, posterior pharyngeal wall, and tongue are easily seen. The use of barium contrast is particularly helpful in defining small gaps in the valve. In cases of small gaps, without contrast, if the palate comes close to the posterior pharyngeal wall, the shadows from each structure may blend together to make it appear as if the two structures are in approximation. With a barium coat, if there is an insufficiency, air bubbles will be seen in the barium, signalling an air leak through the valve.

The barium coat will also allow the tonsils to be visualized if they are positioned posteriorly in the airway (Fig. 11-37). In this projection, it can be determined if the tonsils are interfering with velopharyngeal closure, or if they are in a position dangerous to airway maintenance.

Viewing the articulators in lateral view is very important to understanding the scope of the speech problems related to VPI. For example, in the presence of an oronasal fistula, adjustments in tongue position can be seen and understood in lateral view. Fig. 11-38 shows a lateral view videofluoroscopic study of a patient with a fistula at the junction of the hard and soft palate. The frame shown in Fig. 11-38 is during phonation of the /t/ sound in the word *two* during counting. Note that rather than making

lingua-alveolar contact, the dorsum of the tongue is contacting the middle of the palate in its mid-dorsal segment. This articulatory adjustment cannot be seen at all in nasopharyngoscopy, or any other diagnostic technique for that matter.

Base view

In one of his initial reports on multi-view videofluoroscopy, Skolnick described the use of the base view, which he described as an "en face" view of the pharynx (Skolnick, 1970). In essence, the base view is an axial, or transverse view of the pharynx (Fig. 11-39). The x-ray beam is oriented vertically through the pharynx by placing the patient in a sphinx-like, slightly

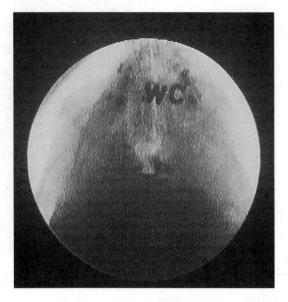

Fig. 11-39 Base view fluoroscopy.

hyperextended position on the fluoroscopic table (Fig. 11-40). Many clinicians have found the base view an appealing view of the velopharyngeal mechanism without really recognizing its drawbacks and difficulties. Furthermore, if nasopharyngoscopy is being performed for the same patient, the endoscope provides a better "en face" view than the fluoroscopic procedure. Therefore, the base view becomes unnecessary in patients for whom nasopharyngoscopy is also obtained.

There are several problems with the base view. First, positioning the patient for the base view is difficult because pharyngeal angulation varies significantly from person to person and with age (Siegel-Sadewitz and Shprintzen, 1986). In young children, velopharyngeal closure occurs between the velum and adenoid so that the point of contact is well anterior to the posterior pharyngeal wall (Fig. 11-41). Lateral pharyngeal wall motion occurs in the "dead space" behind the velum and adenoid (Siegel-Sadewitz and Shprintzen, 1986). Therefore, velopharyngeal closure is happening in several different locations and at different vertical levels. In the base view, vertical levels of the pharynx are superimposed one over the other. If motion is seen, it is difficult to interpret at which vertical level that movement is occurring. Fig. 11-42 shows a diagram of a frontal view and base view in the same patient. The frontal view shows that the lateral walls are moving at two different vertical planes, which resulted in an insufficiency. However, the base view shows closure

because the higher plane of movement (which is also more vigorous) occurs above the level of the movement of the opposite lateral wall. If the lateral view provides all the information necessary regarding palatal, tongue, and posterior wall motion, and frontal view provides all necessary information regarding lateral pharyngeal wall motion, does the base view provide any information worth the radiation exposure to the patient? Probably not. However, following pharyngeal flap surgery, base view does become an important radiographic projection. Because the pharyngeal flap is oriented horizontally in the pharyngeal airway, an axial or transverse view will accurately represent what is occurring to the lateral ports at the level of the flap (Fig. 11-43).

Another potential problem with the base view is that placing the patient in a hyperextended position may alter the movements of the velopharyngeal valve. Hyperextension has been noted to create small gaps in the velopharyngeal valve that were not present in the neutral head position (McWilliams and Musgrave, 1968). It has been hypothesized that patients with marginal velopharyngeal closure may develop insufficiencies when the mechanism is stressed by extending the neck, which angulates the posterior wall away from the velum.

Towne's view

Some clinicians have advocated the Towne's view as a replacement for the base view (Stringer and Witzel, 1986), especially in cases where adenoids are present and change the angulation of closure within the nasopharynx (Fig. 11-44). In Towne's view, the patient is positioned either erect or supine and the head is deflected downward, with the chin closer to the chest (Fig. 11-45). At present, the effect of head position on Towne's view is not well understood. More importantly, however, is the same argument as presented for base view. Because it is advocated that all patients have both nasopharyngoscopy and multi-view videofluoroscopy (Golding-Kushner et al., 1990), and endoscopic views duplicate the Towne's view, it may be better to avoid the extra radiation exposure.

Oblique views

Over 15% of patients with velopharyngeal insufficiency have asymmetric velopharyngeal closure (Argamaso et al, 1994; D'Antonio et al., 1988). Oblique views may be utilized to observe the velopharyngeal sphincter from two aspects, which permit observation of the interaction between the lateral pharyngeal wall and edge of

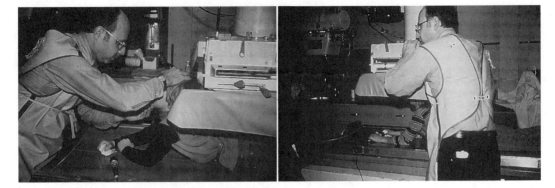

Fig. 11-40 Positioning a patient for base view.

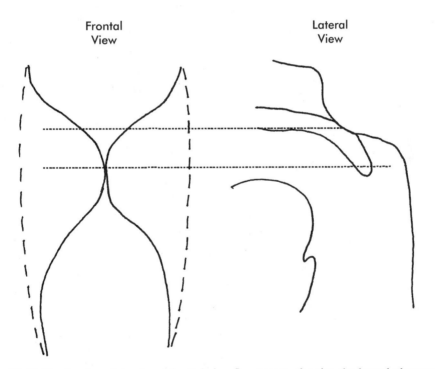

Fig. 11-41 Tracing from lateral and frontal view fluoroscopy showing the lateral pharyngeal walls moving behind the velum in the "dead space" created by velar-adenoidal contact.

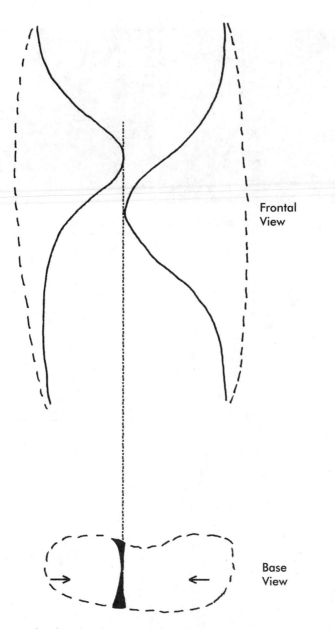

Fig. 11-42 Diagram showing that in frontal view, there are two vertical levels of lateral pharyngeal wall motion which is not perceived in base view where there appears to be contact of the lateral walls.

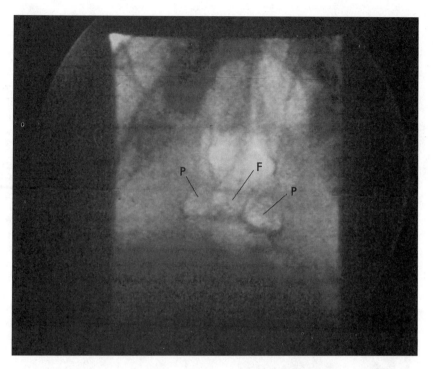

Fig. 11-43 Base view of pharyngeal flap (F) with large lateral ports (P).

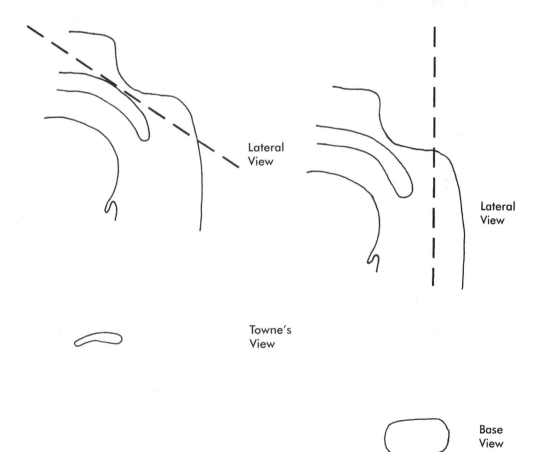

Fig. 11-44 Towne's view angulation (left, A) which for this type of velar-adenoidal closure shows a more accurate representation of the degree of closure than the base view (right, B).

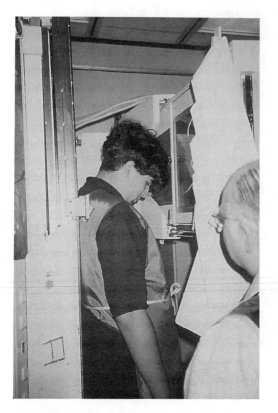

Fig. 11-45 Patient position for Towne's view.

the velum on the same side (Fig. 11-46). To obtain oblique projections, the patient is turned approximately halfway between the position for a lateral and frontal view (Fig. 11-47). Oblique projections can be difficult to interpret because of the superimposition of multiple structures over the field of interest. However, brief samples obtained in oblique projection with a good barium coat may be useful in determining the extent of asymmetry and unilateral insufficiency, especially in disorders where there is marked asymmetry, such as oculo-auriculo-vertebral dysplasia (Shprintzen et al, 1980). While it is true that the frontal view will show asymmetry in lateral wall movement, it does not show asymmetry well. Experienced clinicians will be able to see asymmetry in palatal movement by seeing a double barium line in the velum in lateral projection (Fig. 11-48), but the side of the poorer movement cannot be determined because one side is superimposed over the other. Oblique projections will help to define the source of velar asymmetry.

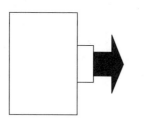

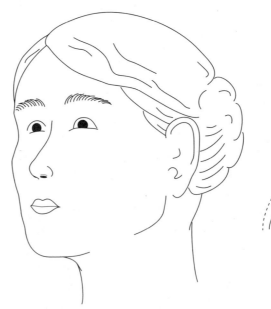

Fig. 11-46 Oblique projection.

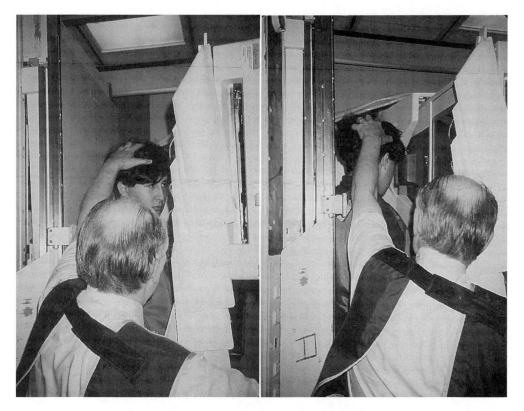

Fig. 11-47 Position for oblique projection.

SPEECH SAMPLE FOR NASOPHARYNGOSCOPY AND MULTI-VIEW VIDEOFLUOROSCOPY

In radiographic procedures, studies must be kept short to limit exposure to ionizing radiation. Nasopharyngoscopic studies can be prolonged to include a more varied and extensive speech sample. However, it is essential to utilize at least some common utterances for both studies for the sake of comparison. All phonemic contexts should be explored, but certain minimum requirements should be included in the studies. The following types of speech samples have been recommended by an International Working Group (Golding-Kushner et al., 1990) and should be obtained:

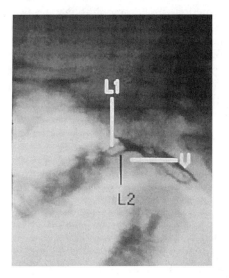

Fig. 11-48 Lateral view videofluoroscopy showing a double barium line along the nasal surface of the velum.

Repetitions of at least four different consonant-vowel combinations, including both nasal and non-nasal utterances. Both high and low vowels should be used. An example would be /ma-ma-ma/, /pa-pa-pa/, /ta-ta-ta/, /ka-ka-ka/, /mi-mi-mi/, /pi-pi-pi/, /ti-ti-ti/, /ki-ki-ki/.

Production of at least two sustained fricatives (preferably both voiceless and voiced) such as /sssss/, /fffff/, /zzzzz/, and /vvvvv/. This is an extremely important sample. Experience has shown that if phoneme-specific closure occurs, it is an extremely important prognostic finding for successfully resolving VPI with speech therapy alone, or speech bulb reduction (see chapters 14 and 16).

Phrases involving connected speech with varying phonemic contexts. Prepared phrases such as "stop the bus," "catch a fish," "Gerry's slippers" and others may be used. Counting to 10 (i.e., 1-2-3-4-5-6-7-8-9-10) is very useful as a way of getting a varied phonemic sample with nasal to non-nasal transitions and voiced-voiceless transitions.

Using this type of sample can be done while limiting fluoroscopic examinations to under 2 minutes, even using three views.

Nasopharyngoscopy can be done for several minutes so that there are essentially no limits on the ability to vary the speech sample. In cases where some variability has been noted, it is suggested that the clinician try to manipulate the speech sample to get the best possible idea of the potential in the valve for closure. Whispering is one stimulus that might be applied because it removes the voicing component, and it has been noted that some patients show much better movement of the valve while whispering.

The extended time available during nasopharyngoscopy also allows the clinician to vary the examination by closing fistulae, if present, with some chewing gum. Patients with speech bulb appliances can be examined with the appliance both in and out of the mouth. In other words, the endoscopic examination should be used to its maximum potential by using the additional time available for experimentation with speech production and stimulability.

REVIEWING STUDIES AND REPORTING RESULTS

To date, there has been no uniform agreement on how nasopharyngoscopic and videofluoroscopic studies should be reviewed and reported. D'Antonio et al (1989) found that group reviews of endoscopic studies were the most reliable way to report the results of such studies. The value of having multiple individuals from a variety of disciplines discuss and approach the studies from different bases of knowledge is a valuable mechanism for ensuring that every detail of the studies is reported.

Golding-Kushner et al. (1990) reported on the results of an International Working Group, which convened to implement some type of standardized procedure for the analysis and reporting of both nasopharyngoscopy and multi-view videofluoroscopy. The system devised a ratio system that rated each component of velopharyngeal closure separately. This procedure holds promise and has been found to be a reliable system in clinical application. Agreement on this type of system will need to wait until there are additional validation studies in the future.

WHY BOTH PROCEDURES?

One outcome of the International Working Group's report was the strong recommendation that all patients with VPI be studied with both multi-view videofluoroscopy and nasopharyngoscopy. In an earlier report, Shprintzen (1987) indicated a 30% rate of disagreement between endoscopic and fluoroscopic studies. The disagreement is attributed to the different kinds of information provided by each examination and the limitations of each. Nasopharyngoscopy is the best procedure for obtaining information about structure. Function can also be observed, but there are limitations on the observation of some of the movements. The tongue cannot be seen articulating except at its very posterior end, and lateral wall motion may often be obscured by other structures such as the velum. Compliance may be a problem in young children, and there is the risk of some discomfort. Videofluoroscopy provides the best information regarding the function of the velopharyngeal valve over the entire vertical and horizontal area of the pharynx. Compliance is excellent and there is no discomfort. However, structure is difficult to interpret, and the patient must be exposed to ionizing radiation. Utilizing the two procedures together overcomes the weaknesses of each while enhancing the strengths of both.

REFERENCES

Argamaso RV, Levandowski GT, Golding-Kushner KJ, Shprintzen RJ: Treatment of asymmetric velopharyngeal insufficiency with skewed pharyngeal flap, *Cleft Palate-Craniofacial J* 31:287-294, 1994.

Astley R: The movements of the lateral walls of the nasopharynx: a cineradiographic study, *J Laryngol Otol* 72:325-328, 1958.

Barclay AE: The normal mechanism of swallowing, *Br J Radiol* 3:534-546, 1930.

Bluestone CD: Eustachian tube obstruction in the infant with cleft palate, *Ann Otol Rhinol Laryngol* (St. Louis), 80 (suppl. 2):1-30, 1971.

Croft CB, Shprintzen RJ, Ruben RJ: Hypernasal speech following adenotonsillectomy. *Otolaryngol Head Neck Surg,* 89:179-188, 1981a.

Croft CB, Shprintzen RJ, Daniller AI, Lewin ML: The occult submucous cleft palate and the musculus uvuli, *Cleft Palate J,* 15:150-154, 1978.

Croft CB, Shprintzen RJ, Rakoff SJ: Patterns of velopharyngeal valving in normal and cleft palate subjects: a multi-view videofluoroscopic and nasendoscopic study, *Laryngoscope,* 91:265-271, 1981b.

D'Antonio L, Marsh JL, Province M, Muntz H, Phillips C: Reliability of flexible fiberoptic nasopharyngoscopy for evaluation of velopharyngeal function in a clinical population, *Cleft Palate J* 26:217-225, 1989.

D'Antonio LL, Muntz HR, Marsh JL, Marty-Grames L, Backensto-Marsh R: Practical application of flexible fiberoptic nasopharyngoscopy for evaluating velopharyngeal function, *Plast Reconstr Surg* 82:611-618, 1988.

Dickson DR: Anatomy of the normal and cleft palate Eustachian tube. *Ann Otol Rhinol Laryngol* (St. Louis) 85(suppl. 25):25-29, 1976.

Dickson DR, Dickson WM: Velopharyngeal anatomy, *J Speech Hear Res* 15:372-381, 1972.

Gereau SA, Shprintzen RJ. The role of adenoids in the development of normal speech following palate repair, *Laryngoscope* 98:99-303, 1988.

Gereau SA, Stevens D, Bassila M, Sher AE, Sidoti EJ Jr, Morgan M, Oka SW, Shprintzen RJ: Endoscopic observations of Eustachian tube abnormalities in Children with palatal clefts. In Lim DJ, Bluestone CD, Klein JO, and Nelson JD, editors: *Symposium on otitis media.* Toronto, 1988, B.C. Decker. pp. 60-63.

Golding-Kushner KJ et al: Standardization for the reporting of nasopharyngoscopy and multi-view videofluoroscopy: a report from an international working group. *Cleft Palate J* 27:337-347, 1990.

Harrington R: (1944). A study of the mechanism of velopharyngeal closure, *J Speech Hear Dis* 9:325-345, 1944.

Henningsson G, Isberg A: Velopharyngeal movements in patients alternating between oral and glottal articulation: a clinical and cineradiographical study, *Cleft Palate J* 23:1-9, 1986.

Hilton W: Case of a large bony tumour in the face completely removed by spontaneous separation. Observations upon some of the functions of the soft palate and pharynx, *Guys Hosp Rep* 1:493-506, 1836.

Hoch L: Golding-Kushner KJ, Sadewitz V, and Shprintzen RJ. Speech Therapy. In McWilliams BJ, editor: *Seminars in speech and language: current methods of assessing and treating children with cleft palates,* New York, 1986, Thieme Inc.

Isberg A, Julin I, Kraepelien T, Henrikson CO: Absorbed doses and energy imparted from radiographic examination of velopharyngeal function during speech, *Cleft Palate J* 26:105-109, 1989.

Kaplan EN: The occult submucous cleft palate, *Cleft Palate J* 12:356-368, 1975.

Lewin ML, Croft CB, Shprintzen RJ: Velopharyngeal insufficiency due to hypoplasia of the musculus uvulae and occult submucous cleft palate, *Plast Reconstr Surg,* 65:585-591, 1980.

MacKenzie-Stepner K, Witzel MA, Stringer DA, Lindsay WK, Munro IR, Hughs H: Velopharyngeal insufficiency due to hypertrophic tonsils. A report of two cases, *Int J Pediatr Otorhinolaryngol* 14:57-63, 1987a.

MacKenzie-Stepner K, Witzel MA, Stringer DA, Lindsay WK, Munro IR, Hughs H: Abnormal carotid arteries in the velocardiofacial syndrome: a report of three cases, *Plast Reconstr Surg* 80:347-351, 1987b.

Maue-Dickson W, Dickson DR, Rood SR: Anatomy of the Eustachian tube and related structures in age-matched human fetuses with and without cleft palate, *Trans Am Acad Ophthal Otolaryngol,* 82:159-163, 1976.

McWilliams BJ, Musgrave RH: The influence of head position upon velopharyngeal closure, *Cleft Palate J* 5:117-124, 1968.

Moll KL: Cinefluorographic techniques in speech research, *J Speech Hear Res* 3:227-241, 1960.

Paradise JL, Bluestone CD, Felder H. The universality of otitis media in 50 infants with cleft palate, *Pediatrics* 44:35-42, 1969.

Pigott RW: The nasendoscopic appearance of the normal palatopharyngeal valve, *Plast Reconstr Surg* 43:19-24, 1969.

Pigott RW, Makepeace AP. Some characteristics of endoscopic and radiological systems used in elaboration of the diagnosis of velopharyngeal incompetence, *Br J Plast Surg* 35:19-32, 1982.

Reath DB, LaRossa D, Randall P: Simultaneous posterior pharyngeal flap and tonsillectomy, *Cleft Palate J* 24:250-253, 1987.

Rich AR: Physiological study of the Eustachian tube and its related muscles, *Bull Johns Hopkins Hosp* 31:206-214, 1920.

Scheier M: Die Bedeutung des Röntgenverfahrens fur die physiologie der sprache und der Stimme, *Archiv Laryngol Rhinol* 22:175-179, 1909.

Schwartz RH, Hayden GF, Rodriguez WJ, Shprintzen RJ, Cassidy JW: The bifid uvula: Is it a marker for an otitis-prone child? *Laryngoscope* 95:1100-1102, 1985.

Shprintzen RJ: Hypernasal speech in the absence of overt or submucous cleft palate: the mystery solved. In Ellis R, Flack R, editors: *Diagnosis and treatment of palato glossal malfunction,* London, 1979, College of Speech Therapists.

Shprintzen RJ: Palatal and pharyngeal anomalies in craniofacial syndromes, *Birth Defects* 18(1), 53-78, 1982.

Shprintzen RJ: An invited commentary on the preceding article by Ibuki, Karnell and Morris. *Cleft Palate J,* 20, 105-107, 1983.

Shprintzen RJ: *Nasopharyngoscopy.* In Bzoch K, editor: Communication disorders related to cleft lip and palate, 3rd ed, Boston 1989, College-Hill.

Shprintzen RJ: Evaluation of velopharyngeal insufficiency. In Brodsky L, editor: *Multidisciplinary approach to craniofacial disorders,* Toronto, 1992, B.C. Decker.

Shprintzen RJ, Croft CB: Abnormalities of the Eustachian tube orifice in individuals with cleft palate, *Int J Pediatr Otorhinolaryngol,* 3, 15-23, 1981.

Shprintzen RJ, Croft CB, Berkman MD, Rakoff ST: Pharyngeal hypoplasia in the Treacher Collins syndrome, *Arch Otolaryngol* 105, 127-131, 1979a.

Shprintzen RJ, Croft CB, Berkman MD, Rakoff ST: Velopharyngeal insufficiency in the facio-auriculovertebral malformation complex, *Cleft Palate J* 17: 132-137, 1980.

Shprintzen RJ, Goldberg RB, Lewin ML, Sidoti EJ, Berkman MD, Argamaso RV, Young D: A new syndrome involving cleft palate, cardiac anomalies, typical facies, and learning disabilities: velo-cardio-facial syndrome, *Cleft Palate J* 15, 56-62, 1978.

Shprintzen RJ, Golding-Kushner K: Evaluation of velopharyngeal insufficiency, *Otolaryngol Clin N Am* 22:519-536, 1989.

Shprintzen RJ, Lewin ML, Croft CB, Daniller AI, Argamaso RV, Ship A, Strauch B: A comprehensive study of pharyngeal flap surgery: tailor-made flaps, *Cleft Palate J* 16, 46-55, 1979b.

Shprintzen RJ, Schwartz R, Daniller A, Hoch L: The morphologic significance of bifiduvula, *Pediatrics* 75:553-561, 1985.

Shprintzen RJ, Sher AE, Croft CB: Hypernasal speech caused by hypertrophic tonsils, *Internat J Pediatr Otorhinolaryngol* 14:45-56, 1987.

Siegel-Sadewitz VL, Shprintzen RJ: Nasopharyngoscopy of the normal velopharyngeal sphincter: an experiment of biofeedback, *Cleft Palate J* 19: 194-201, 1982.

Siegel-Sadewitz VL, Shprintzen RJ: Changes in velopharyngeal valving with age, *Int J Pediatr Otorhinolaryngol,* 11:171-182, 1986.

Skolnick ML: Video velopharyngography in patients with nasal speech, with emphasis on lateral pharyngeal motion in velopharyngeal closure, *Radiology* 93:747-755, 1969.

Skolnick ML: Videofluoroscopic examination of the velopharyngeal portal during phonation in lateral and base projections - a new technique for studying the mechanics, *Cleft Palate J* 7:803-816, 1970.

Stool SE, Randall P: Unexpected ear disease in infants with cleft palate, *Cleft Palate J* 4:99-103, 1967.

Stringer DA, Witzel MA: Velopharyngeal insufficiency on videofluoroscopy: comparison of projections, *Am J Radiol* 146:15-19, 1986.

Subtelny JD: Physio-acoustic considerations in the radiographic study of speech, *Cleft Palate J* 1:402-410, 1964.

Warren DW, DuBois AB: A pressure-flow technique for measuring velopharyngeal orifice area during continuous speech, *Cleft Palate J* 1:52-71, 1964.

Warren DW: *The determination of velopharyngeal incompetency by aerodynamic and acoustical techniques.* In Hogan VM, editor: *Clinics in plastic surgery,* Philadelphia 1975, WB Saunders.

Williams ML, Shprintzen RJ, Rakoff SJ: Adenoid hypoplasia in the velo-cardio-facial syndrome, *J Craniofac Genet Devel Biol* 7:23-26, 1987.

12 The Use of Information Obtained from Speech and Instrumental Evaluations in Treatment Planning for Velopharyngeal Insufficiency

Robert J. Shprintzen

It is obvious that diagnostic accuracy is critical to consistently good treatment outcomes. Though it is certainly true that the treatment of velopharyngeal insufficiency (VPI) and resulting hypernasality can be successful by applying many different types of procedures, consistently successful outcomes depend on an accurate diagnosis guiding the surgeon, dentist, or speech pathologist who will be applying the potential remedy. For example, pharyngeal flap surgery has been reported to be successful approximately 80% of the time when applied in a random manner to patients with hypernasality who have not had advanced diagnostic tests applied (Shprintzen et al., 1979). However, the success rate was increased to 97% when the same surgeons applied their operations based on diagnostic information provided by nasopharyngoscopy and multiview videofluoroscopy (Shprintzen et al., 1979; Argamaso et al., 1980). As shown in Chapters 11, 16, and 17, indications for speech therapy, placement of a speech bulb appliance, and surgery depend on proper diagnostic indications from endoscopic and fluoroscopic examinations. Also important to successful patient management is the expertise of the clinicians. Expertise is not limited to the surgeon's or dentist's manual dexterity or the speech pathologist's ability to apply reinforcers. A major element in the capability of the clinician is the ability to apply proper judgment. Between the ability to collect data from instrumental examinations and the application of treatments is the thought process of the clinician who must interpret diagnostic data so they are relevant to the success of the treatments.

FACTORS TO CONSIDER

In reviewing endoscopic and fluoroscopic studies for the purpose of recommending treatment, the following factors must be noted and analyzed in detail.

Anatomy

As discussed in Chapter 11, the major advantage of nasopharyngoscopy is the ability to observe the anatomy of the nose, pharynx, and larynx in detail. Decisions regarding the advisability of surgery, the choice of operation, and other treatment alternatives are often influenced by observations of the anatomy of the velopharyngeal (VP) valve and surrounding structures. Of particular interest would be the following:

1. The structure of the nasal passages, including the position of the nasal septum, the size of the turbinates, the patency of the nasal airway, and the state and color of the nasal mucous membrane
2. The size, position, and shape of the lymphoid tissue (tonsils and adenoids)
3. The structure of the palate, with special emphasis on the presence or absence of the musculus uvulae
4. The appearance of the pharyngeal mucous membrane
5. The width of the pharynx
6. The vasculature

The structure of the nasal passages. Nasal resonance can be altered significantly by the internal structure of the nose. A deviated septum, enlarged nasal turbinates, constricted nasal passages, or polyps or other growths all can prevent nasal air escape and some degree of resonance even when the VP valve is not functioning properly. Therefore the endoscopic examination must take into account the patency of both nasal passages in relation to the acoustic description of the speech symptoms by the speech pathologist. For example, VPI may be present, but there may be no detectable nasal air escape and nasal resonance may be described as having a mixed hypernasal and hyponasal resonance or a cul-de-sac resonance (see Chapter 9). The structures of the nasal passages may contribute to this problem either singly or in combination. It is also true that adenoid or tonsil enlargement can cause nasal airway obstruction, but the resonance characteristics of lymphoid tissue enlargement are different. Enlarged adenoids tend to cause a hyponasal resonance pattern because of their posterior position and ability to block the entire choanal space. Their position just above the palate places them directly in the position where VP closure occurs, so enlarged adenoids tend to work to the advantage of individuals with a dysfunctional VP valve. Adenoid enlargement does not typically result in either a mixed resonance pattern or cul-de-sac resonance.

The reason that a narrow nasal passage, enlarged turbinates, and septal deviation cause abnormal resonance characteristics is that the obstruction in the nasal passage is anterior to the VP valve. Therefore, if the VP valve dysfunctions, sound or air will escape into the nasal chamber. In the case of mixed hypernasal and hyponasal resonance the degree of nasal obstruction causes the hyponasality, but the obstruction is not complete, so some sound and air can escape anteriorly, resulting in perceived hypernasality, nasal turbulence, or nasal emission. In cul-de-sac resonance the anterior obstruction is complete, or near complete, so resonance can escape into the nasal cavity but not out of the nares. The resonance trapped in the nasal cavity results in the cul-de-sac phenomenon.

Treatment of VPI when there is an anterior blockage of airflow becomes a complicated problem, and decisions should obviously be considered by several different specialists familiar with the associated problems. The surgeon, otolaryngologist, and speech pathologist should all contribute to the discussion of the case. It must be determined if elimination of the VPI will have a significant effect on the acoustic quality of speech after surgery. Similarly, it must be determined if resolution of the nasal obstruction will have a significant effect on speech production. In mixed hypernasality and hyponasality elimination of the VPI without elimination of the cause of the hyponasality will leave the patient with complete hyponasality. Although hyponasality is always a potential complication of surgery to the VP valve, it is not a normal state and should be avoided if at all

possible. If the hyponasal component is caused by enlarged turbinates, chronic nasal obstruction, or polyps, it is recommended that the nose be treated medically before any consideration for VP surgery. Topical steroids are able to shrink the turbinates or nasal mucous membranes, thereby temporarily resolving problems of nasal obstruction, which may then unmask the true extent of the severity of resonance disorder and assist in the process of deciding if surgery to the VP valve is indicated. In the case of a severe septal deviation, which often accompanies complete clefts of the lip and palate (both unilateral and bilateral), nasal surgery is typically deferred until teen years. In cases where the extent of the speech abnormality cannot be determined to be related solely to the VP valve (i.e., independent of the septal blockage), the severity of the hypernasality may be the determining factor for recommending pharyngeal surgery. The size of the VP gap should not be the deciding factor. In the past, it has been our clinical experience at the Center for Craniofacial Disorders that the size of the VP gap is not necessarily related to the severity of the perceived hypernasality. We have seen hundreds of patients with very small gaps but severe hypernasal resonance and, conversely, hundreds of patients with large gaps and minimal hypernasality. Therefore the determining factor for recommending treatment in cases where there are complicating factors such as nasal obstruction must be the judgment of the speech pathologist.

The size, position, and shape of the lymphoid tissue (tonsils and adenoids). Tonsils and adenoids represent a particularly interesting challenge to clinicians involved in the treatment of the VP valve. As discussed in Chapter 11, many clinicians mistakenly group the adenoids and tonsils together in terms of their importance to normal speech production. The adenoids are extremely important to normal speech production and are essentially always the primary site of VP closure in young children (see Chapter 11) (Croft et al., 1981; Siegel-Sadewitz and Shprintzen, 1986; Williams et al., 1987; Gereau and Shprintzen, 1988). Their position in the nasopharynx places them in the vector of movement the velum takes during speech (see Fig. 11-29). The tonsils, however, normally sit in the posterior oral cavity, below and anterior to the VP valve. In some cases the tonsils can be hypertrophic and intrude into the pharyngeal cavity, interfering with VP closure by obstructing the movements of the velum and/or lateral pharyngeal walls (see Fig. 11-23) (Shprintzen et al., 1987). The adenoids are essentially always important to the development of normal speech and may be a liability to normal speech production only if they are so large that they fully obstruct the posterior aspect of the nasal chamber, causing denasality (see Fig. 11-22). Tonsils are virtually never an asset to normal speech production and are often a liability if they are hypertrophic, frequently causing a muffled oral resonance ("potato in the mouth") and possibly causing VPI and hypernasality. Because hypertrophic tonsils may intrude into the nasopharynx or be accompanied by hypertrophic adenoids, mixed hypernasality and hyponasality is a common feature of lymphoid tissue hypertrophy.

In cases where the adenoids are hypertrophic in individuals with clefts, they should be left completely intact unless airway obstruction is compromising health. Adenoidectomy is contraindicated even if the adenoids are causing some degree of hyponasality. Though hyponasality is not normal, it is certainly preferable to hypernasality because the overwhelming number of phonemes in English (and all other languages as well) have no nasal resonance. Adenoidectomy might cause hypernasality (Croft et al., 1981). Partial adenoidectomy, such as lateral band adenoidectomy, might seem a logical approach if the adenoids are obstructive, but this procedure is unpredictable in long-term effect (the adenoid often grows back to its original state), and it would be difficult to predict what degree of removal would be safe without causing VPI. An exception would be removal of the anterior aspect of the adenoid if the tissue is intruding into the choanae. The tissue obstructing the postnasal space can be removed while leaving the tissue in the posterior corner of the nasopharynx intact. Thus the contact point for the velum is not altered while the portion of the adenoid obstructing the nasal airway is removed. Complete adenoidectomy should be contemplated only if there is evidence of obstructive sleep apnea and the entire adenoid is hypertrophic (however, clinicians must also be aware that the tonsils also contribute to apnea and are a more likely source of the problem). The degree of nasal obstruction by the adenoid must be assessed by endoscopic examination, which can successfully visualize the entire choanal space to determine the amount of adenoid filling it (see Fig. 11-22). Lateral view radiographic procedures are also helpful to determine the anterior and posterior structural relationship of the adenoid to the vector of palatal motion (Fig. 12-1).

Chronic middle ear disease is not a legitimate reason for adenoidectomy in children

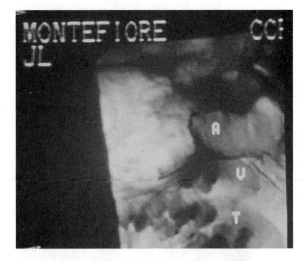

Fig. 12-1 Lateral view fluoroscopy during speech of patient with adenoid (A), filling the choanae while the palate (V) contacts only the posterior aspect of the adenoid along the posterior pharyngeal wall. The tongue (T) is in a normal position.

with clefts, since they are more likely to have persistent otitis media because of Eustachian tube dysfunction. Thinking that adenoidectomy may help to resolve middle ear disease (as it may in some children who do not have clefts) is inappropriate when there is a source for Eustachian tube dysfunction that is independent of the adenoid tissue. Children with cleft palate have structural eustachian tube malformations (Dickson and Dickson, 1972; Dickson, 1976; Maue-Dickson et al., 1976; Shprintzen and Croft, 1981; Gereau et al., 1988) that will not be relieved by adenoidectomy. Eustachian tube anomalies can also be seen endoscopically (Fig. 12-2).

Tonsils are an important structural component to be assessed in individuals with clefts because they may contribute to both speech and respiratory problems. Assessment of the size and position of the tonsils is best done by a combined endoscopic and radiographic approach, as is true of the adenoids. There are clear indications for tonsillectomy based on the combined data derived from speech assessment, nasopharyngoscopy, and videofluoroscopy. If speech is entirely within normal limits, the tonsils are not chronically infected, and there is no evidence of respiratory obstruction, removal is contraindicated, even if they appear very large. However, if there is evidence of hypernasality, endoscopic and fluoroscopic examination become critical.

Because the tonsils normally sit in the oral cavity between the faucial pillars, tonsillar tissue

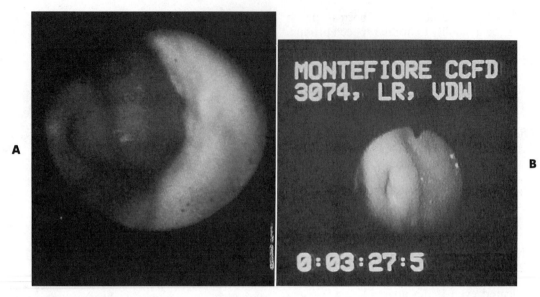

Fig. 12-2 Nasopharyngoscopic view of a normal eustachian tube orifice in a 10-year-old girl who does not have cleft palate *(top)* and a hypoplastic eustachian tube orifice in a 10-year-old girl (bottom) with a cleft palate.

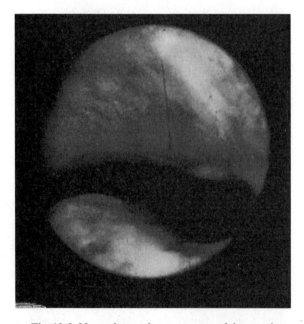

Fig. 12-3 Normal nasopharyngoscopy of the oropharynx showing no evidence of tonsillar tissue.

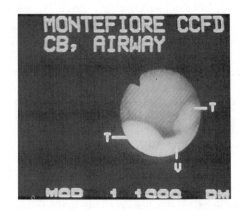

Fig. 12-4 Endoscopy showing tonsils (T) intruding abnormally into the opharyngeal and nasopharyngeal airway behind the velum (V).

should not be visible on nasopharyngoscopic examination (Fig. 12-3). In some children with hypertrophic tonsils, the tonsils extend posterior to the faucial pillars and intrude into the pharyngeal airway (Fig. 12-4), sometimes growing upward into the nasopharynx, sometimes downward toward the hypopharynx. When the

tonsils are observed in the pharyngeal airway in a patient being considered for secondary surgery to resolve the VPI, tonsillectomy (but not adenoidectomy) is always indicated as a procedure separate from pharyngeal flap for the following reasons:

1. The presence of tonsils may cause VPI and hypernasality. It is possible that tonsillectomy alone may resolve the VPI and therefore eliminate the need for a pharyngeal flap (Shprintzen et al., 1987).
2. If a pharyngeal flap is done with the tonsils intruding posteriorly into the pharyngeal airway, they will be positioned beneath the

lateral ports of the pharyngeal flap and be a potential source of obstructive sleep apnea (OSA) postoperatively (see Chapter 5).

3. Though bleeding complications are relatively infrequent in both tonsillectomy and pharyngeal flap, doing the two procedures together would significantly increase the risk (Argamaso et al., 1988). Also, because the operative fields for the tonsillectomy and pharyngeal flap are in close proximity, it would be difficult to isolate the source of bleeding should the complication arise.

Müller maneuver. Nasopharyngoscopic examination of patients being considered for pharyngeal flap surgery should include a procedure known as the Müller maneuver (Sher et al., 1985). This procedure is reported to be predictive of the predisposition toward obstructive apnea and upper airway collapse. The Müller maneuver is designed to introduce a small negative pressure into the airway during nasopharyngoscopic examination to observe if the upper airway collapses during the procedure. The maneuver should be performed on multiple occasions with the endoscope positioned in the nasopharynx, oropharynx, and hypopharynx. With the endoscope in place to observe as much of the pharynx as possible, the examiner gently occludes the patient's nostrils by pinching the sides of the nose. The patient is then asked to breathe deeply through the nose with the lips closed at least 3 or 4 times in a row. Pinching the nose gently increases the resistance of airflow through the nose so that less air is pulled into the nasal cavity. As the diaphragm continues to pull down, the lack of air filling the airway causes a negative pressure. The degree of collapse is typically rated on a five-point interval scale: 0, 1+, 2+, 3+, 4+ (Fig. 12-5). It has been observed that, in patients with a predisposition to obstructive sleep apnea, the airway collapses during the Müller maneuver at 3+ and 4+ levels (Sher et al., 1985). Therefore, if a patient is noted to have a strongly positive Müller response, the advisability of pharyngeal flap must be questioned.

Assessment following tonsillectomy. It is always recommended that speech evaluation and nasopharyngoscopy be repeated approximately 4 weeks after tonsillectomy. This allows sufficient time for the VP valve to adapt to the new physical environment without the tonsils. If it is observed that there has been a change in the VP valving pattern following tonsillectomy, it may be advisable to defer the pharyngeal flap. There are indications from the postoperative endoscopy and perceptual speech assessment that should prompt a recommendation for speech therapy rather than additional surgery. Specifically, if closure is observed to occur on any single phoneme or class of phonemes (such as sustained sibilants or fricatives), even if intermittent, speech therapy should be implemented (see Chapter 16) before considering pharyngoplasty. Intermittent closure would also present an opportunity to utilize speech bulb reduction (see Chapter 17). If closure does not occur but variation is seen in the degree of closure or pattern of closure, speech bulb reduction should be considered before a definitive surgical correction. Of course, the status of the patient's articulation will greatly influence this decision. If articulation is disordered, particularly in terms of the presence of compensatory articulation (such as glottal stops), speech therapy with or without bulb reduction is indicated before additional surgery.

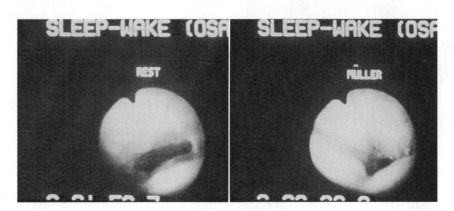

Fig. 12-5 Endoscopic view of a 4+ Müller maneuver in a patient with obstructive sleep apnea.

The structure of the palate, with special emphasis on the presence or absence of the musculus uvulae. Perhaps the greatest advantage of endoscopic procedures is the ability to precisely define the anatomy of the velum, which has diagnostic significance for both speech disorders and the possible diagnosis of primary diseases and syndromes. Repaired palatal clefts have a midline deficiency in muscle because of both absence of the musculus uvulae and contracture along the midline scar. Endoscopic examination often reveals small midline gaps in the VP valve, even when there is excellent movement of the lateral pharyngeal walls and velum (Fig. 12-6). The same problem may occur in submucous cleft palate, where there is separation of the palatal muscles and absence of the musculus uvulae (Fig. 12-7). Patients who have oral signs consistent with submucous cleft palate, such as bifid uvula, an obvious separation of muscle fibers, or a notch in the posterior border of the hard palate, all have obvious midline deficiencies on the nasal surface of the soft palate that endoscopically appears as a concave depression or notch in the midline of the velum. Occult submucous cleft palate (Croft et al., 1978) refers to the muscle abnormalities associated with submucous cleft palate but without that disorder's typical oral stigmata (Calnan, 1954), such as bifid uvula, a marked midline separation of muscles (zona pellucida), and notching of the posterior border of the hard palate. As described in Chapters 1 and 11, there is congenital absence of the musculus uvulae in occult submucous cleft palate, which is not detectable on oral examination because the musculus uvulae is the muscle closest to the nasal surface of the velum, sitting atop all of the other palatal

muscles, and the hard palate and other palatal muscles may be largely intact.

Videofluoroscopic assessment may be helpful in anatomic assessment in cases of submucous or occult submucous cleft palate. It has been shown that, when a normal musculus uvulae is present, the velum thickens considerably on elevation during speech (Croft et al., 1981). This is related to the shortening and thickening of the musculus uvulae when it contracts during speech. Patients with clefts (overt, submucous, or occult submucous) do not display thickening of the velum during the elevation of the palate for speech (Fig. 12-8). The velum in individuals with submucous clefts and occult submucous clefts also looks very short in lateral projection compared to a normal palate (Fig. 12-9).

Another videofluoroscopic clue for determining the presence of a midline concavity in the dorsum of the velum is a double barium line in lateral projection (Fig. 12-10). The double barium line occurs because barium coats each lateral aspect of the velum where muscle fibers are present (Fig. 12-11). If the barium coat used for fluoroscopy is heavy, the same concavity may be seen in frontal projection, often as a V-shaped barium line in the center of the pharynx (Fig. 12-10).

Evidence of a midline muscle deficiency resulting in a consistent gap in the VP valve during speech on endoscopic and fluoroscopic examination is an indication that surgical treatment is necessary to resolve the VPI. Although it is true that the majority of individuals with submucous clefts have normal speech (Shprintzen et al., 1985), in some individuals the anatomic and physiologic circumstances related to VP valving are such that a midline gap cannot be overcome during speech. In these cases, where there is no phonemic variation and no evidence of occasional closure, it becomes essential to fill the midline gap physically with some type of tissue obturator. Although prosthetic obturation with a speech bulb will certainly be successful in these types of cases, it is only a desirable permanent solution for patients who cannot have surgery or who decline surgery. The best solution for small central gaps in the VP valve is a narrow centrally placed pharyngeal flap. Narrow flaps will not impede nasal airflow for respiration but will resolve the VPI when lateral wall motion is good.

The appearance of the pharyngeal mucous membrane. In some cases the appearance of the pharyngeal mucosa may indicate potential problems for surgical candidates. Endoscopic examination is the only diagnostic procedure to reveal

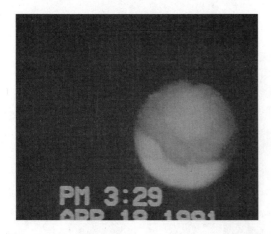

Fig. 12-6 Endoscopic view of repaired cleft with midline gap.

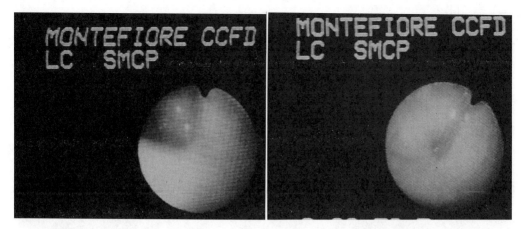

Fig. 12-7 Endoscopic view of submucous cleft palate at rest (A) and during speech (B) with VPI.

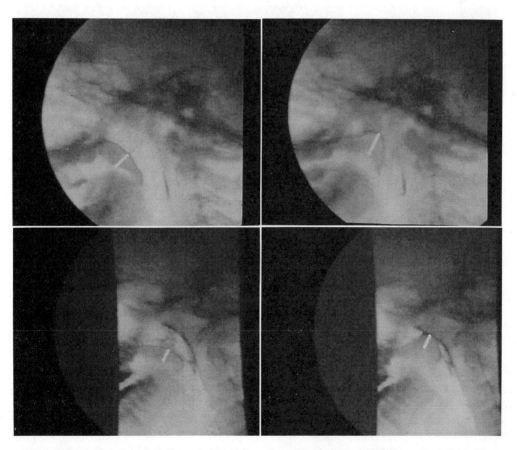

Fig. 12-8 Lateral view videofluoroscopy of the velum at rest *(left)* and during speech *(right)* in an individual with a normal palate *(top)* and an individual with a submucous cleft palate *(bottom)*, showing that the velum thickens during speech in the normal palate but not the cleft palate.

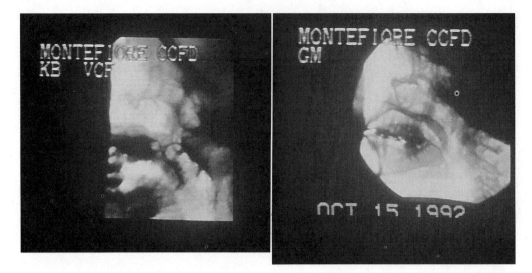

Fig. 12-9 Lateral view of an occult submucous cleft palate *(left)* compared with a normal palate *(right)*, showing the difference in length.

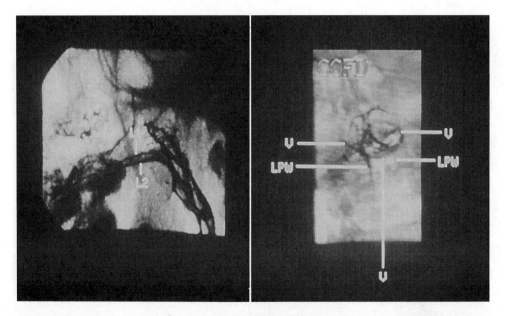

Fig. 12-10 Lateral view videofluoroscopy *(left)* of an individual with a submucous cleft palate showing a double barium line on the dorsum of the velum, indicative of a midline concavity. With a heavy barium coat, frontal view will also show this concavity *(right)*. *(right)*, showing the difference in length.

abnormalities in the mucosa that might indicate possible complications associated with pharyngeal surgery. Four factors in particular that may be encountered in patients with VPI are scarring, mucosal atrophy, papillae, and abnormal growths.

Scarring of the posterior pharyngeal wall may result from adenoidectomy or previous pharyn-

goplasty. In most cases scarring per se is not a contraindication to additional pharyngeal surgery; adenoidectomy leaves a scar high in the nasopharynx above the level of the donor site for a pharyngeal flap. However, scars from previous pharyngoplasties will certainly be in the field of secondary operations. Barone et al. (1994) reported that secondary pharyngeal flaps could

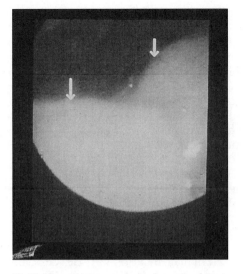

Fig. 12-11 Nasopharyngoscopic view of a submucous cleft palate showing where barium would cling *(arrows)* to produce a double barium line in lateral view videofluoroscopy.

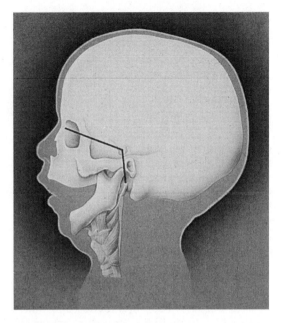

Fig. 12-12 Drawing of the pharynx suspended from the skull base, indicating that platybasia will result in an abnormally large pharyngeal airway.

be done without complication in patients who had had previous vertical pharyngeal flap procedures. Following the raising of a first flap, the pharynx heals by circumferential contraction, which leaves sufficient muscle and mucosa for raising a second flap. Other pharyngoplasties may leave horizontal scars, which could be sources of difficulty for raising a secondary flap or for healing of a secondary pharyngoplasty. Though it is unusual, we have seen several cases of patients who had multiple attempts at pharyngoplasty and had little usable tissue on the posterior pharyngeal wall for additional reconstructive procedures. Nasopharyngoscopic examination of the quality of the posterior pharyngeal tissues is essential in patients who have had previous pharyngoplasties.

Mucosal atrophy is common in patients who have received radiation therapy. The quality of the posterior pharyngeal wall mucosa may indicate potential sources of problems in healing for the surgeon in patients who have had irradiation for tumors of the head and neck. Because many patients who have had radiation therapy may have also had ablative surgery, which would lead to VPI, it is not uncommon for such patients to seek treatment at centers specializing in the care of individuals with clefts. The quality of the tissues of the pharynx is important for proper healing after pharyngeal surgery for the treatment of VPI. Extensive scarring should prompt the recommendation for prosthetic treatment rather than surgical man-

agement, unless a source of healthy tissue can be identified and utilized in a reconstructive procedure.

The width of the pharynx. Pharyngeal width can be indicative of a number of potential problems, as well as a possible diagnostic sign of a number of syndromes. Shprintzen (1982) reported that a number of syndromes included wide pharyngeal spaces, which are typically indicative of a flat skull base (platybasia). When the skull base is flat, the posterior pharyngeal wall, which is suspended from the posterior aspect of the skull base, is drawn away from the palate, which is attached to the anterior skull base (Fig. 12-12). Velo-cardio-facial syndrome, in particular, has been demonstrated to include a flat skull base resulting in a large, often more horizontally oriented nasopharynx, which contributes significantly to the high prevalence of VPI in this common disorder. Because the palate is further from the posterior pharyngeal wall in velo-cardio-facial syndrome, palate repair in such individuals almost invariably provides poor speech results (also affected by pharyngeal hypotonia) (Arvystas and Shprintzen, 1984). The width of the pharynx cannot be measured in absolute terms by endoscopy because the distance of the lens from the object being viewed is unknown and there are no known size referents for comparison. However, there are sufficient visual cues for judging relative width of the pharynx, such as the width of the epiglottis, the amount of the pharynx that can be seen within a single visual field of the pharynx, and the degree of pharyngeal illumination

Of more significant concern is an extremely narrow pharynx because of the potential for obstructive apnea following pharyngeal or even palatal surgery. Because absolute pharyngeal size cannot be measured endoscopically, the examiner must rely on visual cues to judge if the pharynx is narrow and then to explore further using additional procedures. The two visual cues that provide good evidence of narrowing of the airway are (1) the amount of the pharynx seen within the visual field of the endoscope and (2) the amount of light saturation in the pharynx during the examination.

When the pharynx is of normal width, it is difficult or impossible to see both lateral aspects in the field of view of the endoscope (Fig. 12-13). This is because fiberoptic endoscopes have limitations in terms of the cone of acceptance of the lens, usually in the 55- to 65-degree range. Therefore, when the pharynx is extremely wide, the lateral pharyngeal walls fall outside of that cone of acceptance and it becomes necessary to move the endoscope from side to side to visualize the entire pharynx during a single examination. When the pharynx is narrow, both lateral walls can be seen in a single field of view (Fig. 12-14) without moving the endoscope laterally in either direction. It is also often the case that the pharynx is narrowed anteroposteriorly in patients with small upper airways, which can also be detected clinically with fiberoptic endoscopy.

If the clinician feels that the airway is narrow, the issue of the potential for upper airway obstruction must be considered. A higher degree of diagnostic accuracy can be obtained by using a standardized procedure such as cephalometry with barium contrast in the pharynx (Laniado, 1987). By coating the lateral pharyngeal walls, velum, and posterior pharyngeal wall with a thin coat of barium in the same way contrast is used in multiview videofluoroscopy (see Chapter 11), accurate linear measurements of the distance between pharyngeal structures can be made.

The vasculature. One ultimate goal of endoscopic examination of the pharynx in patients with cleft palate or hypernasal speech is to determine if a patient may be a candidate for surgical management of VPI. Besides defining the nature of the VPI, clinicians (surgeons in particular) should be aware of potential sources of complications. One recently detected problem is that of abnormal neck vessels, which might pose risks during surgery. First reported by MacKenzie-Stepner et al. (1987), abnormal medial displacement of the internal carotid arteries has been found as a common feature in velo-cardio-facial syndrome. A more recent study using the state-of-the-art procedure of magnetic resonancy angiography (MRA) has found significant abnormalities in other major neck vessels in velocardiofacial syndrome (Mitnick et al., 1995). Suspicion of vascular abnormalities was first aroused by arterial pulsations in the posterior and lateral pharyngeal walls as detected endoscopically. Normally the pharynx should have no evidence of vascular pulsations

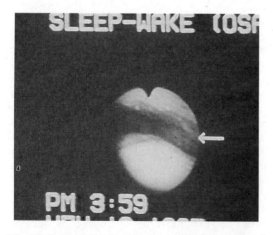

Fig. 12-13 Endoscopic view of a pharynx of normal width from a level approximately 1 cm above the palate. Note that only one lateral pharyngeal wall *(arrow)* can be seen in the field of endoscopic view.

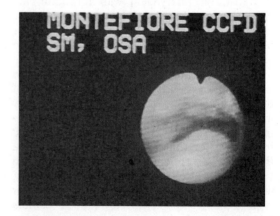

Fig. 12-14 Endoscopic view of a narrow pharynx from a level approximately 1 cm above the palate. Note that both lateral pharyngeal walls can be seen in the endoscopic field of view. The same endoscope was used in the examinations shown in Fig. 12-12 and 12-13.

because the major neck vessels, including the common carotid arteries, the internal carotid arteries, the external carotid arteries, and the vertebral arteries are deep enough in the pharyngeal soft tissues that their pulsations cannot be detected. Therefore observing the pulsations in the pharynx implies that vessels are closer to the surface than normal (and therefore potentially in the surgical field) or that the pharyngeal walls are thinner than normal.

Because pulsations of the pharynx have been found in 50% of a prospectively obtained sample of velo-cardio-facial syndrome patients and an abnormally medial course of the internal carotids has been found in over 50% (Mitnick et al., 1995), it has been recommended that all patients with this syndrome undergo MRA before pharyngeal flap surgery to identify those at risk for severing of the internal carotid artery during surgery. In their prospective MRA study Mitnick et al. (1995) found that not all patients who had an abnormal medial course of the internal carotids had endoscopically evident pulsations. Therefore the absence of pulsations on endoscopic examination does not necessarily rule out the possibility that the internal carotid arteries could be in the surgical field and pose a significant risk. Conversely, not all patients with observed pulsations have medially displaced internal carotid arteries (Mitnick et al., 1995). Therefore the endoscopic observation of pulsations in the posterior pharyngeal wall does not rule out the ability to perform pharyngeal flap surgery in that patient. Experience has shown that patients with severely abnormal neck vessels are rare. Therefore, although applying state-of-the-art diagnostic procedures is always advised, clinicians should not preclude patients from surgery unless there is evidence the patients are at risk.

Function

As mentioned previously and elsewhere in this text, the combined use of nasopharyngoscopy and multiview videofluoroscopy is essential for the complete physiologic assessment of VP function. The specification of treatment for VPI depends on information from these combined examinations, which provides the following detail:

1. The ability to observe the movements of *all* of the structures contributing to VP valving (the soft palate, the lateral pharyngeal walls, and the posterior pharyngeal wall)
2. The ability to observe *where* (i.e., at what location) the structures are moving

3. The ability to observe all movements under *all* types of phonemic conditions
4. The ability to assess consistency
5. The ability to relate the movements to the rest of speech production

The ability to observe movements of all structures contributing to VP valving. Effective physical management of VPI depends on the ability to obturate the VP port during speech. Therefore, it would be ideal to utilize the visual information obtained from endoscopic and fluoroscopic studies to precisely locate an obturator, whether it be a tissue or prosthetic one. An important component necessary to precisely prescribing the obturator is understanding how the procedure works. For example, though the palate plays an important (though not exclusive) role in normal VP closure, it plays little or no role in VP closure following pharyngeal flap surgery (Skolnick and McCall, 1972; Shprintzen et al., 1979; Argamaso et al., 1980; Argamaso, 1990). Therefore, if pharyngeal flap surgery is being considered, the degree, place, and consistency of lateral pharyngeal wall movement become critical in predicting success and prescribing surgery. Because the tissue obturator used in a pharyngeal flap connects the palate to the posterior pharyngeal wall, the movement of the palate or posterior wall is negated. This is not, however, the case with other treatments, such as a speech bulb obturator or sphincter pharyngoplasty, where velar motion can contribute to closure against an obturator that does not tether two structures together.

Patients who have good or excellent lateral pharyngeal wall motion are excellent candidates for pharyngeal flap surgery, even if the palate is not moving at all. Therefore recommending the treatment of VPI based solely on palatal motion is not advisable. Patients who have gross absence of movement in the VP valve from all of its components require maximum obturation, unless the absence of movement is related to other articulation disorders (see below). In such cases the method of obturation of the VP port must meet the criterion of completely or nearly completely occluding the valve.

It has been estimated that approximately 15% of all cases of VPI are asymmetric (Argamaso et al., 1994). Such cases emphasize the importance of assessing *all* components of VP valving. Cases with asymmetric VPI often require treatment skewed to one side of the valve. Centrally placed pharyngeal flaps often fail in such cases (Skolnick and McCall, 1972; Shprintzen et al., 1979; Argamaso et al, 1980; Shprintzen et al., 1980). Therefore, it is essential to see the full extent of lateral pharyngeal wall motion bilaterally to prescribe treatment. The only technique that allows the complete assessment of lateral wall motion for both amount and location is frontal view videofluoroscopy.

The ability to observe where the structures are moving. Because the goal of physical management of the VP valve is to obturate the port during speech, it is not sufficient to know the degree of motion of each of the structures; it is essential to know where they are moving, especially with reference to the vertical height of the pharynx. It is typical for the lateral pharyngeal walls to be moving high in the pharynx, at or slightly below the level of the hard palate. Therefore most surgeons who utilize pharyngeal flaps try to get them as high as possible (because they cannot really be con-

structed higher than the palatal plane). However, there is considerable variation in the place of velar motion and posterior pharyngeal wall motion, when present. In some cases the velum has been seen to move essentially straight upward toward the skull base with relatively little posterior motion (Fig. 12-15). In others the velum may move posteriorly or posterosuperiorly (Fig. 12-15). The velum has also been seen to move only its posterior tip in some cases (Fig. 12-15). This pattern of motion and place of elevation may significantly alter treatment plans because the type of velar movement may not be useful to a particular type of planned obturation. For example, if only the posterior tip of the velum is elevating, this type of motion would have little relevance to either speech bulb placement or sphincter pharyngoplasty, where

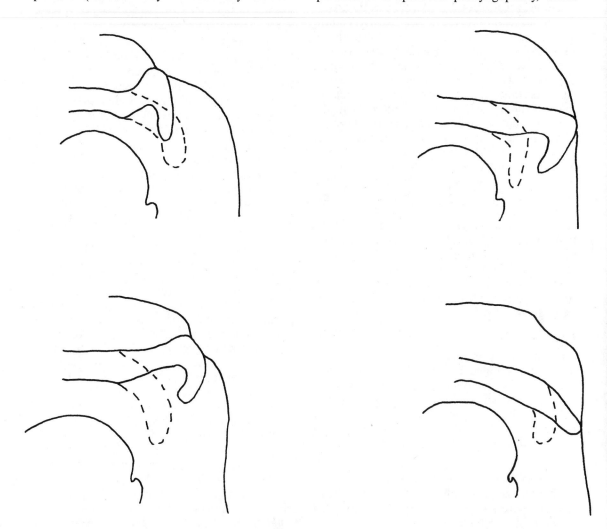

Fig. 12-15 Tracings from lateral view videofluoroscopy showing varying patterns of velar motion during speech, including straight upward *(upper left)*, straight backward *(upper right)*, posterosuperior *(lower left)*, and elevation of just the posterior tip of the velum *(lower right)*.

the obturation depends on the bulk of the midline of the palate.

Movement of the posterior pharyngeal wall, if present, also varies in location (Glaser et al., 1979). In most cases the area of movement on the posterior wall is part of a continuous ring of muscular contraction around the entire pharynx, but, as discussed in Chapter 11, the vertical level of that motion can vary from person to person, sometimes being at a level well below the palatal plane. The direction of the movement of Passavant's ridge, for those who have it, also varies from individual to individual. The presence of Passavant's ridge is of no consequence to treatment with pharyngeal flap, except to indicate that there is active sphincteric movement in the VP valve. Passavant's ridge may, however, be an important component in the treatment of VPI with a speech bulb appliance. The vertical height of the ridge would be important to note so that the bulb could be positioned properly to take advantage of the movement, as well as the movements of all of the other components of VP closure. When Passavant's ridge is present, the bulb should be positioned so that it is not flush against the posterior wall. In this way the bulb can use the pharyngeal wall movement while not applying constant pressure to the pharynx, which can cause pressure sores.

The ability to observe all movements under all types of phonemic conditions. A major mistake often made in assessments of VP valving is the failure to note if there is any variation in function under a variety of phonemic circumstances. It is extremely important to utilize a speech sample for both nasopharyngoscopy and multiview videofluoroscopy that includes sustained fricatives, including /s/ and /f/ (in other words, /ssss/ and /ffff/). As described in Chapter 11, speech samples should include the use of both voiced and voiceless phonemes, both in isolation and in the context of short phrases. It has been observed frequently that some individuals who have VPI during connected speech can achieve closure or at least increased motion on the voiceless sustained phonation /ssss/ or /ffff/. In such cases the surgical option should not be immediately exercised. Instead, speech therapy alone or speech bulb reduction should be employed. In cases where closure is obtained during some speech samples, there is a possibility that surgery can be avoided completely (see Chapter 16).

Another phenomenon that can be encountered is occasionally referred to as the "pulsing palate." This valving problem is one of timing

and coordination and can occur in individuals with or without cleft palate. It often accompanies dysarthria and other neurologic problems but may also occur as an isolated idiopathic disorder. This phenomenon can be detected only by direct visualization of the VP valve by endoscopy and fluoroscopy. The hypernasality caused by this phenomenon is indistinguishable from hypernasality caused by anatomic defects. However, during this type of abnormal VP function the valve may actually close at least intermittently during each production of a nonnasal consonant.

Normally during VP closure the palate and pharyngeal walls start to move toward closure just before the onset of phonation. By the time the production of the speech sample has begun, the valve is closed. The valve will reopen only during the production of a nasal consonant (/m/, /n/, or /ŋ/) or at the conclusion of the phonation of a nonnasal phrase. The valve opens only very slightly during the transition to a nasal consonant. If it were to open wide, the amount of movement necessary to close again could not occur rapidly enough to avoid hypernasal resonance. At the conclusion of an utterance, the valve opens only after speech has ceased. If the valve closes late or opens early, hypernasality is perceived by the listener. This is the root of the perceptual speech impairment in the pulsing phenomenon. The pulsing phenomenon is characterized by persistent closing and opening of the VP valve during normally nonnasal speech. For example, during the phrase "stop the bus" VP closure is initially achieved on the /st/, but the valve then opens on the vowel phoneme /ɑ/ (the o in *stop*). The valve then closes for /p/ and /ð/ and opens again on the next vowel. In some respects the pulsing phenomenon seems to be largely related to either transitions between voiced and voiceless sounds (all vowels are voiced, whereas many consonants such as /p/, /t/, /s/, and /ʃ/ are not) or between pressure consonants and vowels. Therefore individuals who display this phenomenon will often achieve strong, sustained closure on the production of /ssss/ or /ffff/, but during spontaneous conversation the same /s/ or /f/ sounds may be perceived as hypernasal because of the transitional opening and closing of the valve.

Treatment of this type of rhythm or coordination problem is difficult and points out the need for accurate diagnostic data. Physical management by surgical means is strongly contraindicated in these cases. Because the problem is one of a rhythm disorder where the valve is constantly opening and closing, obturating a portion of the valve has no beneficial effect because the valve will continue to function spasmodically even after partial physical obturation has been achieved. The only way surgical obturation would be able to eliminate hypernasal resonance is if an operative procedure completely obstructed the VP orifice. There are, however, alternative treatment options.

In cases where the VP disorder is related to dysarthria, the recommended treatment is speech therapy to eliminate the dysarthria or at least improve the rhythm of articulation. Resolution of the disjointed rhythm associated with all of the components of articulation in individuals with dysarthria almost always results in the simultaneous resolution of resonance disorders, including hypernasality. In some cases nasopharyngoscopic biofeedback may prove useful (Siegel-Sadewitz and Shprintzen, 1982; Witzel et al., 1989).

Speech bulb obturators may be a valuable treatment option in individuals with dysarthria and also in cases of idiopathic or cleft-related rhythm disorders. In such cases it is best to start by making the speech bulb as large as possible to obturate the entire VP port. This negates the tendency for the port to open during normally nonnasal utterances. After several months of reinforcement with nonnasal speech it may then be possible to reduce the appliance. Speech bulb reduction is ideally suited to individuals in whom occasional closure is obtained during speech, which is the case in this particular disorder.

The ability to assess consistency. It is possible that failure to assess the consistency of movement in the VP valve can result in the delivery of unnecessary treatment. To assess consistency, it is essential to directly view the movements of the VP valve and to do so under all phonemic conditions. The selection of the speech sample therefore becomes critical, especially for fluoroscopic studies where the time of exposure must be more tightly controlled. The two types of consistency disorders have been described elsewhere in this text but are repeated here to illustrate that the temptation to treat all forms of VP malfunction by surgery may lead to unnecessary treatments. Consistency problems are of three basic types: phoneme-specific closure, phoneme-specific insufficiency, and posterior nasal fricatives.

Phoneme-specific closure represents a positive sign that patients may be able to improve VP valving dramatically throughout speech, even if they have a gross insufficiency during the majority of speech. It is most common to see phoneme-specific closure on /s/ or /f/. The rea-

son for this is unclear, but there are two possible explanations. First, it may be that the pressure demands for sustained production of /s/ or /f/ are so great that, to produce any type of recognizable sound, the VP valve is forced to function more efficiently. The second possible explanation relates to the timing of phonemic acquisition. Fricatives are learned relatively late in speech development, so they may be learned at a time when motor coordination in general is better and the individual better understands the goal of speech production. These hypotheses are purely speculative, but each may have some element of truth and they are not mutually exclusive. When phoneme-specific closure occurs, surgery should be deferred until speech therapy is utilized to prompt additional movement in the valve. Both speech bulb reduction therapy and nasopharyngoscopic biofeedback therapy may prove useful adjuncts to speech therapy in these cases. Nasopharyngoscopic biofeedback in particular may prove an effective method for obtaining a rapid result in generalizing occasional VP closure throughout speech production.

Phoneme-specific VPI may occur on any single sound or class of sounds. In cases where the error occurs on fricatives (including sibilants), such as /s/ or /f/, it is often found that the individual can achieve closure on sustained production of those sounds, but they have an insufficiency in running speech. Even when tongue placement is normal, the method of production is abnormal in this type of phoneme-specific error. This problem is easily remediable by speech therapy, and surgery should never be considered as a treatment option. Although speech bulb reduction may be effective for phoneme-specific insufficiency, it is not necessary and the cost and difficulty involved are unwarranted. However, nasopharyngoscopic biofeedback can be very effective in resolving phoneme-specific VPI within very few sessions (usually three to five).

The posterior nasal fricative is really an articulatory substitution (see Chapters 8 and 16) during which a sound of frication is made by forcing air through the nose. Although posterior nasal fricatives may occur in association with other abnormalities of VP closure, they may also occur as an isolated substitution. It is a common abnormal substitution in patients with fistulae in the hard palate. As with phoneme-specific VPI, surgery is definitely contraindicated when the only abnormality of VP function is a posterior nasal fricative. Because the aim of this substitution is to produce a fricative sound through the nose, no matter what reconstruction is done to the VP valve, the patient will find a way to force air out of the nose to create that sound. If the patient cannot get air out of the nose, no sound will be produced. In fact, in patients with posterior nasal fricatives clinicians can easily see the nature of the substitution by asking the patient to say a word with /s/ in the initial position or a sustained /s/ and occluding the nostrils during the speech sample. The patient will literally become speechless, unable to produce any substitution for the /s/ because the escape route for the air and sound (the nostrils) has been shut off. Unlike phoneme-specific errors, speech bulbs would not resolve the problem because of the patient's need to push air through the nose to produce sound. Therefore, when posterior nasal fricatives represent the only error of VP valving, the only appropriate treatment is speech therapy. If a fistula is present, it should be obturated or surgically closed.

When posterior nasal fricatives occur in association with consistent VP insufficiency, the observed pattern on endoscopic and fluoroscopic examination is far different from that found in consistent VPI. In such cases there is typically some movement of the lateral pharyngeal walls and palate for all sounds except /s/. During production of /s/, however, the lateral walls may be seen to move outward, away from the midline, probably as a passive response to the pressure of the airflow being directed through the nose. Although treatment of the VPI may be successful with surgery or prosthetics, the posterior nasal fricative will not respond to physical management, and speech therapy will still be required.

The ability to relate the movements to the rest of speech production. Nasopharyngoscopic studies have a limitation that can lead to misinterpretation of the study. With the endoscope positioned above the palate and the oral cavity obscured by the palate, tongue movements are not visible. In cases where patients are utilizing compensatory articulation patterns with tongue backing, the tongue may often push the velum upward in an attempt to occlude the VP port. This maneuver cannot be detected by endoscopy (Fig. 12-16) In fact, the endoscopist will see only the velum elevating (because it is being pushed by the tongue) and may interpret this incorrectly as being a VP movement intrinsic to the palate. This reinforces the recommendation that videofluoroscopy be performed in all patients, regardless of the quality of the nasopharyngoscopy.

Videofluoroscopy allows the clinician to fully assess all speech movements (tongue, lips, teeth, VP mechanism) and relate the movements of the VP valve to the rest of speech production. The association between VP valving disorders and articulation problems is well known and points out the need to recommend treatment based on a more global picture of speech development.

The association of gross VPI with glottal stop articulation patterns has been well documented (Henningsson and Isberg, 1986; Hoch et al., 1986). In the presence of gross glottal stop substitutions for nonnasal consonants the VP valve typically does not function. Because airflow is being cut off at the level of the glottis, well below the VP port, there is no need for the VP valve to move. However, as will be demonstrated in Chapter 16, elimination of the glottal stop pattern often results in a marked increase in movement of the VP sphincter. Therefore it is advised that surgery be deferred in the presence of gross glottal stop substitutions (as well as other compensatory articulation patterns) until articulation therapy has had an opportunity to increase the movement in the VP valve. Speech bulb reduction therapy may be applied in these circumstances to remove hypernasality from the perceived polyglot of cleft palate speech.

WHAT AFFECTS DIAGNOSTIC JUDGMENT AND INTERPRETATION?

A number of factors can influence how a clinician utilizes data obtained from diagnostic examinations. These factors fall into four broad categories: training, treatment options, the number and type of specialists involved in the diagnostic procedure, and personality.

Training

It is undeniable that there is enormous variation in the method of training, the quality of the individuals who provide training, and the extent of training from institution to institution. This is true for all disciplines, professions, and specialties. For example, Clinician A is trained at an institution with a large and active craniofacial unit where hundreds of patients are seen every year. There are frequent opportunities to observe diagnostic procedures, including weekly sessions of nasopharyngoscopy and multiview videofluoroscopy. The people who perform these procedures and who are responsible for the training of Clinician A have performed and interpreted thousands of these procedures. They have published many papers on the subject and are considered experts in their fields. Clinician A becomes familiar with the process of direct visualization of the VP valve using state-of-the-art procedures from the beginning of

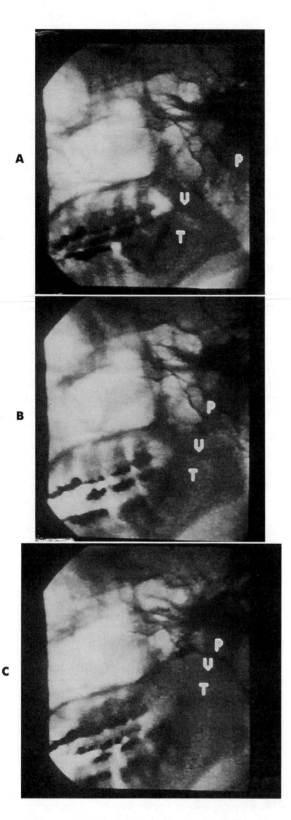

training. Clinician A also receives an extensive background in the anatomy and physiology of the VP valve from a professor who has a strong interest in speech and pharyngeal finction. Combining these two components of training, Clinician A is well prepared to implement these procedures following graduation when employment begins elsewhere.

In contrast, Clinician B is trained at an institution where there is a small cleft palate center which registers only 20 new patients per year. Nasopharyngoscopy is done very infrequently and, when done, is performed by someone who is not adept at the technique. The surgeons at this center believe that nasopharyngoscopy is sufficient for diagnosing VPI, and therefore videofluoroscopy is not done. Because nasopharyngoscopy is done infrequently, the equipment used is not up to date or sophisticated. Nasopharyngoscopic examinations are done without a video system. Clinician B must look over the shoulder of the examiner, catching only brief glimpses of the examination through the endoscope, rather than seeing the entire examination on a television monitor. The interpretation of the examination depends on the examiner making a clinical description based on events that no one else really sees. There has been no strong emphasis on anatomy and physiology of the VP valve. The person teaching anatomy and physiology has little interest in this region of the body so that the explanations provided are those gleaned from old texts and are provided secondhand with no personal

Fig. 12-16 Lateral view videofluoroscopy showing the tongue pushing the velum posteriorly toward the velopharyngeal port.

experience to support the material taught. Though the people providing the training to Clinician B are clearly not providing a comprehensive background, they will not admit so, and they impart a false sense of expertise to Clinician B. Clinician B leaves the program thinking that this clinic is practicing state-of-the-art care. Clinician B is unaware of the advantage of doing both nasopharyngoscopy and multiview videofluoroscopy for all patients because the absence of any experience with the radiographic procedure.

Because there is no standard curriculum for any clinical specialty, the range of experience is quite variable. As a result, there may even be some dispute over the nature of how *state of the art* is defined. Standardizing a curriculum may prove to be difficult because so many different specialists are involved in studying VP function, and certain diagnostic methods may be outside of the capabilities of a particular discipline. For example, speech pathologists have an obvious interest in VP function but cannot personally perform fluoroscopic procedures because the use of radiation makes the technique invasive. There is some dispute over the capacity of speech pathologists to perform nasopharyngoscopy because of the use of topical anesthesia, the risk of causing bleeding or discomfort, and the possibility that an inexperienced examiner could pass the instrument into the glottis and prompt laryngospasm, which could prove fatal. A vasovagal response may also occur, prompting fainting which, if not managed properly, could also prove dangerous to the patient. Therefore at this time it is not recommended that all speech pathologists be given permission to perform endoscopic procedures.

Treatment options

The manner in which one interprets diagnostic data is strongly influenced by the treatment options available for VPI. If a particular center applies surgical treatment to nearly every case and the surgical treatment is essentially the same for each case, then the diagnostic data will not have as dramatic an influence on treatment recommendations compared to centers that provide multiple treatment options. For example, in Center A the head surgeon has been trained to perform a particular pharyngeal flap operation for any case where VPI has been diagnosed. This particular surgeon has read about and been trained to do the lateral port control operation advocated by Hogan (1973). The hypothesis behind this operation is to control the size of the lateral portals on either

side of the pharyngeal flap by sizing them with catheters so that the total area of the opening is no greater than 20 mm^2. This port area is based on the hypotheses of Warren (Warren and DuBois, 1964; Warren, 1975), who utilized pressure flow procedures to calculate that VP gaps of under 20 mm^2 do not result in perceived hypernasality. It should be mentioned that this hypothesis has never been confirmed by direct visualization procedures, and most clinicians who perform endoscopic and fluoroscopic procedures would vigorously dispute Warren's contention. However, this particular surgeon believes that this single pharyngeal flap procedure will resolve all problems of VPI. Therefore the diagnostic data derived from nasopharyngoscopy are important only for a decision about surgery. If VPI is present, the lateral port control operation will be done. If VPI is not present, no operation will be done.

At Center B multiple procedures are performed to treat VPI. When pharyngeal flap is recommended, the surgeon at Center B varies flap width and location as advocated by Argamaso (Argamaso et al., 1980, 1994; Argamaso, 1990). They also have a variety of other operations they might use, such as palatal lengthening procedures and posterior wall augmentations. In some cases speech bulb reduction might be recommended based on the input of the speech pathologist (see Chapter 17). The therapy applied at Center B depends on the information derived from endoscopic and fluoroscopic procedures after review by several team members, including both the surgeon and speech pathologist. Unlike Center A, not only does the information derived from diagnostic procedures indicate if treatment will be applied, but the treatment is chosen to take advantage of the types of movements seen on direct visualization diagnostic procedures.

Specialists involved in the diagnostic procedure

It is important for as many specialists as possible to be involved in the review of the data obtained from endoscopic and fluoroscopic procedures to obtain the most useful information possible from the diagnostic process. Each specialist brings a different perspective on the same data, which is enhanced by an accumulated experience matching diagnostic findings to treatment results. D'Antonio et al. (1989) advocated the concept of several specialists reviewing nasopharyngoscopic studies *and* discussing their reviews of the study to enhance the reliability of the diagnosis. Several actual cases can help to illustrate the importance of group review and discussion.

In the first case a patient is referred to a cleft palate clinic with hypernasality as diagnosed by a speech pathologist within a public school system. That speech pathologist did everything within appropriate professional standards and capabilities in the school setting, including peroral examination, perceptual analysis, mirror testing, and articulation testing (along with other diagnostic procedures not specifically designed to detect nasal emission or nasal resonance, such as language testing). No cleft or submucous cleft was present, but the patient had had a recent adenotonsillectomy. The school speech pathologist recognized the importance of specialized tests that could be applied by an experienced cleft palate team, such as nasopharyngoscopy and multiview videofluoroscopy. In the center to which the referral was made, nasopharyngoscopy was done by the surgeon who did the operations to resolve VPI. The surgeon understood a good deal about VP anatomy and physiology but very little about speech. The surgeon did not know the difference between pressure demands of various phonemes (in fact, the surgeon could not define phoneme) and used a speech sample consisting of vowel sounds, a few isolated words, and repeated syllables, such as pa-pa-pa and ka-ka-ka. The endoscopic examination was not videotaped, and the only record of the examination was a brief note made by the surgeon simply stating that VPI was present and that surgery would be necessary to correct it. No one else was present during the examination (even if someone had been, it would not have made much difference because there was no video system used to allow more than one person to see the examination). The surgeon was also convinced that nasopharyngoscopy represented a definitive diagnostic procedure so that other examinations of the VP valve (such as videofluoroscopy) were not necessary. The other team members had no reason to doubt the surgeon. The recommendation for surgery was made to the mother of the patient, who was compelled by her insurance carrier to seek a second opinion. She therefore contacted a second cleft palate team in a nearby city. At this second team both nasopharyngoscopy and multiview videofluoroscopy were used to assess VP function. In addition, at all diagnostic procedures for VP function a speech pathologist was present and was personally reponsible for administering the speech sample. During the nasopharyngoscopy the speech pathologist used a comprehensive speech sample, which included sustained fricatives such as /ssss/ and /ffff/. It was noted that, during the utterance of the sustained fricatives, the patient achieved a tight VP seal. With a little manipulating of the patient's speech during endoscopy, the speech pathologist was able to get the patient to close the valve on /t/ sounds. Videofluoroscopy confirmed inconsistent closure during speech. A review of the patient's medical records from the admission for adenotonsillectomy indicated that the adenoid was extremely large preoperatively, filling the entire choanal space so that no movement of the velum or lateral pharyngeal walls was necessary to prevent air from escaping through the nose (because the nose was fully blocked by the adenoids). The speech pathologist from the second team hypothesized that the patient was having intermittent VPI caused by the sudden removal of the adenoid. Because the palate and lateral pharyngeal walls did not need to move before the surgery for the patient to prevent air and sound from escaping through the nose, after surgery the palate and pharynx remained motionless. However, when pressure demands were high, as for sustained /s/ and /f/, it became necessary for the VP valve to function for the sound to be produced. This is not an uncommon phenomenon in young children where phoneme-specific VPI or phoneme-specific closure is simply a type of articulation error. The speech pathologist recommended speech therapy, which was supplemented with occasional nasopharyngoscopic biofeedback. The problem was resolved within 4 weeks after 12 sessions of speech therapy, three sessions of which were combined with nasopharyngoscopy.

In the second case a child with a repaired cleft lip and palate had persistent VPI with hypernasal resonance. At the first center a team of a plastic surgeon, speech pathologist, and orthodontist evaluated the child. The speech pathologist utilized nasometry to assess VP function. Neither nasopharyngoscopy nor videofluoroscopy were used, and no otolaryngologist was available to assess the patient. Based on nasometric findings, which indicated constant hypernasal resonance, and because the patient had a repaired cleft, the surgeon recommended a pharyngeal flap. By seeking a second opinion the child was evaluated by a more comprehensive team, which included endoscopic, fluoroscopic, and otolaryngologic examination. On endoscopy, prominent tonsils could be seen in the oropharyngeal airway, interfering with lateral pharyngeal wall motion on both sides and preventing the palate from moving posteriorly to the posterior pharyngeal wall (see Fig. 12-4). This was confirmed on fluoroscopic examination, which showed the tonsils interfering with VP closure (Shprintzen et al., 1987). The otolaryngologist questioned the patient's mother carefully and elicited a history of upper airway obstruction, including occasional episodes of apnea, constant snoring, and difficulties with swallowing large pieces of food. The speech pathologist with this second team noted that there were articulatory errors consistent with tonsillar hypertrophy, including tongue fronting, vowel distortions, and a "potato in the mouth" resonance pattern. A tonsillectomy was recommended as a first stage in treatment followed by speech therapy to eliminate the pattern of articulatory abnormalities. Speech therapy would be followed by repeat endoscopy to determine if there were changes in VP valving. After tonsillectomy and approximately 6 weeks of speech therapy, nasopharyngoscopy showed normal VP function with no evidence of VPI or hypernasal resonance. The otolaryngologist pointed out that, had a pharyngeal flap been done as suggested by the first team, the patient would have been at high risk for severe obstructive apnea (see Chapter 5).

As pointed out by these two cases, it may not be sufficient for teams to be multidisciplinary or even interdisciplinary. The concept of transdisciplinary teams as discussed in Chapter 15 is one which deserves mentioning (LeBlanc, 1994). Transdisciplinary teams not only have representatives of many disciplines (multidisciplinary) who work together (interdisciplinary); they also have learned something of each other's disciplines (transdisciplinary). Shared knowledge across disciplines makes it less likely that potential errors such as those illustrated in these two cases will occur.

Personality

The personalities of the individuals involved in the assessment is a factor not often discussed because of the personal nature of the subject. However, there is no doubt that the type of individual involved in assessment will affect the manner in which a decision is made. People who are easily threatened by other team members may reach decisions that have less to do with the clinical picture and more to do with proving a point. Personality is an intangible factor but one that certainly needs to be addressed by teams. Because individual personalities can have an effect on decisions, it is often advisable for teams to have multiple individuals from a single discipline to counterbalance the personality effect.

Most teams have a dominant personality. There is nothing wrong with a team member trying to assert an opinion considered by that person to be correct. The problem with a dominant personality is when that personality is the one given the most weight because the individual is in a position of authority. In my opinion team directors may best be individuals who have no vested interest in treating the patient or asserting a treatment option. In other words, clinicians should try to ensure that the team operates in a manner such that the patient's interest is the sole determining factor in making a decision regarding treatment.

REFERENCES

Argamaso RV: The pharyngeal flap in cleft lip and palate. In Kernahan DA, Rosenstein SW, editors: *Cleft lip and palate: a system of management,* Baltimore, 1990, Williams & Wilkins.

Argamaso RV, Shprintzen RJ, Strauch B, Lewin ML, Daniller A, Ship AG, Croft CB: The role of lateral pharyngeal wall motion in pharyngeal flap surgery, *Plast Reconstr Surg* 66:214, 1980.

Argamaso RV, Bassila M, Bratcher GO, Brodsky L, Cotton RT, Croft CB, Greenberg LM, Laskin R, MacKenzie-Stepner K, Meyer CM III, Rakoff SJ, Ruben RJ, Sher AE, Shprintzen RJ, Sidoti EJ, Singer L, Strauch B, Witzel MA: Tonsillectomy and pharyngeal flap should not be performed simultaneously, *Cleft Palate J* 25:176, 1988.

Argamaso RV, Levandowski GJ, Golding-Kushner KJ, Shprintzen RL: Treatment of asymmetric velopharyngeal insufficiency with skewed pharyngeal flap, *Cleft Palate-Craniofac J* 1994 (in press).

Arvystas M, Shprintzen RJ: Craniofacial morphology in the velo-cardio-facial syndrome, *J Craniofac Genet Dev Biol* 4:39, 1984.

Barone CM, Shprintzen RJ, Strauch B, Sablay LB, Argamaso RV: Pharyngeal flap revisions: flap elevation from a scarred posterior pharynx, *Plast Reconstr Surg* 93:279, 1994.

Calnan J: Submucous cleft palate, *Br J Plast Surg* 6:264, 1954.

Croft CB, Shprintzen RJ, Ruben RJ: Hypernasal speech following adenotonsillectomy, *Otolaryngol Head Neck Surg* 89:179, 1981.

Croft CB, Shprintzen RJ, Daniller AI, Lewin ML: The occult submucous cleft palate and the musculus uvulae, *Cleft Palate J* 15:150, 1978.

D'Antonio L, Marsh JL, Province M, Muntz H, Phillips C: Reliability of flexible fiberoptic nasopharyngoscopy for evaluation of velopharyngeal function in a clinical population, *Cleft Palate J* 26:217, 1989.

Dickson DR: Anatomy of the normal and cleft palate eustachian tube, *Ann Otol Rhinol Laryngol* 85(suppl 25):25, 1976.

Dickson DR, Dickson WM: Velopharyngeal anatomy, *J Speech Hear Res* 15:372, 1972.

Gereau SA, Shprintzen RJ: The role of adenoids in the development of normal speech following palate repair, *Laryngoscope* 98:99, 1988.

Gereau SA, Stevens D, Bassila M, Sher AE, Sidoti EJ Jr., Morgan M, Oka SW, Shprintzen RJ: Endoscopic observations of eustachian tube abnormalities in children with palatal clefts. In Lim DJ, Bluestone CD, Klein JO, and Nelson JD: *Symposium on otitis media,* Toronto, 1988, BC Decker.

Glaser ER, Skolnick ML, McWilliams BJ, Shprintzen RJ: The dynamics of Passavant's ridge in subjects with and without velopharyngeal insufficiency—a multiview videofluoroscopic study, *Cleft Palate J* 16:24, 1979.

Henningsson G, Isberg A: Velopharyngeal movements in patients alternating between oral and glottal articulation: a clinical and cineradiographical study, *Cleft Palate J* 23:1, 1986.

Hoch L, Golding-Kushner KJ, Sadewitz V, and Shprintzen RJ: Speech therapy. In McWilliams BJ, editor: *Seminars in speech and language: current methods of assessing and treating children with cleft palates*, New York, 1986, Thieme.

Hogan VM: A clarification of the surgical goals in cleft palate speech and the introduction of the lateral port control (LPC) pharyngeal flap, *Cleft Palate J* 10:331, 1973.

Laniado N: *Cephalometric analysis of adult obstructive sleep apnea*, Unpublished thesis, Division of Orthodontics, Department of Dentistry, Montefiore Medical Center, 1987.

LeBlanc E: Personal communication, 1994.

MacKenzie-Stepner K, Witzel MA, Stringer DA, Lindsay WK, Munro IR, Hughes H: Abnormal carotid arteries in the velocardiofacial syndrome: a report of three cases, *Plast Reconstr Surg* 80:347, 1987.

Maue-Dickson W, Dickson DR, Rood SR: Anatomy of the eustachian tube and related structures in age-matched human fetuses with and without cleft palate, *Trans Am Acad Ophthalmol Otolaryngol* 82:159, 1976.

Mitnick RJ, Bello JA, Golding-Kusher KJ, Argamaso RV, Shprintzen RJ: The use of magnetic resonance angiography prior to pharyngeal flap in patients with velo-cardio-facial syndrome, *Plast Reconstr Surg* 1995 (in press).

Sher AE, Thorpy MJ, Shprintzen RJ, Spielman AJ, Burack B, McGregor P: Predictive value of the Müller maneuver in the selection of patients for uvulopalatopharyngoplasty, *Laryngoscope* 95:1483, 1985.

Shprintzen RJ: Palatal and pharyngeal anomalies in craniofacial syndromes, *Birth Defects* 18(1):53, 1982.

Shprintzen RJ, Croft CB: Abnormalities of the eustachian tube orifice in individuals with cleft palate, *Int J Pediatr Otorhinolaryngol* 3:15, 1981.

Shprintzen RJ, Sher AE, Croft CB: Hypernasal speech caused by hypertrophic tonsils, *Internat J Pediatr Otorhinolaryngol* 14:45, 1987.

Shprintzen RJ, Lewin ML, Croft CB, Daniller AI, Argamaso RV, Ship A, Strauch B: A comprehensive study of pharyngeal flap surgery: tailor-made flaps, *Cleft Palate J* 16:46, 1979.

Shprintzen RJ, Croft CB, Berkman MD, Rakoff SJ: Velopharyngeal insufficiency in the facio-auriculo-vertebral malformation complex, *Cleft Palate J* 17:132, 1980.

Shprintzen RJ, Schwartz R, Daniller A, Hoch L: The morphologic significance of bifid uvula, *Pediatrics* 75:553, 1985.

Siegel-Sadewitz VL, Shprintzen RJ: Nasopharyngoscopy of the normal velopharyngeal sphincter: an experiment of biofeedback, *Cleft Palate J* 19:194, 1982.

Siegel-Sadewitz VL, Shprintzen RJ: Changes in velopharyngeal valving with age, *Int J Pediatr Otorhinolaryngol* 11:171, 1986.

Skolnick ML, McCall GN: Velopharyngeal competence and incompetence following pharyngeal flap surgery: a videofluoroscopic study in multiple projections, *Cleft Palate J* 9:1, 1972.

Warren DW, DuBois AB: A pressure-flow technique for measuring velopharyngeal orifice area during continuous speech, *Cleft Palate J* 1:52, 1964.

Warren DW: The determination of velopharyngeal incompetency by aerodynamic and acoustical techniques. In Hogan VM, editor: *Clinics in plastic surgery*, Philadelphia, 1975, WB Saunders.

Williams ML, Shprintzen RJ, Rakoff SJ: Adenoid hypoplasia in the velo-cardio-facial syndrome, *J Craniofac Genet Dev Biol* 7:23, 1987.

Witzel MA, Tobe J, Salyer KE: The use of videonasopharyngoscopy for biofeedback therapy in adults after pharyngeal flap surgery, *Cleft Palate J* 26:129, 1989.

13 Secondary Surgery for Velopharyngeal Insufficiency

Janvsz Bardach

Among the many complications and secondary problems related to cleft palate treatment, it is well established that velopharyngeal insufficiency (VPI) is one of the most complex because it affects the ability of the patient to communicate coherently with other people. According to our long-term clinical observations, VPI is viewed by patients and their families as more debilitating than secondary lip and nose deformities, which affect only physical appearance but do not interfere with verbal interaction.

Though there has been definite improvement in both the surgical techniques and the level of surgical skill, the overall results reported from various centers in primary palate repair are similar enough to indicate that other factors may influence speech results, including the anatomy of the nasopharynx and oropharynx, the movement of lateral pharyngeal walls, the mobility and length of the soft palate, the distance between the posterior edge of the soft palate and the posterior pharyngeal wall, the anterior movement of the posterior pharyngeal wall, the presence and degree of protrusion of the Passavant ridge, the presence or absence of adenoid tissue, and the status of the nasal passages, particularly nasal septal deviation and hypertrophy of the lower turbinates. Oronasal fistulae may also affect speech production by causing hypernasality, velopharyngeal (VP) valving failure, and compensatory articulation.

A question that often arises when planning cleft palate repair is how to create the conditions in each particular case that will result in optimal VP closure and normal speech production. This question can be answered on an individual basis only, following careful diagnostic evaluation and taking into account all factors that may influence the outcome. However, the present state of the art of multidisciplinary treatment of cleft palate does not allow for precise prediction of the outcome because all phases of surgical treatment cannot be controlled to a degree that ensures successful results in every case. The main problem is that

cleft palate is only one contributing factor to VPI, and even this single problem cannot be managed optimally in every case because of the various forms and degrees of severity of clefts, different surgical techniques, different surgical skills, and different healing processes and scar contracture. Thus, even though we may do our best to optimize the results in the surgical treatment of palatal clefts, in some cases the outcome may still be unsatisfactory.

During primary evaluation of the cleft palate, we attempt to establish the basic parameters that will allow for the planning of treatment strategies. The results of cleft palate repair must be judged with regard to two factors: surgical outcome and speech outcome. An optimal surgical result is not always equivalent to an optimal speech result. A palatal cleft can be perfectly closed in the first operation without any resulting oronasal fistulae. As a result of surgery, the palate may be adequately long and mobile, but there may be lack of closure of the VP sphincter that normally separates the oropharynx from the nasopharynx resulting in hypernasality or nasal air escape.

The VP sphincter includes the soft palate and its musculature as well as the superior constrictor muscle of the pharynx. The simultaneous function of these muscles determines the effectiveness of the sphincter. The presence of adenoid tissue on the posterior pharyngeal wall as well as movement of Passavant's ridge may influence VP closure.

Hypernasality and nasal air emission during speech are the most typical features of cleft palate speech and the only indications for pharyngoplasty. When making decisions about surgery to improve speech production, it is necessary to establish the reliability of the diagnosis and to select the surgical procedure most appropriate to each individual case. Decisions regarding the appropriateness of secondary pharyngeal surgery must be made in close conjunction with the speech pathologist, whose assessment of speech production is essential to establishing a diagnosis and prognosis. In recent years more and more plastic surgeons have actively participated in the assessment of VP function by performing or reviewing nasopharyngoscopy. The assessment of the VP structures and function should include intraoral examination of the speech mechanism, examination of the nasal airways, a complete speech and language evaluation, nasopharyngoscopy, and multiview videofluoroscopy. Other assessments, such as aerodynamic measurements, may also be of value. The findings of the speech pathologist and the surgeon serve as the basis for discussion in selecting the most appropriate treatment approach and, when necessary, the surgical procedure.

As indicated in the chapter on cleft palate repair, our experience and the results of clinical studies reveal that the goals of primary cleft palate repair are the following:

1. Complete closure of the entire palatal cleft with special attention paid to closing the anterior palate; this closure must be done in two layers in the area of the hard palate and in three layers in the area of the soft palate
2. Creation of a mobile soft palate to enhance normal function of the VP sphincter and subsequently normal speech production
3. Some lengthening of the soft palate due to detachment of the muscles of the soft palate from the posterior edge of the hard palate and from the periosteum on the nasal surface

It is critical to achieve complete cleft palate repair in the first surgical procedure. With some surgical techniques, postsurgical oronasal fistulae commonly occur as a result of the design of the operation. Since van Langenbeck palatoplasty and four-flap Wardill-Kilner technique (also known as the Oxford technique) both prevent precise closure of the cleft in the most anterior area of the palate entering the alveolar ridge, an anterior oronasal fistula next to the alveolar ridge is present in most patients. In contrast, in two-flap palatoplasty the anterior palatal cleft is closed precisely in two layers, thus avoiding oronasal fistula in this area. Proper surgical technique exercised at the time of cleft palate repair also successfully prevents the formation of oronasal fistulae between the hard and soft palates; fistulae often occur in this area, due to insufficient release of tension of the mucoperiosteal flaps on the oral and nasal sides and lack of proper two-layer closure when both layers are tightly approximated.

In cases when the first operation is not fully successful and closure of the cleft palate is not complete, secondary palatal surgery is more difficult due to wide scarring and subsequent bleeding. The presence of oronasal fistulae, which is the major indication for secondary corrective surgery, can be minimized. If the incidence of oronasal fistulae is higher than 10%, the surgeon must reevaluate the surgical technique and pay more attention to the details of repair in the areas where fistulae are most common. There is one other problem with repeated surgical procedures in the palate: the amount of tissue in this area is limited and outside tissue is not easily supplemented. For this reason repeated surgical procedures cause increased scarring in the area of the hard and soft palates. Severe scarring in the area of the hard palate may lead to severe midfacial growth aberrations; heavy scarring in the area of the soft palate affects its mobility and function.

For a long time there was a widespread opinion among surgeons and speech pathologists that the length of the soft palate was an essential factor in establishing normal VP function. The truth is that the soft palate is only one component of the VP valve. The remaining components are the lateral pharyngeal walls and the posterior pharyngeal wall. Therefore there may be cases in which the palate seems long enough but complete closure of the valve is not achieved due to sluggish movement of the lateral pharyngeal walls or lack of contact between the posterior edge of the soft palate and the posterior pharyngeal wall. On the other hand, the palate may seem short, but when it is functioning well and in combination with vigorous movements of the lateral pharyngeal walls, complete closure may be achieved, resulting in normal speech production. Inadequate functioning of the soft palate, which may be sluggish due to heavy scarring after repeated surgical procedures, usually results in failure to achieve complete closure.

Even with the many advances in surgical techniques for treatment of cleft palate, the problem of subsequent VPI continues to exist. In most cleft centers in this country the percentage of patients who require additional surgical treatment following cleft palate repair ranges anywhere from 20% to 30%. In several clinical studies evaluating the late results of cleft palate repair in cases of unilateral and bilateral complete cleft of the lip, alveolus, and palate, we found the success rate to be 75% to 80%. These findings, as well as findings from other cleft palate centers, indicate a need for subsequent surgical treatment in a substantial number of cleft patients.

TIMING OF SECONDARY PHARYNGEAL SURGERY

Precise assessment of VPI must be obtained with enough certainty to justify indications for surgery. In young patients (2 to 3 years of age) it may be difficult for the speech pathologist to draw definite conclusions about VP dysfunction and recommend surgical treatment. The severity of VPI in addition to the results of examination and testing may lead the speech pathologist and surgeon to choose nonsurgical treatment as a primary course of rehabilitation. The patients selected for nonsurgical treatment (speech therapy) usually exhibit marginal VPI. However, even in cases of moderate but intermittent incompetence, speech therapy may be recommended. Surgical treatment is usually recommended when the velopharyngeal dysfunction is consistent or determined to be related to an anatomic problem. Secondary pharyngeal surgery is indicated when there is definite VPI with hypernasal speech and nasal air emission as determined by the speech pathologist's listener judgment.

Another problem in treatment planning is timing of secondary surgery. Surgery should not be planned until the assessment of the patient's speech can be considered reliable and consistent. According to our experience, this judgment is not possible until 4 to 5 years of age. Shprintzen (1990) has emphasized that pharyngeal flap surgery should not be performed in children below the age of approximately 4 ½ years. He specified four reasons for delaying the surgical procedure: language development, articulation development, assessment of VPI, and compliance and morbidity.

Currently the diagnosis and planning of surgical procedures for treatment of VPI are highly advanced, employing not only acoustic examination but also nasoendoscopy and multiview videofluoroscopy. Both techniques play a special role in the physiologic and anatomic description of the VP mechanism. After examining the patient, the speech pathologist and the surgeon can specifically define the area of deficient closure and plan the surgical procedures most appropriate for the individual patient. With the precision of current diagnostic tools and the ability to plan the surgical procedure according to findings, it would seem that the problem of VPI can be successfully solved in every patient. However, it is necessary to admit that any type of pharyngeal surgery chosen for a particular patient, even when highly successful in terms of speech results, may cause annoying complications for the patient or even present a health risk.

Some cases of severe VPI can be recognized at an early age. However, it may be prudent to delay pharyngoplasty until an age when precise examination can be performed, allowing for functional and anatomic findings to facilitate the planning and performing of the surgical procedure.

In borderline cases the speech pathologist and the surgeon may have great difficulty deciding the timing of surgery and the selection of the surgical technique. In such cases speech therapy must always be recommended before decisions are made about the surgical procedure. In some cases the use of a temporary speech bulb obturator to improve speech production and stimulate pharyngeal movements may result in normal speech without surgical treatment.

A speech bulb obturator occludes the VP space sufficiently to produce normal speech. After it has been worn for several months, it is reduced in size and worn for another month (see Chapter 16). The bulb is reduced on a monthly basis until it can be eliminated, or hypernasality returns. This is called speech bulb reduction. However, in some cases a prosthesis is used to permanently occlude the VP space. I have often treated patients who, after many years of using a prosthesis, requested surgical treatment because they could no longer tolerate the appliance. In light of the current advances in surgical techniques for cleft palate repair, I consider the use of protheses as permanent therapy to be totally unacceptable.

A decision must be made about surgery as soon as possible when (1) VPI is verifiably diagnosed, and (2) nonsurgical treatment has not been recommended. Secondary pharyngeal surgery performed at an early age (4 to 5 years) is often more successful than when performed at a later age because of habitual compensatory speech patterns. The indications for surgery are basically limited to VPI. However, some indications are controversial or highly questionable.

A classic example of controversial and questionable indications can be seen in the case of submucous cleft. There are surgeons who perform an early pharyngeal flap procedure on these patients, a highly questionable approach based on the erroneous assumption that each submucous palatal cleft will lead to VPI and subsequent speech impairment. Some specialists use this assumption as an indication for surgery at approximately 1 year of age. However, both the assumption and the decision to perform a pharyngeal flap procedure are definitely erroneous; and both indicate a lack of understanding of the overall implications following pharyngeal flap surgery.

First of all, there is no justification for assuming that every case of submucous palatal cleft will result in VPI. It is well known that speech is not impaired in most cases of submucous cleft, and the cleft may remain undetected for many years. Second, if there is a submucous cleft that causes speech impairment due to hypernasality, palatoplasty may suffice before considering a pharyngeal flap procedure. Soft palate function may be improved and VPI eliminated by joining the divided muscles of the soft palate after detaching them from the posterior edge of the hard palate. Finally, performing pharyngeal surgery during the first year of age without proper assessment and without establishing a precise diagnosis is inappropriate, professionally erroneous, and, considering the possible complications, potentially dangerous to the child's health. The decision to perform pharyngeal surgery can be justified only when (1) a diagnosis of VPI is established without any doubt, (2) speech therapy proves unsuccessful, and (3) a palatoplasty procedure fails to result in marked speech improvement.

Another questionable indication for pharyngeal flap surgery when a child starts talking unintelligibly at (2 to 3 years of age). Although it is true that hypernasal speech may be detected at this age by the speech pathologist, there is still a need for a more detailed diagnosis as well as consideration of early speech therapy. Choosing surgery at an early age without establishing a precise diagnosis and exploring the possibility of nonsurgical treatment is premature. In cases of VPI the application of surgical treatment must follow a detailed examination and attempts to use speech therapy as a primary approach, with surgical treatment reserved as a secondary approach.

Primary pharyngeal flap at the time of primary cleft repair has been and is still advocated by some surgeons and speech pathologists. During the 1950s and 1960s this approach was quite popular in a number of centers, and it is currently being used in a few American and European centers. The concept of performing primary pharyngeal flap surgery at the time of cleft palate repair was an attempt to create optimal conditions for the development of normal speech. This idea reflected the assumption that pharyngeal flap surgery performed in each patient with palatal cleft will result in perfect speech. However, this concept has never had a solid scientific basis. Furthermore, not all patients with cleft palate require secondary pharyngeal surgery following palatoplasty. It is true that in the past a much higher percentage of patients (over 60%) required pharyngeal flap

surgery due to VPI. At the present time the average success rate following palatoplasty is 75% to 85%. For this reason I consider performing pharyngeal flap or any other type of pharyngoplasty at the time of primary palate repair to be scientifically, medically, and ethically unjustified. At the present time only 15% to 25% of palatoplasty patients require subsequent pharyngeal flap. Therefore the remaining 75% to 85% of patients receive a procedure that is not indicated. In my opinion primary pharyngeal flap surgery is indicated only during primary palate repair in adolescents and adults with unrepaired wide palatal cleft.

CHOICE OF SURGICAL PROCEDURE

It is important to realize that secondary pharyngeal surgery and, specifically the pharyngeal flap, are not physiologic procedures, since they both create an anatomic structure that normally does not exist. Although that structure may be beneficial to speech production, it may also be harmful with regard to other functions, or at least annoying to the patient. For this reason pharyngeal flap surgery should be used only after exhausting all other options to improve speech production without the harmful or annoying affects that may result from pharyngeal surgery. Before using a pharyngeal flap, it is logical to explore any surgical procedure that might alleviate the impact of VPI.

Technologic advances, especially the development of nasoendoscopy and improvements in videofluoroscopy, allow for precise diagnosis of the degree of insufficiency of VP sphincter function. These findings, along with the results of other examinations, may serve as the basis for selection of the surgical technique and the type of pharyngoplasty.

The search for an optimal surgical procedure to treat VPI led to proposals that, when implemented, proved to be more complex than expected (Fig. 13-1). Hogan was one of the first to introduce the concept of controlled lateral ports, based on the assumption that a lateral port of 20 mm^2 created by a pharyngeal flap will result in the ideal condition for normal speech production. This idea sounded as promising as the tailored pharyngeal flaps described by Shprintzen and Argamaso, Salyer, and others. These authors attempted to tailor the size of the flap and the level of the flap base according to the findings from nasoendoscopy, videofluoroscopy, and local conditions of the velopharynx and the soft palate. Following this approach, narrow, moderate, and wide pharyngeal flaps were used with varying modes of insertion.

Tailoring pharyngeal flaps and creating con-

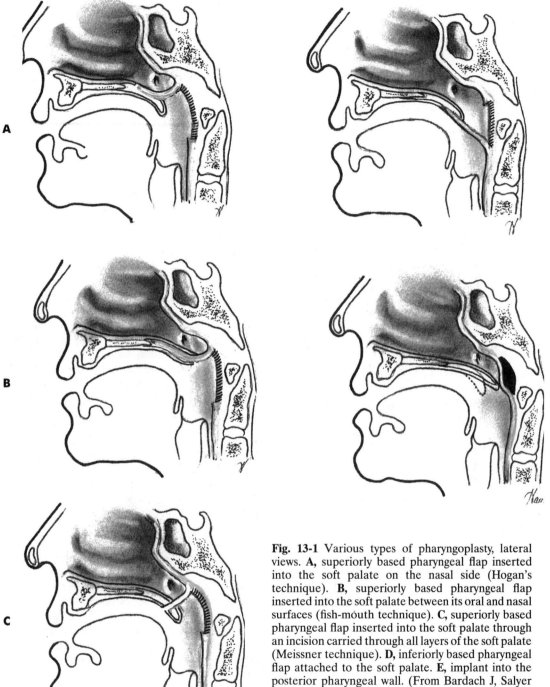

Fig. 13-1 Various types of pharyngoplasty, lateral views. **A,** superiorly based pharyngeal flap inserted into the soft palate on the nasal side (Hogan's technique). **B,** superiorly based pharyngeal flap inserted into the soft palate between its oral and nasal surfaces (fish-mouth technique). **C,** superiorly based pharyngeal flap inserted into the soft palate through an incision carried through all layers of the soft palate (Meissner technique). **D,** inferiorly based pharyngeal flap attached to the soft palate. **E,** implant into the posterior pharyngeal wall. (From Bardach J, Salyer K: *Surgical techniques in cleft lip and palate,* ed 2, St. Louis, 1991, Mosby.)

trolled lateral ports are both based on concepts which assume that the flaps and the ports will remain unchanged following the surgical procedure. In reality this does not happen, since the lateral ports are surrounded by raw edges, and scar contracture during healing cannot be controlled. Lined pharyngeal flaps also have a tendency to contract during the healing process, thus changing their width and thickness. Since the healing process and tissue contracture cannot be controlled, and since the postoperative changes in the size and shape of the ports and pharyngeal flaps are unpredictable, this approach cannot be considered perfectly reliable. However, there is some validity in the idea of tailoring pharyngeal flaps, depending on the findings of the examination by a speech pathologist and surgeon.

A definite diagnosis of VPI is based on objective and subjective findings. Examination of the patient's speech leads primarily to subjective findings. More objective information is provided by the following examinations and findings:

1. Nasoendoscopy
2. Videofluoroscopy
3. Oronasal fistulae in the hard or soft palate
4. Function of the soft palate
5. Presence of Passavant's ridge
6. Size and status of the tonsils
7. Presence and amount of adenoid tissue on posterior pharyngeal wall
8. Function of the lateral pharyngeal walls
9. Width of the nasopharynx

The technique, interpretations, and findings of nasoendoscopy and videofluoroscopy are described in Chapter 11. When examining the palate, attention must be paid to *oronasal fistulae,* which are most commonly found in the anterior portion of the palate, or between the hard and soft palate. On many occasions fistulae in the anterior portion of the palate appear only after maxillary expansion is performed by an orthodontist. Before this procedure the maxillary segments may be approximated so closely that the fistula is virtually invisible and may be detected only by precise probing. The question of whether an invisible oronasal fistula has to be closed remains controversial. In my opinion the existence of communication between the oral and nasal cavities must be considered an indication for surgical closure to prevent fluid and air leaks as well as food retention in the case when the fistula enlarges as a result of orthodontic treatment or growth processes. The oronasal fistula may vary in size and location. Fistulae also may appear as a result of primary cleft palate repair or secondary corrections. A fistula of any size that results in leakage of air and fluid may affect speech.

When the patient exhibits VPI and oronasal fistulae are present in the hard or soft palate, closing the fistulae must be considered before proceeding with the pharyngeal flap. Many surgeons decide to simultaneously close oronasal fistulae and the pharyngeal flap, although staging the procedures and closing the fistulae first may, in many cases, result in such speech improvement; pharyngeal flap then becomes unnecessary.

Examination of the soft palate should focus on function and the distance between the posterior edge of the soft palate and the posterior pharyngeal wall. On some occasions the soft palate may appear short, but when it functions well in combination with vigorous movements of the lateral pharyngeal walls, it may provide for closure of the VP sphincter. In contrast, sluggish movements of the soft palate in a patient with VPI usually indicate the need for pharyngoplasty, since there is little hope of developing better motion of the soft palate and achieving improved closure of the sphincter. Short palate is not always an indication for using pharyngeal flap. Other techniques can be employed to lengthen the short palate and approximate its posterior edge to the posterior pharyngeal wall. One example is a pushback technique, which must be performed with dissection of the muscles of the soft palate and mucosa from the posterior edge of the hard palate, thus allowing the entire soft palate to be pushed back, while achieving only one-layer closure by suturing the mucoperiosteal flaps on the oral side. Another technique that I suggest be used before pharyngeal flap is the Furlow technique of palate lengthening, using an opposing Z-plasty procedure. If these techniques do not provide improvement in speech production, some type of pharyngoplasty is indicated, and my choice in such cases is a superiorly based pharyngeal flap.

When examining the distance between the posterior pharyngeal wall and the posterior edge of the soft palate, consideration must be given to the *presence and location of Passavant's ridge,* which may contribute to better contact between those two anatomic structures. Later in this chapter are techniques for increasing the bulk of the posterior pharyngeal wall, thus creating better conditions for speech production.

The size and status of the tonsils must be taken into account in every patient in which pharyngoplasty is considered. Large tonsils that can occlude the pharyngeal flap ports or the oropharyngeal airway must be removed before pharyngoplasty, especially if pharyngeal flap is used as the mode of treatment. When a wide pharyngeal flap is planned, large tonsils also must be removed before surgery, since the combination of a wide pharyngeal flap with large tonsils may cause airway obstruction. Chronic tonsillitis is another indication for removal of the tonsils.

The question of whether the *adenoid tissue* must be removed still remains controversial. Serious arguments support the benefits of this procedure. Arguments against performing adenoidectomy include the fact that adenoid tissue undergoes spontaneous involution in adolescence, and therefore there is no need to remove adenoid tissue before pharyngeal flap surgery. For this reason adenoidectomy at an early age may be considered unnecessary. The claim that removing adenoid tissue has beneficial effects on ear disease in cleft patients has not been sufficiently proved to justify this approach. The final argument against performing adenoidectomy before pharyngoplasty is the possibility of producing scar tissue in the area selected for pharyngeal flap, which may impair the viability of the flap.

The arguments supporting adenoidectomy must be considered when discussing this procedure in patients with clefts. Removal of the adenoid tissue allows for better design and execution of the surgical procedure, since the operating field is clean and bleeding is minimal due to removal of the adenoids. Removing adenoid tissue also allows for more precise prediction of the surgical results because it eliminates a factor that could lead to recurrent hypernasality at a later age. The primary justification for removing adenoid tissue is that involution at a later age may change the size and shape of the velopharynx and may result in VPI and hypernasal speech if the adenoids occluded the pharynx.

The function of the lateral pharyngeal walls is of primary importance with regard to closure of the VP sphincter. Vigorous movement of the lateral pharyngeal walls may be essential for closure of the VP sphincter, even in cases when the soft palate is short and does not participate in closure. Vigorous movement of the lateral pharyngeal walls in patients with VPI is also an indication to choose a conservative surgical approach, such as a narrow pharyngeal flap. Sluggish movement of the lateral pharyngeal walls always indicates a need for a more radical approach, which usually involves a relatively wide superiorly based pharyngeal flap. Establishing *the width of the nasopharynx* is also necessary, since a wide nasopharynx requires a different pharyngeal flap design than when the nasopharynx is narrow.

When choosing the most appropriate surgical procedures, every individual case must be analyzed in terms of nasopharyngoscopic and videofluoroscopic findings, as well as in terms of the anatomic conditions and function of the VP sphincter.

Speech pathologists and surgeons must consider pharyngoplasty (particularly pharyngeal flap surgery) only after serious evaluation of all other available options and with full understanding of the complications that may result, especially following pharyngeal flap surgery. When analyzing the various options that may be used to correct VPI, priority must be given to the concepts and techniques that avoid serious postoperative complications. These concepts primarily relate to nonsurgical treatment, which includes speech therapy and prosthetic treatment. With regard to surgical options, priority must be given to procedures that avoid the creation of a pharyngeal flap, thus preventing severe airway obstruction. However, as mentioned, the choice of surgical procedure must be based on individual findings and anatomic conditions specific to each patient.

Pharyngoplasty procedures, including the classic operation designed by Orticochea and its modification by Jackson, as well as suturing the posterior tonsillar pillars, are alternatives to pharyngeal flap. However, despite recent advances and new techniques developed in this area, speech results following pharyngoplasty procedures are not always highly satisfactory, and secondary operations may be required. In contrast, the pharyngeal flap procedures, especially when superiorly based, provide more consistently successful speech results than pharyngoplasty.

SURGICAL TECHNIQUES

The various surgical techniques of pharyngoplasty are designed to eliminate VPI following cleft palate repair. VPI of other than cleft palate etiology can also be managed in this way. The basic goal of any pharyngoplasty is to decrease the size of the VP sphincter to allow for complete closure, thus eliminating hypernasality. Various treatment concepts described in the literature aim toward creating the proper anatomic and functional conditions for normal speech production. As indicated previously, the selection of the surgical technique is difficult, since it is based on objective and subjective findings and the outcome of the surgical procedure is not precisely predictable. It would be fair to state that the choice must be based primarily on objective findings, careful examination, as well as the surgeon's experience with a specific surgical procedure. At present there are no clinical data to support using any specific surgical technique as an optimal choice for a particular form of VPI.

The following surgical techniques of pharyngoplasty are now in use and must be considered as options in cases of VPI:

1. Inferiorly based pharyngeal flap (Schöenborn-Rosenthal)
2. Superiorly based pharyngeal flap (Sanvenero-Rosselli)
3. Hogan modification of superiorly based pharyngeal flap
4. Transverse pharyngeal flap (Kapetansky)
5. Sphincter pharyngoplasty (Orticochea, Jackson)
6. Posterior tonsillar pillars pharyngoplasty (Bardach)
7. Augmentation of the posterior pharyngeal wall (Hynes, Blocksma, Bluestone, McCabe, Brauer)

Inferiorly based pharyngeal flap

Inferiorly based pharyngeal flap was initially performed by Schöenborn and was described in 1876. It was refined and popularized in Germany by Rosenthal. This technique requires adequate exposure of the posterior pharyngeal wall. A mouth gag is used to retract the tongue, and a special hook is used to retract the soft palate. The flap is designed on the posterior pharyngeal wall, with the width varying according to anatomic conditions. A local injection is helpful not only in decreasing bleeding in the area, but also in establishing a plane of dissection on the level of the prevertebral fascia.

The operation starts with two parallel incisions on both sides of the designed pharyngeal flap. The incisions are carried through mucosa and muscle to the level of the prevertebral fascia, which can be easily detected by its whitish color. Using curved scissors or pharyngeal flap elevators, the flap can be readily dissected from the fascia. Attention must be paid to avoid performing these incisions in the groove between the posterior pharyngeal wall and the superior pharyngeal constrictor muscle, since in this area it is easy to injure the internal carotid artery, which could lead to profuse hemorrhaging.

After the flap is elevated according to the design, one may determine whether the level of the designated cranial end of the flap is adequate for tension-free insertion of this end into the posterior edge of the soft palate. In cases when it seems that the flap may be too short to insert, it is easy to extend the vertical incisions upward or downward to lengthen the flap.

The soft palate is incised transversely, and the nasal and oral layers are dissected, creating a fishmouth-like defect. The free edge of the pharyngeal flap is inserted into the defect, with its raw surface sutured to the nasal layer of the open defect of the soft palate. The oral layer of the soft palate is sutured to the raw surface at the end of the pharyngeal flap; 3.0 chromic catgut vertical and horizontal mattress sutures are used for attachment of the flap. Special attention must be paid to precisely suture the upper corners of the flap to maintain its width. However, after suturing the flap in place, the major portion of the raw surface of the flap facing the posterior pharyngeal wall remains exposed, which subsequently leads to tubing of the flap during the healing process. This decreases the flap width and increases the size of the lateral ports. To prevent tubing and scar contracture, many surgeons line the raw surface of the flap with free skin grafts. When successful, this technique partially prevents postoperative contracture of the flap. Lining the raw surface of the inferiorly based pharyngeal flap with free skin grafts is not highly successful, not only in terms of the skin graft taking, but also as a preventive measure for scar contracture and narrowing of the flap.

This flap requires secondary correction to achieve a good speech result more often than any other pharyngoplasty technique. On many occasions the inferiorly based pharyngeal flap pulls the soft palate inferiorly and posteriorly, thereby decreasing its mobility. Randall et al. have reported that in their series the inferiorly based pharyngeal flap was found to be as beneficial in the treatment of VPI as the superiorly based flap. The inferiorly based pharyngeal flap is used much less frequently than the superiorly based flap.

Superiorly based pharyngeal flap

The superiorly based pharyngeal flap was designed and described by Sanvenero-Rosselli in 1935. Another design was described by Meissner in 1952 and more recently by Black. The pharyngeal flap described by Sanvanerro-Rosselli is used by the vast majority of surgeons who operate on patients with VPI. The other technique is only used sporadically, in a very few centers.

The basic design of this operation is more logical than the design used for inferiorly based pharyngeal flap. First, the superior flap can be designed at a length that ensures tension-free insertion and fixation of the flap into the bed created in the soft palate. The width of the flap may vary, but it is possible to use a very wide flap if necessary, including the entire width of the posterior pharyngeal wall. Proper allocation of the base of the pharyngeal flap at a level that is higher than the posterior edge of the soft palate is possible, thus avoiding downward pull of the soft palate, which occurs when the flap base is lower than the posterior edge of the soft palate. High positioning of the flap base also allows for closure of the entire raw surface of the flap by mucosal flaps raised from the soft palate.

When the pharyngeal flaps are designed according to the considerations of the anatomic structures and the assessment of VP function, the flap width can be accurately designed. The approach used by Shprintzen and Argamasso is described as effective in 97% of cases. In Salyer's series VP closure was achieved in approximately 95% of patients when a tailored pharyngeal flap was used on the basis of preoperative findings. The tailored pharyngeal flap technique increases the probability of establishing adequate VP closure and minimizes the risk of obstruction, which could lead to hypernasality or denasality. All of these authors rely on the results of objective findings using nasoendoscopy, videofluoroscopy, speech assessment, and physical examination.

In this operation the soft palate may be split transversely or longitudinally to allow for insertion of the superiorly based pharyngeal flap. The raw area on this flap creates the same problem as in the inferiorly based pharyngeal flap, since the postoperative healing process results in unpredictable scarring and flap contracture. This unpredictability of the flap width at the end of the healing process stimulated a search for ways to prevent scarring and contracture of the flap by lining the raw surface with a free skin graft or creating additional mucosal flaps on the soft palate to cover the raw area. This later technique, introduced by Hogan, is described in the next section.

The surgical procedure is performed using a mouth gag to expose the velopharynx and especially the posterior pharyngeal wall. The soft palate is lifted with a special hook, which allows for wide visualization of the entire operating field on the posterior pharyngeal wall. A local anesthetic is used to decrease bleeding, but mainly to facilitate dissection of the pharyngeal flap from the prevertebral fascia.

The cranial base of the flap is designed higher than the posterior edge of the soft palate, which allows for a tension free insertion of the pharyngeal flap into the soft palate. When the base of the inferiorly based pharyngeal flap is designed at the level of the posterior edge of the soft palate or even lower, the superiorly based flap often transfers into the inferiorly based flap after the healing process is completed. This is the reason that some surgeons and speech pathologists are often surprised when they examine a patient who had a superiorly based pharyngeal flap procedure and then discover that the flap has become inferiorly based. Therefore the proper design of the flap width, length, and especially the placement of its base are essential to a successful performance of this procedure.

The width and the length of the flap and the shape of its caudal end must be decided before surgery. Determination of the width of the pharyngeal flap depends on the findings of nasoendoscopy, videofluoroscopy, physical examination of the nasopharynx, and functioning of the lateral pharyngeal walls and the soft palate. The length of the pharyngeal flap depends on the distance between the posterior pharyngeal wall and the posterior edge of the soft palate, as well as the technique of inserting the caudal end of the flap into the soft palate. The caudal end may be designed in a straight transverse line when the fishmouth insertion technique is used. Designing the caudal end in a triangle or semicircle is preferable when the longitudinal split of the soft palate technique is used for insertion.

The fishmouth insertion technique starts with a transverse splitting incision on the posterior edge of the soft palate, thus opening a raw surface shaped like a fishmouth (Fig. 13-2). By splitting the soft palate transversely, upper and lower mucomuscular flaps are created. The lower end of the superiorly based pharyngeal flap is inserted and sutured into this wound, with the upper flap covering the raw surface and the lower flap attached to the mucosa of the pharyngeal flap. Usually, five to seven mattress sutures are used to secure the pharyngeal flap into position. The upper flap covers only a part of the raw surface of the pharyngeal flap. During the healing process the remaining portion usually undergoes unpredictable changes due to tubing of the flap and contracture caused by scarring. These changes may detract from the effectiveness of the operation by altering the size of the ports.

To increase the efficiency of the superiorly based pharyngeal flap, the transverse incision may be carried *not* on the posterior edge of the soft palate, but further down along the nasal surface. By placing the incision here the superior flap of the split soft palate may cover a larger portion of the pharyngeal flap, thus largely preventing tubing and scar contracture. This technique allows for better prediction of the pharyngeal flap stability.

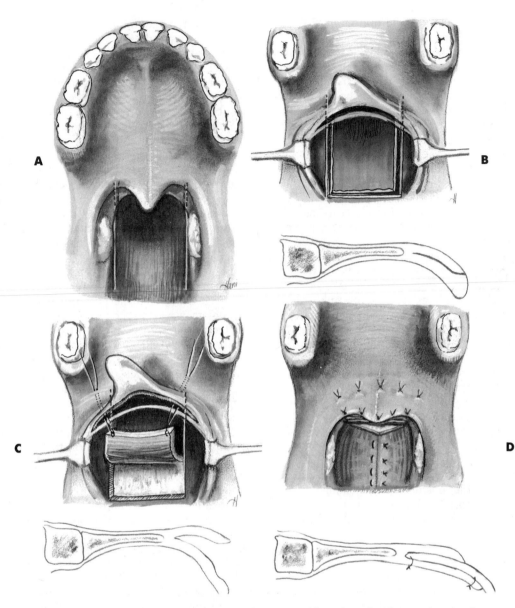

Fig. 13-2 A-D, superiorly based pharyngeal flap inserted into the soft palate so that the tissue of the soft palate covers most of the raw surface of the pharyngeal flap to prevent its contracture. (From Bardach J, Salyer K: *Surgical techniques in cleft lip and palate,* ed 2, St. Louis, 1991, Mosby.)

Lining the superiorly based pharyngeal flap with a free skin graft to prevent changes in flap size and shape during healing is not effective enough and thus is not widely used. The free skin graft often fails to take; when it does take, it does not prevent scar contracture. Inserting the end of the flap onto the nasal surface of the soft palate often allows for adequate closure of the raw surface. One of the most effective techniques is Hogan modification of the superiorly based pharyngeal flap.

Hogan modification of the superiorly based pharyngeal flap

To solve the problem of lining the raw surface of the superiorly based pharyngeal flap, Hogan introduced a procedure aimed at preventing postoperative changes in the size and shape of the pharyngeal flap and lateral ports. Hogan's idea was to raise mucosal flaps on the posterior surface of the soft palate and use them to cover the entire raw surface of the pharyngeal flap after its insertion into the soft palate. To achieve this goal, the mucosal flaps were raised on each side of the longitudinally split soft palate and based on the posterior edge of the soft palate, which allows for transposing the mucosal flaps downward to achieve complete closure of the raw surface of the pharyngeal flap.

In addition to this valuable modification of the pharyngeal flap technique, Hogan also introduced the concept of lateral port control. This concept was based on the premise that creating a port of 20 mm^2, which is approximately the same size as the 14 French catheter, facilitates the creation of conditions for normal speech production.

Hogan's concept of lining the pharyngeal flap with mucosal flaps from the nasal surface of the soft palate is sound and definitely improves the efficacy of the superiorly based flap (Figure 13-3). This is the only technique that, when well executed, successfully prevents drastic changes in the size and shape of the superiorly based pharyngeal flap. The same cannot be claimed for the concept of lateral port control. Postoperative scar contracture cannot be controlled to a degree such that the permanent size and shape of the port can be maintained in the same shape as structured during surgery.

The operation starts with a midline split incision of the soft palate. Both sides of the soft palate are raised and spread apart, thus allowing excellent exposure of the posterior pharyngeal wall where the pharyngeal flap has been designed. In this operation the lower end of the pharyngeal flap is cone shaped, and the upper end, which is the base of the flap, is designed on the level of the posterior edge of the hard palate. This design of the flap and especially of its base allows for tension-free insertion of the lower end into the tip of the wound created by the medium split incision of the soft palate.

The objective and subjective findings by the speech pathologist and surgeon serve as the basis for designing the size of the pharyngeal flap, especially its width. The length of the pharyngeal flap is dictated by local conditions. Local anesthesia is always used in this operation, and the flap is raised on the level of the prevertebral fascia.

Two parallel lateral incisions are made through the mucosa and muscle, approximately 5 mm medial to the lateral pharyngeal wall. The incision, when carried into the groove that divides the posterior and lateral pharyngeal walls, leaves enough tissue for closure of the secondary defect after the flap is raised. If the incision is carried too far laterally, the ascendant pharyngeal artery and nerve and even the carotid artery may be injured, causing a severe complication.

Separation of the superiorly based pharyngeal flap from its bed is easily performed, since the fascia is readily identified by its whitish color. After the flap is completely separated and attached only at its base, a 3.0 or 3.5 endotracheal tube is inserted through the nasal passages to help determine the size of the lateral ports. The surgeon inserts the pharyngeal flap and closes its raw surface with mucosal flaps from the soft palate. Before a bed for the pharyngeal flap is formed, and before the mucosal flaps are raised, the defect on the posterior pharyngeal wall created after raising the pharyngeal flap may be closed using 3.0 chromic mattress sutures. When closing the defect on the posterior pharyngeal wall, it is necessary to include the prevertebral fascia in each suture. By doing so, one may avoid leaving a dead space between the prevertebral fascia and the mucomuscular flaps, which close the defect on the posterior pharyngeal wall. Closure of the defect on the posterior pharyngeal wall results in constriction of the pharynx, which may also be helpful in decreasing the size of the lateral ports and improving conditions for speech production.

The lining for the raw surface of the pharyngeal flap is created on the nasal surface of the soft palate. The mucosal flaps based on the posterior edge of the soft palate are raised, then turned backward and downward. In this way the raw surface on the nasal side is increased to accommodate the raw surface of the superiorly based pharyngeal flap. The mucosal flaps turned backward and downward extend the length of the soft palate, which allows complete closure of the raw surface of the pharyngeal flap. After suturing the pharyngeal flap into the nasal surface of the soft palate and closing the remaining raw surface of the flap with mucosal flaps, the longitudinal incision of the soft palate on the oral side is approximated and closed with mattress sutures. The endotracheal tubes remain in place to allow for formation of the lateral ports. They are usually removed after 48 to 72 hours, thus securing the airway during the adjustment to the postoperative changes.

Transverse pharyngeal flap

Kapetansky introduced another pharyngeal flap modification, which aims to avoid the complications observed in inferiorly and superiorly based pharyngeal flaps. According to his obser-

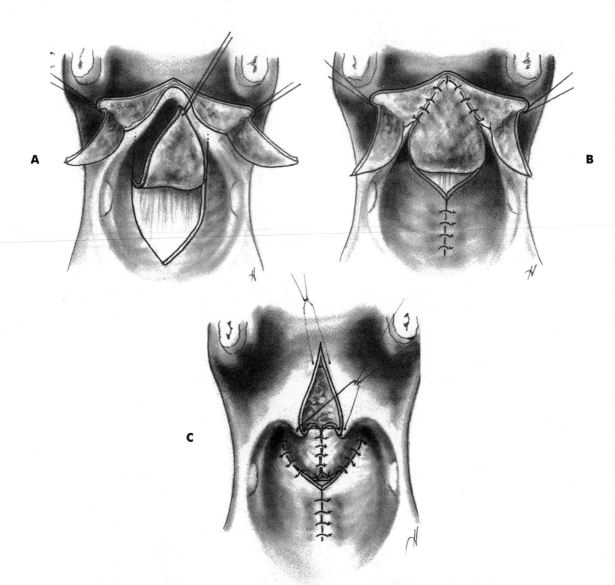

Fig. 13-3 Superiorly based pharyngeal flap: Hogan's technique. **A,** mucosal flaps are raised on the nasal surface of the soft palate to cover the raw surface of the pharyngeal flap, which is raised from its bed and elevated to be inserted into the gap created in the soft palate. **B,** the pharyngeal flap is sutured to the edges of the soft palate on the nasal side. The defect on the posterior pharyngeal wall is closed by simple approximation of the edges. Vertical mattress sutures are used to approximate both edges to the prevertebral fascia to avoid the "tent" effect and dead space. **C,** mucosal flaps raised on the surface of the soft palate are used to cover the raw surface of the pharyngeal flap between the soft palate and the base of the flap in the posterior pharyngeal wall. (From Bardach J, Salyer K: *Surgical techniques in cleft lip and palate,* ed 2, St. Louis, 1991, Mosby.)

vations, postoperative changes in pharyngeal flaps due to tubing and scar contracture decrease the effectiveness of the flaps, since the port size changes and hypernasal speech may relapse. He also indicated that a serious disadvantage of both pharyngeal flaps is the vertical incision, which denervates the constrictor muscles enclosed in the flap tissue. Therefore in his design motor innervation of the pharyngeal flaps is preserved: the flaps remain functional and do not lose their shape and size, since no raw surface is exposed.

In Kapetansky's procedure an S-shaped incision is carried on through the posterior pharyngeal wall. This allows two laterally based transverse pharyngeal flaps to be raised. These flaps are made long enough to reach the end of the soft palate and include the posterior wall muscles down to the cervical fascia. The flaps are sutured together at the midline so that no raw area is left. This tissue is then attached to the raw surface of the wound created in the medial split incision of the soft palate. The raw surface between the two transverse pharyngeal flaps and the posterior pharyngeal wall is used for a nasal respiratory passage after surgery. As this decreases with healing, the subsequent scar formation will open the two lateral ports for breathing and speech.

Several studies were conducted to assess the results of this technique. In the vast majority of patients, it was found that 6 months after the surgery there was consistent lateral wall motion, indicating that innervation of the pharyngeal flaps was intact.

Sphincter pharyngoplasty

The problems with pharyngeal flaps primarily concern postoperative changes in the flap size and shape, which lead to changes in the size and shape of the lateral ports and inadequate speech results. To prevent these changes, various new pharygoplasty techniques have been introduced.

The new techniques aim to substitute two lateral ports with one median port, using mucomuscular flaps that allow the creation of a functional sphincter. These techniques also aim to eliminate or at least minimize airway obstruction and allow for easy elimination of mucus. However, the speech results following superiorly based pharyngeal flap technique are more consistent than the speech results obtained with pharyngoplasty techniques. Further perfection of pharyngoplasty techniques and more clinical studies are needed to establish pharyngoplasty as the leading technique in the treatment of

VPI. The majority of surgeons and speech pathologists now use superiorly based pharyngeal flap.

Orticochea introduced and popularized the sphincter pharyngoplasty in 1968 (Fig. 13-4). He performs the sphincter pharyngoplasty procedure at 2 ½ to 5 years of age. In Orticochea's description of this procedure he indicates that the newly created sphincter functions due to simultaneous contraction of its four walls: the soft palate moves upward and backward; the lateral walls formed by the palatopharyngeus muscles move toward the midline; and the circular or angular posterior border formed by the union of the posterior tonsillar pillars with the posterior pharyngeal wall moves upward and slightly forward. The contractile activity of the pharyngeal muscles remains intact so that the sphincter may regulate the amount of air that passes into the nasopharynx. A short inferiorly based pharyngeal flap is elevated in a standard fashion. Bilateral posterior tonsillar pillar flaps are raised. They are superiorly based and contain the palatopharyngeus muscles. These flaps are sutured to the raw surface of the pharyngeal flap and to the raw surface of the bed created by raising this flap. At the lower end these flaps are sutured to each other so that there is a midline opening instead of lateral ports. Scar contracture during healing makes the median opening narrower, which alleviates hypernasality.

Orticochea emphasizes that, whatever the sphincter's mechanism for closure, its muscular contraction exerts a recurrent centripetal force toward the midline on the oral and nasal mucosa of the transplanted posterior pillars and on the scar tissue that occludes the lateral oronasal passages. This force gradually stretches these structures and increases their size until they become a true membrane or diaphragm with a central sphincteric orifice.

In 1977 Jackson and Silverton presented their modification of the Orticochea technique. The authors attempted to eliminate the problems encountered in the surgical technique described by Orticochea, which had too many raw areas left for healing by secondary intention.

In Jackson and Silverton's pharyngoplasty the design shows the transverse incision on the posterior pharyngeal wall and the lateral pharyngeal flaps consisting of the posterior tonsillar pillars. The lateral flaps are elevated, including the palatopharyngeus muscles. A transverse incision has been made on the posterior pharyngeal wall. Because of muscle contraction, the wound on the posterior pharyngeal wall pre-

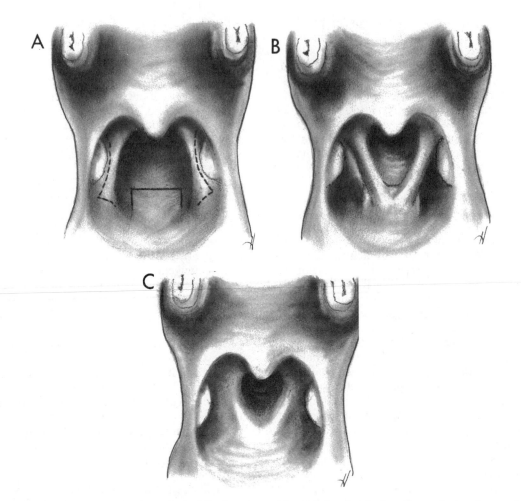

Fig. 13-4 Orticochea pharyngoplasty. **A,** design of two lateral flaps. A flap is raised on the posterior pharyngeal wall. **B,** both flaps are transposed and sutured into the posterior pharyngeal wall. **C,** the pharyngeal port after healing. (From Bardach J, Salyer K: *Surgical techniques in cleft lip and palate,* ed 2, St. Louis, 1991, Mosby.)

sents a wide, raw surface. Following these preparations the medial edge of the posterior tonsillar pillar, including the palatopharyngeus muscle, is sutured to the superior edge of the transverse pharyngeal incision. After the superior edges of the posterior tonsillar pillar have been sutured to the superior edge of the posterior pharyngeal wall defect, the palatopharyngeus muscles are sutured end to end, and the lower edges of the flaps are sutured to the lower edge of the defect.

Following the approximation and positioning of the lateral pharyngeal flaps, both lateral defects created on the posterior pharyngeal wall are sutured together. The medial opening can be made to the desired size by controlling the length of the lateral flaps. At the end of the procedure the lateral flaps, which include the

palatopharyngeus muscles, lie in a transverse direction, creating a port that essentially remains of the same size as the one created during surgery, since there are no raw surfaces to cause changes in size and shape during healing.

Posterior tonsillar pillars

In a further search to solve the problem of surgical treatment of VPI, as well as to avoid complications caused by pharyngeal flaps and some types of pharyngoplasty, Bardach proposed a new approach. The procedure proposed by Orticochea creates one central port instead of two lateral ports. However, it does not alleviate the problem of variance in port size and evacuation of mucus. Bardach's concept of pharyngoplasty, which leaves the posterior pharyngeal wall untouched while minimizing the

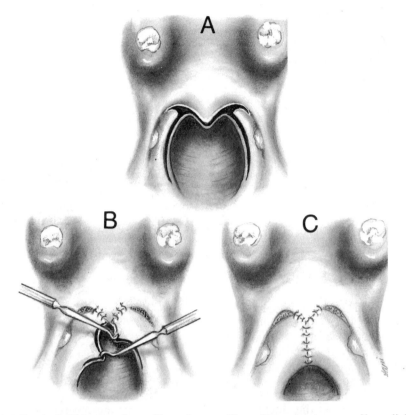

Fig. 13-5 Bardach Pharyngoplasty. Posterior tonsillar pillars are transposed medially to achieve tension-free approximation in the midline. They are sutured together in two layers. Due to transposition, some raw area may retain laterally from the uvula. **A-C,** anterior view. (From Bardach J, Salyer K: *Surgical techniques in cleft lip and palate,* ed 2, St. Louis, 1991, Mosby.)

VP space anterior to it, is based on clinical observations and long-term experience.

The main cause of complications in the surgical treatment of VPI is a pharyngeal flap that can obstruct the airway. When the pharyngeal flap is too wide, partial or total airway obstruction and hyponasality or denasality results; when too narrow, hypernasality is present. Other complications that may be greatly annoying to patients include snoring, retention of mucus, and in extreme cases sleep apnea. Considering all of the surgical techniques and the complications encountered, Bardach introduced a technique in which no flaps are raised to achieve VP closure (Fig. 13-5).

The technique is simple and straightforward. The incisions are carried along the posterior edges of the soft palate and the lateral edges of the posterior tonsillar pillars. Two lateral semicircular incisions at the tip of the posterior tonsillar pillar create two semicircular flaps that can be easily transposed medially to reach the midline of the posterior edge of the soft palate.

Further approximation of the posterior tonsillar pillars is done in two layers, posterior and anterior, which ensures better healing and prevents dehiscence. Depending on the age of the patient and size of the velopharynx, as well as the presence of tonsils and adenoids and movements of the lateral pharyngeal walls, the size of the port can be easily controlled. This operation does not require adenoidectomy prior to pharyngoplasty. However, in patients with large tonsils a tonsillectomy must be performed. This technique does create a central port with no obstruction for evacuating mucus and no danger of airway obstruction.

Augmentation of the posterior pharyngeal wall

Augmentation of the posterior pharyngeal wall presents another option in the treatment of VPI. This procedure moves the posterior pharyngeal wall forward so that the mobile palate can make contact with the posterior wall, thus directing the airflow out of the mouth and preventing its escape into the nose. This procedure appears to be the most appropriate choice for marginal VPI, since it is relatively simple.

The most serious problem with this procedure is finding the optimal material to use for augmentation. Over the years a variety of materials have been used for this purpose. Autogenous and homogenous cartilage were used with limited success. More success was reported with autogenous cartilage, since the homogenous cartilage underwent rapid resorption. The use of various types of Silastic was reported in several studies; however, the success rate was quite limited. Teflon injections were used in several centers, with a large successful series reported by McCabe and Smith. However, Furlow et al. reported obstructive sleep apnea following treatment of VPI by Teflon injection. Brauer described the use of Dacron-wrapped silicone gel implants. In his series the results of the augmentation of the posterior pharyngeal wall were successful in 75% of patients.

Brauer also indicates certain criteria for the use of this technique. One main criterion is good movement of the soft palate; another is the size of the gap between the posterior pharyngeal wall and the posterior edge of the soft palate. If this gap is 6 mm or less, the augmentation technique proves to be successful.

Complications

Various pharyngoplasty procedures have been developed to improve speech in cleft patients. However, surgeons as well as speech pathologists realize that successful treatment of VPI often leads to postoperative complications, ranging from annoyance to definite health and life risk. Because of a larger number of clinical observations and studies, an awareness of these complications is growing among surgeons and speech pathologists. For this reason, new surgical procedures have recently been designed to alleviate the serious problems experienced by patients treated with traditional pharyngeal flap surgery. Furlow's opposing Z-plasty palatoplasty is one of the best examples of a surgeon's attempt to maximize closure of the VP sphincter without employing pharyngeal flap or other techniques of pharyngoplasty.

Pharyngeal flap is definitely a beneficial procedure with respect to speech production, but the quite commonly encountered problems related to airway obstruction must be taken into consideration with regard to the patient's health and well-being. These problems may occur whether the flap is superiorly or inferiorly based. They may relate to partial or complete obstruction, which appears in acute form immediately after an operation, or in chronic form, which lasts for a long time following the pharyngeal flap procedure. Acute airway obstruction results from a sudden change in anatomic structures in which the newly created pharyngeal flap is combined with postoperative edema of the surrounding structures. Patients must suddenly adjust to the results of this condition, i.e., the change in breathing pattern from nasal to oral. Some children experience serious difficulty when adjusting to oral breathing, especially during sleep. Many patients who undergo a pharyngeal flap procedure are at risk for some degree of airway obstruction following the operation.

When planning the procedure, the surgeon must take into account the possibility of airway obstruction and should perform preoperative tonsillectomy and/or adenoidectomy when indicated. This preparation decreases the likelihood of airway obstruction. It is also important to secure nasal breathing through tubes inserted into the nasal passages and the ports, especially during the first 24 to 48 hours after surgery.

According to Gray it is probable that a pharyngeal flap procedure is the most common cause of airway obstruction in cleft patients. Although the incidence of pathologic airway obstruction in cleft patients is not known, nearly all cleft surgeons are aware of this complication. Gray also emphasizes that "it is likely that partial airway obstruction and apnea is underrecognized and undertreated, because the emphasis of treatment of clefts has historically been on the correction of speech, often at the expense of the airway." The consequences of chronic airway obstruction resulting from pharyngeal flap surgery may lead to many symptoms associated with chronic hypoxia, such as failure to thrive, chronic fatigue, inattentiveness, and irritability.

The complications following acute and chronic airway obstruction have not been investigated enough; few data have been compiled to assess the type, frequency, and severity of complications that follow pharyngeal flap surgery. In two investigations, Shprintzen (1988) and Shprintzen et al. (1992) studied the frequency of obstructive sleep apnea following pharyngeal flap. They found that 10% of patients had intermittent sleep apnea in the immediate postoperative period. A protocol was developed for postoperative management and modifications made in operative technique, which have successfully eliminated the risk factors. This area requires more attention and more clinical research from surgeons, speech pathologists, and pediatricians involved in the treatment of cleft patients.

The ability to control the size of the pharyngeal ports is critical at the time of the surgical procedure. According to our experience, precise port control is not possible due to postoperative scar contracture, which can change the size and shape of the ports created during surgery. As mentioned, the unpredictability of the effects of scar contracture may affect the size and shape of the pharyngeal flap as well as the size and shape of the ports. On some occasions it may lead to the recurrence of hypernasality or to more airway obstruction than expected, which subsequently results in hyponasality or denasality.

A VP port that is too large results in hypernasality. In these cases correction is necessary, since the basic goal of creating a pharyngeal flap—improvement of speech—was not obtained. Depending on the size and shape of the pharyngeal flap as well as the size of the lateral ports, the corrective procedure may involve partial or complete reoperation, with the creation of a new pharyngeal flap when the flap is too narrow, undergoes partial or total necrosis, or fails to heal after insertion into the soft palate. The creation of a new pharyngeal flap must be delayed for at least 6 months to have enough tissue for reconstruction. Another solution is to decrease the size of the lateral ports by freshening the edges at the upper portion and suturing them together in two layers. In certain cases two additional pharyngeal flaps can be raised and added to the side of the existing narrow flap. The choice of the procedure to decrease the size of the lateral ports and eliminate hypernasality depends on the local conditions and the surgeon's experience.

A VP port that is too small will lead to hyponasality, snoring, obstructed nasal breathing, and possibly sleep apnea. Patients often complain of loud and persistent snoring, difficulty in evacuating mucus from the nasopharynx, difficulty in breathing, symptoms of fatigue following physical exercise, headaches, and the most severe complication—sleep apnea. These symptoms may appear immediately after surgery due to a change in the anatomy and physiology of the VP mechanism. However, after time some symptoms may subside and others may totally disappear following adjustment to the new conditions, which may not only allow for normal speech production but also for normal function of the VP sphincter. All of these symptoms may be present with differing

degrees of severity, and some may present a serious risk. If persistent snoring and obstructed nasal breathing are present, or if there are any clinical symptoms of sleep apnea, such as struggling for breath, restless sleep, persistent mouth breathing, and chest wall retractions, a sleep study must be performed.

In cases of severe airway obstruction with symptoms of sleep apnea, the problem of the airway must take priority over speech problems. Several techniques may be used to create an airway sufficient for normal breathing in patients with ports that are too small or with total airway obstruction. In all cases of airway obstruction, when the ports are too small or nonexistent, the patient's speech may be very good, often without any sign of denasality. Despite very good speech, it is our strong opinion that continuing partial or total airway obstruction is more detrimental to the general health than hypernasality, which may appear after corrective surgery.

One of the techniques used to create ports of adequate size is port enlargement by excising an appropriate amount of tissue and lining the raw edges of the wound with four mucosal flaps folded downward. This technique is often successful if enhanced with nasopharyngeal port dilation or placement of a stent for a period of several weeks. Another surgical technique includes excising a lateral portion of the pharyngeal flap on each side, thus increasing the size of the ports. The mucosa on the inside and outside of the flap is sutured together, thus preventing postoperative adhesion of the edges. A stent or dilation may be helpful in sustaining the size of the ports.

In severe cases, when none of the above techniques result in improvement of the airways, the pharyngeal flap has to be disconnected from the posterior pharyngeal wall. The flap is detached in a way such that a ridge of tissue remains on the posterior pharyngeal wall. The major portion of the flap remains attached to the soft palate. Detachment of the pharyngeal flap from the posterior pharyngeal wall usually produces good results in terms of the airway and may not affect speech production. In these cases a pharyngeal flap was performed a long time before its detachment, and the speech pattern was well established. However, there were also cases in which detachment of the pharyngeal flap caused recurrent hypernasality, which required further treatment.

There is a dramatic change from the state of hypoxia which results from ports that are too small or totally occluded, to a state in which a normal breathing is restored after the pharyngeal flap is detached. Most of the symptoms observed previously, such as mouth breathing, loud and severe snoring, difficulty in evacuating mucus, headaches, tiredness, inability to do physical exercise, and sleep apnea, may totally disappear in a short time. I have observed adolescents who were passive and lethargic due to chronic hypoxia, who became active and joyful after the airway was opened for normal breathing.

The most severe complication experienced following pharyngeal flap surgery is obstructive sleep apnea, defined as cessation of respiratory airflow. A wide pharyngeal flap as well as large tonsils and adenoid tissue may lead to obstructive apnea. In many patients partial airway obstruction becomes worse during sleep because the pharyngeal musculature relaxes. During the daytime these patients compensate quite well with oral breathing.

A sleep study combined with careful physical and nasopharyngoscopic examination allows one to obtain a precise diagnosis of apnea. If partial or total obstruction of the airway is present and symptoms of hypoxia and apnea are observed, immediate surgical intervention is necessary to restore normal patency of the airway. Objections by speech pathologists that surgical intervention may ruin speech are totally unfounded, because the consequences of chronic hypoxia and apnea are much more dangerous for the patient's general health than slightly hypernasal speech. In these circumstances general health must be the primary concern, and speech secondary. Being more concerned about normal speech than about normal breathing patterns without airway obstruction must be avoided in view of the possible serious consequences of chronic hypoxia and sleep apnea. Speech pathologists who observe symptoms of these disorders must immediately contact the surgeon who performed the operation or refer the patient to a pediatrician.

SUGGESTED READING

Bardach J, Salyer K: Cleft palate repair. In Bardach J Salyer K, editors: *Surgical techniques in cleft lip and palate,* ed 2, St Louis, 1991, Mosby.

Bardach J, Salyer K: Pharyngoplasty. In Bardach J Salyer K, editors: *Surgical techniques in cleft lip and palate,* ed 2, St Louis, 1991, Mosby.

Brauer RO, Fox DR, Humphreys D: Augmentation of the posterior pharyngeal wall. In Bardach J Morris HL, editors: *Multidisiplinary management of cleft lip and palate,* Philadelphia, 1990, WB Saunders.

Gray S: Airway obstruction and apnea in cleft palate patients. In Bardach J, Morris HL, editors: *Multidisiplinary management of cleft lip and palate,* Philadelphia, 1990, WB Saunders.

Jackson IT: Pharyngoplasty: Jackson technique. In Bardach J, Morris HL, editors: *Multidisiplinary management of cleft lip and palate,* Philadelphia, 1990, WB Saunders.

Kapetansky DI: Bilateral transverse pharyngeal flaps for hypernasal speech. In Bardach J, Morris HL, editors: *Multidisiplinary management of cleft lip and palate,* Philadelphia, 1990, WB Saunders.

Orticochea M: The dynamic muscle sphincter of the pharynx. In Bardach J, Morris HL, editors: *Multidisiplinary management of cleft lip and palate,* Philadelphia, 1990, WB Saunders.

Shprintzen RJ: Conceptual framework for pharyngeal flap surgery. In Bardach J, Morris HL, editors: *Multidisiplinary management of cleft lip and palate,* Philadelphia, 1990, WB Saunders.

Shprintzen RJ: Pharyngeal flap surgery and the pediatric upper airway, *Int Anesthesiol Clin* 26:74, 1988.

Shprintzen RJ, Singer L, Sidoti EJ, Argamaso RV: Pharyngeal flap surgery: postoperative complications, *Int Anesthesiol Clin* 30:115, 1992.

Trier WC: Pharyngoplasty. In Bardach J, Morris HL, editors: *Multidisciplinary management of cleft lip and palate,* Philadelphia, 1990, WB Saunders.

14 Orthodontic Treatment of Children with Cleft Lip and Palate

Karin Vargervik

The orthodontist and speech pathologist usually monitor orofacial and speech development throughout the growth period of a child with a cleft. In general, these two specialists interact with cleft patients and with each other more often and over a longer period of time than other specialists participating in the multidisciplinary care. As a member of the cleft palate team, the orthodontist participates in the evaluation and planning of the multidisciplinary treatment, with special focus on dentition, occlusion, and facial growth.

Normal speech can be produced only within an adequate oral environment. The presence of cleft lip, alveolus, and palate or cleft palate only is associated with varying degrees of structural abnormality, which may affect speech production. Also, surgically treated cleft patients may exhibit structural abnormalities, including palatal and alveolar fistulae, a narrow and shallow maxilla, missing and misplaced teeth in the maxilla, disproportion in the maxillary-mandibular relationship, and inadequate velopharyngeal (VP) function. To produce speech in an abnormal oral environment, many patients develop various compensatory mechanisms, some of which may increase speech adequacy, but often speech production remains distorted and speech intelligibility is reduced.

The oral environment undergoes changes throughout the growth period due to normal developmental changes and the treatment received. Therefore the speech pathologist must reevaluate the child with particular focus on stages of development when changes are likely to occur. Most of these stages are also important from the orthodontist's point of view, in terms of treatment procedures employed at various stages of growth and development, as well as before and after surgical procedures. For optimal care it is highly beneficial for the speech pathologist and the orthodontist to examine the patient together so that treatment recommendations and therapy may be coordinated.

The speech pathologist and the orthodontist, who is generally the orofacial growth specialist, interact closely with surgical specialists to determine indications for and timing of surgical procedures. Because intraoral surgical procedures (cleft palate repair, pharyngoplasty, closure of oronasal and nasolabial fistulae, premaxillary retropositioning) and orthodontic treatment may affect speech, the speech pathologist's input is essential to determine the timing and type of surgical procedure. Due to the wide variation of structural abnormalities present in different cleft types and numerous factors influencing the effectiveness of treatment procedures, multidisplinary planning must be tailored to each individual case and adjusted according to the child's developmental and growth characteristics.

Orthodontic treatment in patients with cleft lip and palate includes any treatment modalities performed by an orthodontist at any stage of individual growth and development. Nonsurgical manipulation of the maxillary segments is often referred to as orthopedic rather than orthodontic treatment. The most common use of this procedure takes place in unilateral and bilateral complete cleft of the lip, alveolus, and palate and aims to reposition the maxillary segments into proper alignment. The orthodontist obtains appropriate records, such as cephalometry and panoramic radiograph, dental casts, and photographs at intervals through growth and during treatment periods. These records and the orthodontist's expertise in evaluating them are considered by other team members in determining the timing and design of therapeutic measures. The orthodontist should also be actively involved with health care providers outside of the cleft palate team and should be available for presentation of treatment results.

This chapter focuses on describing typical morphologic findings at five developmental stages and on providing an overview of the orthodontist's assessment and treatment approaches at these stages. An attempt has been made to relate various treatment modalities and intraoral findings to hazards for normal speech production.

Orofacial structures and various orthodontic treatment procedures are described for the stages of early infancy (up to 12 months), primary dentition (1 to 6 years), early mixed dentition (6 to 9 years), late mixed dentition (9 to 12 years), and adolescence (12 to 18 years).

INFANT STAGE (UP TO 12 MONTHS)
Cleft morphology

There is wide variation in the morphology and position of the maxillary segments in unilateral and bilateral complete clefts.

Presurgical orthopedics

Various types of intraoral molding plates can be used to reposition the maxillary segments. Some orthodontists and surgeons use the plates routinely, but there is substantial evidence that on many occasions presurgical orthopedics is not indicated and is not helpful in aligning the maxillary segments. For this reason we do not recommend using this procedure in all cleft patients with complete unilateral and bilateral clefts.

Presurgical retropositioning of the protruding premaxilla may be indicated in bilateral clefts. A so-called feeding plate to cover the palatal cleft and enhance feeding in infants is rarely, if ever, indicated.

Dental characteristics

Primary incisors usually erupt by 12 months.

Cleft lip and palate surgery

Primary surgical procedures for cleft lip and palate repair performed in our cleft palate center are done according to the following schedule:

- Lip surgery is usually performed at approximately 10 weeks of age.
- In bilateral clefts it may be indicated to close one side at a time.
- Cleft palate repair is usually performed between 8 and 12 months of age.
- Cleft palate surgery may be delayed if the mandible is very small or if there is significant developmental delay (for example, Pierre Robin sequence; developmental delay due to the multiple malformation syndromes).

In the newborn with a complete cleft, unilateral or bilateral, the maxillary segments are separated and may be displaced in various dimensions (Fig. 14-1, *A* and *B*). The tissue deficiency between the maxillary segments is determined by displacement of the maxillary

segments, which may vary a great deal, resulting in a wide spectrum of cleft abnormalities observed in infants with clefts.

Surgical restoration of soft tissue continuity of the lip and palate results in approximation of the maxillary segments (Fig. 14-1, *C*). This usually occurs regardless of surgical technique. Realignment of the maxillary segments following the surgical procedure and consequent reduction in the maxillary width depend on several factors, including surgical technique, the surgeon's skill, the individual's response to the operation, the initial degree of tissue deficiency, and the timing of surgical procedures.

Different treatment scenarios have been devised to manipulate the position of the maxillary segments preoperatively and to control the position of the segments postoperatively. One purpose of repositioning the maxillary segments before lip repair is to facilitate surgical lip closure. This may be necessary with a protruding premaxilla, which may also be vertically and horizontally displaced (Fig. 14-2). Retropositioning of the premaxilla can be achieved using an extraoral device, which may or may not be combined with an intraoral appliance. In some cleft palate centers active or passive molding plates are used to reposition the premaxilla into proper alignment within the alveolar arch. At the present time, however, data are not available to demonstrate the efficacy or usefulness of such treatment. Until it has been shown that this type of treatment results in better functional or aesthetic outcomes, molding plates for the cleft infant are not recommended as a routine procedure.

In most centers the general rule is to perform primary cleft lip repair at approximately 10 weeks of age. When continuity of the lip has been restored, the underlying bony structures will be molded by pressure of the functioning lip. The molding effect can also be advantageous in patients with bilateral clefts, repositioning the premaxilla into a more proper alignment. However, a lip that is heavily scarred and tight will have a detrimental effect on maxillary growth, will constrict the maxilla, and will contribute to growth inhibition and unfavorable growth patterns of the dentoalveolar complex.

Graber's study (1949) indicated that the later palate repair could be done, for example, at 4 to 5 years of age, the less would be the detrimental effect on maxillary growth and development. Quite obviously the palate cannot be left open during this period, which is crucial for speech development. Therefore several different treatment scenarios have been developed in attempts

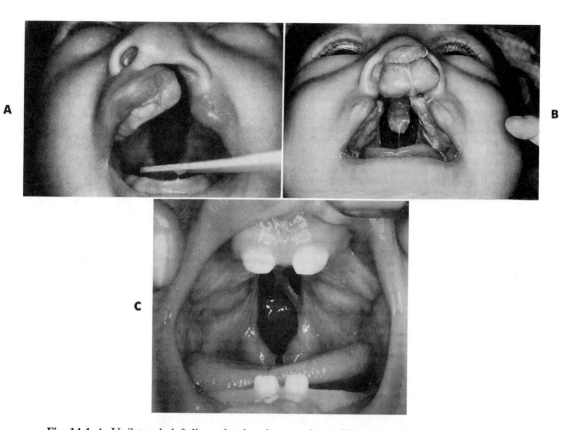

Fig. 14-1 A, Unilateral cleft lip and palate in a newborn. The columella and the large right segment containing the premaxilla are deviated to the noncleft side; the alar cartilages on the cleft side are malformed. **B,** Bilateral cleft iip and palate. Both lateral segments are separated from the premaxilla and are rotated medially behind the premaxilla. The protrusive premaxilla is large, indicating the presence of several tooth buds. The prolabium is attached at the tip of the nose. **C,** Same patient as shown in *B,* after lip repair and before palate surgery. The premaxilla has been molded back farther after restoration of the orbicularis oris muscle.

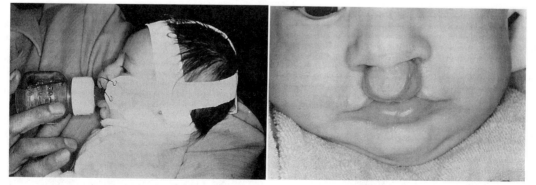

Fig. 14-2 A, Same infant as shown in Fig. 14-1, *B,* with a retraction device in place. A small appliance has been fabricated on a plaster cast of the premaxilla. Traction is being applied by rubber bands between the arms of the appliance and buttons on a custom-made headgear (or bonnet). **B,** After retraction, immediately before lip closure.

to create acceptable conditions for speech development while minimizing interference with maxillary growth. One such approach has been to repair the soft palate early, leaving the hard palate open, while obturating the palate defect with a removable acrylic plate. Reports in the literature indicate, however, that speech results are not as good and maxillary growth not significantly better following this treatment approach (Ross, 1987).

Most centers follow the principle that surgical repair of the cleft palate should be done early enough to provide the child with the adequate structural and functional conditions needed to develop appropriate speech sounds with normal articulation. The majority of primary cleft repairs are currently done between 8 and 12 months of age. It is essential for optimal maxillary growth and development that palatoplasty result in minimal scarring, particularly avoiding scar bands extending across the entire palate and reaching close to the alveolar ridge.

We strongly object to performing primary pharyngeal flap at the time of the primary cleft palate repair. There are two important reasons to object to this procedure at an early age: (1) continuous scar tissue extending from the posterior pharyngeal wall forward to the incisive foramen has been seen to cause significant maxillary growth inhibition in the anteroposterior dimension (Fig. 14-3); and (2) it is impossible to predict that a particular child will be among the 20% to 25% of children who will not develop an adequate VP mechanism as a result of cleft palate repair and will require a pharyngeal flap.

We do not use and do not recommend obturators for the palatal cleft in the time interval after the lip is repaired and before the palate is operated. On rare occasions a feeding plate may be used, but this is not routinely recommended.

PRIMARY DENTITION (1 TO 6 YEARS)
Palate morphology

The maxillary segments in the area of the alveolar ridge are usually in close contact as a result of lip and palate repair. This eliminates air escape in this area. An oronasal fistula in the palate may be present and may allow significant air escape. Even a small fistula localized in the midpalate region may result in marked hypernasal speech and abnormal articulation. Palate morphology is usually adequate for normal tongue placement. In cases when the maxilla is severely constricted or the palate is shallow, the tongue will be displaced and speech may be affected.

Dental characteristics

The primary dentition is usually complete except for the absence of teeth in the cleft area. Supernumerary teeth occur frequently in this stage.

Teeth on the cleft margin may be displaced palatally or sometimes labially, with the crown pointing toward the opposite cleft margin. If aberrant tooth position results in a wide space in the dental arch, speech may be affected.

In unilateral clefts, the primary cuspid on the cleft side is usually in crossbite. Crossbite of the anterior teeth and molars occurs less frequently. A functional protrusive or lateral shift of the mandible may be present. In bilateral clefts both maxillary segments may be approximated toward the midline. This may severely reduce the space for the protruding premaxilla as well as the tongue. The large gap between the teeth in

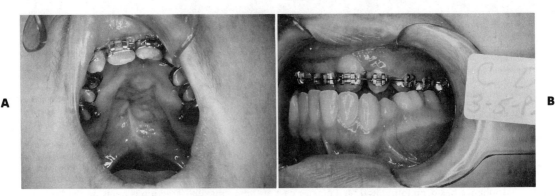

Fig. 14-3 A, Primary pharyngeal flap was done in this child. The flap is tight, in a low position, and has impeded forward growth of the maxilla. **B,** Maxilla is retruded, resulting in class III jaw and dental arch relationship.

the premaxilla and in the lateral maxillary segments may affect speech production.

Treatment

Dental care to maintain all primary teeth is essential. Selective grinding of teeth or orthodontic treatment may be indicated to eliminate a functional shift of the mandible. Temporary placement of a small plate to obturate a palatal fistula may be indicated. In cases when the maxilla is severely collapsed, early maxillary expansion may be started at 4 to 5 years of age.

In our cleft palate center additional surgical procedures performed at this stage may include correction of the secondary cleft lip and nasal deformity (4 to 6 years of age) closure of palatal fistulae, and pharyngeal flap or pharyngoplasty.

The timing and sequence of eruption of primary teeth usually follow the norms established for children born without clefts. The

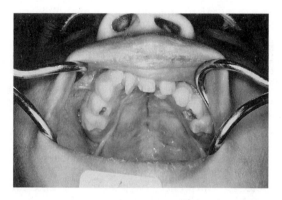

Fig. 14-4 In this bilateral cleft there is a supernumerary tooth mesial to the primary cuspid on the right side. The right lateral incisor is present but is rotated 90 degrees. On the left side the primary lateral incisor is missing, but there is a supernumerary tooth in a palatal position.

exception is the area on the cleft margins where the lateral incisor may erupt ectopically and where often there is also a supernumerary tooth erupting on the cleft margin of the lateral maxillary segment (Fig. 14-4).

The surgically repaired lip and palate approximate normal lip and palate morphology; however, the repaired lip and palate may not necessarily continue to develop favorably in either morphology or function because of neuromuscular abnormalities and growth distortions caused by scar tissue or poor alignment of the lip or palatal segments. The positive molding effect of the surgically restored muscular balance of the lip on the protruding large maxillary segment has been well documented by several researchers.

Close approximation of the maxillary segments, particularly in the area of the alveolar ridge, is a consistent finding subsequent to lip and palate repair. The maxillary segments usually have close contact in the alveolar region at age 4 or 5 (Fig. 14-5,*A*). This contact prevents further approximation of the segments toward each other, unless there is a loss of teeth at the cleft margin with subsequent resorption of the bone. The degree of maxillary width reduction is consequently closely related to the development of the alveolar process, and this in turn is determined to a large extent by the number, position, size, and shape of the teeth in that area (Vargervik, 1983). Early removal of the teeth in the cleft area is therefore contraindicated.

The alveolar process is usually well developed and stable as long as the primary dentition is intact. Crossbite of one or more teeth on the cleft side is the most usual deviation from a normal dental arch formed during this stage (Fig. 14-5, *B*).

Orthodontic treatment may be initiated in the stage of primary dentition. A partial crossbite in

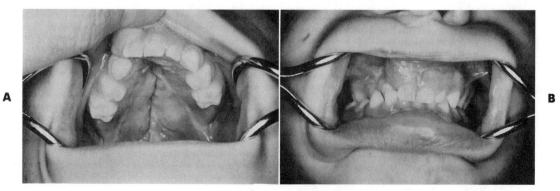

Fig. 14-5 A, Typical arch form in a repaired unilateral complete cleft. The lesser maxillary segment has moved medially; the primary lateral incisor is missing.**B,** Teeth in the lesser maxillary segment are in crossbite.

the cleft segment may be left untreated until the permanent incisors erupt in the maxilla. However, if there is significant collapse of the lesser maxillary segment, and particularly if there is a shift of the mandible into an occlusal relationship, most orthodontists would suggest starting treatment to correct maxillary width and to eliminate the shift of the mandible.

Severe collapse of the maxilla does not allow normal tongue position in the palate, thus predisposing for articulation errors. During the primary dentition stage, little change is seen in dental arch form as long as the teeth are maintained. The occlusal relationship between the mandibular and maxillary teeth also usually remains unchanged during these years. The most detrimental finding at this stage, particularly for speech, is a palatal fistula. If the choice is to delay the surgical procedure to close the fistula, it can be obturated by placement of a small plate or temporary material such as strong adhesive (Fig. 14-6).

EARLY MIXED DENTITION STAGE (6 TO 9 YEARS)
Morphology

Changes from the earlier palate morphology may result from orthodontic treatment to widen the maxilla. Palatal fistulae may become evident due to maxillary expansion when the maxillary segments are moved apart. A jaw-size discrepancy may adversely affect positioning of the tongue.

Dental characteristics

The permanent incisors in the maxilla are almost always malpositioned, particularly the incisors on the cleft side. The permanent lateral incisor on the cleft side is usually missing, leaving a space in the dental arch. In bilateral

clefts both lateral incisors are usually missing. The permanent central incisor on the cleft side is approximately 10% narrower than on the noncleft side. In bilateral clefts, both are narrow. The incidence of both lateral and anterior crossbite increases, primarily due to increasing jaw size discrepancy.

Treatment

Orthopedic and orthodontic treatment to correct the position of the maxillary segments and maxillary incisors should be started when the 6-year molars have erupted and the permanent incisors are in the process of erupting. In cases when a palatal fistula becomes evident following maxillary expansion, it may be indicated to place a small plate or add an acrylic extension to the lingual expansion appliance to eliminate air escape that affects speech. Alveolar bone grafting may be indicated at the end of this stage.

The transition from primary to mixed dentition is characterized by an increase in discrepancy between the maxilla and the mandible and between the upper and lower dental arches. The permanent lateral incisor on the cleft side is frequently missing, and there is a high incidence of congenital absence of bicuspids. The central incisor on the cleft side is an average of 10% narrower than the other central incisor, and its shape is often abnormal. The path of eruption of the central incisors is lingual and toward the cleft, and these teeth are usually severely rotated as well. Further medial displacement of the alveolar process on the cleft side and increased incidence of lateral and anterior crossbite usually occur during this stage.

When the maxillary segments are displaced medially, the tongue cannot be accommodated in its normal position in the palate. The positioning of the tongue is one of the factors

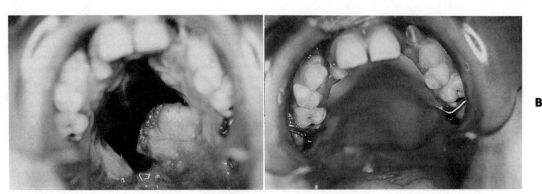

A **B**

Fig. 14-6 A, Extremely large palatal defect that cannot readily be closed surgically. **B,** Plate in place for obturation.

influencing the growth patterns of the maxilla and the mandible. The tongue may be positioned below the maxillary teeth, thus inhibiting alveolar height development. When nasal respiration is impeded, the tongue and mandible may assume a low posture to facilitate oral respiration. If the tongue in this low position does not rest under the occlusal surface of the maxillary teeth, the alveolar height will increase and result in a progressive lowering of the mandible, a more open gonial angle, and a more retruded position of the chin.

Studies on skeletal morphology in unilateral cleft lip and palate have shown few differences from average values for normal subjects in the late primary and early mixed dentition stages. However, the anterior part of the maxilla will become more retrusive while the mandible continues to grow, and generally a significant disproportion starts to appear. At this stage of growth and development orthodontic and orthopedic treatment becomes mandatory.

Orthodontic treatment procedures

The focus of the first phase of orthodontic treatment at the early mixed dentition stage is to create an adequate width of the maxilla and to correct the position of the erupting permanent anterior teeth. The treatment is started after eruption of the permanent maxillary molars and incisors. Most of the central incisors are rotated (Fig. 14-7). Widening of the maxilla is done with a lingual appliance attached to molar bands and sometimes to cuspid bands as well. The device we use most frequently is shown in Fig. 14-8. It consists of a lingual appliance with an auxillary spring that gives more lateral movement of the anterior portion of the segment than the posterior area (Vargervik, 1981). Repositioning of the maxillary segments can usually be achieved

in a few months. After maxillary expansion and straightening of the incisors, the maxillary width and incisor position are retained, preferably with a type of lingual fixed appliance. The child is seen on a regular but infrequent basis during the late mixed dentition as the rest of the primary teeth exfoliate and the bicuspids and permanent cuspids and molars erupt.

The treatment procedures are similar for both unilateral and bilateral clefts. The difference is that in bilateral clefts both lateral segments may be medially collapsed and need to be repositioned. The premaxilla quite often protrudes at an early age but becomes less prominent as mandibular growth tends to catch up. Because of the unique growth pattern of the premaxilla, when it is separated from both lateral segments of the maxilla, as seen in a bilateral cleft, a rather marked protrusiveness is present during the first years of life. This is a normal finding and should not be corrected by a surgical setback. Only in very rare and extreme cases should the premaxilla be reduced surgically.

A frequent consequence of widening the maxilla is uncovering a preexisting palatal fistula. This may become consequential for speech and may require either surgical closure or obturation. In general, it is preferable to surgically close a palatal fistula at the time of alveolar bone grafting. The success in closing the palatal fistula is increased by simultaneous bone grafting. The grafting procedures can be done when adequate maxillary width has been achieved and the maxillary segments are positioned as planned. Most often the optimal time for bone grafting is before eruption of the permanent cuspid. An erupting tooth has an osteogenic effect, and the alveolar contour and height of the alveolar bone are most favorable when the

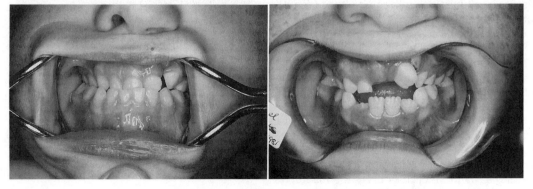

Fig. 14-7 A, Primary incisors are well aligned. **B,** Same child in the early mixed dentition stage, demonstrating malpositioned permanent incisor. Also note that a crossbite is developing at this stage.

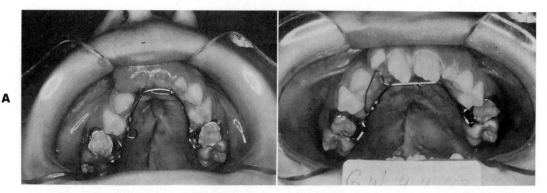

A   **B**

Fig. 14-8 A, Unilateral complete cleft with the medial position of the cleft segment. A lingual appliance has been placed that will move the entire segment laterally. **B,** Outward rotation of the segment has been achieved and the maxillary central incisors and small lateral incisor on the cleft side have erupted.

tooth can erupt into a continuous alveolar process.

LATE MIXED DENTITION STAGE (9 TO 12 YEARS)

The following conditions will be hazards for speech if not corrected by the late mixed dentition stage:

- Constriction of the maxilla (lateral crossbite, shallow palate)
- Disproportion in jaw size (anterior and crossbite)
- Edentulous spaces (missing lateral incisors)
- Presence of palatal fistulae (air escape)
- Short and/or immobile palate (VP insufficiency)

Treatment

Orthodontic widening of the alveolar arch may continue while waiting for the rest of the permanent teeth to erupt. Orthopedic protraction of the maxilla may be indicated if there is a moderate discrepancy of the jaw size. Replacement of missing teeth can be done temporarily using an orthodontic appliance or a plate.

A palatal fistula can be obturated with a plate, but preferably should be surgically closed simultaneous with a bone grafting procedure. Pharyngoplasty may be indicated if VP function is inadequate.

If orthodontic treatment is started at the appropriate time when the permanent incisors are erupting, the orthodontic appliance used during the late mixed dentition is a retention device with a lingual wire usually attached to one molar band on each side. As the mandible continues to grow, and it often grows forward more than the maxilla, periods of additional widening of the maxilla and proclination of

maxillary incisors may be indicated to avoid relapse of lateral and anterior crossbite. Depending on the maxillary size, the presence of teeth, and the position of permanent cuspids, bone grafting of the alveolar cleft is usually performed at 9 to 11 years of age.

When orthodontic treatment has not been started, a child at the stage of late mixed dentition may present with a collapsed narrow maxilla, crossbite, and malposition of teeth (Fig. 14-9). Treatment of these conditions is similar to that used in the early mixed dentition stage.

The main hazards to speech production during the late mixed dentition stage are constriction of the maxilla, edentulous spaces, disproportion in jaw size, and a palatal fistula. The VP mechanism may be compromised by a short palate or a palate that does not function adequately.

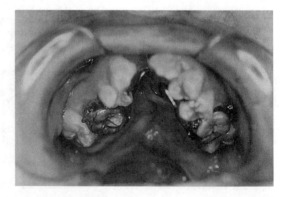

Fig. 14-9 Mixed dentition stage; no treatment has been done. Note severe collapse of the maxilla, irregular dental arches, and malpositioned teeth.

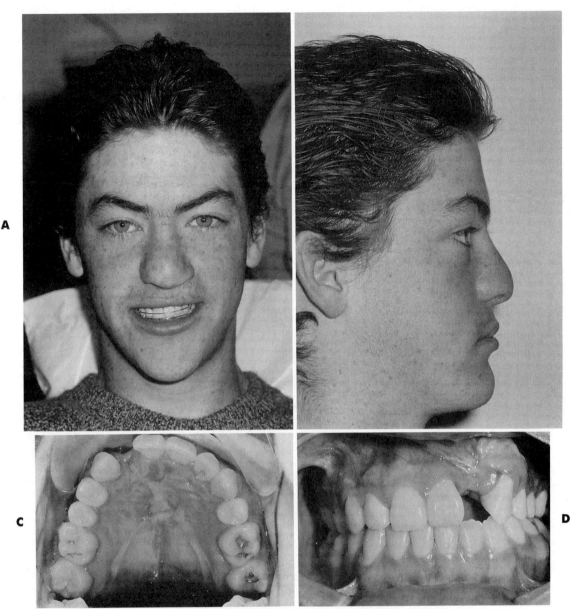

Fig. 14-10 A and **B,** Same patient as shown in Fig. 14-7. Orthodontic treatment has been completed at age 16 years. The alveolar cleft defect (**C** and **D**) has been bone grafted so that the bone is continuous. This provides stability of segment position and also gives adequate bony support for the nose. The missing lateral incisor is temporarily replaced on a retainer. Later it will be replaced permanently on a bridge. Osseointegrated implant replacement can also be considered when there is adequate bone thickness in the area.

ADOLESCENT GROWTH PERIOD (12 TO 18 YEARS)

If appropriate treatment has not been done by this time, all of the unfavorable findings listed for earlier developmental stages may be present, but to a more severe degree. However,

if treatment has proceeded according to protocol, the following would be usual morphologic findings and treatment strategies.

Morphology

During the adolescent growth period the maxilla typically falls behind in growth and development and may become significantly hypoplastic in vertical, sagittal, and transverse dimensions. Adenoid tissue, which may play an advantageous role in speech production in cases of short palate, may markedly decrease in volume at this stage, which in rare cases may cause velopharyngeal insufficiency (VPI). The increasing jaw size discrepancy and the presence of an increased vertical space between the maxillary and mandibular teeth may also be hazardous for normal speech.

Treatment

Bone grafting of the alveolar process should be performed if it was not done at the previous stage. Full orthodontic treatment should be started as soon as the permanent teeth have erupted. If the maxilla cannot be treated orthodontically to achieve adequate size and relationship with the mandible, it should be repositioned surgically by a LeFort I procedure for advancement and lowering.

Surgical advancement of the maxilla may compromise a borderline VP system. If closure was consistently adequate before the procedure, it usually remains adequate. However, in cases when the system functioned in a borderline fashion, it may be expected that speech will be adversely affected and additional surgical procedures will be necessary to improve the VP mechanism.

Missing teeth must be replaced in a more permanent fashion after orthodontic treatment has been completed and after surgical treatment in cases when indicated.

Full orthodontic appliances are placed for final correction after eruption of the permanent teeth. During this stage jaw size discrepancy may increase. If the discrepancy in jaw size cannot be corrected orthodontically, a surgical procedure on either the maxilla or mandible, or both, may become necessary. Most often the maxilla is retrusive and needs to be advanced surgically, although this is necessary in only a small percentage of patients seen.

The final treatment with regard to dentition is replacement of missing teeth on a permanent basis. During growth and treatment phases a missing lateral incisor, which is the most frequently missing tooth, is usually replaced initially on a small retainer and later on by a tooth attached to an orthodontic wire.

The final tooth replacement is usually accomplished by fixed prosthetics or by an osseointegrated implant, which is becoming more common. Treatment of a cleft patient is considered complete at the end of the growth period in the late teens (Fig. 14-10). Regular follow-up visits to the dental specialist and to the general dentist are always encouraged.

Close interaction among various specialists on the multidisciplinary cleft palate team is essential to achieve optimal functional and aesthetic results in an individual born with cleft lip and palate.

REFERENCES

Graber TU: A cephalometric analysis of the developmental pattern and facial morphology in cleft palate, *Augle Orthod* 19:91, 1949.

Ross RB: Treatment variables affecting facial growth in complete unilateral cleft lip and palate, *Cleft Palate J* 24:3, 1987.

Vargervik K: Orthodontic management of unilateral cleft lip and palate, *Cleft Palate J* 18:256, 1981.

Vargervik K: Growth characteristics of the premaxilla and orthodontic treatment principles in bilateral cleft lip and palate, *Cleft Palate J* 20:289, 1983.

SUGGESTED READINGS

Bardach J, Olin WH, Kelly KM: Surgical-orthodontic correction of the protruded premaxilla. In Bardach J, Morris H, editors: *Multidisciplinary management of cleft lip and palate,* Philadelphia, 1990, WB Saunders.

Huebener DV, Marsh JL: Alveolar molding appliances in the treatment of cleft lip and palate infants. In Bardach J, Morris H, editors: *Multidisciplinary management of cleft lip and palate,* Philadelphia, 1990, WB Saunders.

Munro IR, Salyer KE: Orthognathic surgery for patients with cleft lip and palate. In Bardach J, Morris H, editors: *Multidisciplinary management of cleft lip and palate,* Philadelphia, 1990, WB Saunders.

Semb G, Shaw W: Influence of alveolar bone grafting on facial growth. In Bardach J, Morris H, editors: *Multidisciplinary management of cleft lip and palate,* Philadelphia, 1990, WB Saunders.

15 The Dynamics of Speech and Orthodontic Management in Cleft Lip and Palate

Étoile M. LeBlanc and George J. Cisneros

The relationship of the craniofacial complex to the function of speech is extraordinarily complicated. Speech requires physiologic and neurologic control of musculoskeletal valves (lips, tongue, velopharyngeal [VP] muscles, and glottis). This integration of structure and function is a delicate balance that can be at risk for compromise.

The balance can be disrupted by structural malformations, thus fostering a functional compensatory response by the individual that may or may not have an impact on speech production. Extreme examples of this are individuals with cleft lip and palate. The marked variations in dental, occlusal, and maxillofacial growth and harmony (balance) intrinsic to clefting may impede the successful attainment of normal speech acquisition, development, and rehabilitation.

The speech disturbances secondary to the cleft lip and palate malformation are well documented (Morris, 1968; Morely, 1970; Peterson-Falzone, 1975; Bzoch, 1979; Trost, 1981, 1986, 1990, Shprintzen, 1982, 1986; McWilliams, 1984, 1990). In addition to articulation and resonance disorders secondary to velopharyngeal insufficiency (VPI), the structural malformations found in the anterior oral cavity (e.g., dental agenesis, fistulae, alveolar clefting, maxillary hypoplasia) present compounding factors that may also contribute to speech and its existing disorders. Although there is a multitude of published materials on the effects of normal as well as aberrant orofacial structures on the production of speech sounds (Fricke, 1970; Bloomer, 1971; Starr, 1979; Bzoch, 1979; Peterson-Falzone, 1988), minimal attention has been paid to speech disorders in the patient with a cleft lip and palate who is undergoing functional dental rehabilitation. Clearly, assessment and treatment of speech disorders within a malformed structure created by clefting raise unique management issues.

Successful management of clefting relies heavily on the approximation of normalcy whereby the structural, functional, and aesthetic integrity may be brought into better harmony. It has been well established that the management of an individual with cleft lip and palate requires the contributions of many professions. Each specialist has a specific role that helps this synergy.

An interplay between the professions of orthodontics and speech pathology is vital. This relationship requires the speech pathologist and the orthodontist on the craniofacial team to embrace a transdisciplinary approach (LeBlanc, 1994). This approach ensures effective and efficient assessment and treatment of each patient by utilizing the principle of shared understanding. By possessing knowledge and acceptance of each other's specialty, interaction is enhanced.

Without utilizing a transdisciplinary approach the theoretical principles and treatment regimens of orthodontic management may interfere with the conceptual and clinical framework of management of the speech pathologist, the reverse also being true. On the other hand, many theoretical principles of each discipline interrelate with each other and require only delineation of treatment goals, coordination of sequence and timing of treatment, and maintenance of coordinated follow-up to ensure appropriate management.

It is hoped that this chapter will provide an understanding of the dynamics of speech and orthodontic management following a transdisciplinary approach as well as assist in clinical application of assessment and management of a child with cleft lip and palate.

CRANIOFACIAL COMPLEX IN CLEFT LIP AND PALATE

Individuals with cleft lip and palate are influenced by irregularities in the embryonic stage of

305

growth and development. This causes tissue deficiencies and malformations. A cleft of the lip and palate is not solely a cleft of the bony tissue; it is a cleft of muscle as well (Fig. 15-1). Not being able to exert its natural molding influence on the maxillary segments, the incomplete musculature acts in a disproportionate and asymmetric fashion on surrounding bony structures (Subtelny, 1990). Aberrant muscle force tends to pull the palatal segments in a medial direction, causing malformations in growth and development. Individuals with clefts of the lip and palate exhibit marked differences in their maxillofacial growth and development depending on the type and severity of the original malformation (Rosenstein, 1990). A large degree of heterogeneity is involved in clefting, and differences in cleft type and degree of severity of the original malformation can affect management. Also, the manifestations of clefting differ in progressive maturation, as does the stage of development at which judgments and assessments are made. Individuals with bilateral clefts of the palate are most likely to show the greatest degree of tissue

deficiency, followed by patients with posterior clefts, and then those with unilateral clefts (Subtelny, 1990).

The primary bony structure in the craniofacial complex affected by clefting is the maxilla. The maxilla is generally hypoplastic, retruded, and constricted. The resultant concavity or maxillary retrusion varies considerably depending on the severity of the original deformation (Fig. 15-2).

Clefting of the maxillary alveolar processes causes medial collapse of the maxillary arch on the side of the cleft, creating misalignment of the bony maxillary segments (Fig. 15-3). Concomitant anterior crossbites can also occur on the cleft side.

In bilateral cleft lip and palate the premaxilla can be markedly protrusive at birth. This creates complicated management issues because of the number and degree of structures involved.

When the maxillary segments are severely displaced medially, the tongue may not be able to accommodate into a normal position in the cavity. The acquired position of the tongue may influence the vertical development of the max-

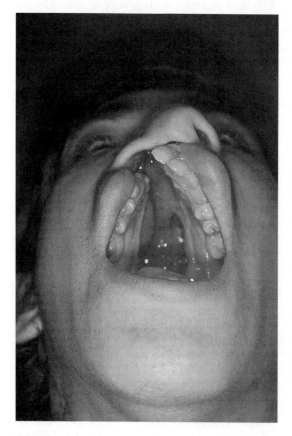

Fig. 15-1 Unrepaired complete cleft lip and palate.

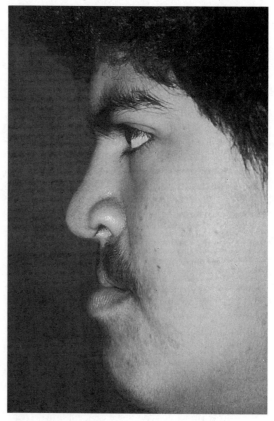

Fig. 15-2 Hypoplastic and retruded maxilla in a cleft lip and palate.

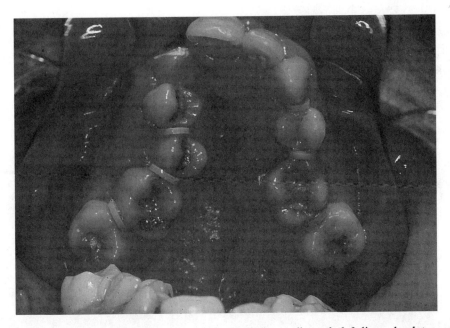

Fig. 15-3 Medial collapse of the maxillary arch in a unilateral cleft lip and palate.

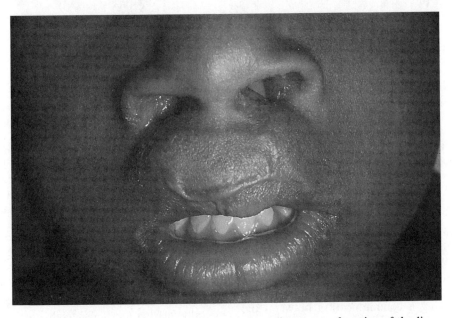

Fig. 15-4 Scar tissue secondary to lip repair impeding range of motion of the lip.

illomandibular relationship. The physiology of the tongue may also be disturbed in the presence of clefting. Very often the tongue positions itself in a posterior position within the cleft, making contact with the upper part of the posterior pharyngeal wall to accomplish swallowing. This has been noted in the fetus during swallowing of amniotic fluid (Malek et al., 1990). The posture of the tongue (passive or dynamic) is more posterior compared with the normal position. As a consequence there is less normal pressure against the maxillary segments. In a unilateral cleft the tongue may assume a lateral position.

A tight, scarred lip and scar tissue bands in the palate can impede the forward growth of the entire maxilla as well as the alveolar process (Fig. 15-4). This reemphasizes the fact that

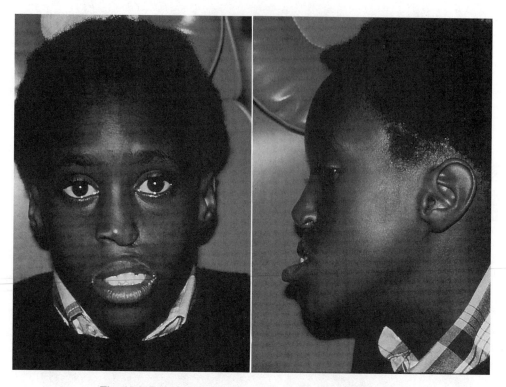

Fig. 15-5 Relative prognathism due to maxillary hypoplasia.

muscle molding action can create a distorted and constricted maxillary alveolar arch and presents the potential for dental malocclusion before palatal surgery.

Mandibular shape varies markedly within the normal population. Its relative position within the face can be affected by the vertical and horizontal position of the maxilla. In the cleft individual the mandible may appear prognathic because of the maxillary deformities. However, this is a relative prognathism (Fig. 15-5).

The alveolus is often an affected site of clefting. Alveolar clefting may have significant impact on occlusal and dental development. Oronasal fistula is tissue dehiscence of the palate causing a communication between the nasal and oral cavity. Fistulae are usually noted in the junction of the hard and soft palate (the most common location), the labial vestibule, the hard palate, the soft palate, and the alveolus (Fig. 15-6). Besides the location, the size of the fistula is important to note. Relatively hidden or small fistulae may have symptoms that are absent or extremely subtle.

Dental deviations inherent in the cleft palate patient are often the same deviations found in the noncleft structure. The differences in both relate to the degree of severity of the dental anomalies and their frequency and location. There is a high correlation between the number and severity of dental deviations and the type and severity of the cleft. They may be attributed to clefting itself or may be secondary to the surgical correction of the primary defect. The primary and permanent maxillary incisors may demonstrate numerous anomalies of tooth morphology, including enamel hypoplasia, macrodontia or microdontia, and aberrations in crown shape. The teeth usually involved are lateral and central incisors on the cleft side. Dental malformations found in the cleft and noncleft population follow (Fig. 15-7):

Anodontia: There is a high incidence of congenitally missing teeth, especially during primary dentition within the cleft population. The lateral incisor adjacent to the cleft is the most commonly affected in permanent dentition. However, there is also a high incidence of congenitally missing bicuspids on both the site of the cleft, the contralateral side, and the opposing arch in complete unilateral clefts.

Natal teeth: Natal or neonatal teeth are common and usually occur in the maxillary incisal area of patients with bilateral cleft lip and palate.

Delayed eruption: Delayed eruption of teeth, especially the maxillary canine on the cleft

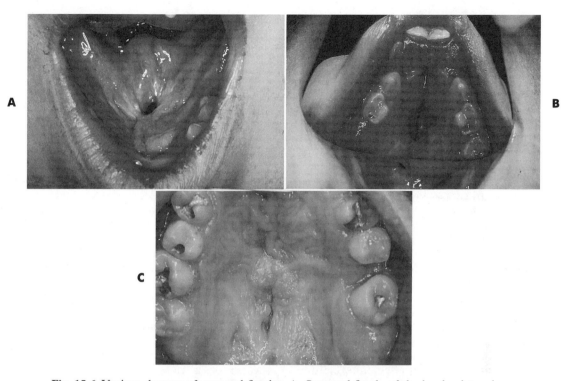

Fig. 15-6 Various degrees of oronasal fistulas. **A,** Oronasal fistula of the hard palate where there is complete communication between the oral and nasal cavity. **B,** Fistula of the hard palate demonstrating evidence of the vomer. **C,** Slit-like fistula of the hard palate.

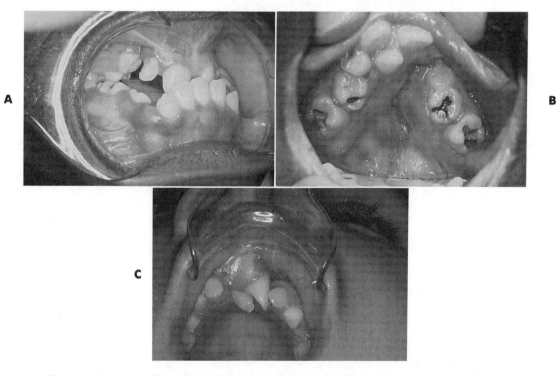

Fig. 15-7 Dental malformations often found in the cleft palate population. **A,** Anodontia of lateral maxillary incisor and irregularly shaped first bicuspid. **B,** Ectopic tooth, malpositioned rotated, delayed erruption, supernumerary teeth. **C,** Malpositioned, rotated.

side, is common. It is not uncommon to observe the eruption of the primary incisor near the margin of the cleft at birth or shortly after. The teeth are ectopic in nature, smaller and expendable. Overeruption of the mandibular teeth is common.

Ectopic teeth: Ectopic teeth are those which erupt out of normal position. Primary lateral incisors commonly erupt adjacent to or within the cleft site. The permanent canine may erupt palatally into the cleft. Permanent teeth that erupt adjacent to a cleft usually have a deficiency in supporting bone and are more susceptible to periodontal disease and premature loss.

Malpositioned teeth: The permanent central incisors adjacent to a cleft of the alveolus are often found to erupt in a rotated position. There is an increased number of fused teeth and malpositioned teeth. The eruption of the central incisors is usually lingual and in the direction of the cleft. The maxillary lateral incisor area is affected most often, especially when it is in direct line of the cleft. Mandibular teeth are usually not affected by clefting.

Supernumerary teeth: Supernumerary teeth are present in the area of the maxillary lateral incisor in both primary and permanent dentition. Supernumerary teeth in the cleft occur more frequently than do congenitally absent teeth. They are found mainly in the area of the cleft but, may occur in the posterior regions as well as in the maxillary and mandibular arches.

Crossbite: Crossbite of one or more teeth on the cleft side is the most typical deviation from normal dental arch form during primary dentition. Posterior crossbites are frequently seen as a result of medial collapse of the posterior segments of the maxilla. With eruption of the permanent dentition, more crossbite relationships are noted along with inhibition of maxillary growth (Subtelny, 1990). This may involve one tooth, the segment, or the entire maxillary arch and may be unilateral or bilateral and either anterior or posterior.

Fused and irregularly shaped teeth: The maxillary teeth may be larger in width and length than normal. They may present problems with arch length as well as esthetics. Tooth size is probably related to heredity or predisposition and has little to do with clefting. Irregularities of tooth size may also cause arch length discrepancies resulting in malocclusion. Tooth size varies between individuals and within the same individual. Malformed or irregularly shaped teeth are usually present adjacent to the cleft.

Malocclusions of the maxillary and mandibular arches occur both in the normal and the cleft population. The differences relate to the severity, type, and location of the cleft. These relationships may be secondary to dental factors (occlusion), the maxillomandibular relationship, or a combination of both, which is usually the case. Occlusal relationships have been described by Angle (1899) and are presented for easy reference in Fig. 15-8:

Class I occlusion is the preferred dental/occlusal relationship. The mesiobuccal cusp of the maxillary first molar rests in the buccal groove of the mandibular first molar. The maxilla is slightly larger than the mandible (Figure 15-8, *A*).

In *class II occlusion* the mesiobuccal cusp of the maxillary first molar is *anterior* to the buccal groove of the mandibular first molar. Therefore the maxillary teeth are seen as protrusive over the mandibular dentition (Figure 15-8, *B*).

In *class III occlusion* the mesiobuccal cusp of the maxillary first molar is *posterior* to the buccal groove of the mandibular first molar. This is the reverse of a class II malocclusion (Figure 15-8, *C*).

THE DYNAMICS OF SPEECH AND DENTITION

Speech sound production in cleft and noncleft populations is a learned behavior; the learning process is affected by structural environment, neurologic integration of cortical activity, and psychosocial parameters.

Speech sound formation does not consist of fixed, static positions of the articulators (e.g., lips, tongue), but rather of dynamic movements in fairly consistent uniform patterns in properly timed sequences. These movements are highly complicated and extremely variable. Bloomer (1971) described the movements as having "kaleidoscope variability and speed." They rarely follow an identical successive pattern, adding to the variability. No two persons' supralaryngeal vocal tracts are identical, presenting with different sizes, shapes, and normal variances in dentition and occlusion. Thus there are significant variations in the manner in which the same sounds are formed by different people.

Speech sounds can be described according to a basic physiologic framework. They may be differentiated according to *place of articulation* (the specific anatomic site around which movable structures act) and *manner of articulation* (the degree of obstruction or occlusion of outgoing air flow at the site of the articulator).

On the basis of this classification one can infer relationships between articulation and certain

A B C

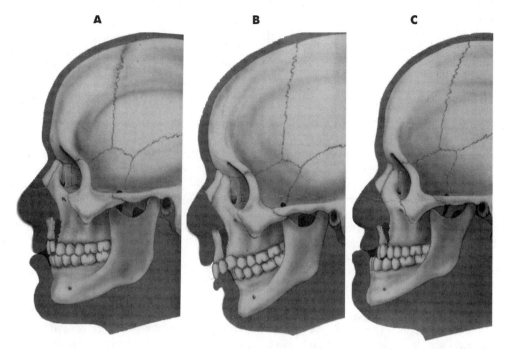

Fig. 15-8 These three figures demonstrate the general dental, skeletal, and soft tissue relationship commonly found with associative malocclusions. **A,** In Class I cleft occlusion, note the upright incisors and deficient upper lip. **B,** In Class II cleft occlusion, note extruded and upright incisors, deficient lip and chin. **C,** In Class III, note deficient lip, and midface (maxilla) and excessive or relative prognathic mandible.

anatomic and physiologic functions. Consonants are formed by a complex series of oral movements utilizing valves that continuously modify air pressure and acoustic output. During speech the tongue changes the shape and size of the oral and pharyngeal cavities to create sound and affect resonance. Vowels, in the traditional sense, are associated with a steady-state articulatory configuration and a particular acoustic pattern. They are produced with various configurations of the oral cavity initiated by changes in lip and tongue shapes. Vowels are rarely affected by dental and occlusal anomalies to such an extent that the auditory and acoustic properties change to impair speech intelligibility.

Production of consonants is determined at least in part by the occlusal relationships of the maxillary and mandibular arch, dentition, and the configuration of the hard palate. The dental arch relationship may be the single most important factor affecting articulation. Nearly 90% of all consonants are made in the anterior portion of the oral cavity. The dental arches (dentition and skeletal arch) act as structural boundaries for lingual placement, are directly involved in the production of phonemes /t,d,n,l/,* assist in the production of many linguopalatal pho-

nemes, and provide a grooving mechanism for production of continuants /s,z,ʃ,tʃ,dʒ/. When a malformation in structure occurs, the chance of disruption of the delicate balance between structure and function in sound production significantly increases. However, the speech mechanism is highly adaptable, and a wide range of compensatory behavior can result in satisfactory sound production.

There are difficulties in any attempt to assess systematically the relationships between dental deviations and speech. One must be aware of inherent methodologic problems, such as the following:

1. The relationship between speech and dentition cannot be assessed until articulation skills are sufficiently advanced.
2. Children go through primary and secondary changes in dentition that might affect speech.
3. The etiology of articulation disorders is multivariant but with significant overlap in clinical features resulting in similarities in presentation.
4. One cannot always assume there is a one-to-one relationship between structural defects and a given articulation problem.
5. One cannot rule out the effects of previous defects that may have been repaired with the habituated articulatory pattern that persists.

---

*In discussing speech sound production, the phonemes are referred to according to IPA format (1989).

6. There is wide variability in the type and degree of variation that may occur in dental and occlusal deviations.
7. The presence of oral habits will affect structure and might affect speech.

Articulatory errors

All too often the term *articulation error* is used to describe a speech sound that is not produced within the realms of expected place and manner of articulation. It is often used with ambiguity within the field of speech pathology so that it is a term not well understood by other professions. Articulatory errors may be differentiated into their etiologic cause (e.g., developmental, phonologic) as well as the type of compensations that are affected.

Obligatory errors. Errors in speech sound production related to structural malformations of the anterior oral cavity are classified as obligatory articulation errors. They have been described as errors in distortion rather than substitutions, omissions, or deletions (Bloomer, 1971; Starr, 1979;). The distortions can be simply characterized into lateral distortions, interdental distortions, and retroflexed distortions. Obligatory articulation errors may co-occur with other articulation disorders, such as functional disorders related to developmental or phonologic processing disorders and maladaptive compensatory articulation patterns consistent with VPI. Obligatory errors are not easily amenable to therapeutic intervention alone and often require assistance of the orthodontist and/or the maxillofacial surgeon to restore the malformation. Obligatory errors are often considered misclassified as compensations.

Compensations. As mentioned, the articulators of the oral cavity are highly adaptable in the presence of a malformation and are capable of movements that retain or maintain the auditory parameters of a sound, minimally affecting intelligibility. The ability to engage in compensatory behavior is heavily reliant on related and unrelated factors, many of which have yet to be identified. Some factors include the following:

1. Effects of concomitant ear disease or ear malformations
2. Severity of the malformation
3. Type of malformation
4. Location of malformation
5. Sound that is specifically affected
6. Phonetic context of the specific sound
7. Level of complexity of speech performance (sound, syllable, word or phrase, or conversational level)
8. Limitations of intellect

Very little is known about the mechanisms driving the process of compensation (Jensen, 1968; Kelso, 1984). There appears to be little information about the processes or systems involved in the initiation of the compensatory behavior. Is there a cause and effect relationship between the type and severity of deformation and the type of compensation used? Do proprioceptive feedback systems play an interactive role? What role do they play? Do individuals with a significant hearing loss and a certain structural malformation present with the same articulatory compensations as a control counterpart? These questions and many more have yet to be answered.

The term *compensation* is frequently used in the literature without a true understanding and definition, consequently leaving much to subjective opinions. The term is used by different professions often within the same field with different connotations. One should be aware of what *compensation* mean to the dental profession (structural compensations of soft and bony tissue) and what is referred to in the speech profession (functional compensations of the articulators).

Compensations may be viewed as *adaptive* (positive) or *maladaptive* (negative), thereby affecting function in both a negative and positive manner. Compensations have the potential to affect the visual parameters as well as the auditory and acoustic parameters, both in an adaptive and maladaptive perspective.

For example, adaptive compensations may be noted in a child diagnosed with ankyloglossia (LeBlanc et al., 1994). Assessment of speech performance may indicate the use of the tongue blade against the dental edge of the maxillary incisors for production of /t/, due to restricted range of lingual movement. Auditory perception indicates correct production of this phoneme. Although the place of articulation was mildly changed, affecting tongue placement, this did not change the identification of the phoneme. Maladaptive compensation in this same individual may be noted in an attempt to produce phoneme /t/. The tongue blade may be placed in an interdental position, producing distortions (interdentalized). The place of articulation is then affected, as are both auditory and visual integrity of the specific phoneme.

Malocclusions

Malformations or malocclusions of the maxillary and mandibular arches have the potential to greatly affect speech sound production. It should be noted that the effect on speech performance is related to many factors that may or may not be directly related to occlusion. The severity of the malformation, the frequency at which the sounds occur, the phonetic context in which the sound is found, and the level of sound production (isolated sound, syllable, word, phrase, and conversational speech) are factors that could change the causal relationship. Within the same individual a combination of several occlusal, dental, and speech anomalies may co-occur, affecting the total outcome of that individual.

The phonemes most affected by malocclusions are /t,d,f,v,s,z,ʃ,tʃ,dʒ/. One of the most difficult sounds to produce is the unvoiced linguopalatal /s/ (Bloomer, 1971). Production of /s/ requires precise placement and function of both the tip and blade of the tongue as well as enough space anterior to the tip of the tongue in the most anterior portion of the palate. The bilabials /p,b/ can be affected to a degree, whereas the phonemes /k,g/ are the least affected.

The contribution of malocclusions and malpositioned teeth to articulatory defects are of special interest because of the complexity of the relationship between occlusal development and the motor aspects of speech.

Malocclusions involving the maxilla (class II, division I or II, with or without crossbites or lateral or anterior open bites) may affect almost all the sounds produced in the anterior oral cavity. Excessive maxillary protrusion has the potential to affect bilabial closure for production of /p,b/ because the upper lip may have difficulty achieving a labial seal. Clinical observations have noted that minimal difficulty is noted in bilabial closure for /m/ when severe class II occurs. This may be due to the nature of the nasal sound, i.e., it is produced with a difference in manner of articulation, requiring no intraoral airflow, whereas /p,b/ require a certain degree of intraoral pressure to produce the plosive feature with the ability to maintain strong, complete bilabial seal. Adaptive compensations may occur for the production of bilabial phonemes in the presence of malformations. Contact for production of /p/ or /b/ may be made with the lower lip with the dental edge of the central and lateral incisors. The plosive feature may be weak with mild distortions noted in the auditory perception of the sound. Mild visual distortion may also be noted.

The production of labiodental phonemes /f,v/ may be minimally affected. Adaptive compensations usually occur, although rarely affecting the auditory properties. However, the visual properties may be affected; exaggerated lip excursion may be noted in attempts to achieve

proper articulator position and to direct airflow. This may be further complicated by the coexistence of an incompetent or shortened upper lip due to malformation or scar tissue. Maxillary protrusion can also affect the ability to direct airflow appropriately for production of sibilants /s,z/ and affricates /ʃ,tʃ,dʒ/. Lingual protrusion can occur at the site of maxillary protrusion, changing the grooving mechanism of the tongue's lateral edges placed against the dental edges of the arch, thus affecting placement and manner of articulation of sibilants and affricates. However, adaptive compensations can also occur when utilizing the maxillary or mandibular lip to create the air turbulence for auditorily correct production of sibilant consonants.

Restricted maxillary arch width will affect lingual contact around the alveolar borders of the maxillary teeth and prevent the correct grooving of the tongue, which may affect sibilant and affricate production (Fig. 15-9). In such cases maladaptive compensations may occur where articulation is attempted in a protruded position against the maxillary dental edge (causing lingual protrusion and sound distortions) or in lingual retraction (in a posterior position) in an attempt to achieve a grooving mechanism. This changes both the auditory and visual integrity of sound production.

Palatal height rarely affects articulation, although if limited range of lingual movement occurs, adaptive compensations usually take place.

Mandibular protrusion (class III) may affect the same phonemes and the integrity of sound production in essentially the same manner as maxillary protrusion, with slight differences. Relatively mild mandibular prognathism causes no difficulty in speech performance. Adaptive compensations can occur with minimal or no auditory changes noted. Visual differences may be noted in lingual protrusion during production of certain plosives and construents. Linguoalveolar consonants /t,d/ may be produced with the lingual blade instead of the lingual apex, often maintaining the appropriate acoustic properties. Sibilant production of phonemes /s,z/ may be produced with lingual protrusion, causing sound errors of interdental distortions. Affricate production of /ʃ,tʃ,dʒ/ can also be affected by lingual protrusion of which lateralized and retroflexed distortions may be made.

Maxillary and mandibular protrusion can be complicated by open bites and crossbites. Lateral and anterior open bites (failure of the maxillary and mandibular teeth to make contact) involving the central and lateral incisors of both

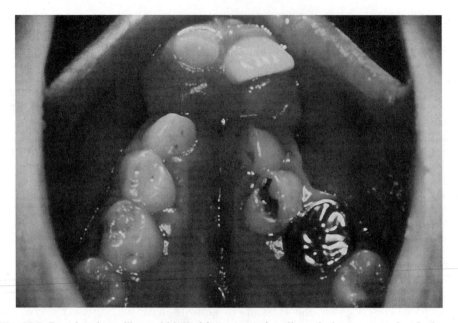

Fig. 15-9 Restricted maxillary width limiting appropriate lingual placement and articulatory strength of contact for lingualveolar sound production.

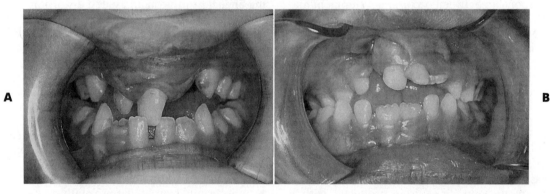

Fig. 15-10 A, Lateral open bite affecting an appropriate seal for production of sibilants and allowing a free space for lingual protrusion during production of sibilants. **B,** Anterior open bite accommodating lingual protrusion during production of sibilants, site for lingual blade contact against dental edge as well as lingual protrusion at rest.

dental arches provide open freeway space for lingual protrusion (Fig. 15-10). These open spaces allow for greater escape of airflow during sound production as well as increasing the difficulty for the individual in being able to successfully trap the airflow to affect a grooving mechanism. Location of the open bite (anterior or lateral) may determine differences in the type of distortion error made. Anterior open bites may facilitate an interdental distortion, whereas lateral open bites may facilitate lateralized and retroflexed distortions. Both anterior and lat-

eral open bites create discrepancies in dental edge occlusion, restrict linguoalveolar contact, and change the dynamics of airflow affecting sibilance. This causes distortions in visual and auditory properties and ultimately will affect speech intelligibility.

Extreme forms of crossbites (right or left lateral shift differences between either the arches or dentition) may be mandibular or maxillary. The tongue is placed in a mechanically unfavorable position for sibilant production and linguoalveolar contact (Fig. 15-11).

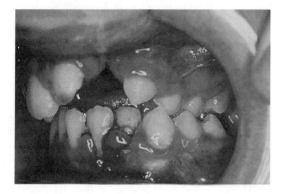

Fig. 15-11 Maxillary dental crossbite.

Dentition

A major factor in assessing the importance of dental variations to consonant productions is the wide variability in type and degree in which they occur. Few dental conditions are so severe that the individual is prevented from acquiring accurate speech. Dental deviations occurring without the presence of complicating factors seldom impose severe problems on articulation. When dental deviations occur in conjunction with arch malformations, VPI, neuromuscular deficits, hearing loss, intellectual deficiencies, or other articulation disorders, their potential effect on speech is greatly enhanced. Although one cannot define the manner in which these diverse problems interact with dental deviations, it appears their significance increases as their number, type, and severity increase (Bankson, 1962; Subtelny, 1964; Laine, 1988). The presence of dental deviations in a person who has previously acquired adequate articulation is of less significance than in a child who is in the process of speech sound development.

Anomalies of tooth position that prevent normal valving contacts of the tongue and lips have the potential to affect speech performance, usually in the form of adaptive compensations rather than obligatory errors. The condition, size, and texture of individual teeth probably have relatively little direct influence on speech. The presence or absence of teeth and their position in the dental arches are the influential factors.

Ectopic eruption and its direct effect on sound production depends on a large extent on the location of the tooth or teeth. Very often incisor teeth are found displaced posteriorly in the palate, which can interfere with lingual placement in the production of linguopalatal phonemes. The number of teeth displaced to a certain area is also a factor. The grooving mechanism of the tongue for production of sibilants and affricates may also be disrupted. The result may be direct, as with obligatory distortions, or adaptive compensations may occur in an attempt to maintain the auditory and visual parameters of the particular sound. Supernumerary teeth or diastema (abnormal spacing), especially in the anterior cavity, can result in lingual protrusion and an anterior lingual resting position if the spaces are substantially large. Such lingual postures result in interdental, lateralized, and at times retracted distortions.

Anodontia (missing or nonerupted teeth) or congenitally absent teeth and oligodontia (presence of only a few teeth) will affect speech sound production much as supernumerary teeth do (depending on the severity of the dental deviation). Anterior teeth in linguoversion, especially when they distort the shape of the anterior alveolar arch of the maxilla, making it particularly difficult for the speaker to produce sibilant consonants. Irregularly shaped or fused teeth rarely affect speech to the extent that auditory and visual integrity is compromised.

ARTICULATION AND RESONANCE IN CLEFTING

Speech disorders in the cleft lip and palate population can be highly complex, in part due to the anterior structural environment in which speech is performed, the functional integrity of the VP mechanism, and their synergistic interaction. The primary disorders that may be found in cleft lip and palate involve resonance, voice, and articulation disorders. The primary resonance and articulation disorders associated with cleft lip and palate are hypernasality and maladaptive compensatory articulation patterns, respectively. The incidence of hypernasality in the cleft lip and palate population is high, but the incidence of compensatory articulation patterns is a surprising 20% (Hall and Golding-Kushner, 1989). Chapter 8 provides a complete account of resonance and articulatory disorders found in cleft lip and palate.

When speaking about the dynamic interaction of speech, occlusion, and dentition in cleft lip and palate, one must have a clear understanding of the speech disorders found in an individual with a cleft lip and palate and how each may or may not be related to occlusal and dental malformations. The two primary articulation disorders found in this population are obligatory and maladaptive compensatory articulation patterns (although, functional articulation disorders may occur within the cleft population as in the noncleft population). The physiology of these disorders differs. Compensatory articulation primarily involves VPI and errors in learning involving VP musculature and place of articulation. Significant physiologic differences and changes occur within compensatory articulation patterns. Many of these differences and changes depend on the type and degree of severity of the maladaptive compensatory pattern, as well as the level at which an individual is in articulatory rehabilitation. The tongue and the VP mechanism are two of the most vital structures for speech and are most affected by dental and occlusal abnormalities.

In a child who is engaged in compensatory articulation patterns, certain differences occur in the movements of the tongue and the vocal tract. When the place of articulation is disrupted and displaced, the tongue is often also displaced in a posterior and sometimes superior or inferior position. This may result in minimal anterior movement of the lingual blade and apex within the anterior oral cavity.

As illustrated, there are degrees of severity in maladaptive compensatory articulation patterns with the type and degree of severity playing a significant role in how occlusal and dental malformations will affect sound production. At the present time there are no standard methods of determining degree of severity. As noted above, in the most severe compensatory articulation pattern one may see little or no movement of the lingual apex during production of linguopalatal sounds /t, d, s, z, tʃ, ʃ, dʒ/ and no labial movement for bilabial phonemes /p, b/. Minimal movement of both articulators (tongue and lips) can also be accompanied by weak intraoral airflow or in many cases none at all. In cases where there is a severe compensatory articulation pattern with no lingual movement (the tongue is in total posterior position during speech), the occlusal and dental malformations of the anterior oral cavity have little effect. However, in a child who demonstrates minimal or inconsistent lingual and bilabial movement in the oral cavity in the presence of maladaptive compensatory articulation patterns, articulator contact may be weak with little or no intraoral airflow and pressure. The occlusal and dental malformations may affect how well the tongue contacts the dentopalatal border to facilitate plosive features and how well the lateral edges make contact with the dental edges of the maxillary arch grooving mechanism to assist in construent features for sibilants, fricatives, and affricates.

Besides the type and severity of the articulation pattern, the individual's level of speech performance in therapeutic remediation of the maladaptive compensatory disorder is a factor. The more anterior the articulations (appropriately utilizing the proper articulators and correct manner and placement of articulation), the more occlusal and dental malformations have the potential to affect speech sound production.

The contribution of unilateral and bilateral alveolar clefts to the degree of hypernasality perceived is minimal (Isberg and Henningsson, 1987). A unilateral or bilateral alveolar cleft will have little effect on the production of sounds unless the degree of the malformation is so significant that it affects place of articulation. Malformations caused by alveolar clefting have the potential to affect the placement of the tongue tip and, in cases of bilateral cleft lip where the premaxilla is severly protruded. The ability of the individual to achieve an adequate bilabial seal for production of bilabials /p,b,m/ and interdentals /f,v/.

The presence of oronasal fistulae and their contributions to articulation and resonance disorders in the cleft lip and palate depend on many factors. The location, size, etiology, and how long they have been present can affect both the degree of hypernasality and speech sound production. Oronasal fistulae at the junction of the hard and soft palate may produce a compensatory substitution pattern called middorsal palatal stops (Trost-Cardamone, 1990) (Fig. 15-12). This pattern changes the perceived acoustic output of the phonemes /t,d,k,g/. Oronasal fistulae due to dehiscence (breakdown of tissue) at the surgical site or because of expanding the maxillary palatal shelves for orthodontic and maxillary surgical treatment may contribute to increased perception of hypernasality and may interfere with correct lingual placement. Lingual compensations may occur in an attempt to locate another site on the anterior palate to facilitate contact for sound production. These compensations may be either maladaptive, in which auditory and visual distortions occur, or adaptive, in which appropriate auditory parameters are maintained. Dental obturators or plates have been used for oronasal fistulae; however, these appliances change the sensory feedback, making sound production difficult. Also, if the child is noncompliant in using the appliance, its intended purpose is defeated.

The same effects of malocclusion and dental deviations described in the noncleft nonsyndrome patient may also occur in the nonsyndrome cleft patient.

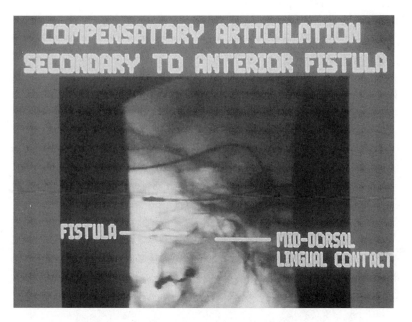

Fig. 15-12 Middorsal palatal stop substitution at site of oronasal fistula.

TRANSDISCIPLINARY MANAGEMENT OF CLEFT LIP AND PALATE

Management of the individual with a cleft lip and palate involves a multitude of professions. Treatment begins immediately at birth and continues well into adulthood. The type and degree of severity of the cleft, as well as the age of the presenting individual, determine to a great extent the type and timing of treatment the individual will require.

Phase I: birth to 2 years

Delays in the onset of language skills and the increased risk for the development of abnormal speech patterns demand the attention of the speech pathologist very early in the life of a child with a cleft lip and palate. Utilizing a preventive approach the initial assessment of a child should begin at 3 to 6 months of age, accompanied by parent counseling or training, if necessary, to assist in speech and language development (LeBlanc, 1994).

Orthodontic intervention may begin much earlier (weeks of age) in certain children with the use of infant orthopedic and feeding appliances. There is much controversy surrounding the use of such appliances. A significant amount of literature advocates the use of infant appliances (Rehrmann, 1970; Latham, 1980; Gruber, 1990; Huebner, 1990; Rosenstein, 1990) but there are those who disagree (Robertson, 1968, 1971; Skoog, 1974; Fara et al., 1990). Both orthopedic and feeding appliances *have the*

potential to interfere with the onset of speech development and the integrity of speech performance. However, little research has been conducted to date in this area.

Depending on the cleft type and the degree of severity, certain orthopedic appliances may be used before lip repair (usually performed at 3 months of age). The misaligned maxillary segments are manipulated in the complete unilateral and bilateral clefts of the lip, alveolus, and anterior palate to create a bony continuum. Premaxillary repositioning is performed with extraoral elastic bands or adhesive facial straps (Fig. 15-13). At times an intraoral appliance is used in conjunction with extraoral premaxillary appliances to align the segments (Fig. 15-14). It is felt by some who advocate this procedure that orthodontic appliances in infancy will stabilize the lesser and greater segments from collapse, place them in alignment, and prepare the structures to enhance the integrity of the arch. This alignment usually occurs between 3 and 9 months of age. Short-term as well as long-term effects are not always positive. Its efficacy in terms of later outcome is now widely doubted. In an increasing number of centers and teams, orthodontists are confining the employment of orthopedic plates to bilateral and wide unilateral complete clefts or discontinuing their use altogether.

Although minimal attention has been paid to the effects of such appliances on speech and language development, their immediate short-term effects raise doubts about their potential to affect lingual placement and manner of articulation at a stage of speech development that is so crucial to the appropriate sequence and timing of sound acquisition. As can be noted in Fig 15-14, the appliance is placed in the anterior oral cavity at the site of the lips and alveolar bone. Intraorally, the palatal appliance is often thick in vertical dimension and can be fairly extensive. This has the potential to negatively affect proprioceptive feedback at a time when the child is beginning to perceive, discriminate, and attempt various sound productions through imitation and play. The infant from 3 to 9

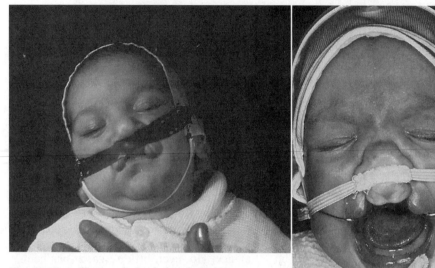

Fig. 15-13 A, Extraoral elastic bands acting as premaxillary repositioners. B, Extraoral elastic band in combination with wire premaxillary positioner.

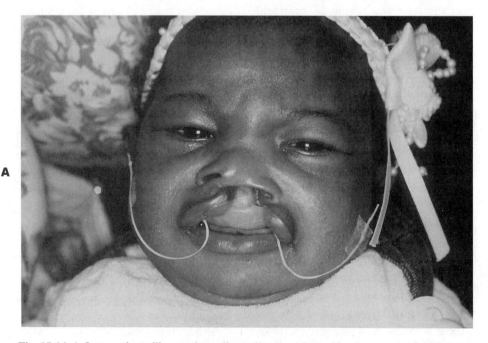

Fig. 15-14 A, Intraoral maxillary orthopedic appliance with significant amount of thickness in the vertical dimension.

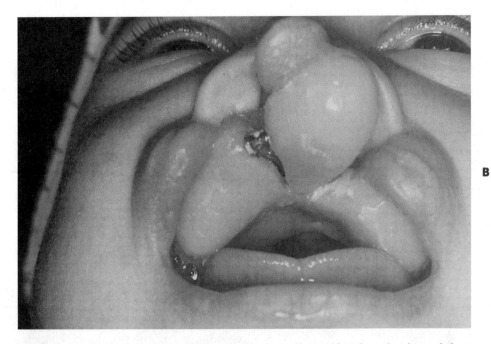

Fig. 15-14, cont'd. B, Intraoral maxillary orthopedic appliance. Note how the size and shape of the appliance have the potential to affect bilabial closure.

months of age transcends a period of rapid sound production via differing levels of babbling with a determined sequence of sounds being developed. The bilabials /p,b,m/ are usually the first phonemes to be acquired. However, a maxillary appliance may delay onset of such production because it restricts and limits bilabial closure and strength of contact. Linguoalveolars /t,d/ are produced at the site of the appliance (alveolar ridge), which affects lingual placement, degree of articulatory contact, and intraoral air pressure. The potential for such appliances to delay the onset of speech, increase the occurrence for development of maladaptive compensations, and subsequently facilitate delays in receptive and expressive language development is a realistic concern.

Whether an orthopedic appliance is used or not, it is advisable for the orthodontist to see children during this age group to answer any questions the parents may have on growth and development and to monitor growing craniofacial structures. Frequently photographs (extraoral and intraoral) and maxillary molds are taken. Very rarely is active, direct orthodontic treatment initiated in primary dentition. Historically, the use of feeding appliances in the early years of cleft palate management was adamantly supported (Kelly, 1971; Razek, 1980; Jones et al., 1982; Fleming et al., 1985). However, support for feeding appliances has significantly abated (Singer and Sidoti, 1992 LeBlanc, 1994); much to the chagrin of many professionals, these appliances are still used today. In the vast majority of children with *isolated cleft lip and palate,* few changes to the normal method of feeding need to be instituted. Position feeding schedule changes and modifications in the nipple cut are often the only adaptations required (Singer and Sidoti, 1992). Very little need for specialized nipples and bottles is required.

Lip repair is essential at an early age. It not only presents the child with a improved appearance, but also the reconstructed lip musculature creates a compressive force on the displaced bony segments, initiating a molding action that serves to bring the alveolar segments closer together (Pruzansky, 1955). Lip closure also restores the structure of the lips for sound production. The earlier these articulators are restored to their normal structure, the earlier function will be restored for feeding and speech sound production.

Phase II: 2 to 4 years

Orthodontic and speech management within this age group requires a more interactive treatment plan than phase I. Appropriate sequencing and timing of the treatment options are necessary. During this period the orthodontist may obtain additional dental models and

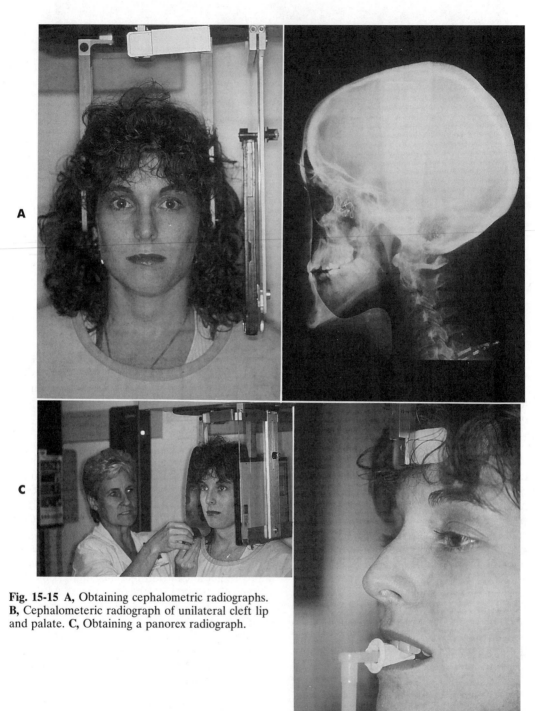

Fig. 15-15 A, Obtaining cephalometric radiographs. **B,** Cephalometeric radiograph of unilateral cleft lip and palate. **C,** Obtaining a panorex radiograph.

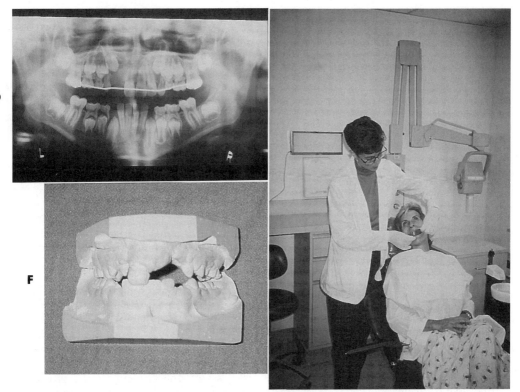

Fig. 15-15, cont'd. D, Panorex radiograph of unilateral cleft lip and palate. **E,** Obtaining impressions of the maxillary and mandibular dental arches. **F,** Model of dental arches of a bilateral cleft lip and palate obtained from the impressions.

photographs (intraoral and extraoral). Cephalometric radiographs provide information on the growth of the cranial base, maxilla, mandible and their relationships to each other, and dental panoramic radiographs are taken to assist in planning the individual treatment plan (Fig. 15-15). These provide a baseline profile and also identify any abnormalities of the primary dentition that can be treated by the pediatric dentist. In addition, this information can be very useful to the speech pathologist and physiologist in providing information on the anatomic sites such as tonsils, adenoids, and cranial base measurements.

Between 2 and 4 years the development of speech and language moves at such a rapid rate that one expects the necessary skills for effective communication to be well instituted by the end of this period. It is also during phase II that initiation of speech rehabilitation begins, if necessary. Treatment of compensatory articulation patterns secondary to VPI can be conducted by therapeutic, prosthetic, and surgical means. Therapeutic treatment is the preferred option of treatment (Chapter 16).

Phase III: 4 to 6 years

The therapeutic process of eliminating compensatory articulation patterns secondary to VPI may continue during this period. However, it is during this time that an increasing degree of interaction between professionals is demanded. A transdisciplinary approach is often seen in this phase because interaction is required by the orthodontist and speech pathologist to establish an integrated treatment plan and then implement the plan.

It is usually within this age group that other treatment options are utilized. Palatal appliances and speech bulb reduction appliances (see Chapter 17) provide passive and active means to facilitate VP closure. As noted in Chapter 17, very specific criteria are required for this treatment option to be successfully implemented. Often the integrity of speech proficiency is the primary concern, since other surgical procedures (pharyngeal flap) are deferred until the individual has achieved anterior, oral articulation (LeBlanc, 1992, 1994). Other procedures also are necessary, such as maxillary expansion prior to alveolar bone grafting, which may have to be deferred until speech proficiency has been achieved. This is an example of the transdisciplinary approach in action. Through discussion of all professionals involved, the orthodontist and maxillofacial surgeon will defer respective treatment until the speech pathologist has achieved the desired goal. In many instances the speech pathologist will adjust desired goals because intraoral appliances may affect lingual placement and subsequently prolong the therapeutic process.

Dental appliances to obturate oronasal fistulae are often used in children ages 4 to 6 years. The purposes of such an appliance are to prevent direct communication between the nasal and oral cavities (eliminating hypernasality), to provide stability for surrounding tissue, and to reduce the effect of further dehiscence in fresh breakdowns (Fig. 15-16).

Appliances can cause sufficient change in the size and shape of the oral cavity, creating a new intraoral structural environment. They may have negative effects on articulation and oral resonance. Slight variations in oral resonance may be related to the presence of an appliance and how the articulators (tongue and lips) adjust. The degree of change depends on the location, size and shape of the appliance. Articulation patterns that existed before the appliance may be changed but not necessarily improved. Thickness of the appliance serves to limit vertical space for tongue movements during speech, creating difficulty for the individual to achieve appropriate place and manner of articulation. If the alveolar ridges are not well delineated, lingual contacts are not made well. Intraoral appliances may present with transient maladaptive compensations that last from days to weeks before adaptive compensations develop or the articulators have accommodated to the presence of the appliance. Extraoral appliances may restrict jaw movement for speech but are not clinically significant.

Phase IV: 6 years to adolescence

Speech management continues and may involve intensive articulation therapy, direct visualization techniques to monitor progress, or surgical and prosthetic management (see Chapter 12). Orthodontic treatment is usually performed on a cleft palate patient in two phases. In the early mixed dentition stage, before full eruption of the permanent incisors, orthodontic therapy is begun to correct anterior and posterior crossbites, major malalignments prior to alveolar bone graft. After or prior to the eruption of the permanent dentition, the second (fixed appliance) phase begins. The timing generally correlates with the circumpubertal growth spurt, which assists with anteroposterior alignment of the maxilla and mandible.

In the majority of the children with complete clefts, presurgical orthodontic therapy before alveolar bone graft is necessary. It often is necessary to expand the palatal arch transversely before bone grafting is conducted. Max-

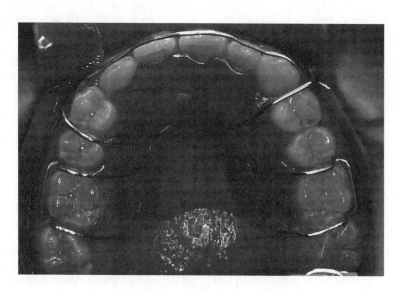

Fig. 15-16 Oronasal fistula obturator.

illary expanders are used in children with cleft lip and palate, particularly where the maxillary arch has collapsed or narrowed (Fig. 15-17). They are positioned inside the dental arch, often fitting across the hard palate. Slight steady pressure provided over time will result in tooth movement or arch expansion. Various mechanisms are used, depending on individual need. One or 2 months after the arch is expanded, braces may be placed on the maxillary teeth to facilitate alignment of the teeth adjacent to the expanded cleft. Arch wires of increasing size are placed over a period of several months until they are of sufficient dimension. The palatal appliance is subsequently removed and a fixed retainer placed (Fig. 15-18). The bone graft is then performed. At times bone grafting is deferred for a short period. Placement of a

palatal appliance to obturate the fistula is often performed.

Expanders have the potential to affect sound production as well as resonance quality. The nature, size, and shape of the expander, as well as the length of time inserted, are factors that may affect speech integrity, the progression of therapy, and the amount of progress attained while the expander is in place. This again illustrates the need for transdisciplinary management. Resonance may be affected because fistulae can be exposed by the lateral movement of the palatal segments. Depending on the size, shape, and location, these fistulae may contribute to the perception of increased hypernasality and facilitate reduced intraoral airflow, affecting strength of articulatory contact. Oronasal

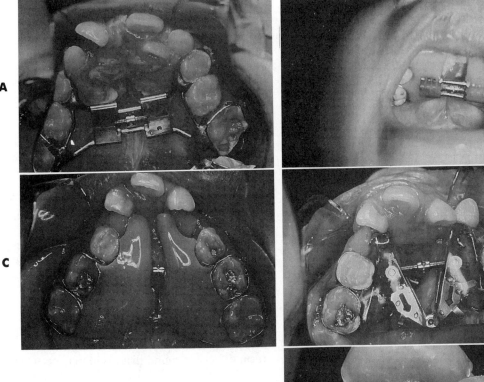

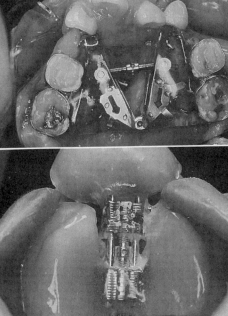

Fig. 15-17 Various types of maxillary expansion appliances (**A-D**). The site of such appliances may affect placement of lingual contact for production of linguoalveolar phonemes (tongue-tip and sibilant). Presurgical orthopedic device used to retract the maxilla (**E**).

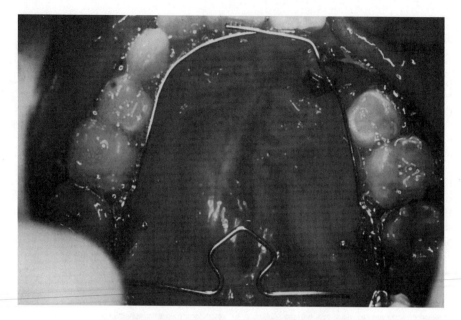

Fig. 15-18 Fixed retainer after maxillary expansion.

fistulae are often the site for compensatory articulation error (middorsal palatal stop) secondary to VPI. The effectiveness of lingual placement on the anterior palate for production of linguoalveolars may be weak and distorted, and adaptive and maladaptive compensations may develop.

Bone grafting of a maxillary alveolar cleft is usually performed during mixed dentition. The timing is determined by dental development to avoid tooth loss and is not judged according to chronologic age. The bone graft is placed before eruption of the permanent tooth into the cleft, usually the lateral incisor if present, or later prior to canine eruption. This eliminates the possible negative sequela of the permanent tooth erupting into the unrepaired cleft, which could lead to tooth loss and probable prosthetic replacement. The eruptive process enhances graft stability and results in a more vertical growth of the alveolar bone. Bone grafting around a partially exposed tooth usually results in marked bone absorption and negative outcome.

The speech therapeutic process is temporary interrupted while the individual is undergoing surgery. It is usually 3 to 6 weeks after surgery before the child is entered into speech therapy. The procedure of bone grafting the alveolar ridge does not produce negative effects on speech production or its rehabilitation.

Once maxillary expansion and bone grafting have been completed, classic orthodontic treatment can be instituted. Banding and other related techniques are effective in moving individual teeth but are not always useful in changing skeletal relationships. Therefore they are limited when there is marked skeletal malocclusion between maxillary and mandibular arches. Surgical orthodontics are used to advance, retrude, and realign the maxilla or mandible and sometimes, with appropriate bone grafts, to provide supplemental bony tissue.

The final phase of treatment consists of adjusting the alignment of teeth with conventional labial orthodontic appliances. If the lateral incisor is missing, a decision needs to be made whether to maintain space for prosthetic replacement or to move the cuspid and the rest of the teeth in the cleft segment forward to close the space. Subsequently, retainers are placed until the final prosthetic replacements can be made.

Bands and brackets rarely have long-term effects on sound production. Temporary, short-term effects of sound distortion may occur due to changes in the structural environment, changes in proprioceptive feedback, and the discomfort often felt when bands and brackets are initially placed. The effects are transient and one should expect accommodation to occur in a short time (time varies by individual).

Phase V: adolescence to adulthood

Speech management (direct therapy and/or monitoring) will be maintained well into adulthood.

The retention of orthodontic treatment is often noted as a significant problem (Little, 1988). Once fixed appliances are removed, natural muscular forces acting on the teeth are no longer opposed. As a consequence relapse may ensue. Few studies have looked at the effects of retention on speech sound performance in the noncleft population and essentially none in the cleft population. It appears that many factors are involved in whether speech sound production and resonance are affected, such as whether a maxillary or mandibular retention is used or both and the size and thickness in the vertical dimension.

CONCLUSIONS

Three to four decades ago the management of an individual with cleft lip and palate was often conducted with a multidisciplinary approach. Interdisciplinary approaches were introduced as a means of better facilitating management. A transdisciplinary approach encompassing the principles of a multidisciplinary approach and an interdisciplinary approach as well incorporating a new framework of shared management will greatly enhance the treatment of these individuals.

REFERENCES

Angle EH: Classification of malocclusion, *Dental Cosmos* 41:248, 1899.

Bankson NW, Byrne MC: The relationship between missing teeth and selected consonant sounds, *J Speech Hearing Disord* 27:341, 1962.

Bloomer HH: Speech defects associated with dental malocclusions and related abnormalities. In Travis LE, editor: *Handbook of speech pathology and audiology,* Englewood Cliffs, NJ, 1971, Prentice-Hall.

Bzoch KR: Etiological factors related to cleft palate speech. In Bzoch KR, editor: *Communicative disorders related to cleft lip and palate,* Boston, 1979, Little, Brown.

Bzoch KR: *Measurement and assessment of categorical disorders related to cleft lip and palate.* In Bzoch, editor: *Communication disorders related to cleft lip and palate,* Boston, 1979, Little, Brown and Co.

Coupe TB, Subtelny JD: Cleft palate—deficiency or displacement of tissue? *Plast Reconstr Surg* 26:600, 1960.

Fára M, Müllerová, Smahel Z: *Presurgical orthopedic treatment in unilateral cleft lip and palate.* In Multidisciplinary management of cleft lip and palate, Bardach J and Morris HL, editors: W.B. Saunders, 1990.

Fleming P, Pielou WD, Sounders DF: A modified feeding plate for use in cleft palate infants. *J Ped Dent,* 1:61-64, 1985.

Freide H, Johanson B: A follow-up study of cleft children treated with primary bone grafting. I. Orthodontic aspects, *Scand J Plast Reconstr Surg* 8:88, 1974.

Fricke JE, editor: *Speech and the dentofacial complex: the state of the art,* ASHA Report No.5, 1970.

Gruber H: Presurgical maxillary orthopedics. In Multidisciplinary management of cleft lip and palate. Bardach J and Morris HL, editors: W.B. Saunders, 1990.

Hall C, Golding-Kushner KJ: *Long-term follow-up of 500 patients after palate repair performed prior to 18 months of age.* Sixth International Congress on Cleft Palate and Related Craniofacial Anomalies, Jerusalem, Israel, June, 1989.

Huebener DV, Marsh JL: *Alveolar molding appliances in the treatment of cleft lip and palate infants.* In Multidisciplinary management of cleft lip and palate, Bardach J and Morris HL, editors: W.B. Saunders, 1990.

Isberg A, Henningsson G: Influence of palatal fistulas onvelopharyngeal movements: a cineradiographic study, *Plas Reconst Surg,* 79:525-530, 1987.

Jenson R: Anterior teeth relationship and speech. *Acta Radiol* (suppl) 276:1, 1968.

Jones JE, Henderson L, Avery DR: Use of a feeding obturator in infants with severe cleft lip and palate, *Spec Care Dent* 2(3):116, 1982.

Kelly E: Feeding cleft palate babies, *Cleft Palate J,* 8:61-64, 1971.

Kelso JAS, Tuller B, Vatikiotis-Bateson E, Fowler CA: Functionally specific articulatory cooperation following jaw pertubations during speech: evidence for coordinative structures, *J Exp Psychol (Hum Percept)* 10:812, 1984.

Laine T, Warren DW, Dalston RM, Hairfield WM, Morr KE: Intraoral pressure, nasal airflow and airflow rate in cleft palate speech, *J Speech Hear Res* 31:432, 1988.

Latham RA: Orthopaedic advancement of the cleft maxillary segment: a preliminary report, *Cleft Palate J,* 17:227, 1980.

LeBlanc EM, Barone C: Quantitative analysis of ankyloglossia, *J Pediatr,* 1994.

LeBlanc EM: The role of speech language pathology in management of cleft lip and palate. In Cleft palate treatment from birth to adolescence: a primer for parents, Berkowitz S, editor: (in press).

LeBlanc EM: *Fundamental principles in speech language management from birth to adolescence.* In Cleft palate treatment from birth to adolescence, Berkowitz S, editor: 1994.

LeBlanc EM: *Oral facial defects and speech production,* New York, 1992, State Association of Pediatric Dentistry.

LeBlanc EM: Fundamental principles in speech pathology management in the cleft lip and palate from birth to adolescence. In Berkowitz S, editor: 1994.

Little RM, Riedel RA, Artun J: An evaluation of changes in mandibular anterior alignment from 0-20 years postretention, *Am J Orthod Dentofac Orthop* 93:423, 1988.

Maddieson I: Report on the 1989 Keil Convention, *J International Phonetic Association,* 19:2, 1989.

Malek R, Martinez H, Mousset M-R, Trichet C: *Mulidisciplinary management of cleft lip and palate in Paris, France.* In Multidisciplinary management of cleft lip and palate, Bardach J and Morris HL, editors: W.B. Saunders, 1-10, 1990.

McWilliams BJ, Morris HL, Shelton RL: *Cleft palate speech,* Philadelphia, 1984, BC Decker.

McWilliams BJ, Morris HL, Shelton RL: Cleft palate speech, ed 2, Philadelphia, 1990, BC Decker.

Morely ME: *Cleft palate and speech,* London, 1970, Longman Group.

Morris HL: Etiological bases of speech problems. In Spriestersbach DC, Sterman D, editors: *Cleft palate and communication,* New York, 1968, Academic Press.

Peterson-Falzone SJ: Nasal emission asacomponent of the misarticulations on sibilants and affricates, *J Speech and Hear Dis* 40:106, 1975.

Peterson-Falzone SJ: *Speech disorders related to craniofacial structural defects.* In Lass NJ, McReynolds LV, Northern

JL, Yoder DE: Handbook of speech-language pathology and audiology. Philadelphia, 1988, B.C. Decker.

Pruzansky S: Factors determining arch form in clefts of the lip and palate, *Am J Orthod* 41:827, 1955.

Razek MKA: Prosthetic feeding aids for infants with cleft lip and palate, *J Prosthet Dent* 44:556-561, 1980.

Rehrmann A, Koberg WR, Koch H: Long term postoperative results of primary and secondary bone grafting in complete clefts of lip and palate, *Cleft Palate J* 7:206, 1970.

Robertson NRE, Jolleys A: Effects of early bone grafting in complete clefts of the lip and palate, *Plast Reconstr Surg* 42:414-421, 1968.

Robertson NRE: The changes produced by pre-surgical oral orthopaedics, *Br J Plast Surg* 24:57, 1968.

Rosenstein S: *Early maxillary orthopedics and appliance fabrication.* In Kernahan DA, Rosenstein SW, editors: Cleft lip and palate: a system of management, Baltimore, 1990, Williams and Wilkens.

Rosenstein SW: Facial growth and development in cleft patients. In Kernahan DA, Rosenstein SW, editors: *Cleft lip and palate: a system of management,* Baltimore, 1990, Williams & Wilkins.

Shprintzen RJ: Palatal and pharyngeal anomalies in craniofacial syndromes, *Birth Defects* 18:53, 1982.

Shprintzen RJ: Surgery for speech: the planning of operations for velopharyngeal insufficiency with emphasis on both pharyngeal physiology and articulation, *Proceedings of the British Craniofacial Society,* Manchester University Press, 1986.

Singer L, Sidoti EJ: Pediatric management of Robin sequence, *Cleft Palate J,* 29:3, 220, 1992.

Skoog T: *Plastic Surgery: new methods and refinements.* Stockhom: Almqwist-Wiksell International, 1974.

Snidecor JC, Kaires AK: A speech corrective prosthesis for anterior open bite malocclusion and its effect on two postdental fricative sounds, *Prosthet Dent* 15:779, 1965.

Starr CD: Dental and occlusal hazards to normal speech production. In Bzoch KR, editor: Communicative disorders related to cleft lip and palate, ed 2, Boston, 1979, Little, Brown.

Subtelny JD, Mestre JC, Subtelny JD: Comparative study of normal and defective articulation of /s/ as related to malocclusion and deglutition, *J Speech Hear Disord* 46:138, 1964.

Subtelny JD: Orthodontic principles in treatment of cleft lip and palate. In Bardach J, Morris H, editors: *Multidisciplinary management,* Philadelphia, 1990, WB Saunders.

Trost-Cardamone JE: Effects of velopharyngeal incompetency on speech. In Coston G, editor: Velopharyngeal incompetence and communication, *J Childhood Commun Disord* 10:(31-49), 1986.

Trost J: Articulatory additions to the classical descriptions of the speech of persons with cleft palate, *Cleft Palate J* 18:193, 1981.

Trost J, Cardamone JE: The development of speech: assessing cleft palate misarticulation. In Kernahan DA, Rosenstein SW, editors: *Cleft lip and palate: a system of management,* Baltimore, 1990, Williams & Wilkins.

16 Treatment of Articulation and Resonance Disorders Associated with Cleft Palate and VPI

Karen J. Golding-Kushner

Approximately 80% of children born with non-syndromic cleft palate who undergo palate repair by 18 months of age develop speech free from compensatory errors without any type of therapeutic intervention (Hall and Golding-Kushner, 1989). However, for the other 20% of these children, and for the many others with syndromes associated with clefts or with velo-pharyngeal insufficiency (VPI) related to other causes, the road to normal speech often seems long and arduous. Compensatory speech errors (glottal stops, pharyngeal fricatives, nasal snorting, and others), are often thought to be resistent to speech therapy, so the goal of normal speech often seems elusive. This need not be the case. The purpose of this chapter is to describe therapeutic principles and techniques that have proven very effective in eliminating articulation errors associated with VPI. Alternative and complementary treatment modalities for articulation and resonance problems, including speech bulb appliances and nasopharyngoscopic biofeedback are also discussed briefly. Speech bulb reduction is discussed in more detail in Chapter 17. The important issue of the timing and sequencing of multiple treatment modalities is addressed.

ARTICULATION DISORDERS

Individuals with cleft palate or other craniofacial disorders may exhibit articulation disorders related to a variety of causes including, but not limited to VPI, palatal fistulae, malocclusion, fluctuating or chronic hearing loss, and tonsillar hypertrophy. They may also have the same phonologic and developmental articulation disorders found in patients without clefts. Errors may be developmental, compensatory, or obligatory. Obviously, effective treatment depends on accurate diagnosis and the selection and sequencing of appropriate therapy modalities.

Developmental articulation errors

Children with cleft palate are susceptible to the same developmental speech disorders and phonologic and linguistic delays as their noncleft peers. The term *delayed articulation* indicates that phonetic proficiency is at a level considered normal at an earlier stage of development. Errors result in production of a sound as it might be produced by an otherwise normal child at an earlier age. Interdental lisps and blend reductions are examples of such errors, which are usually the result of placement errors or omissions. If speech errors produced by a child with a cleft palate are developmental, they are unrelated to the presence of the cleft and should be treated in the same manner as if the cleft were not present. No special approaches or techniques are indicated.

Certain populations of children with clefts are at very high risk for speech and language delays in addition to severe compensatory articulation disorders. Examples of such groups are children with velo-cardio-facial syndrome, in which cognitive deficits are found in nearly all affected individuals, and Treacher Collins syndrome, in which moderate to severe hearing loss is common (Shprintzen et al., 1978; Golding-Kushner et al., 1985; Golding-Kushner, 1991). It is appropriate to establish home stimulation and early intervention programs for them as would be appropriate for linguistically delayed infants without cleft palate.

Compensatory articulation errors

There are several published compendiums describing compensatory errors associated with cleft palate and VPI (Morley, 1970; Peterson, 1975; Trost, 1981). Unfortunately, the term *compensatory* has been used to describe errors associated with both VPI and palatal fistulae, which may cause confusion. For example, the middorsal palatal stop may be produced by

Table 16-1 Anatomic or physiologic defect usually associated with some common compensatory articulation errors

	Associated problem		
Compensatory errors	VPI	Fistula	Malocclusion
Middorsal palatal stop		X	X
Pharyngeal stop	X	X	
Glottal stop	X		
Pharyngeal fricative	X	X	
Nasal snort	X		
Laryngeal fricative	X		

speakers with palatal fistulae or by some individuals with severe orthodontic abnormalities but is not generally caused by VPI. On the other hand, glottal stops occur in the presence of VPI but do not generally develop in speakers with good VP closure even if multiple fistulae are present. So even though all of the errors are referred to as compensatory, they are not all associated with the same underlying anatomic or etiologic base. The more common errors and the anomaly with which they are usually associated are listed in Table 16-1.

Obligatory articulation errors

A distinction should be made between compensatory errors and obligatory errors. Compensatory errors, which are usually substitutions, are errors in learning that affect place of articulation (e.g., glottal stop for bilabial stop) and/or manner of articulation (e.g., /s/ produced on inhalation). Compensatory errors can be corrected only by speech therapy. In contrast, obligatory errors, usually distortions, result directly from an anatomic defect, are not easily amenable to therapy, and often self-correct when the underlying structural cause of the error is corrected; compensatory errors do not (Philips and Kent, 1984; Golding-Kushner, 1990, 1991). Obligatory errors include nasal emission and reduced intraoral pressure related to VPI or fistulae, and certain articulation distortions related to palatal fistulae and malocclusion. For example, a speaker with severe crossbite or absent teeth at the alveolar cleft site may use correct tongue placement and emit an oral air stream (Fig. 16-1). However, an *oral* sibilant distortion may be unavoidable because of the occlusal abnormality. Tongue tip protrusion may be obligatory for some speakers with severe class III malocclusions. Further correction of obligatory distortions may be impossible until the malocclusion is corrected, at which time the distortion might resolve without

therapy. On the other hand, abnormal structure does not necessarily explain an articulation error or preclude therapy. Nasal snorting in a patient with the identical malocclusion seen in Fig. 16-1 *must* be targeted in speech therapy and should not be deferred until completion of orthodontic management. However, it is important for the therapist, patient, and family to realize that the immediate goal is elimination of the compensatory error, and a mild *oral* distortion may be unavoidable (i.e., obligatory) until the structural abnormality is corrected.

Compensatory adaptations

Another category of errors may be referred to as compensatory *adaptations,* which include errors that are the closest possible approximation to a sound in the presence of an anatomic deviation. Examples of this type of error are inversion of /f, v/ (i.e., use of the upper lip and mandibular teeth) or substitution of a labiodental plosive for bilabial plosive by an individual with a severe class III malocclusion. Articulation placement errors in this category may or may not resolve spontaneously when the anatomic deviation is corrected, but may be a reasonable, functional compensation until correct placement is possible.

General categorization of errors as developmental, compensatory, or obligatory is important for decisions regarding the timing of therapy and selection of appropriate targets in therapy. Phonetic distinctions among errors of the same category, such as a pharyngeal fricative versus a laryngeal fricative, are less important in planning therapy because the focus of therapy is on how to produce the target sound correctly and not on the error.

Visual distortions

Certain compensatory errors and compensatory adaptations produced by individuals with structural abnormalities or following surgery result in

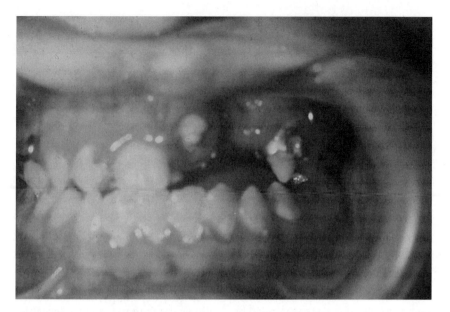

Fig. 16-1 Patient with class III malocclusion and absent teeth at the site of the alveolar cleft. A mild oral sibilant distortion may be considered obligatory and treatment may be deferred. However, nasal snorting in this patient should be treated with aggressive speech therapy.

visual but not auditory speech distortions. Common visual distortions are inversion of labiodental fricatives /f, v/ in the presence of a severe class III malocclusion, and use of the tongue blade instead of the tongue tip for linguoalveolar sounds /t, d, n/ following release of a glossopexy (LeBlanc and Golding-Kushner, 1992). The decision to treat these errors in speech therapy must consider the extent of the structural abnormality, whether the error is obligatory, adaptive, or compensatory, and the degree to which the visual distortion is distracting during conversation.

Velopharyngeal insufficiency and speech

VPI* may give rise to two types of speech disorders: hypernasality (a resonance problem) and articulation errors, including obligatory and compensatory errors. VPI *does not* cause developmental articulation errors or speech delay. Most speakers with VPI are hypernasal and have the obligatory errors of nasal emission and reduced intraoral pressure. However, not all hypernasal speakers demonstrate compensatory articulation errors. In fact, most do not. This highlights the fact that the nasal resonance

problem and the articulation problem are separate components of the speech disorder, and must be considered separately. It also demonstrates the role that learning plays in the development of these aberrant articulatory gestures. Further evidence lies in the observation that, following successful physical management of VPI with prosthetics or surgery, resonance may be normal, but compensatory articulation errors persist† (Trost, 1981; Croft et al., 1981). Also, compensatory articulation errors do not develop in speakers who had normal speech but acquired VPI following adenoidectomy, head trauma, or other secondary insults.

The most common compensatory speech error is the glottal stop, which is often produced as a substitution for stop-plosive consonants. The glottal stop represents maintenance of the *manner* of articulation, but results from errors in both the place of articulation and the articulators used. A glottal stop is produced by abrupt adduction of the vocal folds and/or ventricular (false) vocal folds in an attempt to briefly interrupt the outgoing airstream. The articulators used are the vocal folds, instead of the lips or tongue, and the place of articulation

---

*Some clinicians and researchers make a distinction among velopharyngeal insufficiency, incompetence, and inadequacy depending on the etiology of the disorder. The difference is unimportant in planning speech therapy. Fortunately, all may be referred to as VPI.

†Shprintzen (1990) correctly points out that it would be less confusing to professionals, less disappointing to patients, and more accurate to refer to a pharyngeal flap as "surgery for VPI" rather than "surgery for speech."

is laryngeal rather than oral. That is, the air is obstructed at an area posterior and inferior to the correct place of articulation before the airstream has reached the VP valve. Attempts to produce *all* plosive sounds present the same problem for the child learning to talk, and the glottal stop substitution is often made for all plosives and often other nonnasal consonants. As a result, production of "pa-pa-pa" sounds the same as production of "ta-ta-ta" and "ka-ka-ka" and all are produced as /ʔa-ʔa-ʔa/. This lack of sound differentiation, not the hypernasality, is responsible for poor speech intelligibility.

Pharyngeal and laryngeal fricatives are often used as substitutions for fricative sounds and, like the glottal stop, represent correct manner of articulation but incorrect place of articulation. During production of nasal snorting, air is actively, although not necessarily consciously, pushed through the nose, often accompanied by tongue backing. This should not be confused with the passive nasal emission or nasal escape that is obligatory with VPI and which disappears when the nostrils are occluded. In contrast, if a speaker is producing a nasal snort and the nostrils are occluded, there will be no outgoing air because the intended exit route of the air has been blocked. Because the tongue is back, a velar sound may be produced. Pinching the nares shut is useful as an initial procedure to elicit oral production of /s/.

Coproduced glottal stops

Some speakers move or even use the lips and tongue simultaneously with a glottal stop, producing the *appearance* of correctly articulated sounds. However, the actual valving of the airstream remains glottal. This is referred to as a coproduced or coarticulated glottal stop (Trost, 1981; Henningsson and Isberg, 1986; Golding-Kushner, 1989) and is often evident in the speech of patients who have been in speech therapy and instructed in correct lip/tongue placement but not in airstream management. A coproduced glottal stop is as incorrect an error as a substituted glottal stop, and should be treated as such, not reinforced. Some patients learn correct production of sounds but continue to insert the error sound after the correct production (e.g. /pʔai/). Therefore care must be taken not to inadvertently reinforce the production of intrusive glottal stops and pharyngeal fricatives. This may be accomplished by avoiding an exclusive focus on lip/tongue placement. The speech pathologist should cue and reinforce airflow manner as well as the place at which the airstream is modified. For example, it is better to elicit the sound /b/ with an instruction such as

"stop the air with your lips," than a statement such as "close your lips." Statements used to elicit and reinforce sound production must be specific.

TREATMENT OF ARTICULATION DISORDERS
Early intervention and home programs in the treatment of compensatory articulation disorders

There is truth to the aphorism that an ounce of prevention is worth a pound of cure. Although it is nearly impossible to make a valid assessment of VP function before age 3½ or 4 years (Shprintzen and Golding-Kushner, 1989), articulation errors associated with VPI can be detected at the onset of speech. A speech evaluation should be accomplished early, by 12 to 15 months of age. Therapeutic intervention should be initiated at the earliest necessary time. For infants and toddlers this intervention often may be effectively provided through the use of supervised and clinician-directed home programs. The goal is to reduce the likelihood of the establishment of a pattern of abnormal compensatory errors.

To be efficient and effective, home programs should include the following components as represented by the following outline:

I.   Evaluation
II. Parent training
  A. Recognizing the difference between oral and compensatory articulation
  B. Application of behavior modification techniques
  C. Troubleshooting
III. Follow-up
IV. Reevaluation

Parents or other caregivers may be trained to recognize the undesirable abnormal compensations such as glottal stops and pharyngeal fricatives. Listener training may be accomplished using audio tapes of contrasting correct and incorrect productions and by helping parents to identify the errors in their own child's babbling or early words. Once the parents are able to recognize a glottal stop, pharyngeal fricative, and nasal snort, they can be trained in behavior modification techniques to elicit certain target sounds and to provide positive reinforcement when the sound is correctly produced in a word or correctly babbled. They should also be trained to troubleshoot and to identify and avoid behaviors in themselves that elicit inappropriate or avoidance responses in their child. After training, the parents should be given a written instruction sheet for reference, such as the one in the box on p. 331.

It is useful to suggest specific activities for the parents to do with the child and ways to ensure that, as the child is babbling and learning the first words, correct patterns of articulation are reinforced and a glottal stop articulation disorder does not develop. Initial target words before palate repair should be nasal loaded (mommy, more). Following palate repair they may be

---

HOME PROGRAM REFERENCE SHEET

Children with cleft palate can learn to talk but they may need some extra stimulation. You have listened to the tape recording and you know which sounds we would like to hear your child making. This program was designed to help you help your baby.
This packet contains:
1. 10 pictures of common words or objects
2. A list of 15 other simple words
3. Record sheets

Instructions
Every day set aside 10 to 15 minutes when you and your child can be alone. Pick any of the pictures (or, if possible, use the real objects) and include any of the other words. Show your child the picture or object, talk a lot about it. Include saying the word, making sure he/she can see your mouth moving. Encourage your child to repeat the practice word.
If your child talks back and makes the sound the way you did, give him/her praise by clapping, smiling, tickling, or kissing.* If your child doesn't talk back or is making the glottal sound, withhold the praise but keep on talking.†

Record keeping
After 5 or 10 minutes, use the record form. Put a check mark in the column if the child correctly produced the target sound (word), or an X if your child used glottal speech.
Don't worry if your child does not talk back right away; he/she is watching and listening to you, and is learning.
We will call you every 2 weeks to discuss the program and to see how things are going. If you have any questions before then, call us right away. We think that with a little work now while your child is young, future speech problems may be avoided. Good luck, and be sure to call with any questions or problems.

Therapist's name:_____

Phone_____

(Golding and Kaslon, 1981.)
*This direction is modified as appropriate for the baby's age, but in most cases edible reinforcers are not appropriate.
†Note that there is not punishment. Rather, negative reinforcement is used: that is, withholding the reinforcer in response to an incorrect production.

plosive loaded (baby, toes, cookies). Parents should be contacted by telephone every 2 weeks, and the infants should be scheduled for clinical reevaluation at least quarterly.

It should be stressed that home programs are *not* necessary for the majority of infants with cleft palate because the majority develop normal speech without intervention. However, our experience with this type of early treatment for children who *are* developing a glottal pattern has been successful, especially with infants in the stages of midbabbling and first words. In most cases trained parents working at home are able to elicit normal sound production patterns in their children so that glottal speech does not become established and subsequent speech therapy is not needed. On the other hand, our home programs have not been very successful with children with a more established phonetic repertoire, even when they were as young as 2 years of age. In most cases, once a child has established a glottal pattern, direct articulation therapy is necessary.

Articulation therapy for compensatory speech disorders

Goals of articulation therapy for compensatory speech disorders. The long-term goals of articulation therapy for speakers with compensatory speech disorders are (1) to eliminate glottal stops and establish correct production of oral stops; and (2) to eliminate pharyngeal/laryngeal fricatives and nasal snorting and establish correct production of oral fricatives and sibilants.

Reduction of nasality and VPI is not listed as a goal of therapy, although this may occur when sound production is correct. This is discussed in more detail in the section of this chapter on pharyngeal flaps. Improvement of intelligibility is also not stated as a goal because it is vague, and progress is not easy to measure objectively.

Basic principles of articulation therapy for speakers with compensatory errors.

1. In selecting and sequencing target sounds, consider consistency of errors noted during the evaluation (including stimulability testing), contexts in which the sounds were correctly produced, and developmental sequence. The patient's speech profile should determine the therapy sequence. In general, the goal is to bring articulation anterior by beginning with front sounds (the errors generally involve tongue backing to some degree). In patients with gross errors affecting all sounds, the initial focus should be on labial and tongue tip sounds, including /f, v, p, b, s, z, t, d, θ, ʃ/ (Hoch et al., 1986).

2. Encourage the use of strong articulatory contacts, especially if there is weak intraoral pressure. The use of light articulatory contacts to decrease the perception of hypernasality has been suggested (McWilliams et al., 1990; Van Demark and Hardin, 1990). However, although an increase in strength of contacts may increase the loudness of nasal turbulence, it is more often associated with improved VP motion and tends to enhance speech intelligibility (Hoch et al., 1986; Golding-Kushner, 1989). Increasing strength of articulatory contacts does not mean increasing volume.

3. Be direct and specific. Tell the patient exactly where to place and what to do with the lips and tongue, and how to direct the outgoing airstream (Golding-Kushner, 1989).

4. Build a repertoire of correctly produced words by using only target words in which all sounds are produced correctly. Untrained listeners (which includes patients and their parents) often have difficulty focusing on a specific target sound within a word. This may cause confusion in the mind of the patient who can hear that a word is not correct even though a particular target sound within that word is correct. For a patient with a severe articulation disorder, the initial word list will be limited and may contain only: /h/ + vowel/nasal words *(hay, he, hi, high, ho, who, ham, hem, him, her, hum, honey)*. Available target words for drill become more diverse as therapy progresses.

Therapy procedures for compensatory errors. At the initiation of therapy, the process of correct speech should be explained to the patient and parent in terms appropriate to the child's level of understanding, and the nature of the error should be defined. Even the youngest children can understand that the "cough sound" or the "throat sound" is incorrect and not to be produced. Directions such as "make the wind come out of your mouth" are useful, especially for fricatives and sibilants. Traditional articulation therapy techniques emphasizing correct place and manner of articulation are often effective. However, the compensatory errors of this population may require some special techniques. Many of the procedures I have used were based on the pioneering work of Morley (1970) and are modifications of procedures described previously (Hoch et al., 1986; Golding-Kushner, 1989).

Glottal stops can easily be eliminated using maneuvers that keep the vocal folds apart, such as gentle whispering, overaspiration, or the use of a sustained /h/. Therapy should begin with /h/ to establish production of an oral airflow with an open glottis. This phoneme is used to break the glottal pattern and may then be used as a facilitator to elicit other sounds. Oral movements may then be overlaid on the outgoing sustained oral airstream to produce other sounds. For example, sustaining /h/ and gently closing then opening the lips will result in production of a bilabial plosive. If the open glottis for the /h/ has been maintained and not interrupted, an oral and aspirated /p^h/ without glottal stop will emerge. It is essential to listen carefully to be sure that a glottal stop has not been inserted at the /p-/ release, or coproduced. This can be ensured by overaspirating the /p-/ release. Easy overaspiration by insertion of a sustained /h/ usually breaks the glottal pattern because it requires an open glottis, which is in physiologic conflict with a glottal stop. This may be presented to the patient as whispering, or doing a "big /h/." As an example, "pie" will sound like /p/ + "*hh*high." The easy overaspiration should be used until voiceless plosive-vowel syllables are correctly whispered with no glottal stop on 10 consecutive trials. The difference between a voiceless and voiced plosive is the voice-onset time (VOT), not the mechanics of the gesture. Therefore voicing may be introduced at the end of the elongated consonant-vowel (C-V) syllable, with VOT gradually brought forward toward the consonant on subsequent trials until the C-V syllable is correctly produced with both voiceless and voiced plosives used. The sequence of trials using successive approximations to establish production of the word "two" might be as follows. Each line is repeated until there are five *consecutive* correct productions. The repeated letters represent elongation of a sound; the underlined segments are voiced:

T^{hhhhhh}UUUUU (fully whispered)

T^{hhhhhh}UUU$\underline{UU}$ (voicing is introduced after the vowel onset)

$T^{hhhhhh}$$\underline{UUUUU}$ (voicing is introduced at the vowel onset)

$T^{hhh}$$\underline{UUUUU}$ (the duration of aspiration is decreased)

$T^h\underline{U}$ (normal production)

Some patients find it easier to learn correct oral plosives in the medial or final word position before the initial position. This should be considered in sequencing target sounds and contexts. In that case the /h/ may be initiated and sustained while lip or tongue movements are overlaid on the sustained egressive airstream. For example, to produce /p/, the patient should be instructed to sustain /h/ while closing then opening the lips. A young child could be told to "keep the wind coming out." As above, VOT is gradually moved toward the consonant release so that the sequence of trials moves from fully whispered to normal phonation. Each step is repeated until correctly produced five consecutive times, as follows. Repeated letters represent elongation of a sound; underlined segments are voiced:

^{hhhhhh}AAAAAA (fully whispered)

^{hhhhhh}AAAP^{hhhhhh}AAAAA (fully whispered, bilabial closure overlaid)

^{hhhhhh}AAP^{hhhhhh}A<u>AAAAA</u> (voicing is introduced after the vowel onset)

^{hhhhhh}AAP^{hhhhhh}<u>AAAAAA</u> (voicing is introduced at the vowel onset)

^{hhhhhh}AAP^{hhh}<u>AAAAAA</u> (duration of p- release aspiration decreased)

^{hhhhhh}AAP^h<u>A</u> (normal duration of p- release aspiration for medial position)

^{hh}AP^h<u>A</u> (decreased duration of "carrier aspiration")

P^h<u>A</u> (normal production in initial position)

The procedure to establish production of oral stop consonants may be summarized as follows:

1. Whisper plosive sounds with overaspiration, then introduce voicing at the end of the syllable with a gradual VOT shift.
2. Sustain /h/ with labial or lingual gestures overlaid.

Some patients have difficulty with velar plosives /k, g/. Therapy for these sounds may begin with production of nasal /ɔ/ in the medial and final positions. Nasal occlusion imposed during production of the sustained velar nasal will elicit a velar plosive. The release should initially be overaspirated using /h/ as described above.

Nasal occlusion and release are useful in the elimination of nasal snorting and in the establishment of oral fricatives and sibilants. As noted earlier, in the case of nasal *emission* or *turbulence** air is orally directed and nasal occlusion eliminates unwanted nasal escape of

air and permits unimpeded oral emission. On the other hand, initial productions of nasal *snorting* with the nares occluded often result in no sound because air is purposely directed nasally, but the nasal exit route is closed. Most patients learn to direct the air through the mouth rather than the nose quickly, within a few trials. A sample sequence of trials follows, with each step repeated until there are five consecutive correct productions.

1. Gently but fully occlude the nares (at the nasal tip); sustain /f/ for 3 to 5 seconds.
2. Occlude the nares, sustain /f/ for 3 to 5 seconds, release nares, then occlude nares while still sustaining /f/.
3. Sustain /f/ for 3 to 5 seconds, then occlude and release nares *after* onset of /f/ as monitoring device.
4. Proceed to C-V syllables and quickly into meaningful contexts (words).

Correctly produced sounds may be used as facilitators to elicit error sounds. For example, if /θ/ is correctly produced, the patient may be instructed to sustain it for five consecutive trials and then to repeat the sound with the tongue *inside* the teeth. Within one to three trials, a correct oral /s/ is usually produced. Retracting the tongue further into the center of the mouth results in /ʃ/. Adding voice (humming) while sustaining voiceless sounds /s, f/ results in production of their voiced cognates /z, v/.

Regardless of the nature of errors produced, multiple types of cues may be provided to elicit production of sounds. Some patients respond best to certain types or combinations of cues. These cues, which should also be used during the stimulability testing portion of speech evaluations, follow:

1. *Auditory cues* including modeling. This is the most common type of cuing whereby the patient repeats a sound or word produced by the clinician.
2. *Phonetic cues.* A sound produced correctly is used as a phonetic facilitator to elicit another sound using a series of successive approximations. Examples are producing /θ/ with the teeth closed to elicit /s/; whispering /ba/ to elicit /pa/.
3. *Visual cues.* The patient watches the therapist's use of articulators directly or in a mirror; the patient uses a mirror, feather, or cotton ball to provide visual feedback of oral air flow. (*Caution!* The feedback device must be held in a position that will prevent its response to nasal airflow, which would inadvertently reinforce incorrect responses.)

---

*Nasal turbulence is noisy nasal emission. It has also been referred to as nasal *rustle.*

4. *Verbal cues.* The therapist provides specific instructions for articulation placement and manner of airstream management (e.g., for /s/: "Put your tongue behind your teeth and make the air come out of your mouth").

5. *Manual cues.* The therapist or patient manipulates the lips, tongue, or nose of the patient. Examples are the use of nasal occlusion to force oral air emission during fricative and sibilant production, or use of a tongue depressor to hold the tongue tip down during production of linguavelar sounds.

6. *Tactile cues.* Touch is used to provide the patient with feedback about some aspect of production, such as feeling a puff of air from mouth on the hand or feeling labial pressure during production of bilabial sounds on a finger.

Phone-specific VPI. In phone-specific VPI complete VP closure is achieved during periods of correct oral articulation. However, during one sound (usually /s/) or group of sounds (usually sibilants or fricatives), VPI is present.

Most cases of phone-specific VPI involve nasal snorting. Production of a nasal snort *must* occur with an open VP port. Even if the port is fully obstructed by a pharyngeal flap or speech bulb, a speaker producing this sound will manage to move the lateral and posterior pharyngeal walls outward so that the nasal exit route is available. This error is most often used as a substitution for sibilant sounds /s, z, ʃ/, but may be a substitute for fricatives /f, v, θ,/ and may occur as an isolated error either in speakers with repaired clefts or in individuals with normal palates.

Some noncleft speakers with this error may have oral apraxia and have difficulty with the coordination of articulatory gestures in the absence of weakness, paralysis, or anatomic defect.* They are often erroneously said to be hypernasal on /s/. As illustrated in the case history that follows, speech therapy for phone-specific VPI is usually quick and highly effective, and recurrence of VPI has not been observed.

Case history 1. The patient was a 4½ year-old girl who had received speech therapy elsewhere for 2 years with no improvement in her production of /s, z/. She was referred to the Center for Craniofacial Disorders of Montefiore Medical Center with a diagnosis of apraxia, VPI, and

---

*Patients with compensatory articulation are often erroneously described as apraxic because it *appears* that they can't move their tongues to execute movements. In most cases they are not apraxic and the problem is *omission* of oral articulation gestures, not inability to produce them.

suspected submucous cleft palate. The referring speech pathologist requested that nasopharyngoscopy be done and suggested that the child needed a pharyngeal flap. Nasopharyngoscopy revealed that the child had a normal palate on both the oral and nasal surfaces but with isolated VPI on /s, z/ only. VP movement and closure were otherwise normal. Articulation was characterized by nasal snorting on /s/ and developmental errors including an /r/ distortion. Nasal flaring was observed.

Articulation therapy was initiated immediately, with the goal to establish oral production of /s/. The first procedure was to use /θ/ as a facilitator to elicit sustained /s/. The child was instructed to sustain /θ/ with the teeth closed and tongue behind the teeth. Within three trials, a correct oral /s/ was produced. Nasal occlusion and release were also used to provide the patient with the ability to easily establish an oral airstream. On the first trials with nasal occlusion, she was unable to produce any sound but she quickly learned to direct the air through her mouth, rather than her nose. She was able to produce /s/ + vowel syllables correctly by the end of the first session.

The patient was seen for 11 sessions over 5 weeks. Each session lasted 20 to 25 minutes. There were three visits per week during the first 2 weeks, and two visits per week for the following 2 weeks. By session 11, nasal snorting was almost completely eliminated and she was able to produce all sibilants orally in all contexts during spontaneous conversation with 90% consistency during therapy and during conversations with her mother outside of therapy. The occasional errors that persisted were on /s/ + nasal blends (sn, sm). The nasal flaring, which was ignored during therapy, disappeared spontaneously once the nasal snorting was eliminated. After 5 weeks there was no further need for intensive therapy and she was referred back to her school system for continued therapy for the /r/ distortion and a mild language delay. Resonance was normal, and VP closure was achieved consistently throughout phonation as visualized on nasopharyngoscopic examination. The child was seen for follow-up 6 months, 1 and 2 years following discharge. All follow-up examinations revealed that she had maintained completely normal articulation and resonance (including during /s/ + nasal blends) with complete VP closure confirmed endoscopically.

Therapy procedures to avoid. The most effective and efficient way to use therapy time is to correct articulation errors and establish strong articulatory contacts. It is a poor and inefficient use of time to teach strategies to improve intelligibility such as rate reduction and the use of light articulatory contacts. The therapy goal is *correct* speech, not just *intelligible* speech. When articulation is correct, speech will be fully intelligible.

Nonspeech lingual and labial exercises or activities intended to increase the strength or range of motion are not among the recommended therapy procedures. Individuals with compensatory speech errors have almost no movement of the oral articulators. However, this is usually due to an error in learning rather than paralysis or weakness. Because the airstream has been stopped or constricted at the glottis or in the pharynx, lip and tongue gestures serve no purpose and may not be learned. Even most patients with very severe glottal stop speech disorders have normal tongue tip activity during production of nasal /n/ and normal bilabial closure for nasal /m/. It should be obvious that if tongue movement/elevation is sufficient for /n/, it is sufficient for the oral cognates /t, d, s, l/. It is a waste of therapy time to try to "strengthen" the tongue before working on production of tongue tip plosives. The problem is not the strength of the tongue, but rather what the speaker has (not) taught the tongue to do during speech. Similarly, there are no speech sounds that require the speaker to protrude and move the tongue from one corner of the mouth to the other, or around the circumference of the lips. Therefore exercises to increase the range of motion of the tongue serve no purpose in articulation therapy for these patients.

Important therapy principles

To be effective, therapy must be direct, intensive, and frequent.

Intensity of therapy. Seventy to 100 correct productions of the target sounds should be elicited at each session (Hoch et al., 1986). The most efficient procedure to accomplish this, especially when targeting sounds at the syllable and word level, is drill. Drill is often regarded as an uninteresting therapy procedure of last resort. However, with motivating stimuli and reinforcement materials, an upbeat clinician attitude, and fast pace, it is highly effective. Prearranged reinforcers should be provided at appropriate intervals, following behavior modification techniques. A frequency count of correct responses at each level of therapy (syllables, words, phrases, sentences, conversation) must be kept. It is appropriate to move from one level to the next when a 70% correct response rate or better during two consecutive sessions is achieved. A patient may be at different levels for

different target sounds, and groups of sounds may be targeted together. For example, a therapy sequence for one patient may be /h/, then /p/ (to establish plosive production), then /b, t, d, k, g/ as a group while introducing /f/ as the first fricative.

Effective use of reinforcers. Reinforcers should be simple, quick, and motivating to be effective without interfering with the flow and focus of therapy. For example, for a toddler the clinician and child can each hold a block or small toy car, and make them "talk" while bouncing or tapping them on the floor or table, saying a target syllable with each tap, such as "pa-pa-pa." The activity is motivating and self-reinforcing when paired with verbal praise and smiling by the clinician. A slightly older child might be expected to repeat target syllables or words. The clinician might hold a large container and place a block into it. The container should be held out of sight during the drill to avoid distraction and be replaced in the child's view while the clinician adds to the collection. At predetermined intervals (5 minutes at first, longer intervals depending on the child's ability to delay gratification), the canister may be given to the child for a minute of free play. Other reinforcement procedures might include permitting the child to make every tenth or twentieth check mark on a data recording sheet, receive a star or sticker for every x number of correct responses, or to color for 1 minute after each 5 minutes of drill. An older patient should be able to defer receipt of tangible reinforcers (such as stickers) until the end of a session, relying on verbal reinforcement at shorter intervals. Verbal reinforcement should be specific (*good /t/, good sound, good talking, good speech, good try*). The phrase "Good boy/girl" should *never* be used as a reinforcer because it implies that on unsuccessful attempts the child is a bad person.

Frequency of therapy. Therapy should initially be individual and frequent. Short sessions are more effective than long ones, especially at the beginning. A sample schedule is 5 days a week for 15 to 20 minutes at each session, or 3 days a week for 20 to 30 minutes. Twice a week is usually not frequent enough, even when appropriate procedures are used, and hour-long sessions are too long, especially for young children. Even for adults, long but infrequent sessions do not provide the necessary practice needed to acquire any new skill.

Hoch (Hoch, 1981; Hoch et al., 1986) described a number of children who received articulation therapy twice a week for several months without substantial progress. Each session was almost like a first visit. By simply adding one session per week, the children progressed rapidly and within 3 months had normal articulation. There are several possible reasons that this made such a difference, including the fact that therapy was more frequent. Because the parent brought the child to the hospital more often, the *parent* made more of a commitment to therapy. To avoid future visits to the hospital for therapy they seemed more willing to keep appointments. As a result of their increased commitment to therapy, the parents were more willing to do homework assignments with the child, so that even though the child was seen at the hospital clinic 3 days a week, he or she had some type of therapy 5 or even 7 days a week. Perhaps most important, more frequent therapy sessions helped the child to understand the importance of therapy and correct speech and made therapy seem less like an optional extracurricular activity, like soccer or piano lessons. This is especially important for children receiving therapy at school. Significantly greater improvement in speech and more consistent maintenance of improved speech following intensive therapy was also reported by Albery and Enderby (1984).

Once the patient is able to produce all phonemes without compensatory errors and is progressing at the sentence level of therapy, frequency of sessions may be reduced to two times per week. More attention can then be given to carryover into limited conversational speech in therapy in the classroom and at home. The patient and a family member should set aside some time each day during which correct speech is expected and during which the patient must correct any errors. The amount of time should be increased each day, starting with 5 to 15 minutes. Some families center this correct speech time around an activity, such as a ride in the car on the way to another activity, or during a trip to the supermarket. These contexts ensure that the conversation during which correct speech is expected will be natural. The child can be reminded that all speech during that time must be correct. The parents should refrain from correcting every speech error at other times or the child will feel hassled and frustrated. Therapy should be phased out gradually as more correct speech time outside of therapy occurs.

Home assignments and carryover. Regardless of where therapy is provided, 10 minutes of home practice should be scheduled on all nontherapy days with homework assignments written into a speech notebook. The tasks sent home should trail therapy by at least one

session. Speech pathologists working in schools should make a special effort to maintain contact with the parents so that home assignments can be effectively managed and carryover of new speech skills can be facilitated. Parental contact may take the form of face-to-face meetings, telephone conversations, letters, or a combination of all three. Tasks to be completed at home should be useful and simple enough to ensure that expectations for their execution are realistic. Recording forms or charts and pictures should be provided so that speech time at home is spent on production of speech targets and does not become busy work for the parents, such as searching through magazines to cut out pictures. Picture cards used by the therapist may be photocopied and carried home by the child in a pocket created by taping an envelope on three sides in the speech notebook. Pictures may be copied twice so that the child and parent can play card games such as Go Fish, Concentration, Old Maid, and others.

Responsibility for therapy and progress: whose fault is it, anyway? If a patient does not respond to treatment, the therapist should examine the way in which he or she has structured therapy, including its goals, procedures, reinforcers, frequency, and home assignments. In almost every case of a compensatory speech disorder, **if a patient's speech does not improve significantly within 3 to 6 months, and compensatory errors are not being replaced by oral speech, it is likely that the problem lies with the therapist and not with the patient.** Elimination of glottal stops and nasal snorting is not dependent on maturity or development, VP closure or lack thereof, or use of a speech bulb. It is the responsibility of the therapist to arrange an appropriate therapy schedule, set appropriate goals, select and use appropriate and motivating procedures and reinforcers. Behavior modification techniques are recommended and include positive reinforcement of correct productions and *verbal* punishment of incorrect productions ("No, that's the bad way"). In other words, if progress is not seen or is very slow, the therapist must review his or her own performance before blaming the child or attributing it to abnormal anatomy. For example, a hyperactive child must have variety of quick drill reinforcers presented in rapid sequence to maintain attention. A different set of reinforcers and different amount of frenetic activity is necessary for different patients.

If the patient is a child, the parent's responsibility is to get the child to therapy. Arranging therapy in the school relieves them of this burden, but adequate therapy is not always available in schools because of fiscal or logistic limitations. The parent should help with home assignments to increase the frequency of therapy, but not all caregivers are willing or able to do so. The therapist must take the responsibility to keep the parent informed about the therapy process and impose involvement in therapy on the parent. This poses a special challenge to speech pathologists in a school setting where contact with the parent is typically infrequent. Parents should always be aware of the current target sounds and contexts and the therapy procedures so that they can adjust their expectations for the child's speech at home. They should be informed, for example, if a particular sound is being targeted at a sentence level and another at a word level. The child has a responsibility to bring his or her speech book to sessions and to do home assignments. The patient's most important responsibility is to participate actively in therapy and home practice tasks. It may be useful to put these responsibilities into writing in the form of a contract, signed by all parties at the beginning of therapy and modified as needed. The contract may be attached to the front page of the speech notebook as an ongoing reminder.

A child who time and again says "I can't" should not have the negative behavior reinforced by a long pep talk or discussion about abilities. The child should not be encouraged or allowed to indulge in self-pitying types of comments or feelings. This serves to waste valuable therapy time and rewards task avoidance strategies. Rather, the therapist should acknowledge the patient's frustration and move directly to task to demonstrate his or her ability to succeed. For example, a child who complains that she absolutely can't imitate /t/ could be told in a matter-of-fact way, "It's hard, but I'll help you; put your tongue...." The negative comments will diminish. A child who persists in refusing to attempt a new task may be trying to tell the therapist that the level of difficulty has increased too quickly. In that case, drop back a level for a few minutes longer, and introduce the next target in smaller steps. Always end the session with a task for which there is already a success record so that the patient leaves with a positive feeling and sense of accomplishment.

Coordination of speech services. Many patients are evaluated and monitored by a specialist on a cleft palate or craniofacial team but receive ongoing speech therapy at another location. This demands close cooperation between the team and treating speech pathologists. Honest misunderstandings may occur, which are easily clarified by close communication. Unfortunately, differences of opinion or "turf" conflicts may lead to problems that impede speech therapy and interfere with the overall multidisciplinary treatment plan set by the team. Those issues may include the recommended frequency of therapy, recommended and discouraged procedures, sequencing of speech and language goals, sequencing of speech therapy and surgery, and use of a speech bulb.

The treating craniofacial team's recommendation for more frequent therapy is often met with resistance because many schools and clinics have a tradition of scheduling visits on a weekly or biweekly basis. However, this may not always be in the best interest of the patient. Block scheduling (Van Hattum, 1974), whereby intensive, individual therapy (3 to 5 days per week) is available to a limited number of patients for 3 to 6 months, should be considered. Following that period, most patients have progressed sufficiently to reduce to a biweekly individual schedule, and a different patient can be "blocked." At that point it may also be possible to schedule two patients in a group. Larger groups do not provide an opportunity for each child to produce the large number of responses needed at each session to ensure adequate rehearsal of new sounds. Sessions should be spaced evenly over the week (e.g., three sessions per week should be on Monday, Wednesday, and Friday, not two visits on Tuesday and one on Wednesday).

Unfortunately, school-based speech and language pathologists are often pressured to abide by a child study team's or school board's opinions about appropriate therapy even though this undermines their own professional expertise and ignores the needs of the child. The unwillingness or inability of a school or clinic therapist to challenge decisions made by administrators and arrange the needed scheduling should be viewed as a failure at two levels. First of all, it perpetuates an impression that speech pathologists are second class professionals, incapable of creating schedules that meet specific patients' needs. Furthermore, maintaining an inadequate therapy schedule reduces the likelihood of success, perpetuating the myth that compensatory errors are difficult to treat. Teachers often protest that speech therapy demands too much out-of-classroom time. Again, 15-minute sessions four times per week are more useful than biweekly 30-minute sessions; they provide the same total minutes of therapy but may be less disruptive.

Some children need both articulation and language therapy. The speech pathologist working outside of the craniofacial team, especially one in a school setting, may prioritize language/learning needs or easier articulation goals. Again, close cooperation between the treating therapist and the team therapist is absolutely essential. In some cases pharyngeal flap surgery or reduction in the size of a speech bulb may depend on the elimination of compensatory articulation errors. The treating therapist must become an auxiliary member of the cleft palate team and maintain a perspective on the interplay of medical, surgical, dental, and prosthetic plans and speech therapy. He or she should try to be flexible enough to defer other speech and language therapy goals, rewrite an individualized educational plan (IEP), and shift the focus to compensatory articulation errors for 3 to 6 months. During that time, language goals may be incorporated into the articulation tasks or addressed directly for a few minutes during each session. For example, articulation target words may include new vocabulary, or a particular syntax goal could be worked in as a carrier phrase. This requires flexibility and creativity on the part of the treating speech pathologist. If this type of coordination is not possible, the parents must be persuaded to seek articulation therapy elsewhere. It is better to have no articulation therapy at school and seek it elsewhere than to have inadequate treatment.

Case history 2. This case represents a situation that had the ingredients for guaranteed failure. The child was a 5-year-old girl with repaired cleft palate and a severe compensatory articulation disorder that had not responded to 4 years of "therapy" in the local community. She was brought to the Center for Craniofacial Disorders on a yearly basis for follow-up. At each reevaluation the child's ability to produce correct fricatives and plosives including /f, p/ with no pharyngeal fricative and no glottal stop was demonstrated during the stimulability testing portion of the speech evaluation, within four to five trials for each phoneme. The correct therapy method was demonstrated for the parent, who watched passively. The parent refused to schedule speech therapy at the hospital because it was inconvenient and returned the child to the local therapist, who had already refused to schedule more than 1 session per week for 2 years because of the child's age, lack of progress, and hypernasality, and his own busy schedule. The child became increasingly frustrated, and the parent became angrier at each yearly visit because the local therapist who "knew the child better" had convinced her that pharyngeal flap surgery was needed before

therapy could proceed. Attempts were made to encourage the therapist's participation with the craniofacial team and to improve coordination of services, but to no avail. Temporary speech bulb placement, which might have been considered to facilitate therapy, was not possible because the parent was noncompliant for multiple visits to the orthodontic department. Though the excuse of convenience was ostensibly the reason for not scheduling therapy at the hospital, the years without proper treatment resulted in a far more damaging inconvenience.

Nasal grimace. Some speakers with VPI have facial or nasal grimacing associated with attempts at nasal constriction to reduce air escape. This usually disappears spontaneously once VPI is completely eliminated and, although it produces visually distorted speech, should be ignored in therapy when VPI is present. If grimacing persists 2 months after complete elimination of VPI (confirmed via direct visualization of VP closure), it may be eliminated easily using behavior modification techniques and a mirror for feedback. As with other compensatory and adaptive behaviors, adults with long-standing grimacing may have more difficulty in eliminating the grimace than children.

TREATMENT OF RESONANCE DISORDERS

Disorders of nasal resonance include hypernasality and hyponasality. Disorders of oral resonance include muffling and potato-in-the-mouth resonance.

Hypernasality

The most common cause of hypernasality is VPI, and for most hypernasal patients correction of VPI requires surgery, usually a pharyngeal flap. However, in some cases the use of therapeutic alternatives may eliminate the need for a pharyngeal flap or decrease the amount of nasopharyngeal obstruction necessary. Selection and sequencing of treatment option(s) must be based on correct application of both clinical (perceptual) and physiologic criteria. This necessitates direct visualization of the VP mechanism during speech, which can be accomplished only via nasopharyngoscopy and multi-view videofluoroscopy. Possible treatment options for VPI include speech therapy, biofeedback therapy, fistula repair, tonsillectomy, speech bulb reduction, and pharyngeal flap.

Speech therapy. Speech therapy should never be undertaken for the treatment of hypernasality unless there is clear evidence that the patient is able to achieve VP closure during a speech task, evidence which can be obtained only through direct visualization of VP closure using nasopharyngoscopy or multi-view videofluoroscopy. Increasing strength of articulatory contacts and increasing mouth opening during phonation may reduce hypernasality. Simple feedback devices that can be used in any therapy setting are discussed in the next section.

Therapy procedures to avoid. Many procedures for speech therapy to eliminate or reduce hypernasality have been published, including the use of nonspeech activities intended to improve palatal elevation and/or VP closure. Though there is strong evidence against their usefulness, some therapists continue to do palatal exercise, massage, blowing, positioning, icing, sucking, swallowing, cheek puffing, gagging, palatal strengthening, stroking, and other nonspeech activities. These are of no value because patterns of VP activity during these tasks is different than during speech, and there is no evidence of any carryover of improved VP closure during these tasks to changes in VP closure during phonation or to reduction of hypernasality (Powers and Starr, 1974; Ruscello, 1982; Starr, 1990; Van Demark and Hardin, 1990). These techniques serve only to frustrate patients, parents, and clinicians, waste time, effort, and money, and delay the application of appropriate treatment. Similarly, neurodevelopmental techniques (NDTs) are not applicable to the treatment of VPI or compensatory speech errors. Reduction of respiratory effort has also been suggested (Dalston et al., 1990). Although making the speech signal less audible may succeed in reducing perceived hypernasality, there is no evidence to suggest that it improves VP closure.

Blowing may have limited usefulness as an introductory activity (not as a therapy goal) for an infant or toddler who does not understand the linguistic concept of making air ("wind") exit through the mouth as opposed to the nose. Easy blowing of bubbles, feathers, cotton balls, or paper with the nose open and closed may help to establish this concept. In this context, blowing may be used as a play activity *for a few minutes,* but a speech sound, such as /h/ or /ɵ/ should be immediately introduced. The speech sound should then be substituted for the blowing, and the movement of bubbles or feathers produced by the sustained fricative or overaspirated plosive may serve as a reinforcement activity because it is highly motivating for most young children. In addition to the visual reinforcement of the bubbles, verbal reinforcement should be specific, for example, "Good, you said

/fffff/. That was mouth wind." Negative practice, or deliberate replication of an error and corresponding correct production, may be useful to reinforce the nasal versus oral concept, and allows for "silly time" for young children. For example, once correct /s/ production is elicited five consecutive times, a child with nasal snorting could be instructed to make the "old, yucky" sound with "nose wind" and then to make the "new, good /s/ with mouth wind."

Blowing with phonation overlaid was suggested by Shprintzen et al. (1975) as a means of improving VP closure in patients who had better closure during blowing than during speech. Shprintzen subsequently noted that the patients with whom this procedure was successful demonstrated good VP closure during production of sustained fricatives (Shprintzen, 1989). That is, they had phonetic differences in VP closure. Unfortunately, sustained fricatives had been omitted from the examination protocol of the original four subjects with whom this procedure had been tested. Shprintzen concluded that the sustained fricatives and/or sibilants during which VP closure was achieved could be used as facilitators in clinical articulation and biofeedback therapy more effectively and more efficiently than blowing. The importance of including sustained fricatives and/or sibilants in the fluoroscopic and endoscopic protocols was also stressed (Shprintzen, 1989; Shprintzen and Golding-Kushner, 1989).

Nasopharyngoscopic and other visual biofeedback. Some individuals are able to learn to increase or change VP closure using fiberoptic nasopharyngoscopy, which allows the patient to visualize VP movements directly during phonation (Siegel-Sadewitz and Shprintzen, 1982; Yamaoka et al., 1983; Hoch et al., 1986; ACPA, 1993). Use of the endoscope allows the patient to visualize VP movements as they occur, and the lack of radiation allows for extended sessions that would not be feasible using videofluoroscopy. As with all therapeutic procedures, patient selection should be based on specific clinical and physiologic criteria. Clinical criteria for the use of visual biofeedback to improve VP closure are unambiguous evidence of nasal escape or turbulence on only one sound or a class of sounds, usually (but not always) sibilants, variable resonance, and adequate patient compliance for repeated and extended endoscopy. Physiologic criteria are the presence of intermittent VP closure, variable VP closure with evidence of stimulability for improvement during the initial examination, phone-specific VPI or phone-specific closure. Multi-view videofluoroscopy, especially the lateral view, is essential for correct interpretation of nasopharyngoscopy in establishing that the physiologic criteria are met because it provides the only clear view of tongue movement. Compensations such as tongue-assisted velar motion may be seen that might otherwise be misinterpreted as good closure (Fig. 16-2).

The advantage of endoscopic biofeedback therapy is that, when effective, treatment is very simple and fast, with results evident in a few sessions. In fact, biofeedback therapy should be discontinued if there is no response to treatment within two or three sessions. The disadvantages include the cost and limited availability of the instrument and personnel for use in many therapy settings.

Procedure for nasoendoscopic biofeedback. The patient is seated facing a television monitor with the endoscope in place (Fig. 16-3). The flexible endoscope should be coupled to a video camera that is mounted on a tripod for stability and to free the clinician to stand near the monitor. Using the image on the monitor, the therapist teaches the patient to recognize the structures

(palate, lateral and posterior pharyngeal walls, adenoid) and movements visualized and to recognize differences in closure on different phonemes or in different phonetic contexts, such as at nasal-oral transitions.

Stimulability testing to establish that there is potential for VP closure will have been done at the time of initial examination because it is the basis for patient selection for this therapeutic procedure. An expanded speech sample is obtained at the first therapy session to determine the specific contexts in which VP closure occurs. This must include observation of VP motion during production of all phonemes in multiple phonetic contexts, as well as consideration of the consistency of timing and synchrony of VP gestures. Some common timing errors are early release of closure at nonnasal to nasal transitions (e.g., "*pan*"), delayed closure at nasal to nonnasal transitions (e.g., "*nap*"), and pulse opening at voice-voiceless and voiceless-voice transitions (e.g., "*vest*"). The clinician should also look for patterns affecting classes of sounds with better or worse closure, bearing in

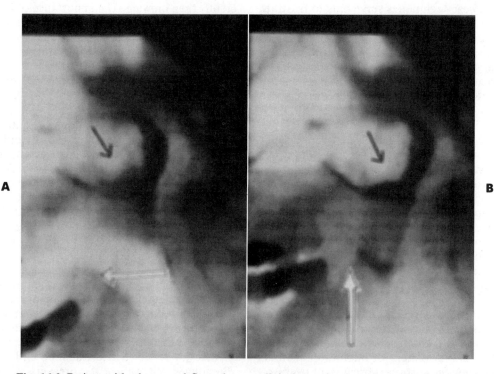

Fig. 16-2 Patient with pharyngeal flap who, on clinical examination of nasal emission and nasopharyngoscopy, appeared to have good velopharyngeal closure only during production of velar plosives /k, g/. Lateral view videofluoroscopy revealed consistent VPI (**A**) with tongue-assisted velar elevation during /k, g/ (**B**), establishing that the endoscopic impression of phone-specific closure was an articulatory artifact.

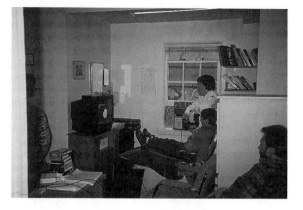

Fig. 16-3 Setup for nasopharyngoscopic biofeedback.

mind that some variation in tightness of closure and velar height is to be expected.* During the first session, an orientation is also given to the patient regarding what is occurring in the VP port. He or she should be able to recognize and identify when VP closure is occurring and when it is not.

Therapy begins with production of VP closure during production of a sound in a known successful context, based on initial probe testing. For many patients this is a sustained isolated /s/ or /f/ or a whispered production of a C-V-C syllable such as /pop/, but could be any sound or syllable. This should be repeated five times to be sure that the patient appreciates that VP closure is occurring. The phonetic string is gradually increased in length and complexity by reduplication of syllables or addition of other sounds.

If VP opening occurs on one sound or class of sounds, that sound should be embedded within a context in which VP closure occurs or placed in the final word position immediately following another consonant. For example, if the VP port opens only during production of /s/, a stimulus word sequence might be "pet, pest, pets," or "pet, pets." The final /s/ would then be sustained ("petsssss"), then followed immediately by the sustained sound repeated in isolation ("petssss ssss").

Difficulty in maintenance of VP closure during transitions between voiced and voiceless sounds may be approached using sustained

---

*Velar height during vowel production is correlated with tongue height (higher elevation on high vowels), and tight closure may not occur during production of isolated low vowels. However, complete VP closure should occur during production of all consonants including liquids and semivowels (/l, r, j, w/), and should be maintained during production of vowels embedded between consonants.

sibilant or fricative sounds. The patient should sustain a sound, for example, /f/ for five repetitions, then introduce voicing during production of the middle segment, producing a continuous voiceless fricative beginning and ending as /f/ but transitioning to /v/ in the middle ("fffvvvfff"). This would be repeated until there are five consecutive correct productions. This could be varied by beginning with the voiced sound /v/ and eliminating voicing midway to embed the /f/, or beginning with the voiceless fricative and embedding voice. In selecting phonetic contexts to manage VP closure problems affected by timing and voicing, it must be kept in mind that all vowels are voiced unless whispered. Whispered word production may be used as a facilitating context with voicing gradually introduced in medial or final word positions.

Patients often begin to self-monitor closure during the first session. Some have the ability to spontaneously effect closure at rest. Caution must be taken to avoid reinforcement of compensatory or aberrant pharyngeal and articulatory gestures, such as breath holding, laryngeal tension, or lingual backing to support the velum giving the false impression from a superior view that VP closure has occurred. Speech tasks involving nasal phonemes are not used during the first two or three sessions unless the only problem is maintenance of VP closure near transitions between nasal and nonnasal phonemes, or abnormally timed closure/opening.

Endoscopic biofeedback therapy must be frequent and intensive, at least three times per week, with sessions lasting from 10 to 20 minutes. If biofeedback therapy is going to be successful, results will be evident quickly, and the therapy program should be completed within several weeks. Single sessions of endoscopic feedback are often useful in conjunction with traditional articulation therapy, especially for patients with nasal snorting of sibilants or other phone-specific errors. Nasopharyngoscopic biofeedback therapy has also been used successfully to resolve residual VPI following pharyngeal flap surgery in some adults (Witzel et al., 1989).

Case history 3. The patient was an 8-year-old girl with repaired cleft palate and history of Robin sequence secondary to Stickler syndrome (see Chapter 2). VP closure improved following a speech bulb reduction program, but progress seemed to plateau and further bulb reduction was not possible because the appliance was as small as possible. She was able to maintain good VP closure during the production of sustained fricatives and during voiceless plosives in some C-V contexts, but throughout most of the speech sample there was evidence of mild VPI. By her fifth session of endoscopic biofeedback, which occurred during the second week of treatment, she was able to maintain closure during production of sentences and her resonance during conversation was normal. She returned for weekly sessions for 2 weeks, then monthly sessions for 3 months for maintenance and was discharged. Follow-up endoscopy 1 year later revealed complete VP closure except for occasional bursts of air, which were asymptomatic as clinical evaluation revealed normal resonance.

Other biofeedback techniques. Visual feedback of nasal airflow may be provided to the patient using simple devices such as a mirror or See-Scape, and a stethoscope may be used for auditory feedback of nasal escape. The availability, low cost, and noninvasive character of these instruments enhance their appeal. Caution must be exercised in interpreting performance measured by these tools because output is affected by factors other than VP closure, such as nasal patency/resistance, congestion, respiratory effort, and placement of the device. Nasal phonemes should always be tested first to ensure that the instrument is positioned properly to respond to nasal escape/nasalization and that the nostrils are patent. If nasal airflow or resonance is not registered, the device should be repositioned and nose cleared. In the case of the airflow devices, multiple repetitions of oral stimuli should be produced successively to avoid intrusive nasal breathing, which might be confused with nasal emission. If the patient has a fistula, care must be taken that its covering is complete and tight, or there will be no way to differentiate between nasal escape related to VPI and that related to the fistula.

The nasometer is a relatively new instrument that may have application for visual feedback of changes in resonance during therapy, although this has not been studied. The appeal of nasometry is its computerization and apparent objectivity. However, it has, at best, a moderate correlation with perceptual ratings of nasality by highly experienced clinicians (Pearson $r = .82$) (Dalston et al., 1991), and a low correlation with nasopharyngoscopy, and even a low correlation with pressure flow estimates of port size (Pearson $r = .32$) (Dalston et al., 1991). Correlations between nasometry and listener judgments of nasality in patients with pharyngeal flaps have not been significant (Hardin et al., 1992; Nellis et al., 1992). Furthermore, the correlation between nasalance scores and perceptual evaluation appears to be influenced by the speech sample used (Dalston and Seaver, 1992), raising further questions about the reliability and validity of the instrument.

It is important to bear in mind that these instruments provide feedback about *consequences* of VP closure and its interaction with other vocal tract events, not about VP closure directly. In contrast, nasendoscopy allows the patient to visualize actual VP movements *as they occur.*

Tonsillectomy. The tonsils are not known to play a role in normal articulation or resonance.* Normally the tonsils are situated in the oral cavity between the anterior and posterior faucial pillars. Sometimes otherwise healthy tonsils are hypertrophied or posteriorly displaced into the oropharynx, where they may have a negative effect on oral and nasal resonance and on articulation (Shprintzen et al., 1987; Henningsson and Isberg, 1988). Tonsil position is more important than tonsil size, and the intruding tonsils may appear unremarkable on oral examination (Traquina et al., 1990). Endoscopic examination is essential in diagnosing speech abnormalities related to tonsils and in determining if tonsillectomy is indicated to improve speech or resonance.

Effect on oral resonance. Hypertrophic and/or retrodisplaced tonsils occupy space in the oropharyngeal area, which is a resonator for speech. The resultant damping, or attenuation, of voice results in a muffled quality, which has been referred to as "potato-in-the-mouth" or "marshmallow mouth" resonance. This posterior muffling is different from the anterior muffling heard in some craniofacial syndromes, such as Apert syndrome, in which alveolar hypertrophy constricts the oral resonator itself. Occlusion of the nostrils does not affect this type of resonance. Oral resonance may be improved by tonsillectomy. Speech therapy is not indicated.

Effect on nasal resonance. Retrodisplaced, hypertrophied tonsils may cause hypernasality by interfering mechanically with VP closure (Shprintzen et al., 1987; Traquina et al., 1990). This may be diagnosed using multiview videofluoroscopy, but is most clearly visualized endoscopically. The tonsils may inhibit mesial movement of the lateral pharyngeal wall and/or elevation of lateral aspects of the velum, or may physically obstruct contact between the velum and posterior or lateral pharyngeal walls (Fig.

---

*The adenoids play an important role in VP closure in children, serving as a focal point for velar and lateral pharyngeal wall contact during phonation.

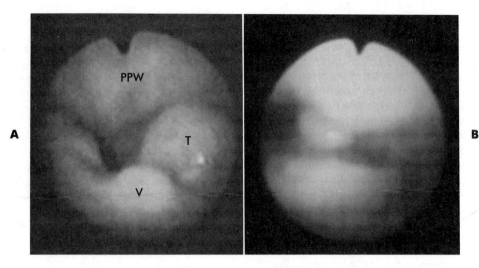

Fig. 16-4 Nasopharyngoscopic view of a tonsil in the velopharyngeal port at rest (**A**) and causing VPI during speech (**B**).

16-4). The resultant VPI is often unilateral or asymmetric and very mild or intermittent.

Suspicion of tonsil-related VPI indicating a need for tonsillectomy should be raised if hypernasality is very mild or intermittent and there are also problems affecting respiration (snoring, mouth breathing), deglutition (picky, slow eater, soft food preference), and articulation (tongue fronting).

Effect on articulation. Tonsillar hypertrophy in a toddler may lead to the development of aberrant articulation patterns characterized by a tongue fronting pattern with substitution of /t, d, n/ for /k, g, ɔ/. In these cases a forward tongue position is often noted at rest, and a diagnosis of tongue thrust may be made when actually the child may be attempting to open or enlarge the airway by keeping the tongue forward. Posterior tongue placement for velar and vowel sounds is difficult because the hypertrophied tonsils occupy the space where the tongue root should be for a back sound, leading to the development of the anterior speech pattern. If tonsillectomy is performed early, the articulation pattern often reverses itself without intervention. However, habit strength may necessitate articulation therapy if early correction of the tonsillar hypertrophy is not undertaken.

To summarize, the clinical indications for considering tonsillectomy to improve speech are mild/intermittent hypernasality and/or muffled or "potato-in-the-mouth" oral resonance, and tongue fronting articulation errors. Respiration and deglutition, which occur in the shared pharyngeal space, may also be affected. Physiologic indications of a need for tonsillectomy

must be obtained endoscopically and include retrodisplacement of the tonsils into the airway, intermittent and/or asymmetric VPI especially affecting lateral pharyngeal wall motion, lateral VP gaps above the tonsillar pillars, or intrusion of the tonsil into the closure plane.

It must be stressed that tonsillectomy does not cause lasting hypernasality, except in very rare cases. Transient hypernasality may occur in normal patients. If hypernasality persists beyond three months, it may suggest that there is scar tissue or additional lymphoid tissue affecting VP movements. If no structural or neurologic problem can be identified, speech bulb reduction or biofeedback therapy may be useful. Hypernasality in patients with VPI may seem to be exacerbated following tonsillectomy if it was being masked by oral muffling.

If oral resonance is muffled and physical obstruction (e.g., tonsils, alveolar hypertrophy) is ruled out or cannot be corrected, therapeutic techniques to improve resonance include increasing mouth opening and eliminating tongue humping or posterior tongue carriage, if it occurs.

Tonsillectomy should also be done at least 6 weeks before pharyngeal flap surgery if the tonsils are endoscopically visualized in the airway, or are moderately large (at least 2+). This is primarily for protection of lateral port patency following pharyngeal flap but also because tonsillectomy may result in increased lateral pharyngeal wall motion. Therefore nasopharyngoscopy should be repeated at least 6 weeks after tonsillectomy for final planning of pharyngeal flap surgery.

Repair of oronasal fistula. Articulation and resonance problems in some patients may be related to the presence of palatal fistulae. Clinical indications suggestive of contribution of a fistula to these problems include tongue backing errors such as k/t, in which the speaker is trying to produce sounds posterior to the fistula to avoid loss of air pressure through it. Compensatory errors often involve tongue backing or palatalization of sounds, including middorsal palatal stops and palatal or pharyngeal fricatives, which are also produced with the tongue retracted behind the fistula. Nasal emission may be more severe on sounds with a place feature anterior to the fistula. Depending on its size, shape, and location, it may be possible to obturate the fistula temporarily with dental wax or sugarless chewing gum to see if reduction or elimination of nasal escape occurs. Nasopharyngoscopy may provide physiologic evidence that an oronasal fistula is contributing to hypernasality by revealing increased VP movement with the fistula occluded (Isberg and Henningsson, 1987). If obturation during nasopharyngoscopy or videofluoroscopy is not possible, very mild or intermittent VPI may suggest a fistula effect.

If articulation errors are directly related to the presence of a fistula, it may be advantageous to have it repaired or obturated before speech therapy. However, if this cannot be done for several months or longer, speech therapy should not be delayed. The compensatory errors can be eliminated even in the presence of the fistula. In fact, the fistula may be used as a placement cue for correct production of anterior sounds. For example, the child may be instructed to "put the tongue in (front of) the hole." As noted in the section on articulation therapy, in the presence of VPI persistent nasal air escape is to be expected, but articulation placement can be corrected.

Speech appliances. Prosthetic speech appliances such as speech bulbs and palatal lifts may be useful in patients with VPI in three ways. First, an appliance may be used as a permanent treatment alternative to surgery if medical or other conditions mitigate against surgical correction of VPI. Many speech pathologists are more comfortable treating articulation disorders of children and adults with VPI **after** the hypernasality component has been addressed. Speech appliances provide the potential for normal resonance and intraoral pressure during articulation therapy. Therefore the second use of appliances is as a temporary adjunct to speech therapy, before definitive surgical treatment. The third use of appliances is for the reduction

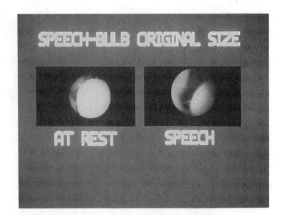

Fig. 16-5 Speech bulb occupying entire velopharynx at rest **(left)** and movement of the velopharynx *outward* from the rest position during nasal snorting of /s/ **(right).**

of VPI. This last application, speech bulb reduction, is discussed in detail in Chapter 17.

The purpose of a speech bulb is to provide obturation of the VP port during phonation. Like a pharyngeal flap, it provides the potential for normal resonance and intraoral pressure but does not alter compensatory articulation errors, not even nasal snorting. As seen in Fig. 16-5, nasal snorting is accomplished by movement of the velopharynx *outward* from the rest position, allowing nasal air escape even in the presence of the largest speech bulb accommodated at rest. Therefore concurrent speech therapy is essential for most speech bulb patients.*

The treating speech pathologist plays an important role in reinforcing the patient's need to wear the bulb during all waking hours and not only during therapy sessions. The therapist should be aware that hypernasality and nasal emission will not be eliminated until construction of the speech appliance is complete, and speech will not be radically improved until the articulation errors have been eliminated. Goals and procedures for speech therapy are the same for patients with speech appliances as for those without appliances. Critical speech changes include eliminating compensatory articulation errors and increasing strength of articulatory contacts. Once it is established that the speech bulb is of adequate size, its presence may be ignored. The appliance should not be removed

---

*McGrath and Anderson in Seattle have reported fitting speech bulbs as early as age 2 years in children with glottal stop speech. They observed resolution of the articulation disorder without speech therapy. We have not obturated children that young and have not observed spontaneous speech improvement in any patient (see Chapter 17).

during therapy unless the manager of the speech bulb program specifically gives instructions to the treating therapist to do so. Removal of the appliance during part of a therapy session may be suggested when the speech bulb has been reduced in size to the point that the next possible reduction is its absence.

There are several benefits to using a speech bulb in conjunction with therapy. Resonance may be normal while the articulation errors are treated, posing less distraction for the therapist, patient, and parents who may find it difficult to focus on resonance and articulation separately. We have also observed that many speech pathologists seem to address articulation disorders more aggressively when VPI is not present. It is not surprising that patient progress is better when the therapist's attitude is positive. Another benefit, discussed more fully in Chapter 17, is increased VP closure.

Speech therapy alone may yield similar results in eliminating articulation errors and increasing VP motion for most patients within 3 to 6 months (Golding, 1981; Golding-Kushner, 1989; Hoch et al., 1986; Ysunza et al., 1992). However, we have observed that in most settings including schools, clinics, and even hospitals, the use of a speech bulb may facilitate articulation therapy. It is not clear whether this is because the port is physically occluded or because the therapist's attitude is more positive.

Pharyngeal flap surgery. In many cases, hypernasality can only be corrected surgically. The sole function of a pharyngeal flap is to eliminate VPI and the only anticipated effects on speech are the elimination of hypernasality and nasal escape of air, enabling the speaker to impound normal intraoral pressure for consonant production.

The relationship between speech therapy and pharyngeal flap surgery. To understand the choice of therapeutic procedures and the rationale for the timing of treatment, it is important to view the speech mechanism as a valving system through which an outgoing airstream passes and is modified. This system includes the laryngeal or glottal valve, the VP valve, and the oral valve, consisting of labial or linguopalatal constrictions and occlusions. When a glottal stop is produced, the vocal folds adduct, blocking the airstream, and creating plosion at the larynx (the inferiormost valve), which will not be affected by VPI. Thus the manner of articulation (plosion) is preserved, but the place of articulation is changed, and the wrong articulators are used. Because the plosive event has already occurred, there is no need to effect a second occlusion at a higher

valve. As a result, correct articulatory gestures are not reinforced and not learned. In fact, as noted earlier, lingual and labial movements are often abandoned altogether. VPI is often exacerbated for the same reason: because the acoustic event (i.e., the plosive sound) has already been produced at the laryngeal valve, there is no real purpose to further modification of the airstream at the VP valve.

It has long been thought that articulation therapy for compensatory articulation should be deferred until VPI is eliminated through surgical or prosthetic management (Brooks et al., 1965; McWilliams et al., 1990; Smith, 1969; Van Demark, 1974). However, there is a growing body of evidence suggesting that articulation therapy should precede pharyngeal flap surgery in most patients.

Individuals with glottal stop substitutions almost invariably have gross VPI. That is, there is little or no movement observed in the velum or lateral pharyngeal walls during speech. However, in those same individuals better movement of the VP valve occurs during their occasional correct production of sounds (Fig. 16-6). Furthermore, elimination of glottal stops, pharyngeal fricatives, and nasal snorting usually increases VP movements, confirming that compensatory errors and VPI have a bidirectional relationship (Golding, 1981; Golding-Kushner, 1989; Henningsson et al., 1986; Ysunza et al., 1992). Presurgical speech therapy, using the procedures described, has proven to be highly successful in eliminating compensatory errors, and VP movements usually im prove* (Fig. 16-7) (Golding, 1981; Tanokuchi et al., 1986; Golding-Kushner, 1989; Ysunza et al., 1992). The therapeutic process is no more difficult than for patients receiving speech therapy following pharyngeal flap surgery. The key difference is that the therapy outcome will be speech accompanied by nasal emission and reduced intraoral pressure. With the nares occluded, articulation of oral sounds will be normal.

In one study Golding-Kushner described changes in VP function in 14 subjects with VPI and compensatory articulation who had articulation therapy before surgery (Golding, 1981; Hoch et al., 1986). There were five subjects who had intermittent VPI, including one with phone-specific VP closure,† three with

---

*Developmental articulation errors are not related to VPI and their elimination does not affect VP function.
†VPI except during production of a single sound during which VP closure is achieved. Phoneme-specific closure, like phone-specific VPI, may occur more frequently on /s/ than on other sounds.

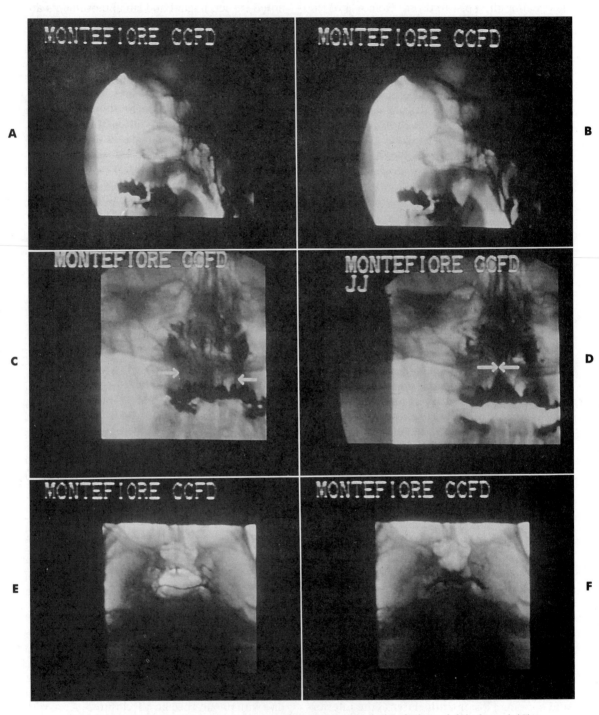

Fig. 16-6 Velopharyngeal closure during glottal stop articulation in lateral (**A**), frontal (**C**) (arrows mark lateral pharyngeal walls), and base (**E**) views, compared to VP closure during oral production (**B, D,** and **F**) for the same sound in the same patient.

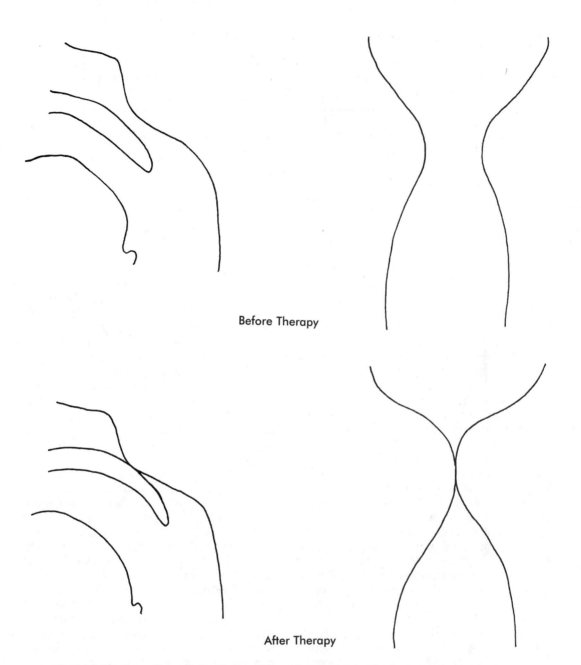

Before Therapy

After Therapy

Fig. 16-7 Tracings of lateral view (left) and frontal view (right) videofluoroscopic examinations of a patient preceding and following articulation therapy to eliminate abnormal compensatory errors.

phone-specific VPI, and one with nonspecific variability (Table 16-2). The VPI of all five resolved completely with *articulation* therapy, and surgery was not needed. This suggests that neurologically intact patients who demonstrate at least *some* ability to effect VP closure, even during production of only one sound, may have the potential to achieve closure when compensatory errors are eliminated. Three other sub-

jects in that study with consistent VPI and very poor lateral wall motion also showed improvement. Following articulation therapy they had better, even excellent, lateral pharyngeal wall motion, so less obstructive pharyngeal flaps were needed. There were four subjects with the consistent presence of VPI but variable degree of VPI, ranging from mild to gross in a single examination. Following articulation therapy,

Table 16-2 Changes in velopharyngeal closure following articulation therapy to eliminate compensatory errors

N	VPI before articulation therapy	VPI following articulation therapy		
		Eliminated	Decreased	Unchanged
5	Intermittent VPI	5/5		
3	Mild VPI w/absent or poor LPW motion		3/3 mild VPI w/good or excellent LPW motion	
4	Variable VPI ranging gross to mild		3/4 mild consistent VPI	1/4
2	Gross VPI			2/2*

LPW, Lateral pharyngeal wall.
*The two subjects with gross VPI also failed to demonstrate improvement in their articulation. One of the subjects had velocardiofacial syndrome; the other was neurologically impaired.

three of them demonstrated persistent but consistently mild VPI. Consistency in the severity of their VPI ensured a better postoperative prognosis and made these subjects candidates for narrower pharyngeal flaps.

The plan for surgical management should be based on the status of the VP valve during correct articulatory placement and production and not on the VP dynamics of glottal speech. Assessment of the VP valve by nasopharyngoscopy and multiview videofluoroscopy should be done when the patient can produce the speech protocol with correct articulation and has at least 70% correct articulation during conversation. This should be about 3 to 6 months after the initiation of intensive and appropriate speech therapy if the compensatory speech disorder was severe. If VP closure is seen to occur even only occasionally, speech therapy should be continued and endoscopy repeated after 3 months. If the presence and size of the VP gap are consistent, plans for physical management of the insufficiency should proceed.

There are several advantages to doing speech therapy before pharyngeal flap surgery. First and most important, when the establishment of normal articulatory placement and production results in improved VP valving, the degree of surgical obstruction of the nasopharynx can be reduced. The benefit of varying the postoperative width of pharyngeal flaps has been described (Shprintzen et al., 1979; Shprintzen, 1989). For an inactive VP valve, very wide pharyngeal flaps are necessary. When the lateral pharyngeal walls move well, a narrower pharyngeal flap can be constructed that may decrease the patient's postoperative discomfort from nasal obstruction and risk of obstructive sleep apnea. Some patients obtain enough motion in the VP valve to avoid surgery altogether.

Another advantage to articulation therapy before pharyngeal flap is immediate appreciation of the surgical result. The sole purpose of the pharyngeal flap is to eliminate VPI, resulting in normalization of intraoral pressure and resonance. When closure of the VP valve is obtained surgically, compensatory articulation errors are barely affected. Hypernasality may be reduced, but glottal stops persist. Patients who go into surgery with glottal speech awaken with the same speech disorder. Even when they have been counseled before surgery that the articulation disorder will persist, the patient and family cannot help but be disappointed at that outcome after a major surgical ordeal to "improve speech." The feeling of failure is reinforced by the fact that after this trauma the patient must still go for intensive speech therapy. Furthermore, it has been our experience that delaying surgery helps the family understand the importance of speech therapy, motivating improved attendance and compliance in most cases.

To summarize, the clinical criterion for articulation therapy before pharyngeal flap is the presence of a compensatory speech disorder in which errors are related to VPI and articulatory contacts are weak. Physiologic criteria are evidence of phone-specific VPI, phone-specific VP closure, variability in VP closure with an identified phonetic pattern, variability in VP closure related to strength of articulatory contacts, or other evidence of potential for increased VP motion that may be of sufficient degree to affect the surgical plan.

Optimum time for pharyngeal flap. Pharyngeal flap surgery may be performed safely and with excellent results in both children and adults (Hall et al., 1991). Clearly, there are psychosocial benefits to normalizing resonance before a child enters school. Therefore the preference is to do surgery at the earliest possible age. However, proper surgical planning is impossible until the child is able to provide an adequate speech sample with oral articulation and cooperate for nasopharyngoscopy and multi-view videofluoroscopy. Most children meet this requirement by age 4 years. Good surgical results may be obtained in adults (Hall et al., 1991). However, adults tend to have more postoperative complaints than children related to changes in nasal respiration, even when the flap is narrow and both lateral ports are widely patent. Adults with poor lateral pharyngeal wall motion who need very wide or subobstructing flaps have difficulty accommodating to the nasopharyngeal obstruction, which will not decrease with time (as it does in children who have growth ahead of them). For some adults it may be necessary to raise a less than optimal flap and counsel the patient that some nasal escape and hypernasality will persist.

Adults with persistent compensatory articulation disorders present a more complex problem. Technically and physiologically, articulation therapy is the same as for children, but the need to eliminate compensatory articulation errors is even greater because of the potential for improved lateral pharyngeal wall motion. Unfortunately, but not surprisingly, adults are often poorly motivated for speech therapy or even resistant to it because of the longevity of their speech problem and history of many years of unsuccessful therapy (Hall et al., 1991; Witzel, 1991). They have no reason to believe that this therapeutic experience will be any different. Ironically, these adults are destined for extreme disappointment if surgery is performed in the presence of their compensatory speech because the surgical "failure" will be apparent to them as soon as they speak after surgery.

Surgical correction of VPI is contraindicated if other aspects of speech and/or language are severely impaired. For example, if child is 7 or 8 years old but has language skills on an 18-month or 2-year level, a pharyngeal flap will do nothing to enhance communication or quality of life. In such cases the hypernasality is not a primary concern, especially if articulation is severely impaired as well.

In summary, pharyngeal flap surgery should be performed when articulation is oral and the primary speech disorder is hypernasality. A screening check for this clinical criterion is to determine if an oral speech sample sounds normal with the nares occluded. Cognitive skills and language development should be functional. Physiologic criteria for pharyngeal flap surgery are based on direct visualization of all components of VP movement at all vertical levels of the vocal tract. This can be obtained only using a combination of lateral and frontal view videofluoroscopy plus nasopharyngoscopy, or multiview videofluoroscopy in three views (lateral, frontal, and en face) (Skolnick, 1989; Golding-Kushner et al., 1990). Surgery is indicated if VPI is consistent in *presence* and *degree*. Surgery is an appropriate option for VPI that is variable in degree if all other treatment options are inappropriate or have been unsuccessful. Pharyngeal flap surgery is absolutely contraindicated for phone-specific VPI, with no exceptions.

Speech therapy following surgery. Patients who continue to need articulation or language therapy may resume treatment as soon after surgery as they feel well enough to do so, usually after 2 or 3 weeks. However, reevaluation of resonance and nasal emission should be delayed until 3 months following surgery. Treatment of nasal emission, nasal grimace, hypernasality, or hyponasality should never be undertaken until the results of the 3-month postoperative nasopharyngoscopic examination are reviewed.

HYPONASALITY

Hyponasality, or denasality, may coexist with hypernasality or may occur as an isolated disorder of nasal resonance. It may be chronic, acute, or transient. Patients with hyponasality should undergo examination to determine the underlying cause and to determine if medical correction of the problem is possible. Nasal and nasopharyngoscopic examinations are necessary to rule out sources of nasal and nasopharyngeal obstruction. Examination and treatment by an otolaryngologist or allergist may be appropriate for some patients who chronically sound congested.

Hyponasality almost always occurs as a sequela to pharyngeal flap surgery but is usually transient and resolves within 6 months. In patients with absent lateral pharyngeal wall motion, a subobstructing, or very wide, pharyngeal flap must be raised to eliminate hypernasality. In those cases hyponasality is a planned surgical outcome and may persist for years, until growth occurs and changes in the pharynx reopen the lateral pharyngeal ports. This allows for adequate nasal respiration and resonance without recurrence of hypernasality (Siegel-

Sadewitz and Shprintzen, 1986). When this surgical outcome is anticipated, the child and parents must be counseled that the child will sound congested for an extended period (depending on proximity to the preteen growth spurt). If hyponasality is expected to persist for a period of several years or more, therapeutic treatment may be appropriate. Procedures might then include increasing the duration of articulatory contacts during production of nasal consonants.

REFERENCES

ACPA: Parameters for the evaluation and treatment of patients with cleft lip/palate or other craniofacial anomalies, *Cleft Palate Craniofac J* 30(Suppl 1): 1993.

Albery L, Enderby P: Intensive speech therapy for cleft palate children, *Br J Disord Commun* 19:115, 1984.

Brooks A, Shelton R, Youngstrom K: Compensatory tongue-palate-posterior pharyngeal wall relationships in cleft palate, *J Speech Hearing Disord* 30:166, 1965.

Croft C, Shprintzen RJ, Rakoff S: Patterns of velopharyngeal valving in normal and cleft palate subjects: a multiview videofluoroscopic and nasoendoscopic study, *Laryngoscope* 91(2):265, 1981.

Dalston R, Seaver E: Relative values of various standardized passages in the nasometric assessment of patients with velopharyngeal impairment, *Cleft Palate J* 29(1):17, 1992.

Dalston R, Warren D, Smith L: The characteristics of speech produced by normal speakers and cleft palate speakers with adequate velopharyngeal function, *Cleft Palate J* 27:393, 1990.

Dalston R, Warren D, Dalston E: Use of nasometry as a diagnostic tool for identifying patients with velopharyngeal impairment, *Cleft Palate J* 28:184, 1991.

Golding KJ: *Articulation and velopharyngeal insufficiency: a rationale for pre-surgical speech therapy,* Paper presented at Fourth International Congress on Cleft Palate and Related Craniofacial Anomalies, Acapulco, Mexico, May 1981.

Golding KJ, Kaslon K: *A home program for infant stimulation,* Paper presented at Annual Symposium of the Center for Craniofacial Disorders of Montefiore Hospital and Medical Center and the Albert Einstein College of Medicine, Bronx, NY, March 1981.

Golding-Kushner KJ: *Speech therapy for compensatory articulation errors in patients with "cleft palate speech,"* Videotape produced by the Center for Craniofacial Disorders, Montefiore Medical Center, Bronx, New York, 1989.

Golding-Kushner KJ: *Craniofacial morphology and velopharyngeal physiology in four syndromes of clefting,* Unpublished doctoral dissertation, The Graduate School and University Center, City University of New York, 1991.

Golding-Kushner KJ et al: Standardization for the reporting of nasopharyngoscopy and multiview videofluoroscopy: a report from an international working group, *Cleft Palate J* 27(4):337, 1990.

Golding-Kushner KJ, Weller G, Shprintzen RJ: Velo-cardio-facial syndrome: language and psychological characteristics, *J Craniofac Genet Dev Biol* 5(3):259, 1985.

Hall C, Golding-Kushner KJ: *Long-term follow-up of 500 patients after palate repair performed prior to 18 months of age,* Paper presented at Sixth International Congress on Cleft Palate and Related Craniofacial Anomalies, Jerusalem, Israel, June 1989.

Hardin MA, Van Demark D, Morris HL, Payne M: Correspondence between nasalance scores and listener judgments of hypernasality and hyponasality, *Cleft Palate J* 29(4):346, 1992.

Henningsson G, Isberg A: Velopharyngeal movements in patients alternating between oral and glottal articulation: a clinical and cineradiographical study, *Cleft Palate J* 23:1, 1986.

Henningsson G, Isberg A: Influence of tonsils on velopharyngeal movements in children with craniofacial anomalies and hypernasality, *Am J Orthod Dentofac Orthop* 94:253, 1988.

Hoch L: *Mass trial articulation therapy in cleft palate: a case study,* Paper presented at 20th Annual Symposium of the Center for Craniofacial Disorders, Montefiore Medical Center, Bronx, NY, 1981.

Hoch L, Golding-Kushner KJ, Sadewitz V, Shprintzen RJ: Speech therapy. In McWilliams BJ, editor: *Seminars in speech and language: current methods of assessing and treating children with cleft palates,* New York 1986, Thieme.

Isberg A, Henningsson G: Influence of palatal fistulas on velopharyngeal movements: a cineradiographic study, *Plast Reconstr Surg* 79:525, 1987.

LeBlanc S, Golding-Kushner KJ: Effect of glossopexy on speech sound production in Robin sequence, *Cleft Palate J* 29(3):239, 1992.

McWilliams BJ, Morris HL, Shelton RL: *Cleft palate speech,* ed 2, Philadelphia, 1990, BC Decker.

Morley ME: *Cleft palate and speech,* ed 7, Baltimore, 1970, Williams & Wilkins.

Nellis J, Neiman G, Lehman J: Comparison of nasometer and listener judgments of nasality in the assessment of velopharyngeal function after pharyngeal flap, *Cleft Palate Craniofac J* 29:157, 1992.

Peterson SJ: Nasal emission as a component of the misarticulation on sibilants and affricates, *J Speech Hearing Disord* 40:106, 1975.

Philips BJ, Kent RD: Acoustic-phonetic descriptions of speech production in speakers with cleft palate and other velopharyngeal disorders, *Speech Lang Adv Basics Res Pract* 11:113, 1984.

Powers G, Starr C: The effects of muscle exercises on velopharyngeal gap and nasality, *Cleft Palate J* 11:28, 1974.

Ruscello DM: A selected review of palatal training procedures, *Cleft Palate J* 18:181, 1982.

Shprintzen RJ: Research revisited, *Cleft Palate J* 26(2):148, 1989.

Shprintzen RJ: Surgery for speech. In Huddart AG, Ferguson MWJ, editors: *Cleft lip and palate: long-term results and future prospects,* vol 1, New York, 1990, Manchester University Press.

Shprintzen RJ, Goldberg RB, Lewin ML, Sidoti EJ, Berkman MD, Argamaso RV, Young D: A new syndrome involving cleft palate, cardiac anomalies, typical facies, and learning disabilities: velo-cardio-facial syndrome, *Cleft Palate J* 15(1):56, 1978.

Shprintzen RJ, Golding-Kushner KJ: Evaluation of velopharyngeal insufficiency, *Otolaryngol Clin North Am* 22(3): 519, 1989.

Shprintzen RJ, Lewin ML, Croft C, Daniller A, Argamaso RV, Ship A, Strauch B: A comprehensive study of pharyngeal flap surgery: tailor made flaps, *Cleft Palate J* 16:46, 1979.

Shprintzen RJ, McCall G, Skolnick ML: A new therapeutic technique for the treatment of velopharyngeal incompetence, *J Speech Hear Disord* 40:69, 1975.

Shprintzen RJ, Sher A, Croft C: Hypernasal speech caused by tonsillar hypertrophy, *Int J Pediatr Otorhinolaryngol* 14:45, 1987.

Siegel-Sadewitz VL, Shprintzen RJ: Nasopharyngoscopy of the normal velopharyngeal valve: an experiment in biofeedback, *Cleft Palate J* 19:194, 1982.

Siegel-Sadewitz VL, Shprintzen RJ: Changes in velopharyngeal valving with age, *Int J Pediatr Otorhinolaryngol,* 11:171, 1986.

Skolnick ML: Commentary, *Cleft Palate J* 26:91, 1989.

Smith J: Contradictions for speech therapy for cleft palate speakers, *Cleft Palate J* 6:202, 1969.

Starr C: Treatment by therapeutic exercises. In Bardach J, Morris H, editors: *Multidisciplinary management of cleft lip and palate,* Philadelphia, 1990, WB Saunders.

Tanokuchi F et al: Articulation training for velopharyngeal reinforcement, *Studia Phonologica* 20:, 1986.

Traquina D, Golding-Kushner KJ, Shprintzen RJ: *Comparison of tonsil size based on oral and nasopharyngoscopic observation,* Paper presented at Society of Ear Nose and Throat Advances in Children, Washington, DC, December 1990.

Trost J: Articulatory additions to the classical description of the speech of persons with cleft palate, *Cleft Palate J* 18(3):193, 1981.

Van Demark D: Some results of speech therapy for children with cleft palate, *Cleft Palate J* 11:41, 1974.

Van Demark DR, Hardin MA: Speech therapy for the child with cleft lip and palate. In Bardach J, Morris H, editors: *Multidisciplinary management of cleft lip and palate,* Philadelphia, 1990, WB Saunders.

Van Hattum RJ: *Clinical speech in the schools: organization and management,* Springfield, Ill, 1974, Charles C Thomas.

Witzel MA: Commentary, *Cleft Palate J* 28:182, 1991.

Witzel MA, Tobe J, Salyer KE: The use of videonasopharyngoscopy for biofeedback therapy in adults after pharyngeal flap surgery, *Cleft Palate J* 26(2):129, 1989.

Yamaoka M, Matsuya T, Miyazaki T, Nishio J, Ibuki N: Visual training for velopharyngeal closure in cleft palate patients: a fiberoptic procedure, *J Maxillofac Surg* 11(4): 191, 1983.

Ysunza A, Pamplona C, Toledo E: Change in velopharyngeal valving after speech therapy in cleft palate patients: a videonasopharyngoscopic and multi-view videofluoroscopic study, *Int J Pediatr Otorhinolaryngol* 24:45, 1992.

17 Speech Bulbs

Karen J. Golding-Kushner, George Cisneros, and Etoile LeBlanc

The concept of applying dental prostheses (obturators) to the treatment of hypernasal speech was introduced by McGrath in 1860 (McGrath and Anderson, 1990), predating Passavant's surgical attachment of the velum to the posterior pharyngeal wall in 1865 in what was the first pharyngeal flap (Stark and Frileck, 1971). The basic principle of both is to create a permanent separation between the nasopharynx and oropharynx when velopharyngeal insufficiency* (VPI) is present. As with a pharyngeal flap, the purpose of speech bulb and palatal lift appliances is to obturate the velopharyngeal (VP) port during speech. This results in the elimination of hypernasality and passive nasal emission/turbulence, and provides the speaker with the ability to impound normal intraoral pressure when other aspects of articulation and voice are normal. The mere presence of a speech appliance does not have any positive effect on articulation. In fact, as with any dental retainer, it may temporarily interfere with articulation when initially placed and for several days until the speaker accommodates to it (McWilliams et al., 1990; Chapter 15). Dental appliances designed to obturate palatal fistulae are also prosthetic speech appliances. However, the focus of this chapter is the use of dental appliances in the treatment of VPI.

TYPES OF SPEECH APPLIANCES

The two most common prosthetic devices used in the treatment of VPI are palatal lifts and speech bulbs (Fig. 17-1). The anterior portion of both appliances, the palatal portion, is a retainer, which can also serve as an obturator of palatal fistulae if present. The appliances differ in their posterior extensions. A palatal lift is a device that, as its name suggests, elevates the soft palate into the velopharynx with a fingerlike extension projecting from the palatal portion (Fig. 17-2). This type of appliance may be useful for cases in which VPI is due to inadequate velar

elevation but in which there is sufficient lateral pharyngeal wall motion to meet the edges of the raised palate, and the palate is of sufficient length and thickness to contact the posterior pharyngeal wall when elevated. A speech bulb consists of a wire extension from the palatal portion that courses behind the palate and terminates in an acrylic ball or elliptical structure, which is adapted in size and shape to the VP gap during phonation (Fig. 17-3).

Success of a speech appliance in eliminating VPI, like success of a pharyngeal flap, depends almost entirely on the ability of the lateral pharyngeal walls to close around the palate or appliance. In most cases of VPI poor lateral pharyngeal wall motion necessitates the choice of a speech bulb, which can be customized to the full width of the pharynx if necessary. A palatal lift cannot, although it may be extended laterally. Construction of speech bulbs is described later in this chapter.

USES OF SPEECH APPLIANCES

Speech appliances have three primary applications in the treatment of patients with VPI. They may be used as permanent obturators, on a temporary basis prior to surgical management, or as a therapeutic technique to reduce VPI. VPI and associated symptoms may be controlled equally well in children and adults with syndromic and nonsyndromic cleft palate, and with neurologic disorders.

Permanent speech appliances

The traditional use of speech appliances is as a permanent treatment alternative to surgery when medical or other conditions contraindicate surgical correction of VPI, or when the patient (or family, if the patient is a child) elects not to have surgery. Patients with degenerative neurologic disorders may be better candidates for permanent use of an appliance than for surgery because a speech bulb can be enlarged if necessary. This is especially true when other aspects of speech such as articulation and laryngeal vocal quality may be expected to

---

*Velopharyngeal insufficiency, incompetency, and inadequacy are used interchangeably in this chapter.

352

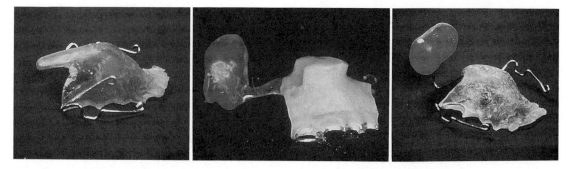

Fig. 17-1 Palatal lift, permanent speech bulb, and temporary/pediatric bulb.

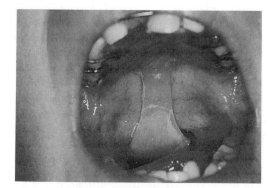

Fig. 17-2 Palatal lift in mouth.

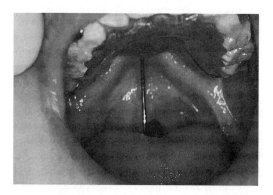

Fig. 17-3 Speech bulb in mouth.

deteriorate and significantly impair intelligibility. Speech appliances are of limited use in managing the hypernasality of severely dysarthric patients in whom articulation is unintelligible, even with the nares occluded.

The primary advantages of a prosthetic appliance over surgery are their noninvasive modifiability and reversibility. However, there are numerous drawbacks. Appliances should be removed during sleep and to be cleaned several times a day, and they may become damaged from frequent manipulation. Speech symptoms related to VPI are present when the appliance is removed. Therefore loss or absence of the appliance may affect social relationships because of speech that abruptly becomes stigmatizing. Retention of a speech appliance during periods of dental exfoliation and eruption poses particular difficulty and may be impossible during active orthodontic therapy.

Temporary speech appliances

Speech appliances may be used as a temporary treatment for VPI when definitive surgical treatment must be delayed for more than a few months. A delay in pharyngeal flap surgery or other pharyngoplasty* may be imposed for a variety of reasons. For example, there may be a need for other necessary medical treatment, such as cardiac surgery, before undertaking an elective (i.e., not life-preserving) procedure. Patients with cleft palate or other craniofacial disorders may have other surgical procedures that should precede a pharyngeal flap in their treatment plan. This might be because of a potential change in VP function following the procedure (e.g., maxillary advancement) or because of the risk of increasing the difficulty of intranasal intubation for anesthesia, especially if a wide pharyngeal flap is planned.

In some neuromuscular disorders and myopathies anesthesia and surgery for VPI, which may affect airway function, must be deferred until respiratory disorders are resolved and stable. Furthermore, VP closure may improve with age

---

*The most common procedure for treatment of VPI is a superiorly based pharyngeal flap. Other procedures include sphincter pharyngoplasty and posterior pharyngeal wall augmentation, discussed in Chapter 5. In this chapter pharyngeal flap is considered, but the discussion for the most part applies to any secondary surgical procedure for treatment of VPI.

in patients with certain unstable neurologic disorders. Pharyngeal flap surgery should also be deferred in patients with an uncertain neurologic diagnosis in whom prognosis for stability of VPI is unknown, or if VP closure might improve as in Prader-Willi syndrome.

Pharyngeal flap surgery is often delayed in patients with compensatory articulation disorders until after articulation therapy (Hoch et al., 1986; Shprintzen, 1990; Golding-Kushner, 1994). It has been suggested that in some cases articulation therapy proceeds more quickly when VP closure is adequate. The temporary use of a speech bulb may therefore facilitate speech therapy without compromising the principle of constructing a pharyngeal flap to suit optimum VP closure during noncompensatory articulation (Chapter 16). In those patients a prosthetic speech appliance provides the potential for normal resonance and intraoral pressure during articulation therapy and may therefore be useful as a temporary adjunct to speech therapy.

Therapeutic use of appliances: speech bulb reduction

Speech appliances may also be useful in some patients in reducing VPI. Harkins and Koepp-Baker (1948) observed that speech appliances seemed to stimulate increased VP motion in some patients. This was considered in earnest in the 1960s and early 1970s, primarily by Blakely (1964, 1969), Shelton et al. (1968, 1971), and Weiss (1971). However, most of the early studies did not provide strong support for the use of speech bulb reduction as a treatment for VPI. At that time construction and placement of speech bulbs were accomplished by trial and error. Effectiveness of treatment was judged according to changes in velar elevation observed using static lateral radiographs (during production of isolated sounds) or lateral cineradiography (during connected speech) and changes in resonance. Although these were state-of-the-art assessment techniques at that time, examination could not be repeated frequently to facilitate speech bulb construction or to monitor change because of the risks of radiation exposure. Another significant limitation is that the size and configuration of the VP gap cannot be fully appreciated from a lateral view alone. Furthermore, improvement in VP motion short of complete closure did not influence surgical decisions because pharyngeal flaps were not intentionally constructed in varying widths. We know now that modifications in VP function can be meaningful even if VPI is not eliminated because surgeons are able to design less obstructive pharyngeal flaps (Shprintzen et al., 1979; Argamaso, 1990).

The availability of multiview videofluoroscopy and nasopharyngoscopy to guide the selection and design of individual speech appliances and to evaluate their effectiveness has led to a renewed interest in including speech bulb therapy among the available treatment options for VPI (Golding et al., 1977; Schechter et al., 1977; McGrath and Anderson, 1990). Our observations suggest that gradual reduction in the size of a speech bulb is often accompanied by increased VP motion in select cases and that these changes are usually primarily in the degree of lateral pharyngeal wall motion (which could not have been appreciated in the earlier lateral radiographic studies). Current clinical practice relies heavily on the use of nasopharyngoscopy at all stages of treatment: diagnosis and patient selection, bulb construction, bulb modification, and ongoing monitoring of VP closure for bulb reduction (Rich et al., 1988; Golding-Kushner, 1988; Golding-Kushner and Cisneros, 1989; McGrath and Anderson, 1990).

PATIENT SELECTION FOR SPEECH BULB REDUCTION THERAPY

Clinical, physiologic, and psychosocial criteria should be considered in determining if a particular patient is an appropriate candidate for speech bulb reduction therapy. Patients and parents/caregivers (if the patient is a child) must be highly motivated and capable of good compliance for the treatment program. Parents and professionals involved with the child, especially speech pathologists, must be supportive and continually provide positive reinforcement. They must understand the goals of treatment and that the speech bulb has to be worn during all waking hours, removed at night, and reinserted in the morning. They must be vigilant about oral and appliance hygiene and about keeping and cooperating during repeated appointments for nasopharyngoscopic examination and modification of the appliance, and for speech therapy if it has been recommended.

Cognitive level and age may affect the length of time to complete treatment, but some very young children and mentally retarded or learning disabled children and adults have successfully tolerated wearing the appliances and have managed speech bulb reduction therapy. Problems encountered by some mentally retarded or learning disabled patients included poor compliance in the dental chair and for nasopharyngoscopy and parental ambivalence about the treatment program because of a strong expectation of failure. A few patients did not adapt to the presence of the appliance and developed an abnormal tongue humping posture, perhaps in an unconscious attempt to hold the appliance in place with the tongue.

Management of VPI, whether surgical or prosthetic, is of low priority in patients with nonfunctional or severely impaired language skills. The physiologic criterion for patient selection is gross or variable VPI,* or intermittent VPI with closure occurring less than 50% of the time. Most patients using a speech bulb also have compensatory speech disorders and receive speech therapy. For them it is as yet unclear if improved VP valving is secondary to the bulb reduction or to the effects of speech therapy. We have seen two or three patients with normal articulation but variable or gross VPI who were fitted with speech bulbs but did not receive speech therapy, yet demonstrated marked improvement in VP closure with bulb reduction.

Patients with VPI and compensatory articulation patterns such as glottal stops should especially be considered for speech bulb reduction therapy if they have a poor or slow response to appropriate articulation therapy. In these patients continued concomitant speech therapy is essential.† However, the use of a speech bulb is strongly contraindicated if VPI is phone-specific (i.e., VPI occurs on only one sound or class of sounds) because it is unnecessary and a poor use of resources. Phone-specific VPI should be treated with speech therapy alone. Speech bulb reduction therapy may not be worthwhile in patients with compensatory errors who demonstrate a good response to articulation therapy and a consistent pattern of mild or moderate VPI but no nasopharyngoscopic evidence of ability to achieve VP closure.

Speech bulbs to be used as permanent obturators for patients in full adult dentition are generally made with a cast metal technique. They snap rigidly into place and, like a denture, require little adjustment and maintenance. Permanent speech bulbs to be used by children are constructed in the same way as speech bulbs to be used temporarily or in speech bulb reduction therapy. Periodic inspection, maintenance, and

adjustment necessitate regular visits to the dental specialist, and long-term pressure of the appliance on the retaining teeth demands rigorous dental follow-up. Thus patient and parent motivation and compliance must be excellent.

CONSTRUCTION OF SPEECH BULBS
First visit: orientation
Speech bulbs are usually constructed by dental specialists (orthodontists, prosthodontists, pediatric dentists) but are sometimes fabricated by general dentists. At the time of the patient's first visit the dental specialist evaluates patient maturity and observes the parents' apparent motivation and attitude about the procedure. The parents' cooperation must be enlisted or chances for successful placement of an appliance in a child of any age will be severely hampered. The procedures for construction, monitoring, and reduction of the appliance, which have been outlined for the family before referral to the dental specialist, are explained once again, and the patient's and parents' responsibilities are reviewed. The patient's age influences the degree of responsibility shifted from the patient to the parents and may affect the time needed for construction. This is because a young child may need more time to adapt to each part of the appliance before construction may proceed. One of the parents' most important roles is to coach the child and encourage wearing the appliance throughout the four stages of construction:

Stage I: palatal appliance
Stage II: velar extension
Stage III: mini-bulb
Stage IV: final bulb

It is also the parents' responsibility, in the case of a young child, to ensure that the appliance is removed nightly for cleaning and replaced in the morning.

Although it seems that daytime wearing and nightly removal of the appliance should be obvious, we have heard parents admit to the opposite. One said she diligently helped the child insert the speech bulb in his mouth every night and remove it upon awakening. The mother was afraid to let the child eat with the appliance and he was unable to insert and remove it independently at school. Once apprised of their particular needs, adults and adolescent patients make their own commitments. Treatment cost should also be explained, if this has not already been done. Oral hygiene must also be reviewed, and patients must be free from any dental decay and disease.

---

*A variable closure pattern is one in which VPI ranges in severity within a single examination but is not related to specific articulation errors, such as nasal snorting. Lateral pharyngeal wall motion may range from absent to excellent. Errors in timing of VP movements may also contribute to variable VPI.

†McGrath and Anderson (1990) have reported resolution of glottal stop speech disorders in some patients younger than 3½ years old, who were fitted with speech bulb appliances but did not have speech therapy. This observation has not been reported elsewhere.

Second visit: preparation of teeth and stage I palatal appliance

At the second visit the teeth are prepared for the appliance. Many patients are in the primary dentition, and the primary posterior molar teeth have few retentive regions. Therefore the dental specialist must create a retentive (undercut) region to secure the appliance in the mouth. This may be done by resin bonded augmentation of the posterior teeth to create undercuts. If the desired material cannot be placed, orthodontic bands can be placed directly onto the teeth with attachments on the outside surface of the band to improve retention.

After the teeth are prepared, an impression is taken of the upper dentition. The impression is sent to the laboratory with the palatal portion of the appliance. The clasps are typically made of .036 orthodontic wire.

Third visit: placement of the stage I palatal appliance

The patient returns when the palatal appliance is ready. The appliance is worn full time, including during sleeping and eating, to allow the patient to accommodate to it. After 2 weeks the patient returns for the next stage.

Stage II: velar extension

A plastic fingerlike projection, shaped to follow the contour of the velum at rest,* is gradually added to the acrylic of the palatal appliance. Light-cured resin compound (Triad) may be used. The plastic extension is taken to the end of the soft palate/beginning of the uvula. If extended fully in a single sitting, the velar extension may elicit gagging, so the velar extension is constructed gradually, usually over two appointments. Between visits the parents must encourage the child to wear it as much as possible. The important change in instructions at this stage and through the remainder of treatment is that the appliance must be removed during sleep to eliminate any risk of obstruction and to reduce tension on the retaining teeth and oral mucosa. Patients may begin by wearing the appliance for 10- to 20-minute intervals several times a day, and increase the amount of time with the appliance in the mouth daily, until it is tolerated full time, except during sleep. At that time the projection may be extended further, and the accommodation process is repeated. The patient must be comfortable with the completed velar extension before proceeding to the next stage. The velar extension stage of treatment may require two to four visits.

---

*Unlike a palatal lift, which is designed to change the position of the velum.

Stage III: mini-bulb

The plastic or resin velar extension is removed and replaced with a wire (we prefer .045). The wire should be contoured to follow the shape of the passive velar extension from its insertion in the palatal appliance for its full length. The wire should extend beyond the soft palate 15 to 20 mm and should, at that point, be bent upward approximately 90 degrees. Retentive helices should be placed at both ends of this wire. At the palatal end the wire is secured to the palatal appliance with orthodontic acrylic resin. A small plastic bulb measuring about 3 to 4 mm in diameter is placed at the free end of the wire, which will extend up into the nasopharynx. This is referred to as the mini-bulb. Pliable material that molds during swallowing should not be used to shape the bulb. VP motion is different during swallowing and speech (Shprintzen et al., 1974), and medial movement of the lateral pharyngeal walls will compress the bulb and prevent it from serving its function as a cork in the VP port during speech. The bulb must be constructed to provide a surface against which VP closure can occur. The gag reflex may be exacerbated during insertion of the mini-bulb, and the parents must coach the patient through this difficult phase. The mini-bulb stage of treatment requires one visit.

Stage IV: final bulb

The patient returns when the mini-bulb is worn full time while the patient is awake. The bulb is enlarged laterally in 4- to 5-mm increments on either side until a change in resonance is noticed during word or phrase production by the speech bulb team.† Changes in nasality are used to monitor construction at this stage because the bulb, which is in the nasopharynx, cannot be seen intraorally. The speech pathologist and dental specialist must work together closely, especially if the dental specialist is unfamiliar with the method for eliciting an appropriate speech sample (see box on p. 357). The number of visits needed to complete construction of the bulb depends on the degree of bulb enlargement tolerated at each visit and the final size needed. Visits for further bulb enlargement should be scheduled at the shortest intervals tolerated by the patient so that the appliance is completed as

---

†The speech bulb team includes the dental specialist, endoscopist, and coordinating speech physiologist or speech pathologist, who actually manages the speech bulb program. The treating speech pathologist who provides ongoing therapy (who may be different from the speech pathologist on the team), patient, and parents are important adjunct team members whose comprehension, support, and cooperation during all aspects of the speech bulb reduction program are essential.

SPEECH SAMPLE TO MONITOR CHANGES IN NASAL RESONANCE

Nasal sample
mama
no no no
new hanger

Oral sample
pa pa pa
baby boy
big girl
kitty cat
table top
stop the bus
fifty five
sustain /sssss/
sustain /fffff/

quickly as possible. No effect on VP motion can be expected until the bulb is fully completed, and hypernasality will not be eliminated until that time. This stage of treatment may require two to four visits.

Completion of the appliance: final modifications

When the dental specialist hears changes in resonance as described or thinks that the speech bulb is large (this is completely subjective), nasopharyngoscopy is performed with the appliance in place. The dental specialist can then be given instructions for further bulb modification needed to establish complete VP closure during speech. These instructions should address the vertical height of the bulb so that it will be at the level of most active VP motion and/or enlargement of specific regions of the bulb. The bulb must be wide enough for contact with the lateral pharyngeal walls during speech, and it must be large enough in its anteroposterior dimension for contact with the velum and posterior pharyngeal wall to avoid air escape around the anterior or posterior aspects of the bulb. It is ideal if the dental specialist is present and able to see the bulb in situ at the time of nasopharyngoscopy or to review the videotape after the examination so that he or she can see the location and size of VP gaps around the bulb. When that is not possible, the endoscopist must provide detailed information, preferably with a sketch. The endoscopist and dental specialist must agree on the orientation of the appliance when applying terms such as right, left, front, and back. Communication must be specific and may be facilitated by using terms corresponding to endoscopic images with the bulb in place (Fig. 17-4).

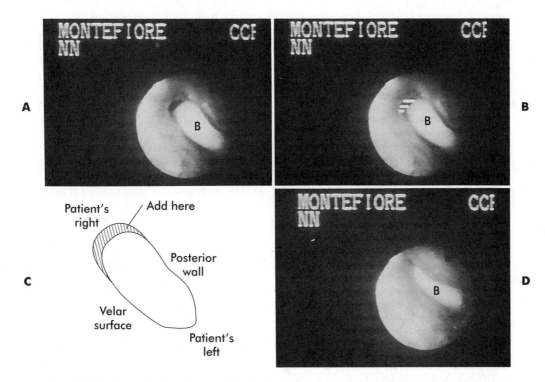

Fig. 17-4 Endoscopic view of a speech bulb showing a gap at the left of the bulb during speech (**A**). The gap is marked for review of the dentist (**B**) and a tracing sent (**C**) and material added so that following modification, complete closure is obtained (**D**).

MAINTENANCE OF SPEECH BULBS

Once the speech bulb is completed and VPI is eliminated during speech, the patient should return to the dental specialist at least at 2-month intervals for maintenance and to ensure proper retention. Wires and clasps are subject to fatigue and distortion with frequent handling and should be inspected. This is especially important when the patient is in mixed dentition. At the dental specialist's discretion, adults wearing a permanent speech bulb appliance may be asked to return for routine examination and adjustment of the appliance less frequently. As noted previously, these appliances are usually made of cast metal and more durable, necessitating less frequent maintenance. On the other hand, more frequent visits (monthly) may be scheduled during the reduction phase of speech bulb reduction therapy, if the appliance has been constructed for this purpose.

REDUCTION OF SPEECH BULBS

The full-size speech bulb is left in place for at least 1 month. In patients with compensatory articulation disorders who are receiving concomitant speech therapy, the bulb should not be reduced until compensatory articulation errors have been eliminated at the phrase or sentence level with at least some carryover into conversation. Specifically, the patient should be able to produce voiced and voiceless plosives, sibilants, fricatives, and affricative sounds with 90% consistency in structured tasks and at least 50% accuracy in conversation.

Complete VP closure with the speech bulb in place should be confirmed endoscopically before reduction. The dental specialist begins this phase of treatment by reducing the bulb approximately 2 mm on each lateral edge. This often results in mild VPI and hypernasality. Nasopharyngoscopy and a brief perceptual speech evaluation should be repeated 2 to 4 weeks later to determine if normal resonance and VP closure around the bulb have returned in spite of the reduction in the size of the bulb. If so, the bulb may be reduced an additional 2 to 3 mm from every surface contacted by pharyngeal tissue. If there is a VP gap at any surface, acrylic should be added to the bulb to establish closure at that site. At each monthly visit endoscopy and a brief perceptual speech evaluation should be done with the speech bulb in place and with it removed. In this way changes in configuration of VP movement can be observed and used to guide further bulb adjustments. For example, the vertical height of maximum lateral pharyngeal wall movement may be at a position higher or lower than it was originally when the amount of movement increases. The width and, when possible, the circumference of the bulb are decreased gradually until treatment is complete.

Gradual reductions in the size of the speech bulb are made following every endoscopic examination that confirms continued VP closure. When endoscopy is not possible, reduction may be based on the speech pathologist's report of perceived normal resonance and absent nasal emission on a mirror test. Bulb reduction results in one of two possible outcomes. In most cases a point will be reached following which additional reduction results in VPI and a return of hypernasality that does not improve after a day or two. One attempt should be made to increase the size of the bulb to reestablish complete closure for 1 month, and then to reduce again. If repeat reduction again results in hypernasality, an assumption can be made that maximum benefit has been achieved, and permanent surgical treatment of VPI should be considered.

The second possible outcome is that the bulb is reduced until the wire retaining the bulb is nearly exposed, and further reduction is not possible, but complete VP closure is maintained during speech with the appliance in place. The bulb should be gradually removed a few hours per day (e.g., at first an hour in the morning and in the evening) until it is no longer needed. This outcome of complete resolution of VPI using speech bulb reduction without surgical intervention is rare, and our experience with long-term maintenance of "cures" has been discouraging, as discussed in later in this chapter.

SPEECH THERAPY

Speech bulb or palatal lift appliances enable a patient to achieve VP closure. Their effect on speech is limited to management of hypernasality and nasal emission/turbulence and to providing the potential for normal intraoral pressure. If articulation is otherwise normal, concurrent speech therapy is not indicated and should not be scheduled.

Most patients with gross VPI or variable VP motion who are being considered for speech bulb reduction therapy *do* have articulation disorders, and the mere presence of an appliance does not affect articulation. Any patient with articulation errors, especially compensatory errors or weak articulatory contacts, must receive concomitant speech therapy. The goals and procedures recommended for patients with speech bulbs are the same as for patients without appliances. In fact, the treating speech pathologist should ignore the presence of the appliance, other than to reinforce its consistent use. Hypernasality will not be eliminated until the appliance is fully constructed. Until that time, speech therapy should target normal articulation placement and oral airstream direction using nasal occlusion as necessary. The most critical speech therapy goals are to eliminate abnormal compensatory errors such as glottal stops and nasal snorting, and to increase the strength of articulatory contacts. This is described in more detail in Chapter 16. If the patient's error pattern includes nasal snorting or posterior nasal fricatives, which are usually accompanied by outward VP motion, correct production of /s/ and /f/ should be early therapy goals (Fig. 17-5). This will facilitate adequate judgment of speech bulb size and readiness for reduction. Under no circumstances should the speech pathologist remove the bulb during therapy unless instructed to do so by the speech bulb team. This may be requested during the final stage of reduction as described in the preceding section, when the appliance is being phased out by removal for designated periods each day.

As discussed in Chapter 16, use of a speech bulb may facilitate articulation therapy because it provides the potential for normal resonance while working on articulation production. This may be less distracting for patients, therapists, and parents who have difficulty focusing separately on resonance and articulation. Obturation of the VP gap also provides the patient with the potential to impound normal intraoral pressure, which may facilitate progress in eliminating abnormal compensatory gestures. Interestingly, some speech pathologists approach articulation disorders more directly and more aggressively, therefore more appropriately, when there is evidence of complete VP closure. Use of a speech bulb may also facilitate generalization of speech improvement to conversation out of the clinic.

THE SPEECH BULB REDUCTION PROGRAM AT MONTEFIORE MEDICAL CENTER
Patient sample

Speech bulb reduction programs are managed slightly differently by different craniofacial teams, and this may affect overall outcome. As an example, the speech bulb reduction program at Montefiore Medical Center is described. Thirty-one patients between the ages of 3½ and 50 years (median age was 6 years 8 months) were

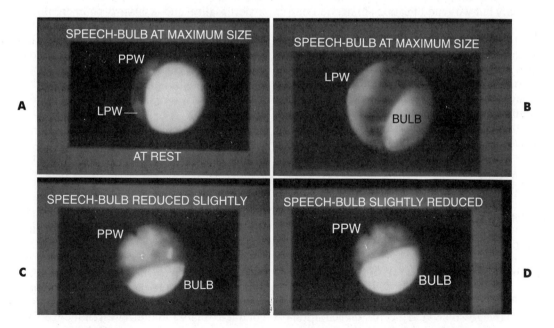

Fig. 17-5 A, At rest with largest bulb in place showing bulb as wide as pharynx. **B,** Nasal snort on /s/ showing movement away from rest position, opening ports around bulb. **C,** Reduced bulb at rest. **D,** Reduced bulb during phonation of correct /s/ showing inward motion and improved VP closure.

referred into the speech bulb reduction program following review of their speech and nasopharyngoscopic and multiview videofluoroscopic examinations. Diagnoses were nonsyndromic and syndromic repaired or submucous cleft palate (Stickler syndrome, velo-cardio-facial syndrome, Robin sequence), neurologic disorders, and idiopathic VPI (in one case 1 year after adenotonsillectomy). Each patient underwent a dentofacial examination in the orthodontic program and did not have any immediate orthodontic needs that would contraindicate placement or retention of a speech appliance. Patients were considered good candidates for the program if they had gross VPI with no lateral pharyngeal wall motion, variable VPI with varying degrees of lateral pharyngeal wall motion, or VPI with a severe compensatory articulation disorder that had been resistant to traditional articulation therapy alone. In addition, each patient had been compliant for all or most of the assessments, kept all appointments, and completed any restorative dental treatments needed. Furthermore, every patient or primary caregiver indicated an understanding of the mechanics of the speech bulb program (e.g., gradual construction of the appliance, monthly or more frequent endoscopy to guide and monitor appliance construction and reduction), the need for concurrent speech therapy in most cases, and the possibility that surgery would still be necessary but with modifications in needed flap width.

Of the 32 patients referred, 17 completed the program. The mean number of visits needed for construction of the appliance was 8.3 (range 4 to 12 visits) depending on patient compliance and rapidity of adaptation to the appliance permitting further enlargement. The number of visits was slightly higher for residents and dental specialists who had limited experience in speech bulb construction than for more experienced dental specialists. Total treatment time, from construction to final removal of the appliance, ranged from 6 months to 3¼ years, except for one patient who was treated over 6 years. Mean treatment time was 21.8 months, and the median treatment time was 22 months. The total number of visits ranged from 9 to 19 (mean = 14.5, median = 14).

Treatment outcome

Nasopharyngoscopic guidance of speech appliance construction ensured that VPI was eliminated in every patient who followed through. That is, with the appliance in place, symptoms of VPI, including hypernasality and nasal emission/turbulence were completely eliminated in every case, regardless of diagnosis. There is no question that speech bulb appliances can be used effectively to manage VPI.

Some reduction in the size of the speech bulb was possible in every patient. However, analysis of the usefulness of this type of treatment to attempt to reduce VPI must consider the degree to which the changes in VP motion affected subsequent surgical needs. There were two patients of the 16 who completed the program who appeared to have been "cured" without surgery. Both had normal hearing, cognition, and palatal morphology. Their case histories follow.

Patient 1 was a 9-year-old boy with hypotonia and normal palatal morphology. He initially presented with intermittent VPI, intermittent hypernasality, and mildly dysarthric articulation. His speech bulb was constructed and reduced over a period of 21 months (13 visits). He received concurrent hospital-based speech therapy. Four months following complete removal of the speech bulb, he had complete VP closure and normal resonance. His dysarthric articulation was unchanged. Unfortunately, we have no information on long-term maintenance of this result because he has not returned for reevaluation.

Patient 2 was a 4½-year-old boy with Aarskog syndrome and normal palatal morphology. He initially presented with gross VPI except for phone-specific closure on sustained /s/, severe hypernasality, and a severe compensatory articulation disorder. In addition to articulation therapy, he was in the speech bulb reduction program for 13 months (10 visits), following which he had intermittent VPI and hypernasality. He continued to receive school-based articulation therapy and demonstrated normal resonance and VP closure after an additional 13 months of treatment. Like patient 1, he has not appeared for subsequent follow-up. Because he was concurrently in articulation therapy and speech bulb therapy, it is impossible to determine the effect of the appliance itself. Similar results have been achieved with speech therapy alone in patients with phone-specific VP closure (Golding, 1981; Golding-Kushner, 1989, 1994).

Two other patients who finished the program had complete VP closure and normal resonance 4 months after the appliance was removed. However, they returned 2½ to 3 years later with complete relapse to their pretreatment VPI and had pharyngeal flap surgery. One had hypotonia and the other had a repaired incomplete cleft palate with history of Robin sequence and airway problems in infancy that necessitated a temporary glossopexy.

There were three patients in whom hypernasality decreased enough that, although there remained some nasality and evidence of VPI following removal of the speech bulb, the families elected not to pursue more definitive surgical treatment. They also were not interested in continuing to use the speech bulb to control their residual VPI.* All three had mild or intermittent VPI at the onset of treatment.

Ten of the 17 patients completing speech bulb treatment needed pharyngeal flaps. Six of them needed a less obstructive pharyngeal flap† than they would have without the speech bulb reduction program and speech therapy. Only four patients needed pharyngeal flaps as wide as they would have without the speech bulb therapy.

In almost every patient for whom improvement occurred, increases in pharyngeal motion obtained over successive reductions were maintained during phonation with the speech appliance removed (Golding-Kushner, 1988; Golding-Kushner and Cisneros, 1989). However, in two patients treated at our center‡ the presence of the bulb was necessary for any movement to occur. Excellent pharyngeal motion closing 95% of the VP port was elicited with appliances in place that had been large at the beginning of treatment but had been significantly reduced until there remained only slightly more acrylic than necessary to cover the supporting wire. However, when the appliances were removed (during the same endoscopic examination), there was a relapse to gross VPI with no pharyngeal or velar motion. In both of these patients the presence of even a very small bulb was enough to prompt excellent VP closure but with the bulb removed there was no motion whatsoever. Excellent motion resumed as soon as the appliance was replaced. In one of the patients gross VPI was present when the speech bulb was

reduced past a particular threshold, but complete closure was elicited by increasing the size of the bulb slightly (Fig. 17-6).

A phenomenon whereby VP gestures appear to be abandoned has been referred to as functional surrender (Hagerty et al., 1968), discouraged motion (Morris, 1968), and palatal surrender (B. J. McWilliams, personal communication, September 3, 1991). This may help to explain the exacerbation of VPI that occurs during glottal stop speech and might also suggest a role for Passavant's ridge in both normal and cleft subjects. The ridge often occurs at a different vertical level than maximum velar movement and often seems not to contribute to VP closure (Glaser et al, 1979). If there is a critical resistance level needed to drive the vocal tract valves, then the ridge may serve an important function, even when not contributing directly to closure. The observation of the two patients described above supports the possibility that nasopharyngeal resistance plays a role not only in the modification of sounds, but actually in invoking pharyngeal motion (Golding-Kushner, 1991).

Speech bulb dropouts

Fifteen patients withdrew from the speech bulb reduction program. They ranged in age from 4 to 28 years, with a mean of 10½ years and a median of 6½ years. Compliance was affected by factors including patient and parent motivation, cost, distance to the treatment center, effort in maintaining and inserting the appliance, and time. Two of the patients had pharyngeal flap surgery, but the other 13 disappeared. They included patients with and without cleft palate. Nine of the patients left as early as the first or second visit or before final bulb placement. Six patients remained in the program from 1 to 3½ years before withdrawing. In a few instances younger patients lost or broke the appliance repeatedly, necessitating reconstruction or replacement at a high cost of time and money. Only one patient had difficulty tolerating the appliance. A common reason for termination of the program was poor compliance among the parents of some patients and among adult patients. Multiple appointments were missed or canceled, and visits were scheduled at intervals that were much longer than recommended (e.g., 6 months instead of 1 month), which prolonged treatment. In some patients the appointments kept were spaced with such long intervals that the appliance needed major reconfiguration to accommodate to changing dentition each time, especially when the appliance had not been worn for weeks or

---

*One of those patients was a moderately mentally retarded adult with repaired cleft palate who was in a sheltered environment, one was an adolescent with fetal hydantoin syndrome, normal palate, and learning disabilities, and the third was a normal boy with submucous cleft palate and severe hoarseness that actually masked his hypernasality, especially to listeners other than speech pathologists. The hoarseness was present before and during the 2 years that his VPI was completely eliminated by the speech bulb. He had vocal fold nodules and a long history of vocal abuse, and his hoarseness was not believed to be related to his VPI.
†At Montefiore Medical Center the surgical procedure for constructing a pharyngeal flap is varied to establish different postoperative widths. Less obstructive means a wide or narrow flap instead of a subobstructing flap, or a narrow flap instead of a wide one.
‡The patients were an 8-year-old boy with generalized congenital hypotonia and normal palate and a 12 year old girl with an occult submucous cleft palate and ptosis but no other apparent neurological problems.

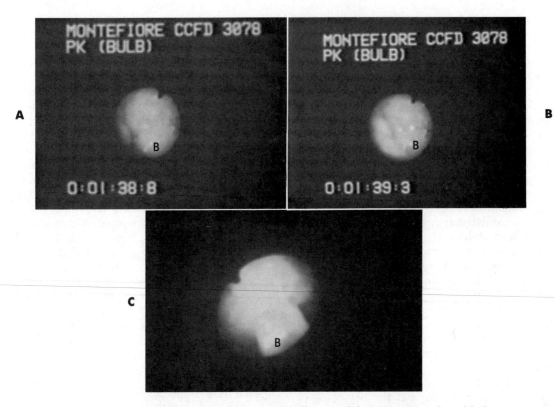

Fig. 17-6 Nasopharyngoscopy showing a speech bulb at rest (**A**), during phonation with closure around the bulb (**B**), and gross VPI with the bulb reduced to its narrowest stage (below threshold of nasopharyngeal resistance, there was an absence of VP motion).

even months at a time. This was often attributed to work and school schedules or to distance to be traveled to the medical center, all of which were known to the families before initiation of treatment. In these cases it seemed true that their path to the hospital was paved with good intentions but the reality of the trip was too complicated.

CONCLUSIONS

Clinical criteria for speech bulb or speech bulb reduction therapy include a poor or slow response to articulation therapy for compensatory articulation errors in a patient with VPI and a need to buy time when there is a medical or psychosocial contraindication to surgery. Physiologic criteria for speech bulb reduction therapy are gross or variable VPI (prior to pharyngeal flap) or intermittent VPI when closure occurs less than 50% of the time but is not phoneme-specific.

Long-term follow-up suggests that complete VP closure achieved following speech bulb reduction is not always maintained, but improved lateral pharyngeal wall motion is maintained if

pharyngeal flap surgery is performed. Following speech bulb reduction therapy, complete resolution of VPI should be anticipated only if there is some evidence of closure during initial evaluation as in intermittent or phoneme-specific VPI. Otherwise, the therapy goal is reduction, not resolution, of VPI. That goal is meaningful only if there are several surgical options to take advantage of varying degrees of VPI. A useful application of speech bulbs may be in facilitating and accelerating the pace of articulation therapy and in improving lateral pharyngeal wall motion so that less obstructive pharyngeal flaps are necessary. Interestingly, temporary obturation with a speech bulb during speech therapy combined with speech bulb reduction to improve the prognosis for success of a pharyngeal flap was proposed by Blakely in 1964.

Speech bulb appliances have advantages over surgery in that they are modifiable if changes in VP motion occur, making treatment fully reversible. They may be used to treat VPI by gradual reduction in their size. On the other hand, disadvantages of a speech appliance include interference with or by other orthodontic treatment, loss of normal resonance when the appliance is out for repair or cleaning or is misplaced, and the potential of long-term wearing of the supporting teeth. Like the pharyngeal flap, their size and placement should be guided endoscopically.

Continued research is needed to determine the value of speech bulb reduction therapy in cases in which VP motion has improved but surgery is still necessary. Furthermore, it is difficult to separate the effect of speech therapy on VP motion from the effect of the speech bulb, because most speech bulb patients also receive speech therapy. Improved VP motion has been observed in many patients following speech therapy to eliminate compensatory errors alone (Golding-Kushner et al., 1990; Ysunza et al., 1992) and, in a few cases, from speech bulb therapy alone (McGrath and Anderson, 1990). Clearly, speech bulb reduction therapy can provide valuable management flexibility by offering an additional treatment modality.

REFERENCES

Argamaso RV: *The pharyngeal flap in cleft lip and palate.* In Kernahan DA, Rosenstein SW, editors: *Cleft lip and palate: a system of management,* Baltimore, 1990, Williams & Wilkins.

Blakely RW: The complimentary use of speech prostheses and pharyngeal flaps in palatal insufficiency, *Cleft Palate J* 1:194, 1964.

Blakely RW: The rationale for a temporary speech prosthesis in palatal insufficiency, *Br J Dis Commun* 4:134, 1969.

Glaser ER, Skolnick ML, McWilliams BJ, Shprintzen RJ: The dynamics of Passavant's ridge in subjects with and without velopharyngeal insufficiency: a multiview videofluoroscopic study, *Cleft Palate J* 16:24, 1979.

Golding KJ: *Articulation and velopharyngeal insufficiency: a rationale for pre-surgical speech therapy,* Paper presented at Fourth International Congress on Cleft Palate and Related Craniofacial Anomalies, Acapulco, Mexico, May 1981.

Golding KJ, Schechter B, Shprintzen RJ, Rakoff S: *A new approach to the placement of prosthetic speech bulbs for velopharyngeal inadequacy,* Paper presented at Third International Congress on Cleft Palate and Related Craniofacial Anomalies, Toronto, Canada, June 1977.

Golding-Kushner KJ: *Speech-bulb reduction in the treatment of velopharyngeal insufficiency,* Paper presented at Society for Ear, Nose, and Throat Advancements in Children, New York, 1988.

Golding-Kushner KJ: *Speech therapy for compensatory articulation errors in patients with cleft palate speech,* Videotape produced by the Center for Craniofacial Disorders, Montefiore Medical Center, Bronx, New York, 1989.

Golding-Kushner KJ: Craniofacial morphology and velopharyngeal physiology in four syndromes of clefting. Unpublished doctoral dissertation. The Graduate School and University Center, City University of New York, 1991.

Golding-Kushner KJ, Cisneros GJ: *Speech-bulb reduction in the treatment of hypernasal speech,* Paper presented at Sixth International Congress on Cleft Palate and Related Craniofacial Anomalies. Jerusalem, Israel, 1989.

Golding-Kushner KJ et al: Standardization for the reporting of nasopharyngoscopy and multiview videofluoroscopy: a report from an international working group, *Cleft Palate J* 27(4):337, 1990.

Hagerty RF, Hess DA, Mylin WK: Velar motility, velopharyngeal closure, and speech proficiency in cartilage pharyngoplasty: the effect of age at surgery, *Cleft Palate J* 5:317, 1968.

Harkins C, Koepp-Baker H: Twenty-five years of cleft palate prosthesis, *J Speech Hear Disord* 13:23, 1948.

Hoch L, Golding-Kushner KJ, Sadewitz V, Shprintzen RJ: Speech Therapy. In McWilliams BJ, editor: *Seminars in speech and language: current methods of assessing and treating children with cleft palates,* New York, 1986, Thieme.

McGrath CO, Anderson MW: Prosthetic treatment of velopharyngeal incompetence. In Bardach J, Morris H, editors: *Multidisciplinary management of cleft lip and palate,* Philadelphia, 1990, WB Saunders.

McWilliams BJ, Morris HL, Shelton RL: *Cleft palate speech,* Philadelphia, 1990, BC Decker.

Morris HL: Etiological bases for speech problems. In D.C. Spriestersbach DC, Sherman D, editors: *Cleft palate and communication,* New York, 1968, Academic Press.

Rich BD, Farber K, Shprintzen RJ: Nasopharyngoscopy in the treatment of palatopharyngeal insufficiency, *Interna J Prosthet* 1(3):248, 1988.

Schechter B, Golding KJ, Shprintzen RJ, Rakoff S: A new approach to the placement of the prosthetic speech bulb in velopharyngeal inadequacy, *Cleft Palate J* 14(4):361, 1977 (abstr).

Shelton RL, Lindquist AF, Chisum L, Arndt WB, Youngstrom KA, Stick SL: Effect of prosthetic speech bulb reduction on articulation, *Cleft Palate J* 5:195, 1968.

Shelton RL, Lindquist AF, Arndt WB, Elbert M, Youngstrom KA: Effect of speech bulb reduction on movement of the posterior wall of the pharynx and posture of the tongue, *Cleft Palate J,* 8:10, 1971.

Shprintzen RJ: The conceptual framework for pharyngeal flap surgery. In Bardach J, Morris H, editors: *Multidisciplinary management of cleft lip and palate,* Philadelphia, 1990, WB Saunders.

Shprintzen RJ, Lencione RM, McCall GN, Skolnick ML: A three dimensional cinefluoroscopic analysis of velopharyngeal closure during speech and non-speech activities in normals, *Cleft Palate J* 11:412, 1974.

Shprintzen RJ, Lewin ML, Croft CB, Daniller AI, Argamaso RV, Ship AG, Strauch B: A comprehensive study of pharyngeal flap surgery: tailor made flaps, *Cleft Palate J* 16:45, 1979.

Stark RB, Frileck S: Primary pharyngeal flap and palatorrhaphy. In Grabb WC, Rosenstein SW, Bzoch SW, editors: *Cleft lip and palate: surgical, dental, and speech aspects,* Boston, 1971, Little, Brown.

Weiss CE: Success of an obturator reduction program, *Cleft Palate J* 8:291, 1971.

Ysunza A, Pamplona C, Toledo E: Change in velopharyngeal valving after speech therapy in cleft palate patients: a videonasopharyngoscopic and multiview videofluoroscopic study, *Int J Pediatr Otorhinolaryngol* 24:45, 1992.

Index

A

Acceptability, speech, 147
Adenoidectomy
  arguments about, 283
  contraindications to, 259
  preoperative, prior to pharyngoplasty, 292
  reason for, 234
Adenoids
  enlarged, resonance affected by, 258
  hypertrophic, pharyngeal obstruction caused by, 161
  hyponasality caused by, 234
  nasopharyngoscopy for examination of, 234-236
  obstructive apnea caused by, 80
  on posterior pharyngeal wall, velopharyngeal insufficiency diag-
    nosis and, 282
  removal of, arguments about, 283
  speech affected by, 277
  velopharyngeal valve treatment and, 258-261
  videofluoroscopy for observation of, 248
Adolescence
  dentition in, 303-304
  personality disturbance in, velocardiofacial syndrome associated
    with, 41
Adrb-2 gene, clefting and, 37
Adult
  compensatory articulation disorders in, 349
  personality disturbance in, velocardiofacial syndrome associated
    with, 41
  pharyngeal flap surgery for, 349
  speech managment for, 324-325
  speech-language screening of, 204
Affricate sounds, formation of, 139
Age
  palate repair and, 10-11
  pharyngeal flap surgery and, 348-349
  two-slap palatoplasty and, 120
  videofluoroscopic examination and, 242
Airflow, nasal, visual biofeedback for, 342
Airstream
  flow of, through vocal tract, 139
  speech development and, 138
Airway
  cleft complications and, 75
  collapse of, Muller maneuver and diagnosis of, 261
  complications in, following surgery, 78-82
  disorders of, multiple anomaly syndromes and, 66
  function of
    speech-language screening of infant and assessment of, 182
    speech-language screening of preschool child and assessment
      of, 185
    speech-language screening of school-age child and assessment
      of, 201
  nasal
    blockage of, 145
    obstruction of, 81
  obstruction of
    causes of, 182
    gastrostomy contraindicated by, 68
    as pharyngoplasty complication, 292
    Robin sequence associated with, 32
    sleep apnea and, 293
  pharyngeal flap surgery effect on, 81
  upper, nasopharyngoscopy for examination of, 234
Alar base, cleft lip and, 3
Alcohol
  cleft lip and palate and mother's use of, 29
  teratogenic disorders associated with, 29

Alveolar arch
  premaxilla placed in, 112
  widening of, orthodontic treatment for, 302
Alveolar cleft; *see* Cleft alveolus
Alveolar process, bone graft and, 304
Alveolar ridge, cleft of, 3
Alveolus
  development of, crossbite and, 299
  embryonic, diagram of, af
American Cleft Palate Association, team treatment concept
    and, 12
Amnion, early tears in, cleft and limb anomalies associated with, 21
Amnion rupture sequence, 32f
Anesthesia
  malignant hyperpyrexia and, 87
  topical, endoscopic examination and, 230
Anesthesiology, craniofacial team inclusion of, 13t
Ankyloglossia, speech affected by, 156
Anodontia
  description of, 308
  sound production affected by, 315
Apert syndrome
  abnormal pitch associated with, 147
  abnormal soft palate in, 158
  autosomal dominant inheritance of, 23
  cleft palate shape in, 158
  hyponasal resonance associated with, 154
  hypoplastic tympanic membrane associated with, 164
  shallow nasopharynx associated with, 160
Apnea
  abnormal nervous system as cause of, 79
  brain malformation as cause of, 79
  central, 73
  holoprosencephaly associated with, 21
  mixed, 73, 79
  obstructive, 73, 79, 80
    tonsils as cause of, 235
  pharyngeal flap surgery associated with, 79-80
  pharyngoplasty and, 78-79
  pharyngoplasty as cause of, 79-80
  sleep; *see* Sleep apnea
  types of, 73
Appliance
  intraoral, 322
  orthodontic
    in adolescent, 304
    prior to cleft lip repair, 317
  orthopedic, maxilla repositioning with, 318
  palatal, 318
    velopharyngeal closure facilitated with, 321
  speech, 344-345; *see also* Speech bulb
    permanent, 352-353
    temporary, 353-354
    types of, 352
    uses of, 352-354
Apraxia, oral, hypernasality and, 334
Arm, short, Robinow syndrome associated with, 20
Arnold-Chiari malformation, syndromes associated with clefting
    and, 164
Artery
  bleeding from, in palatoplasty, 133
  carotid
    abnormalities in, 240
    evaluation of, 266
    in velocardiofacial syndrome, 266, 267
Articulation
  compensatory; *see* Compensatory articulation